P9-DCP-238

Surgical Diagnosis

PHILIP THOREK, M.D., F.A.C.S., F.I.C.S.

Clinical Professor of Surgery (Formerly Assigned to Gross and Topographic Anatomy), University of Illinois College of Medicine; Diplomate of the American Board of Surgery; Professor of Topographic Anatomy and Clinical Surgery, Cook County Graduate School of Medicine; Member of the American Association of Anatomists; Fellow, American College of Chest Physicians; Surgeon-in-Chief of the American Hospital

With Drawings by
CARL T. LINDEN
Formerly Assistant Professor in Medical Illustration, University of Illinois College of Medicine, Chicago

SECOND EDITION

PHILADELPHIA TORONTO

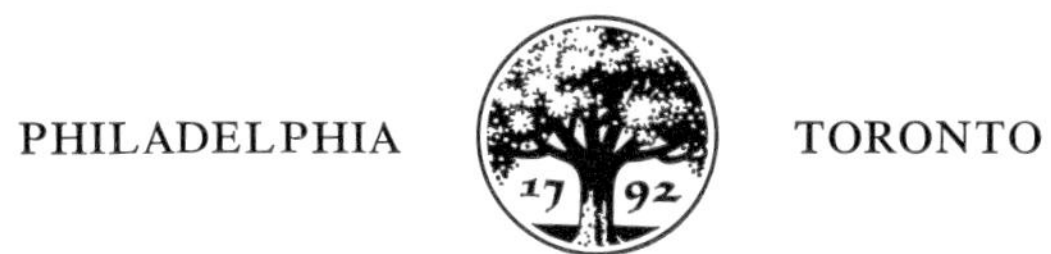

J. B. LIPPINCOTT COMPANY

SECOND EDITION

ISBN-0-397-50139-0
Library of Congress Catalog Card Number 65-11357

Printed in the United States of America

7 6

TO AGNES

Preface to the Second Edition

It has been 9 years since *Surgical Diagnosis* first appeared. Many of the changes that have taken place during the past decade are well known to the medical profession. To attempt to keep up with *all* the advances in any given specialty is a herculean and, in most instances, an impossible task. Progress in cardiovascular surgery is one of the outstanding accomplishments in this era. Hence, a new section has been added dealing with this subject. Needless to say, the material is presented in a simplified version. It is the hope of the author that it will act as a stimulus to some for further study.

Changes in nomenclature also take place from year to year. Particularly in the fields of bile pigments and jaundice, to mention two, has this been true.

In this day of computer medicine greater emphasis has been placed on the laboratory In some areas of surgical diagnosis it is only by means of laboratory data that the diagnosis can be clinched. I do not desire to play down the computer; however, I am a firm believer that the observations made at the bedside by a seasoned clinician constitute the most important phase of diagnosis.

For the past 15 years I have had the good fortune to have access to the skill and talents of the artist, Carl Linden. Much of the success of the first edition was due to his contributions. To him I am especially grateful. A thank-you goes to Stanley A. Gillet for his untiring efforts in editing the manuscript and indexing this work. Finally, I wish to express my gratitude for the continued cooperation of the Medical Department of the J. B. Lippincott Company.

Philip Thorek, M.D.

Preface to the First Edition

Diagnosis is the first and most important part of surgery. Correlation of the reduced morbidity and mortality that accompany an accurate diagnosis certify to this.

The student and clinician should have a plan or method which guides him in his investigation of a medical problem. Such a plan must be simple, concise and workable. A method that satisfies these requisites and has served me well for the past 25 years consists of the following:

1. A well-taken history.
2. A careful evaluation of the present symptom complex.
3. A properly conducted physical examination.
4. Consideration of pertinent laboratory data.

Little can be overlooked or forgotten if such a method is scrupulously followed. The modern approach to diagnosis unfortunately tends to make the laboratory primary. It is not my intent to minimize laboratory findings; indeed, on occasion, they are a vital if not our sole source of information. However, most diagnoses can be made correctly long before such information is available.

In writing this book some dogmatism was inevitable if basic principles were to be retained and properly stressed. Purists and supercritics will frequently censure such pedagogy and offer the rare case or diagnostic minutiae to support their criticism. It is true that exceptions and rare instances must always be kept in mind, but these should be relegated to a secondary place, particularly in a book of this type.

I have made little or no distinction in the method of presenting this material for undergraduate and postgraduate students. The basic principles and practices remain the same for both levels. Constant exposure to clinical material and diagnostic dilemmas are necessary prerequisites for the development of the master diagnostician, and no book can presume to accomplish this.

It is my sincere hope that the method of presenting this material will help my colleagues as it has helped me. I shall be most grateful to those who read this book if they will call to my attention errors and omissions of important items. In this type of presentation, a bibliography and list of references seem redundant, and they have been omitted.

A word of sincere gratitude is due the artist, Carl Linden. His artistic skill and creative execution of the illustrations give clarification to the text.

I wish to thank my chief, Dr. Warren Cole, for the opportunities afforded me at the University of Illinois College of Medicine.

To the J. B. Lippincott Company I wish to say, in this our third venture, "Thank you for your continued co-operation and warm understanding."

PHILIP THOREK, M.D.

Contents

1

Head

SCALP

Anatomy

The scalp consists of 5 layers: skin, subcutaneous connective tissue, epicranial aponeurosis, subaponeurotic areolar layer and pericranium. It is well supplied with blood vessels; hence, it bleeds readily, resists infection and maintains its viability.

Wounds

Scalp wounds do not gape unless the epicranial aponeurosis has been divided; one can tell at a glance the depth of a given wound. A blow on the head may be severe enough to produce a hematoma without causing a scalp wound. When such *closed wounds* are present, the extravasation of blood may take place beneath the loose subaponeurotic layer or beneath the pericranium. A collection of blood (or pus) beneath the epicranial aponeurosis (dangerous area) involves the whole area being limited by the attachments of the occipitofrontalis. On the other hand, a collection of blood beneath the pericranium will be limited by the suture lines, since the pericranium dips into these. Hematomas can be exceedingly deceptive, since their softer centers may be mistaken for a depressed skull fracture. A roentgenogram of the skull will reveal whether or not a depressed fracture is present.

An *open wound* (when the skin is broken) increases the risk of infection.

Cephalhematoma is a collection of blood

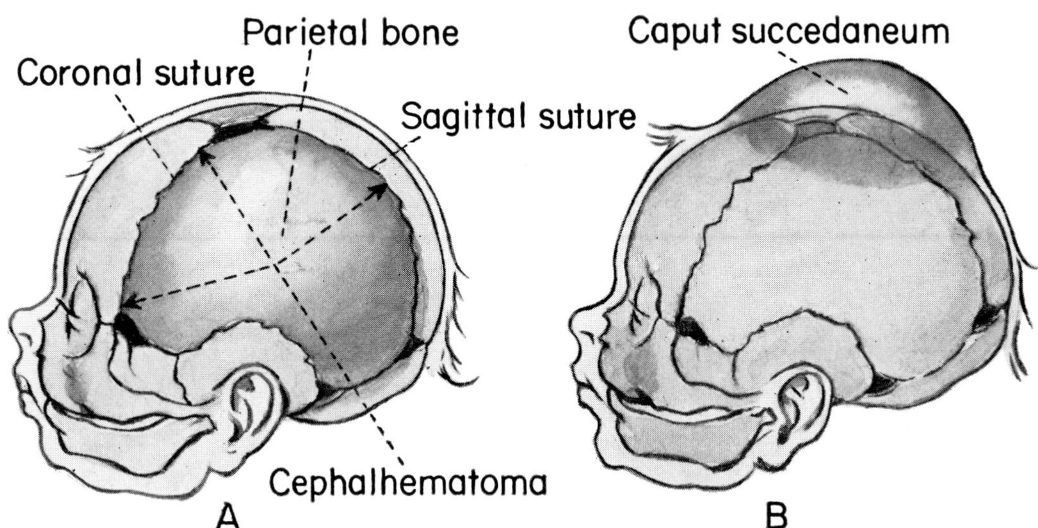

Fig. 1. Cephalhematoma or caput succedaneum? Both may be associated with birth canal trauma. The caput succedaneum is not limited by the cranial sutures.

between the pericranium and one of the cranial bones. The areas most frequently involved are the frontal, the parietal and the occipital. It is the result of birth injury and must be differentiated from a *caput succedaneum.* The latter is a circumscribed edema with ecchymosis which results from prolonged pressure in the birth canal. It is differentiated from cephalhematoma by the fact that a caput is not limited by the cranial sutures (Fig. 1).

Avulsion of the scalp is the tearing away of this structure from the skull. The most common causes in modern times are beauty parlor and industrial accidents. The separation occurs in the subaponeurotic layer; usually the pericranium is left intact.

Infections

Boils and carbuncles of the scalp are extremely painful, since this structure is thick and inelastic. In the aged, the diabetic or the asthenic, serious sequelae can result. The infection penetrates beneath the aponeurosis. In such instances the distribution would be the same as that described under "Hematoma" (p. 1). Erysipelas and cellulitis may follow abrasions or trivial wounds. Pain, edema, fever, regional lymphadenitis and leukocytosis are characteristic. The lymphatics of the scalp drain in the following manner (Fig. 2): The frontal and the anterior parietal regions drain into the preauricular lymph nodes. The midparietal region drains first into the postauricular lymph nodes and then into the nodes of the posterior triangle. The occipital region drains first into the nodes near the insertion of the trapezius muscle and then into the posterior triangle. Enlargement of the lymph nodes in the *posterior triangle* of the neck frequently results from pediculosis capitis.

Cysts

Sebaceous cysts frequently occur in the scalp (wens); often they are multiple. Suppuration, ulceration or epitheliomatous degeneration are sequelae of such cysts. A localized swelling *in* the scalp can be moved on the skull. A swelling which originates

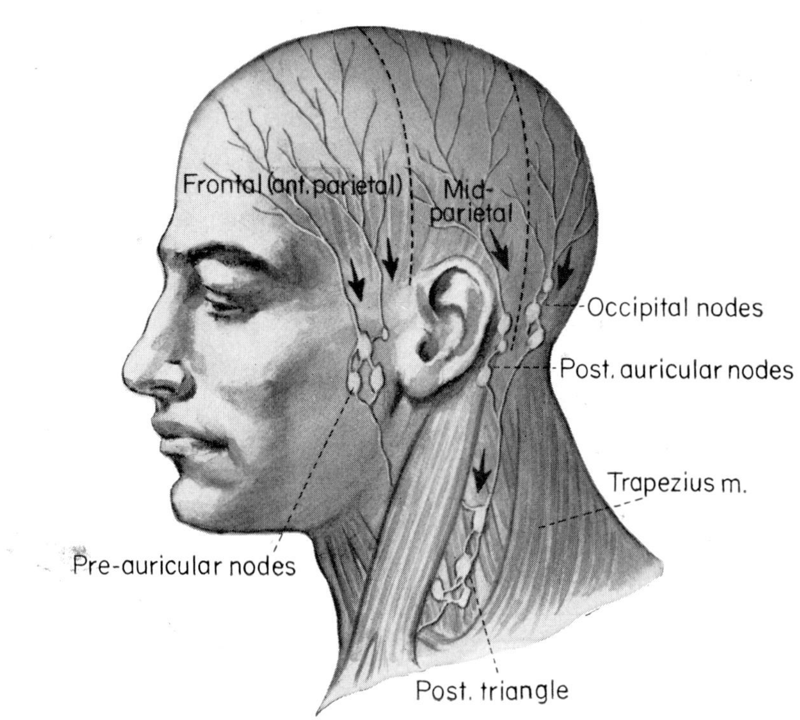

Fig. 2. The lymphatic system of the scalp.

from the bony skull permits the scalp to be moved over the swelling (Fig. 3).

Dermoid cysts are rarely seen. They occasionally communicate by a narrow neck with the subdural space and occur in the skin of the temple.

Tumors

Both benign and malignant tumors can originate from the scalp. These must be suspected when the lesion moves with the scalp over the underlying bone. In this respect the tumor resembles a sebaceous cyst. Secondary tumors also may affect the scalp.

A cirsoid aneurysm occasionally involves the scalp, particularly in the region of the superficial temporal artery. It results from an arteriovenous fistula (congenital or traumatic). Enormous tortuous veins and arteries course over the scalp and the temple of the involved side.

SKULL

The contour of the skull may vary tremendously and still be within normal limits. A definite relationship to race is noted. A *dolichocephalic* skull is elongated. *Brachycephalic* skulls are round. *Megacephalic* skulls have a capacity of over 1,450 cc. and are found in the highly civilized. *Microcephalic* skulls have a capacity of less than 1,300 cc. and are found in the more primitive types.

Diseases

Osteomyelitis may occur as a primary condition, or secondary to furuncles, carbuncles, burns and infected hematomas. This has been alluded to on page 2.

Other diseases which affect the skull are: rickets, syphilis, tuberculosis, Paget's disease and xanthomatosis.

Tumors arising from the skull usually are osteomas. Also, benign giant cell tumors have been reported. Sarcoma may be primary or secondary.

Fractures

Since the skull is not a weight-bearing structure, the fracture per se is unimportant from a structural standpoint. Of great significance is the damage to the vessels, the meninges and the brain (Fig. 4).

These fractures will be discussed as *vault*, *basal* and *depressed* fractures. Any combination of these may occur.

Vault Fractures. Fractures of the vault

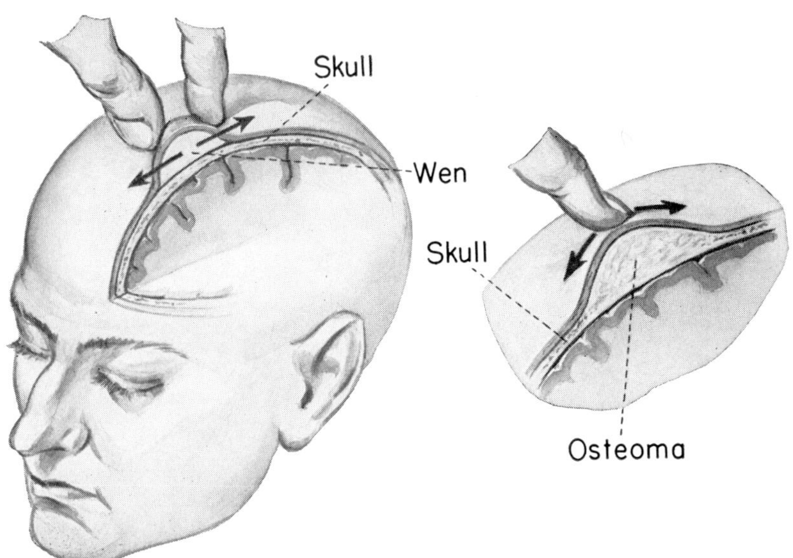

Fig. 3. A sebaceous cyst moves with the scalp over the skull. The scalp moves over an osteoma.

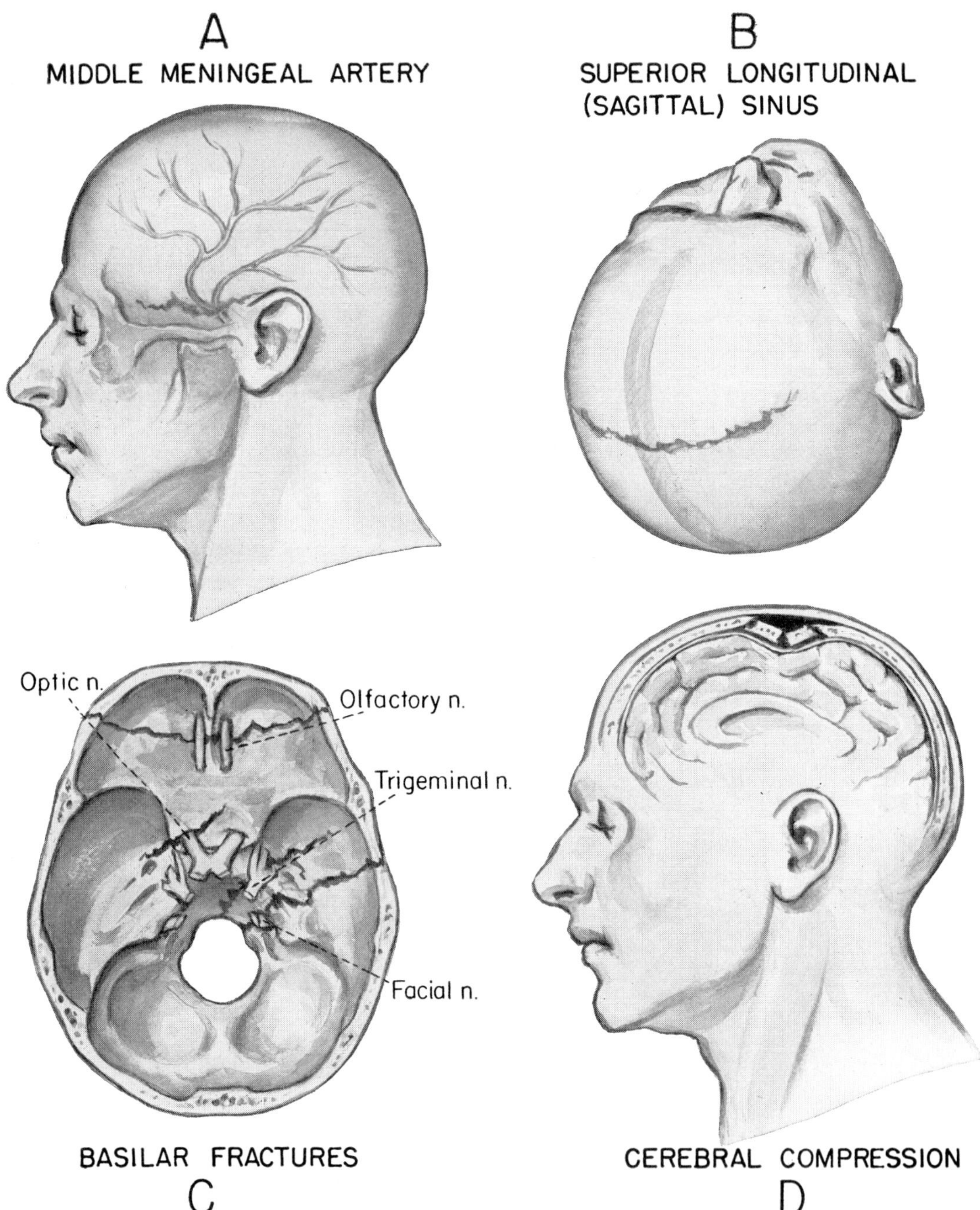

FIG. 4. Soft tissues which may be injured in skull fractures.

are the most common type and are usually *linear*. If uncomplicated, they are of little significance, except that they serve as evidence of injury. *In children* such fractures lead to absorption of the surrounding bone and for some unknown reason may produce a round defect in the bone. The margins of these defects are smooth and regular. Vault fractures which occur in the temporal region may cause a laceration of the middle meningeal vessels (p. 8). Extension of linear vault fractures into the base of the skull is not uncommon. *Healing* of linear fractures usually is complete in normal children from 6 to 12 months of age, but in adults such fracture lines may remain open for years. In the latter instance the edges of the fracture are smoother and round.

Basal Fractures. Basal skull fractures may involve one or more of the 3 fossae (Figs. 4 C, 5). Unlike fractures of the vault, fractures of the base are often overlooked on the roentgenogram; hence, the importance of their clinical evaluation.

Anterior Fossa Fractures. Fractures of the *anterior fossa* often involve the cribriform plates of the ethmoid bone and the paranasal sinuses (Fig. 6). Fractures involving the orbital roof may be associated with intra-ocular extravasation of blood with resultant ecchymosis of the eyelids. A gradual increase in the suffusion of blood in the *eyelids*, particularly the lower lids, in the absence of direct trauma is strongly suggestive of an anterior fossa basal skull fracture. In severe cases exophthalmos may result; this may be severe enough to endanger the eye. Involvement of the paranasal sinuses and/or the cribriform plate is of importance in that they provide an entrance for infection. Fractures of the *cribriform plate* are frequently associated with the escape of blood, cerebrospinal fluid or brain tissue from the nose. A fracture through the frontal sinus also may be associated with a pneumocephalus (air in the cranial cavity). Such air may become encysted in the frontal lobe or enter the ventricular system. Fractures in this fossa may

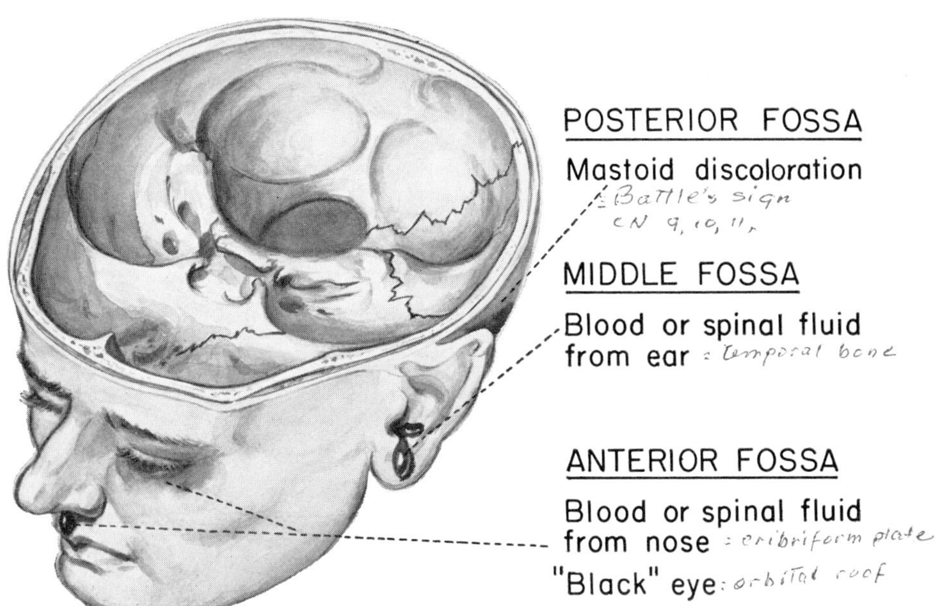

FIG. 5. Basal skull fractures may involve any one or all of the 3 fossae in the base of the skull. The outlet of the anterior fossa is the nose; of the middle fossa, the ear. The posterior fossa has no outlet but must be suspected of having a fracture when a hematoma develops in the region of the mastoid process.

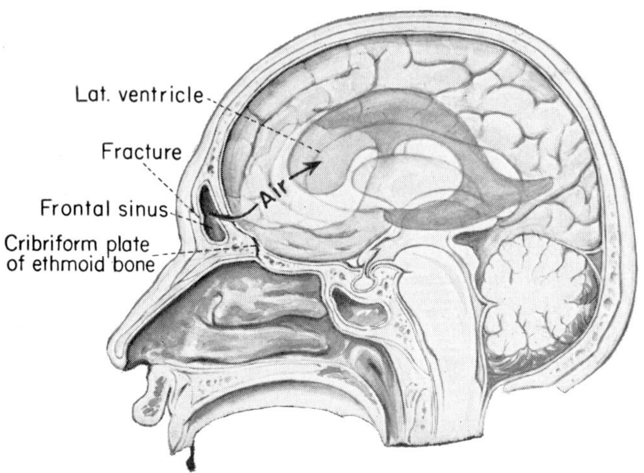

FIG. 6. Basal skull fracture involving the anterior fossa. This illustration depicts a fracture involving the frontal sinus, and air entering the cranial cavity.

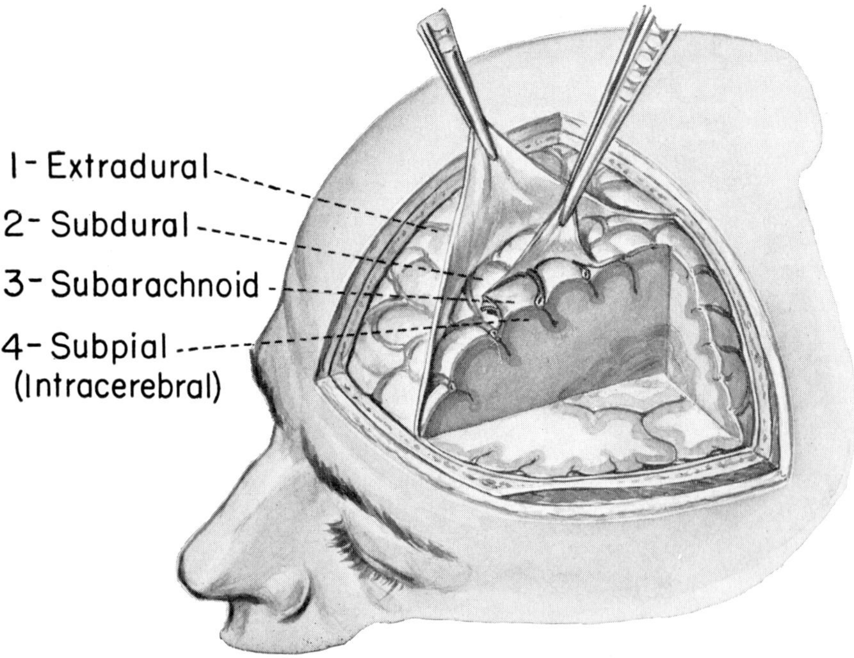

FIG. 7. The 4 intracranial spaces and associated intracranial hemorrhages. Extradural hemorrhage is usually arterial hemorrhage (middle meningeal artery). Subdural hemorrhage originates from the blood sinuses and is therefore venous. Subpial hemorrhage is intracerebral and is associated with hypertension (apoplexy) or ruptured aneurysms of the circle of Willis.

injure the *optic* and the *olfactory* nerves. If the olfactory nerves are involved, a partial or a total loss of the sense of smell may result. If the fracture extends through the optic foramen, usually the optic nerve is injured (p. 12).

Middle Fossa Fracture. These injuries may involve the temporal bone. In such instances blood, spinal fluid or brain tissue may appear at the external auditory meatus. The cranial nerves which can be involved in this fossa are: 3, 4, 5, 6, 7 and 8. The 7th (facial) and the 8th (auditory) are involved most commonly; this results in facial paralysis or auditory-vestibular involvements, respectively.

Posterior Fossa Fracture. When this fossa is involved, blood or spinal fluid may pass into the pharynx. *Battle's sign* (postauricular ecchymosis) is suggestive of a posterior fossa fracture. Unfortunately, this does not appear for 24 to 36 hours. The nerves that may be involved in this fossa are the 9th, the 10th and the 11th (p. 12).

Depressed Fracture. Depressed skull fractures are important, because they may produce brain injury and convulsions. Depressed fractures in the central area over the motor and the sensory zones or in the occipital region over the visual areas are particularly dangerous. Those involving the frontal or temporal region are not as serious.

Contrecoup injury is found at a site away from the direct location of the trauma.

The interpretation and the value of spinal puncture and the study of spinal fluid are discussed on page 9.

MENINGES AND RELATED BLOOD VESSELS

The meninges, the pia, the arachnoid and the dura mater are vulnerable in head and spinal injuries. The pia mater dips into each fissure of the brain, thereby fitting very much as a glove would fit a hand. However, the dura and the arachnoid do not dip into the fissures but rather cover the brain as a mitten would cover the hand.

Clinically, it is helpful to discuss intracranial hemorrhage as related to 4 spaces (Fig. 7):

1. The extradural space
2. The subdural space
3. The subarachnoid space
4. The subpial space

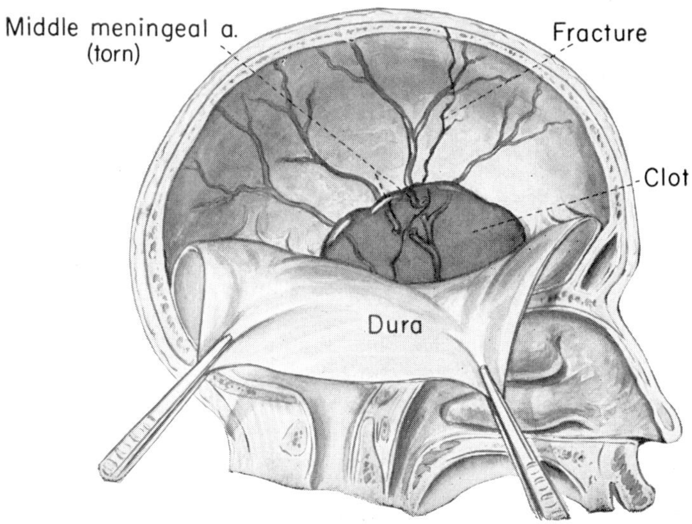

FIG. 8. Extradural hemorrhage (middle meningeal artery hemorrhage). The fracture that produces this type of bleeding involves the temporal bone. As the hemorrhage progresses, the dura is stripped away from the bone.

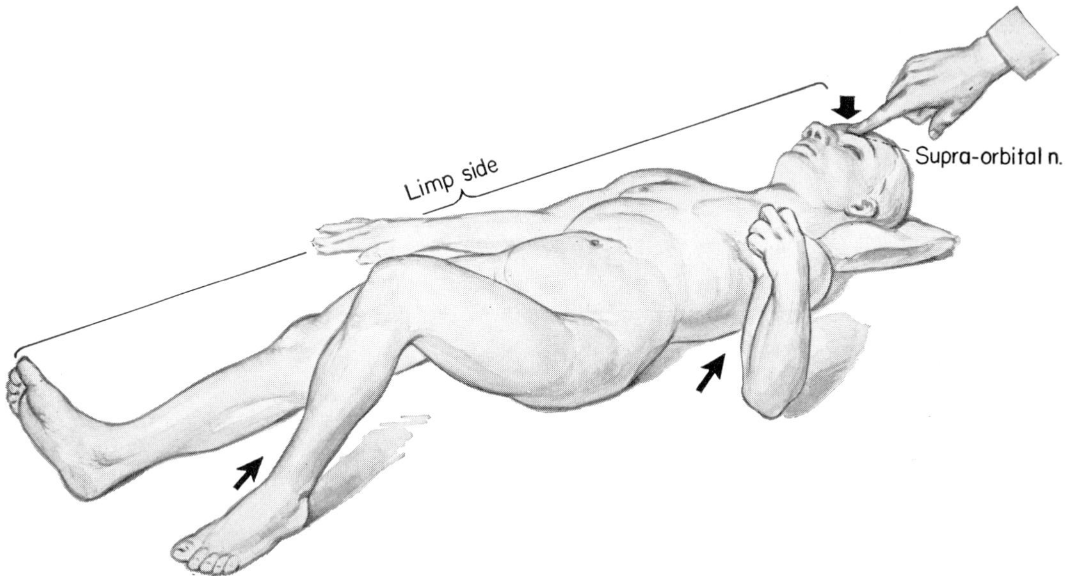

FIG. 9. The supra-orbital test applied to an unconscious patient. If a hemiplegia is present, the patient responds to this painful stimulus by moving the sound side. The affected side remains limp.

INTRACRANIAL HEMORRHAGE

Extradural Hemorrhage. This type of hemorrhage may occur with or without a skull fracture. Fractures involving the vault, particularly the temporal region, cause a laceration of the middle meningeal vessels. Many authorities believe that it is the bleeding middle meningeal artery which strips the dura away from the skull (Fig. 8). In the classic picture the patient becomes unconscious following a blow on the head. He then recovers consciousness (lucid interval), but later becomes drowsy, lapses into coma, and, if untreated, he dies. This clinical picture is subject to the widest of variations, even occurring without a lucid interval.

The clot produces increased intracranial tension with pressure on the brain. *Hemiplegia* in an unconscious patient can be demonstrated by making firm pressure over a supra-orbital nerve (Fig. 9). This produces a painful stimulus to which the patient responds by moving only the sound side. The affected side remains limp. Corroborating signs such as the presence of increased deep reflexes, absent abdominal reflexes and Babinski's sign should be sought on the affected side. A monoplegia may be the first sign of an extradural hemorrhage. The arm is affected more often than the leg.

The *pupils* may be of value in both localizing and diagnosing the lesion. At first the pupil on the involved side is small and reacts to light; however, later it becomes dilated and fixed (Fig. 10). The *spinal fluid* is also a valuable diagnostic aid. Following a head injury an insidious onset of coma and hemiplegia, along with a clear spinal fluid, is suggestive of *extradural hemorrhage.* Any force sufficiently great to rupture the meningeal vessels may rupture cerebral vessels also; hence, both intradural and extradural bleeding may occur together. The differential diagnosis of bloody spinal fluid is discussed on page 9. Increased pressure of spinal fluid suggests increased intracranial pressure, which may be due to one of many causes.

Subdural Hemorrhage. The condition of so-called chronic subdural hematoma is more common than extradural hemorrhage. The trauma responsible for the hemorrhage may be trivial and forgotten. In about a fourth of these patients a history of loss of consciousness is elicited. The condition usually manifests itself 2 or 3 weeks after the head injury. The common complaints are headache and diplopia. Intermittent somnolence and weakness of one side of the body are due to a seepage of blood over the cerebral hemispheres. The superior sagittal sinus is fixed to the skull and is immovable in contrast with the brain, which moves on impact. The superior cerebral veins pass from the superior surface of the brain into the superior sagittal sinus. A blow on the head may tear one or more of these veins (Fig. 11). Examination of the eye grounds will show blurring of the optic disk or papilledema in about half of the cases. Spinal fluid examination reveals an elevated pressure; the fluid has a yellowish tinge (50%). The pupil on one side may become dilated and fixed. Roentgenograms of the skull at times show a shift of a calcified pineal body away from the side of the lesion. Electroencephalograms, pneumoencephalograms and ventriculoencephalograms are helpful if the patient's condition permits.

Chronic subdural hematoma in infants occurs usually between 6 months and 2 years of age. The etiology is obscure; however, some are of the opinion that it is associated with mild head trauma, particularly in children who are malnourished and have a vitamin C deficiency and a bleeding tendency.

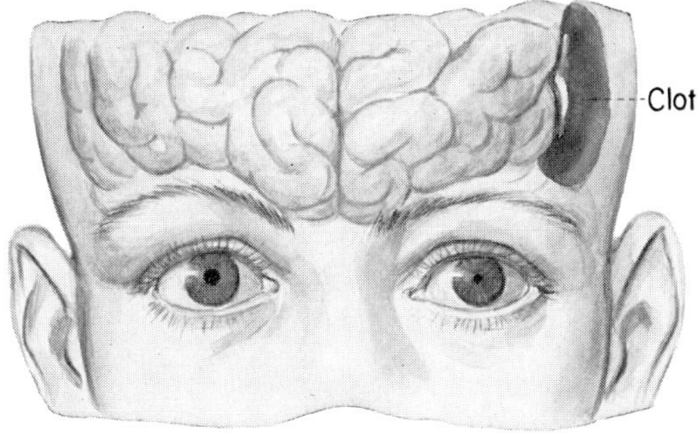

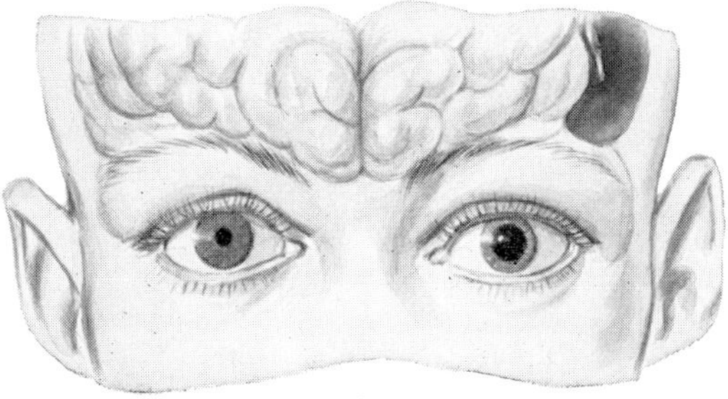

FIG. 10. The pupil is an important diagnostic aid in extradural hemorrhage. In the early stage the pupil on the involved side may be small and react to light. However, the typical finding reveals a pupil on the involved side that is dilated and does not react to light. Prognosis is poor when both pupils are dilated and fixed.

Subarachnoid Hemorrhage. This may or may not be associated with trauma. Its value in traumatic lesions has been discussed under the caption of "Extradural and Subdural Hemorrhages" (p. 8). The condition referred to as *spontaneous subarachnoid hemorrhage* is a vascular accident which occurs in younger and middle-aged people. It is due to a rupture of an aneurysm of the circle of Willis. Such aneurysms are usually congenital but in older people are arteriosclerotic. Severe meningeal irritation with stiff neck and positive Brudzinski and Kernig signs is demonstrable. If the bleeding is massive, deep coma results. A dilated pupil may be present on the side of the hemorrhage; cranial nerve involvement will help to localize the lesion. A final diagnosis is made by the demonstration of frank blood in the cerebrospinal fluid which is under high pressure. The question may arise as to whether or not the blood is due to the spinal puncture. This can be determined in 2 ways: In using the 1st method the bloody spinal fluid should be collected in 3 marked test tubes (about 3 ml. in each); if the blood is due to trauma of the spinal puncture, the fluid becomes clearer and less bloody from the 1st to the 3rd tube. If the blood is due to a head injury, it is intimately mixed with spinal fluid, and the 3 test tubes contain an equal amount of blood and show no color changes. In the 2nd method one permits the collected bloody spinal fluid to stand in a given test tube for 24 hours. In intracerebral bleeding the supernatent fluid is yellow; otherwise, it remains crystal clear.

Cerebral vascular spasm, hemorrhage, thrombosis and embolism also must be considered in the differential diagnosis of spontaneous cerebrovascular accidents

Subpial Space Hemorrhage. This is intracerebral hemorrhage, since the pia is so in-

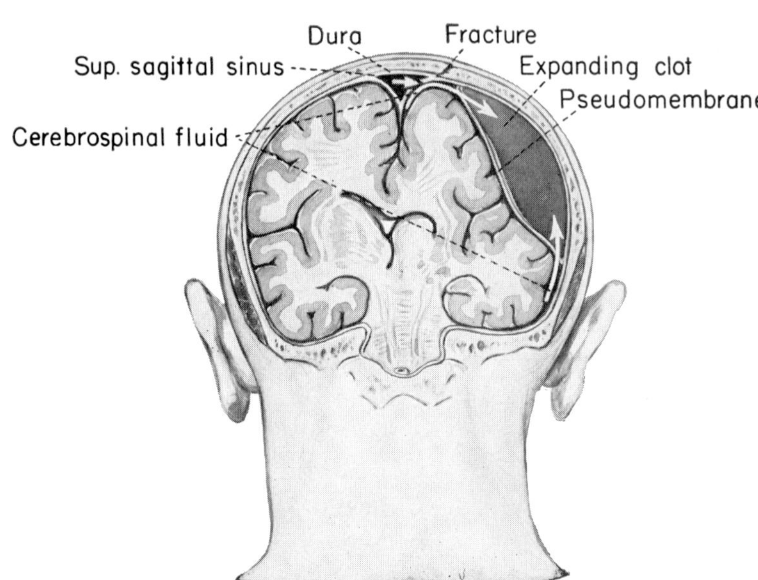

FIG. 11. Subdural hematoma. The superior cerebral veins pass from the superior surface of the brain to the superior sagittal sinus. A blow on the head may tear one of these veins or the sinus.

timately connected with brain tissue that both structures act as one unit.

BRAIN

CONCUSSION

Cerebral concussion is clinically considered to be a transient stage in which consciousness is lost for a brief period of time following trauma to the head. Some authorities consider that further restriction of the definition calls for an accompanying retrograde amnesia; the backward extension in time is roughly proportional to the degree of trauma. It is believed that this state represents a physiologic disruption of neural activity.

CEREBRAL EDEMA AND INCREASED INTRACRANIAL PRESSURE

Brain swelling may be caused by other conditions besides trauma; however, it is the latter that is pertinent to this discussion. Since the brain and the meninges are enclosed within the rigid bony skull, little room is available for expansion. As the brain swells, intracranial pressure increases and presents definite signs and symptoms. These are important guides for the clinician, since prognosis and treatment directly depend on them.

SIGNS OF CEREBRAL "DECOMPENSATION"

The greater the brain swelling the greater is the intracranial pressure. Swollen brains "decompensate." The signs of such "decompensation" are:

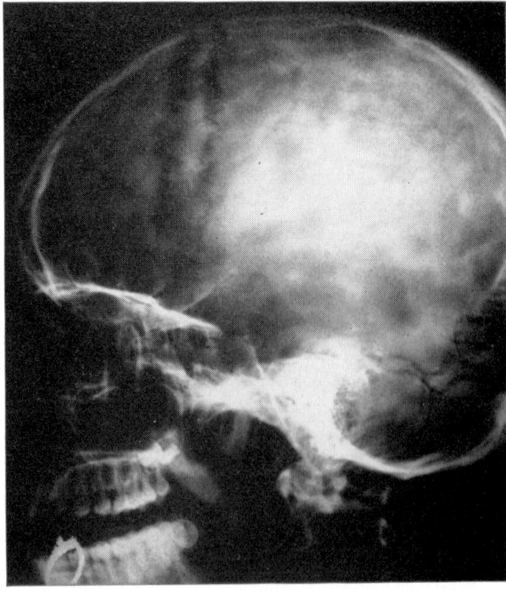

FIG. 12. Roentgenogram revealing typical digital impressions of the skull in a case of brain tumor.

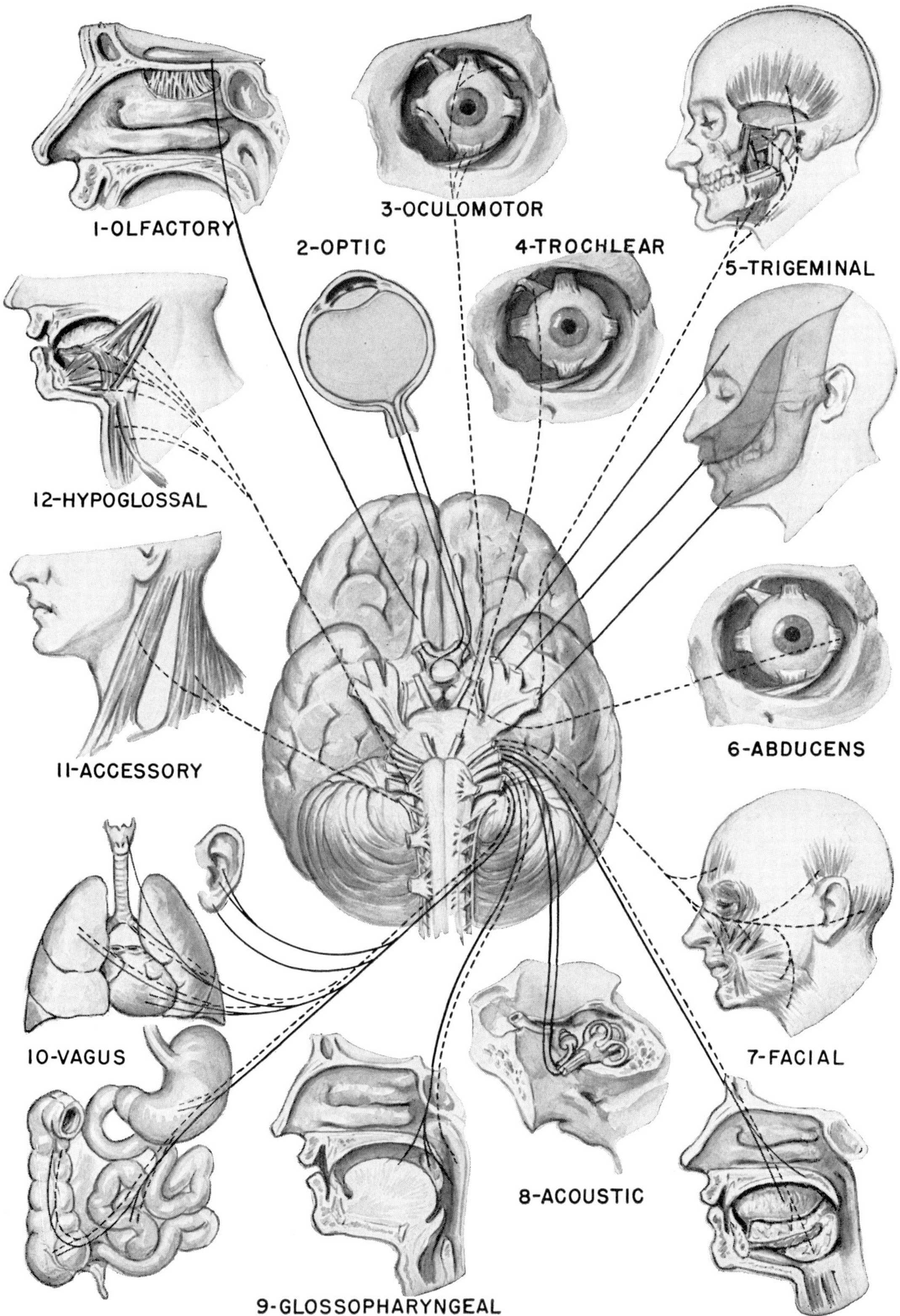

FIG. 13. The 12 cranial nerves. These nerves originate from the base of the brain and therefore are exposed to injury in basal skull fractures. Simple and rapid tests must be utilized to determine such injuries. A test for each nerve is discussed in the text.

TABLE 1. FUNCTIONS AND TESTS IN CRANIAL NERVES

CRANIAL NERVES	FUNCTIONS AND TESTS
1. Olfactory	This nerve governs the sense of smell. *Test:* Partial injury results in hyposmia; complete injury results in anosmia on the corresponding side.
2. Optic	This is the nerve of vision. *Test:* Various degrees and forms of impairment of vision and/or blindness determine the site and the nature of the injury.
3. Oculomotor	This nerve supplies all the ocular muscles except the lateral rectus and the superior oblique. *Test:* Ptosis of the upper lid is due to paralysis of the levator palpabrae superioris; proptosis is caused by paralysis of most of the ocular muscles which normally exert traction on the eyeball; mydriasis is produced by unopposed sympathetic fibers. Loss of accommodation results from paralysis of the ciliary muscle; diplopia and external strabismus are due to the unopposed action of the external rectus and the superior oblique muscles.
4. Trochlear	The 4th nerve supplies the superior oblique muscle; it is rarely involved alone. *Test:* Diplopia and deficiency of movement of the eye in a downward and outward direction result from its injury.
5. Trigeminal	There are 3 sensory branches: ophthalmic, maxillary and mandibular. A motor branch supplies the muscles of mastication. *Test:* Instruct the patient to "clench your teeth" and feel for the contractions of the masseter muscles on the affected side. Sensation may be tested over the sensory distribution.
6. Abducens	This nerve supplies the external rectus muscle. *Test:* Internal strabismus.
7. Facial	Its motor branch supplies the facial muscles; the sensory branch supplies the anterior two thirds of the tongue and the soft palate. *Test:* "Blow out your cheeks"; the involved side remains flat. (Numerous other tests can be utilized.)
8. Auditory	The cochlear division is associated with hearing; the vestibular division controls equilibrium. *Test:* Unilateral deafness and possible impairment of vestibular functions are present.
9. Glossopharyngeal	It supplies taste to the posterior third of the tongue; also has other sensory and motor branches. *Test:* Can a probe be felt on the posterior third of the tongue?
10. Vagus	It supplies sensory fibers to the skin and the thoracic and the abdominal viscera; also contains motor fibers. *Test:* This is accomplished best by ascertaining the condition of the recurrent laryngeal branch. If affected, the vocal cord is immobile and fixed in the cadaveric position on the involved side.
11. Spinal Accessory	This nerve has cranial and spinal portions. The spinal portion sends motor fibers to the upper part of the sternocleidomastoid and the trapezius muscles. *Test:* "Shrug your shoulders." The involved shoulder lags or remains dropped.
12. Hypoglossal	It supplies motor fibers to the strap muscles of the neck and the muscles of the tongue. *Test:* "Stick out your tongue"; the tongue will deviate to the involved side.

1. Deepening coma
2. Increasing fever
3. Slowing of the pulse
4. Irregularities of respiration
5. Elevation of blood pressure

Coma is in direct proportion to cerebral edema. If a patient enters the hospital in coma and later becomes lucid, the brain is "compensating." Should the reverse be true, the brain is "decompensating."

The temperature rises as the brain swells. If the patient is in a state of shock, the temperature will drop rapidly and become subnormal.

The pulse becomes slower as the brain swells. Progressive bradycardia indicates increasing intracranial pressure. If shock is present, this changes to the typical rapid, feeble, thready pulse. The respirations are regular and of normal depth if cerebral edema is not increased. When the respirations become shallow, sonorous, deep or irregular, intracranial pressure is increasing. The systolic blood pressure rises as the brain swells and "decompensates."

The forementioned 5 signs should be *recorded* and *charted* in every head-injury patient every hour on the hour. In this way one can determine readily if a patient is improving or requires surgical treatment.

Tumors

The subject of brain *tumors* is discussed in detail in appropriate texts; however, such lesions also produce signs of increased intracranial pressure and may cause confusion. A classic *triad* is associated with such tumors. It consists of headache, vomiting and choked optic disks. The roentgenogram may be of value in diagnosing increased intracranial pressure. In children there is a separation of the suture lines. In adults erosion of the posterior clinoid processes may be shown. If the pressure is of long duration, the so-called "digital impressions" produce a characteristic blotchy appearance of the calvarium (Fig. 12).

CRANIAL NERVES

Simple, rapid and accurate testing of the 12 cranial nerves should be mastered (Fig. 13). The necessary data for such tests is tabulated. The more detailed examination can be found in texts on neurology.

2

The Oral Cavity

An exact and detailed examination of the oral cavity is essential because of the numerous local lesions that may be present, and the many clues to systemic diseases that can be uncovered. Lips, tongue, oropharynx, tonsillar area and teeth must be studied systematically.

LIPS

The lips should be everted so that the entire mucosal surface can be inspected.

Cleft Lip and Palate. These congenital defects may range from a minute unilateral notch of one lip border to a complete bilateral lip and palate defect. Although the hare has an upper lip cleft in the midline, and the abnormality of the lip occurring in human beings is almost always a *lateral* cleft, we continue to use the inaccurate term "harelip." These defects constitute the most common serious anomalies of childhood. Fifty per cent of cases of cleft lip are associated with a cleft palate. If a cleft palate has not been diagnosed and corrected, permanent speech defects will result. If the palate is repaired before the age of 24 months, excellent results will be obtained in 90 per cent of the cases.

Cancer of the lip occurs predominately in the male; it appears usually after the age of 50. It resembles a superficial "split" or a warty excrescence but feels indurated. The *lower* lip is involved most frequently. This is a fairly common tumor and often is associated with exposure to the sun, preexisting leukoplakia or heavy smoking. Although dermoid in type, it frequently is curable, since it metastasizes to the regional lymph nodes in only 10 to 15 per cent of the cases.

Leukoplakia is a whitish translucent patch that appears at the corners of the buccal cavity.

Primary chancre may simulate cancer but usually involves the upper lip. Diagnosis is established by darkfield demonstration of the *Spirochaeta pallida;* the serologic tests are usually negative in this stage. The submental and the submandibular lymph glands usually become quite enlarged. Bilateral enlargement of these nodes is not infrequent because of the crossed lymphatic drainage.

Herpes labialis appears as a tender, elevated crusted plaque. Absence of ulceration, its short duration and lack of induration are its distinguishing features.

Peutz-Jeghers Syndrome. In 1921 Peutz first described a case of inherited polyposis of the mucous membranes of the intestines and the nasopharynx, attended by "peculiar pigmentations of the skin and mucous membrane" (Fig. 14). When a patient displays multiple pigmented spots, brown and black in color, on and about the vermilion surfaces of the lips, the clinician should think of this syndrome and order a thorough gastrointestinal roentgenographic study. At times pigmented areas are found on the mucous membrane of the inner cheeks. Inquiry should be made regarding any familial tendency toward such "freckles." In this condition the patient suffers frequently from polyps of the gastrointestinal tract, especially in the jejunum and the ileum (See p. 160).

TONGUE

Carcinoma of the tongue is the most common malignant lesion of the oral cavity. A dental ulcer is a frequent precursor of such a lesion. Particular importance should be attached to the cutting edge of a broken tooth or an irregularity on a denture placed directly opposite the lesion. A malignant lesion is hard; frequently it is associated with a necrotizing ulcer. Metastases occur early and usually involve the submental and the submaxillary lymph nodes, when the anterior two thirds of the tongue is involved. If the tumor is located in the posterior third or base of the tongue, the deep cervical nodes are affected.

Fissuring of the tongue should be noted (Fig. 15). Horizontal fissures usually are normal and of no clinical significance; longitudinal fissuring is strongly suggestive of a luetic glossitis.

Tuberculosis produces a very painful yet superficial ulcer of the tongue. It is almost always associated with active pulmonary tuberculosis. The demonstration of the specific bacilli and biopsy determine the diagnosis.

Vitamin deficiencies can be diagnosed by careful inspection of the tongue.

When whitish patches appear, one should suspect Monilia, particularly if vigorous antibiotic therapy has been instituted.

OROPHARYNX

Tonsils. Enlarged tonsils must not be confused with pathologic ones, and detritus in the tonsillar crypts must not be mistaken for pus. Acute tonsillitis is associated with a "sore throat," and the tonsils appear to be swollen and red. Recurrent attacks result in scarring and distortion (chronic tonsillitis). In peritonsillar abscess the involved tonsil appears to be pushed toward the opposite side. Carcinoma, tuberculosis and lymphoma of the tonsils are encountered occasionally.

Retropharyngeal abscess usually affects infants and children. It presents a protrusion of the posterior pharyngeal wall. Palpation of any inflammatory lesion involving this area should be performed with the patient in the Trendelenburg position, because of the danger of aspirating the contents if an abscess is broken inadvertently. Neoplasms that involve this area must be differentiated.

TEETH

Infections arising from the teeth constitute a major cause of swelling about the jaws, the lower two thirds of the face and the upper part of the neck. Odontogenic infections usually spread by direct continuity; the lymphatics assume a place of secondary importance. The extension of dental abscesses follows the lines of least resistance. Location of local swelling is dependent on the situation of the particular tooth involved and its anatomic relationship to bone, fascia and muscle (Fig. 16). If the maxillary teeth

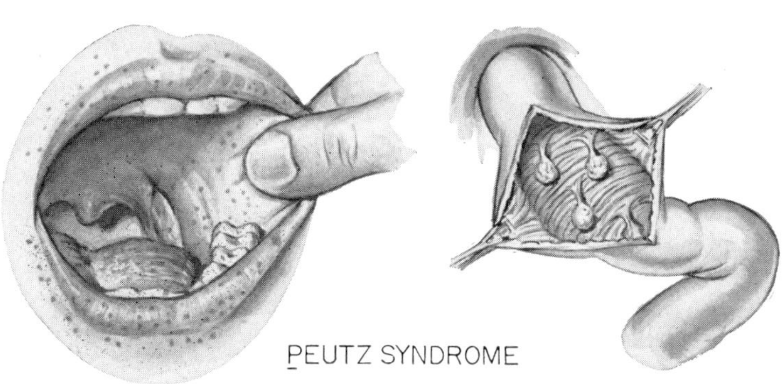

FIG. 14. The Peutz-Jeghers syndrome is characterized by a polyposis of the intestinal tract and pigmentation about the face and the mouth. The letter "P" has been used as a mnemonic.

are involved, an alveolar abcess may perforate into the vestibule, the antrum, the palate, or even regions separated by muscular attachments. A vestibular abscess reveals a shiny, fluctuant swelling in the region of the root apex or slightly below it. When premolars or molars are involved, the submaxillary area is affected, and a swelling appears below the mandible which obliterates the lower mandibular border. This is extremely tender and may be associated with trismus (spasm of the masticatory muscles). The differential diagnosis is concerned primarily with lymphadenitis and sialadenitis. Involvement of submaxillary glands rarely obliterates the line of the jaw; pus may be seen at the opening of Wharton's duct. Submaxillary abscesses can pass into the sublingual space and produce an elevation of the floor of the mouth with displacement of the tongue. The submental area becomes infected when pus burrows past the digastric muscle.

Ludwig's angina is a form of deep infection that involves the floor of the mouth, the submaxillary regions and the deep tissues of the neck as far as the hyoid bone. It is often bilateral; this is in contrast with the unilateral deep cervical abscess. Extensive induration and swelling of the floor of the mouth appears early, and the tongue is pushed upward and backward, thus interfering with swallowing and breathing. Edema of the glottis is a serious complication that can be fatal before redness and fluctuation are apparent in the neck.

SALIVARY GLANDS

Parotid Gland

Inflammation. Acute suppurative parotitis results from an infection which usually spreads via Stensen's duct (Fig. 17); it may be a manifestation of pyemia. It is noted particularly in dehydrated patients and in those who have oral sepsis and duct stasis. So-called "surgical mumps" is a serious postoperative complication. The onset is usually abrupt and is ushered in with chills, fever and a painful, tender parotid gland. Inspection reveals a prominent and red duct orifice from which blood or pus may be expressed (Fig. 18). As a rule only 1 gland is involved, but should the disease continue, the opposite side also can become affected.

The causative agent is usually staphylococcus. Although the parotid capsule is thick, the enlarged gland stands out as a diffuse swelling related to the ear and extending downward and backward over the angle of the jaw. The differential diagnosis between cervical adenitis, preauricular adenitis, and parotitis may be difficult. The loca-

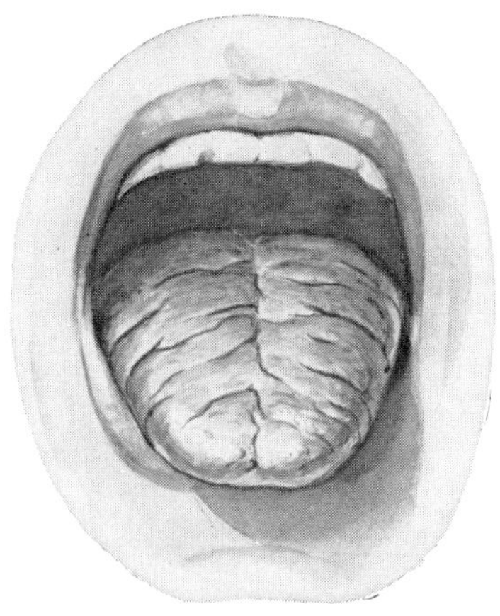

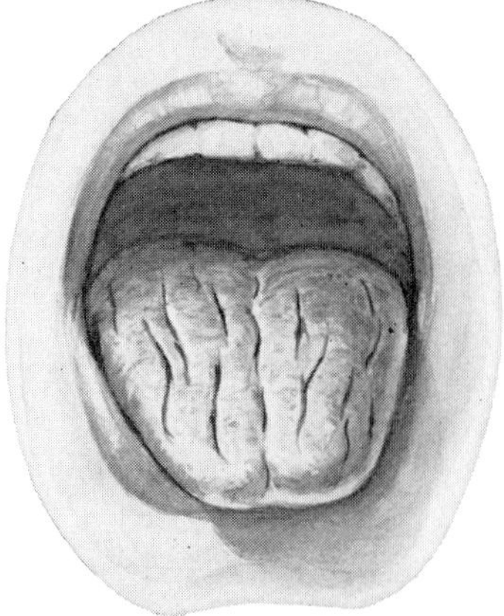

Fig. 15. The diagnostic value of fissures on the tongue. Normal fissures run horizontally; longitudinal fissures suggest lues.

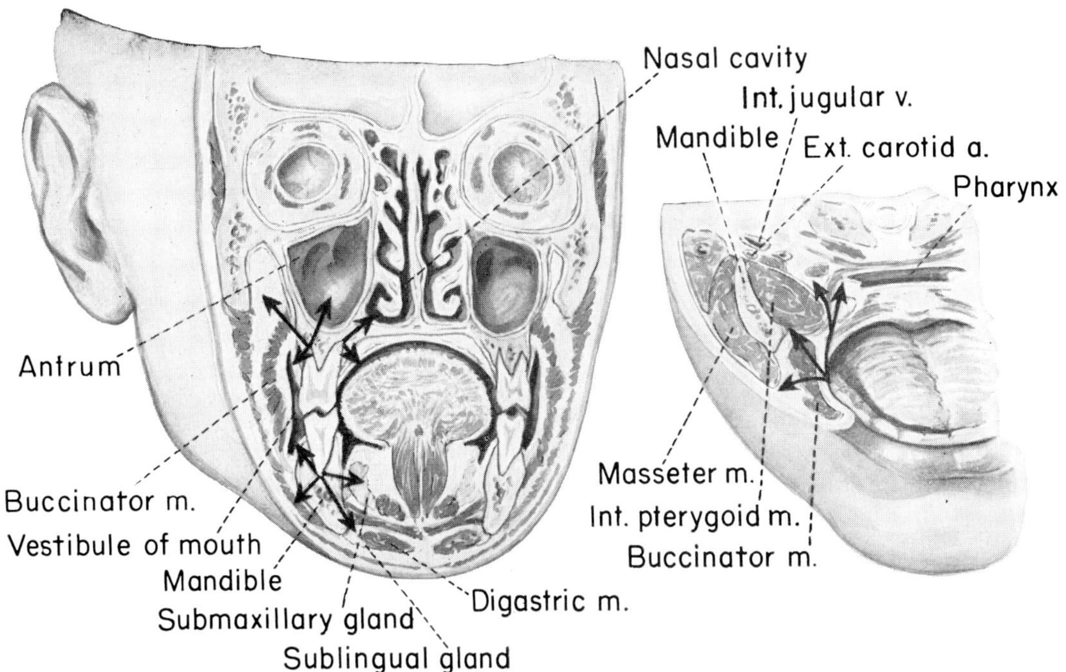

FIG. 16. Odontogenic infections. Infections arising from the teeth produce swellings about the jaws, the face and the neck. They may be confused with and must be differentiated from enlargements of the cervical lymph glands and particularly the salivary glands.

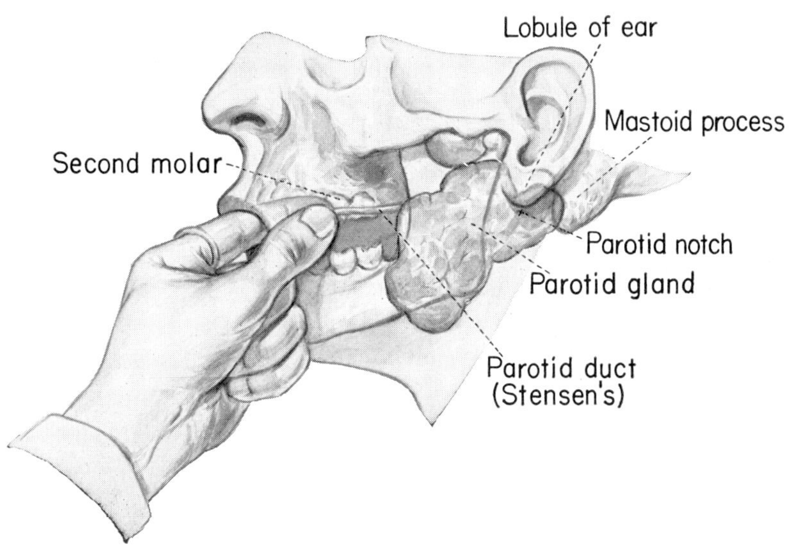

FIG. 17. The parotid gland and Stensen's duct. The duct orifice is opposite the upper second molar. The posterior aspect of the gland is related to the lobe of the ear and is situated between the angle of the jaw and the mastoid process (parotid notch).

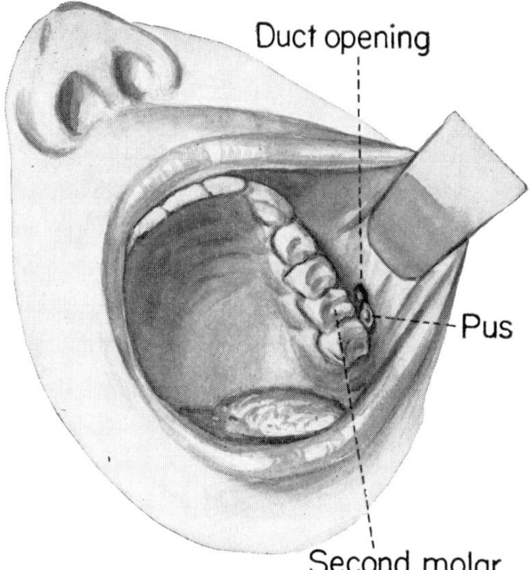

FIG. 18. The orifice of Stensen's duct. Pus may be seen exuding from the opening of the parotid gland.

tion of a lesion associated with lymphadenitis is of great diagnostic importance. When pus or blood is seen at the orifice of Stensen's duct, the diagnosis of parotid involvement is certain.

Tumors. The numerous classifications of salivary gland tumors are of greater value to the pathologist than to the clinician. It is practical to consider such tumors as mixed tumors or frank carcinomas.

A *mixed tumor* is the most common neoplasm of the parotid gland. Some experts consider it to be a carcinoma of low-grade malignancy, whereas others insist that it is benign. Such tumors are apt to recur and to metastasize late. When they do recur, they usually are multicentric. One concept is that long-standing mixed tumors may undergo malignant degeneration.

The space that exists between the tip of the mastoid process and the angle of the jaw is the "parotid notch." This area is filled with the parotid gland, and from here the gland extends in front of and behind the ear (Figs. 17, 19). Since the lobule of the ear covers this notch, *any* parotid swelling involving this region elevates it (Fig. 19).

A *frank carcinoma* of the parotid usually is indistinguishable clinically from a mixed tumor. Involvement of the 7th cranial nerve occurs more frequently in cancer than in benign lesions that affect the gland (Fig. 20). The branches of this nerve must be tested carefully, since only one portion of the nerve may be involved.

Warthin's tumor (papillary cystadenoma lymphomatosum) occurs predominately in males. It is located typically at the posterior margin of the lower pole of the gland and may be bilateral. Since these tumors are soft, encapsulated and cystic, they must be differentiated from retention cysts of ductal origin.

Submaxillary Salivary Gland

Although acute pyogenic inflammation is encountered more frequently in the parotid gland, chronic inflammatory processes affect the submaxillary gland more frequently. These are usually secondary to obstructions of Wharton's duct. Frequently such obstructions are caused by calculi or mucous plugs (Fig. 21). The history is quite stereotyped. The patient complains of a painful mass below and in front of the angle of the jaw;

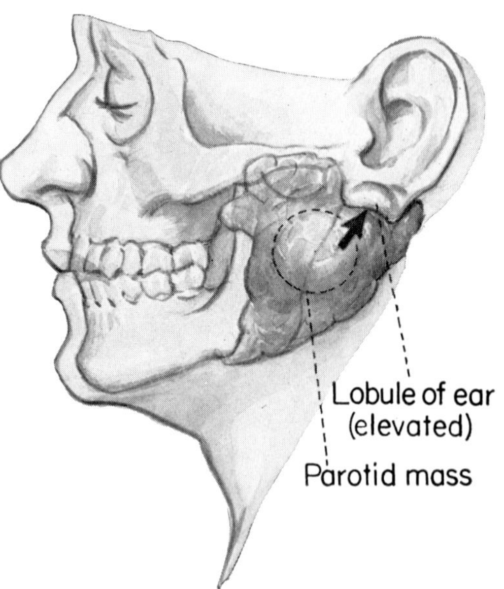

FIG. 19. Relation of the parotid gland to the lobule of the ear. If a parotid mass is located in the region of the ear lobule, the latter is elevated.

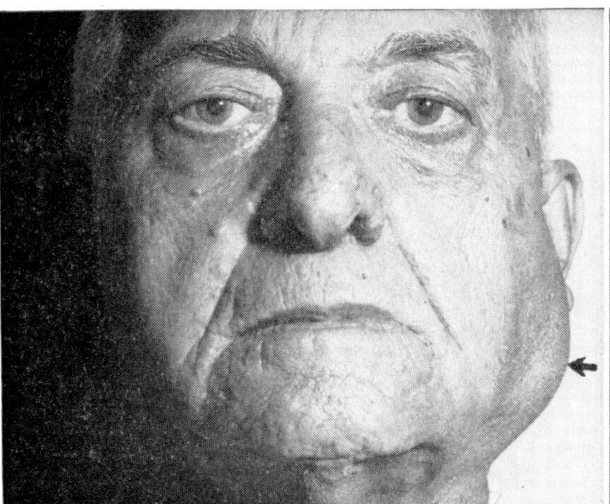

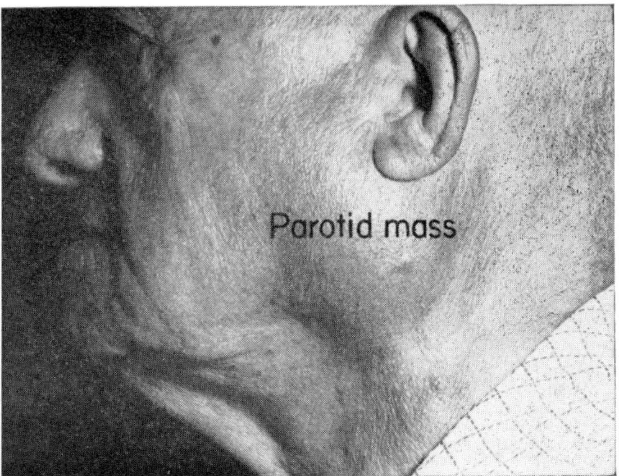

FIG. 20. Retention cyst of the parotid gland. Enlargements of the gland are not always due to tumors. Note the absence of facial nerve involvement.

this is associated with the ingestion of a meal; eating tart foods like lemon and pickles usually is associated with the pain. Inspection of the floor of the mouth reveals a red and edematous orifice of Wharton's duct (Fig. 22). By means of bidigital palpation the course of the duct and the firm calculus usually can be felt (Fig. 23). The roentgenogram corroborates the presence of the stones, since they are rich in mineral salts. The gland is enlarged and tender and may be confused with submaxillary lymphadenitis. It is important to examine thoroughly the mouth and the pharynx for foci of infection that may be associated with

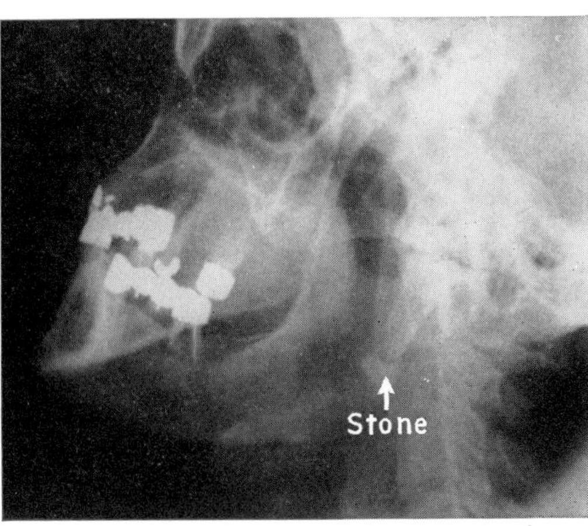

FIG. 21. Roentgenogram revealing a calculus in the submaxillary (Wharton's) duct. Roentgenographic corroboration of such sialoliths is frequently possible, because these stones have a high mineral content.

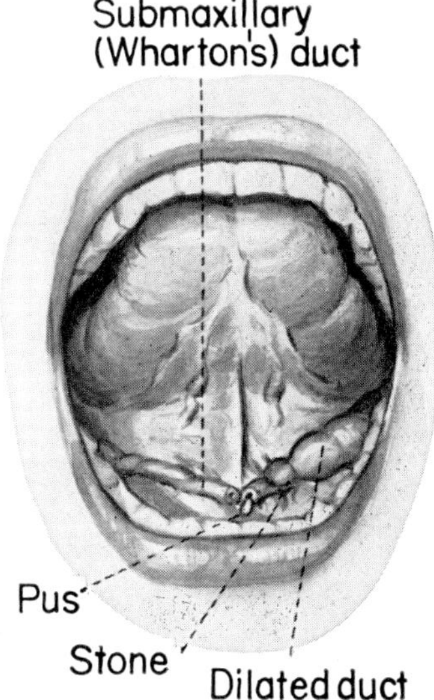

FIG. 22. A calculus in the submaxillary (Wharton's) duct. Examination of the floor of the mouth reveals the edematous duct orifice and a drop of pus which can be expressed easily. The duct is dilated proximal (as the saliva flows) to the stone.

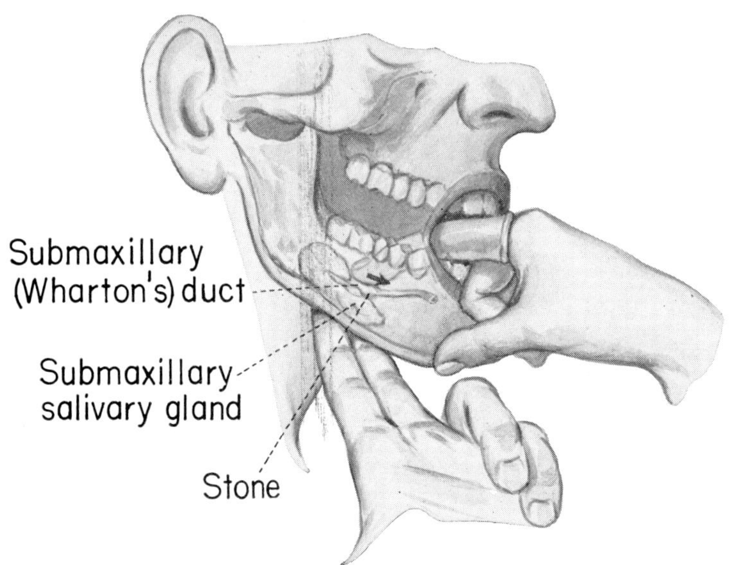

Fig. 23. Palpation of the submaxillary gland and duct. The gloved intraoral finger strokes the duct distally (arrow). This permits an evaluation of the duct and frequently locates the stone and expresses pus.

lymphadenitis. Metastatic tumors also appear in this region.

Mixed tumors and carcinomas of the submaxillary salivary glands do occur but are less common than in the parotid.

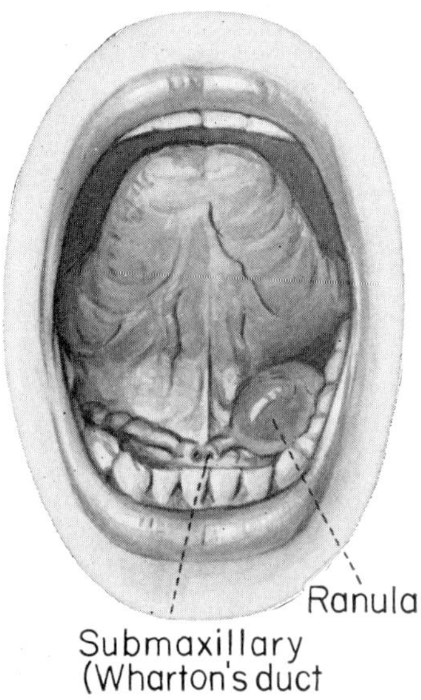

Ranula
Submaxillary
(Wharton's duct

Fig. 24. Ranula. This cystic swelling of one of the sublingual glands is close to the submaxillary (Wharton's) duct but is not connected with it.

Sublingual Gland

The term *ranula* is associated with the sublingual salivary gland. This is a mucous gland that undergoes myxomatous degeneration (Fig. 24). The involved gland is usually the sublingual, but one of the solitary glands that are present over the buccal mucous membrane also may be affected.

A ranula appears as a bluish, unilateral, transparent cystic swelling in the floor of the mouth. It was so named by Hippocrates, since he likened it to the swelling of a frog's belly. Wharton's duct can be identified as an opaque band that traverses the anterior wall of the cyst. Although the cyst displaces the duct, it is in no way directly associated with it. Ranulas may have a cervical prolongation; hence, palpation beneath the jaw and the upper cervical region should be included in the examination.

Mikulicz's Disease

Mikulicz's disease is characterized by a bilateral inflammatory involvement of all or any group of salivary glands, plus involvement of the lacrimal glands. It is relatively uncommon but should be diagnosed easily.

3

Neck

The diagnosis of a neck lesion may be extremely simple or so difficult that a final diagnosis can be reached only by exploration and biopsy. The clinician must be ever mindful of the possibility that the mass may be a *metastatic* node from an intra-oral, an intranasal or a hypopharyngeal tumor; however, it may be a primary tumor or a congenital lesion. Examination of the neck always should be integrated with that of the head, the face and the oral cavity. The muscles, the bone and the cartilaginous structures can mask the lesion or even be mistaken for a pathologic process.

Orientation and relation to the osseocartilaginous framework must be determined. These can be accomplished if the following 5 questions are answered systemically:

1. Is the lesion in the midline?
2. Is the lesion in the anterior or the posterior cervical triangle?
3. What is the relationship of the lesion to the sternocleidomastoid muscle?
4. Is it single or multiple?
5. What are its physical properties?

To obtain proper relaxation for adequate palpation of the neck, the following positions of the head should be utilized (Fig. 25). The anterior triangle of the neck is relaxed if the occiput is pushed forward so that the patient's head is flexed. The posterior triangle of the neck can be felt properly if the patient's head is inclined toward the side that is being examined. The submental region is examined best with the head flexed slightly in the neutral position.

The supraclavicular regions must be palpated carefully in every case. The pulsations

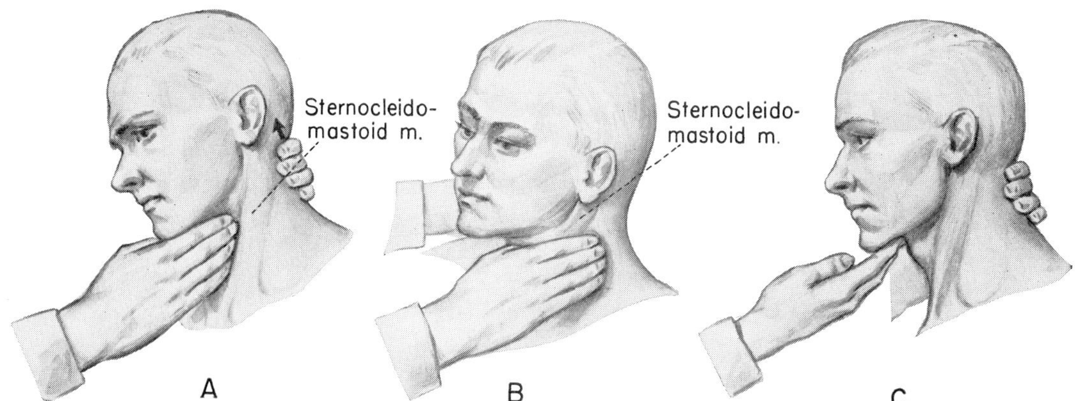

Fig. 25. Palpation of the neck. (A) The anterior triangle of the neck is relaxed if the occiput is pushed forward. (B) The posterior triangle of the neck is felt best if the patient's head is inclined toward the side that is being examined. (C) The submental region should be examined with the head slightly flexed.

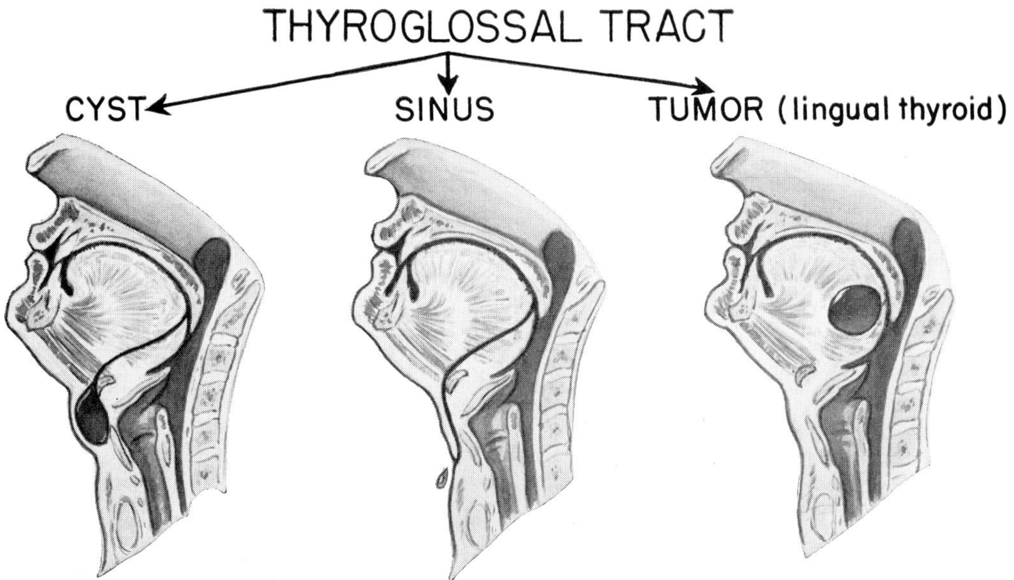

FIG. 26. Anomalies of the thyroglossal tract. Developmental defects affecting this tract may result in a cyst, a sinus or a lingual thyroid.

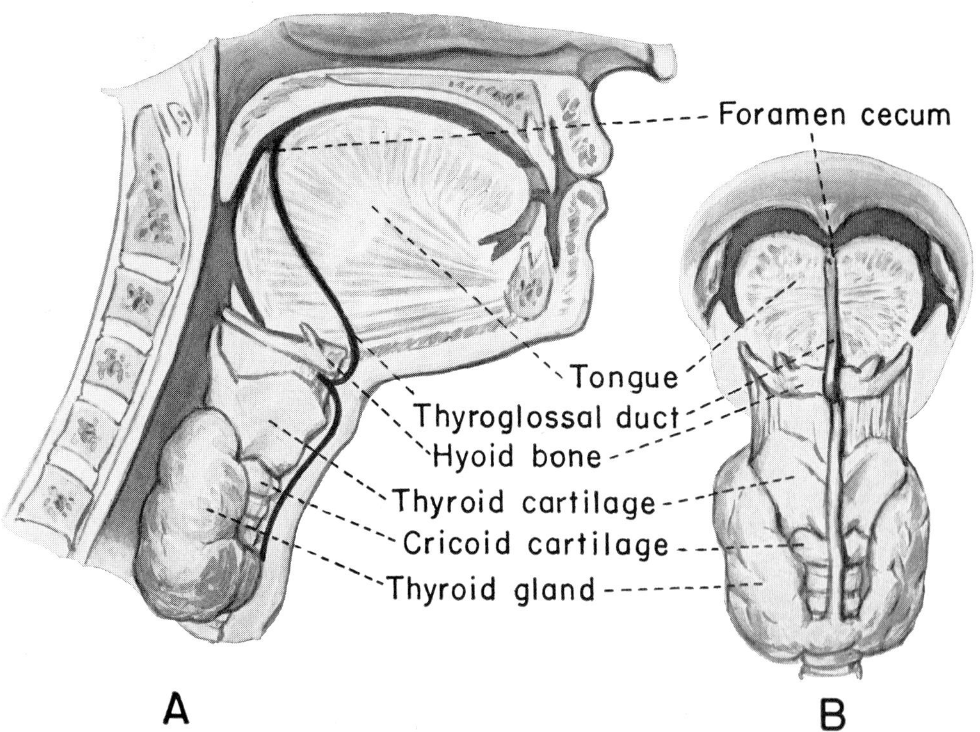

FIG. 27. The thyroglossal tract originates at the posterior aspect of the tongue (foramen cecum), extends downward and ends as the thyroid gland.

of the 3rd portion of the subclavian artery are felt in an angle formed by the clavicle and the posterior border of the sternocleidomastoid. The back of the neck can be relaxed when the patient's head is partially extended.

CONGENITAL DEFECTS

The more important congenital lesions are thyroglossal duct cysts, branchiogenic cysts and sinuses, and cystic hygromas.

Thyroglossal Tract Conditions

Anomalies of the thyroglossal duct arise from a congenital persistence of this tract. They may be divided conveniently into 3 conditions: (1) thyroglossal cysts, (2) thyroglossal sinuses and (3) thyroglossal tumors (lingual thyroid) (Fig. 26).

The thyroglossal tract originates at the foramen cecum, which is located at the posterior third of the tongue (Fig. 27). From this site a solid column of cells grows downward in the fetus; this column becomes canalized and forms the thyroglossal duct, from which the thyroid gland develops. The 3 listed anomalies occur along this tract.

Thyroglossal Cysts. These occur in the *midline* of the neck and usually during childhood. Recurrent inflammatory bouts result in disfigurements. They may appear between the submental area and the suprasternal notch but are found most commonly near the hyoid bone. The cyst may be tiny or as large as a golf ball. If no inflammation is present, it is smooth, round and displaceable, although it is anchored to the deeper tissues and the hyoid bone. It is not attached to the skin; nor is it tender unless inflamed. These cysts move with swallowing and also with protrusion of the tongue (Fig. 28). They represent the most common swellings in the midline of the neck. Although the diagnosis is not difficult, the *differential diagnosis* includes consideration of pyramidal thyroid lobe, lymph nodes, lipomas, sebaceous cysts and branchial cleft cysts.

Dermoids, lipomas and sebaceous cysts can occur also in the midline of the neck.

Thyroglossal Sinuses. These sinuses result from spontaneous perforation of or surgical incision into a thyroglossal cyst. When inflammation or abscess formation is present, redness, pain and heat are noted. Their *midline* position is the most diagnostic feature.

Thyroglossal Tumors. These tumors constitute the so-called lingual thyroids; they are

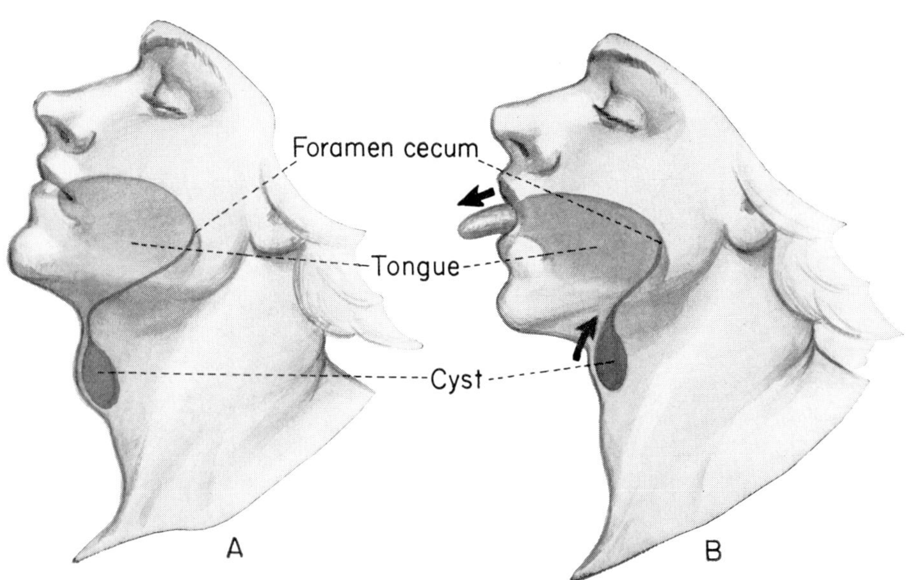

Fig. 28. Thyroglossal cyst. These cysts move with swallowing and with protrusion of the tongue.

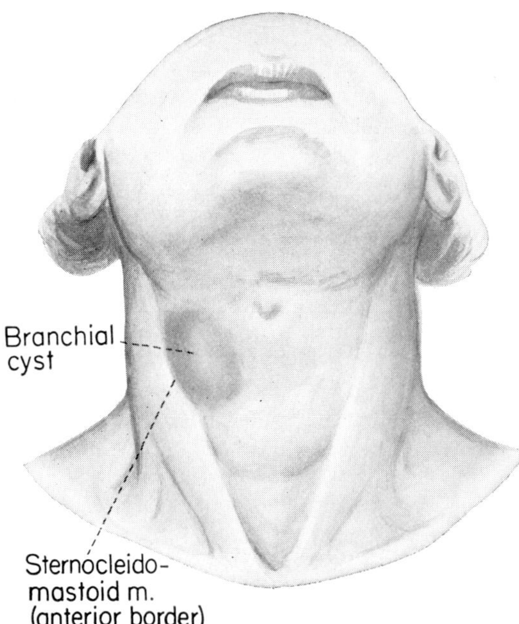

FIG. 29. Branchial cyst. These cysts are congenital and always appear along the anterior border of the sternocleidomastoid muscle.

rare. They usually represent the total thyroid tissue that the patient possesses; if they are removed, they may produce surgical myxedema. Since they are located between the back part of the tongue and the hyoid bone, they resemble thyroglossal cysts. This differential diagnosis is most difficult. It is preferable to explore them rather than to aspirate them; they should be biopsied before removal is commenced.

Differential diagnosis of thyroglossal tract anomalies includes branchiogenic cysts, lymphadenitis, tuberculous lesions, midline cervical clefts and specific granulomas.

Branchial Cysts and Fistulas

Branchial cysts are congenital. They appear in the anterior triangle of the neck. They may be found anywhere along the *anterior border* of the sternocleidomastoid muscle. The usual site is the middle third of that muscle (Fig. 29). They may be unilateral or bilateral. Pain is rarely present. As a rule the diagnosis is easy, but these may be mistaken for tuberculous adenitis, cystic hygroma, carotid body tumor, metastatic glands and thyroid adenomas. Thyroglossal cysts should cause no diagnostic difficulty, since they lie in the midline of the neck. At times it may be necessary to aspirate the cyst; such fluid reveals the typical cholesterol crystals.

Branchial fistulas appear as small dimples or tiny openings closely associated with the *anterior border* of the sternocleidomastoid muscle. The fistula may be complete or incomplete, depending on whether or not there is an internal opening that extends into the pharynx (Fig. 30). This information can be elicited readily by the injection of a radiopaque material into the external opening. The external opening is situated along the lower third of the *anterior* border of the sternocleidomastoid muscle. If the fistula is complete, it dips between the external and the internal carotid arteries before entering the pharynx. A discharge of mucoid material is commonly present. Secondary infection is a frequent complication. When this occurs, the discharge becomes purulent, and signs of inflammation are present. A draining tuberculous sinus may be confused with a branchial fistula. Tuberculosis is suggested by the presence of multiple cutaneous openings and palpable enlarged lymph glands. Other specific granulomas must be differentiated also.

Cystic Hygroma

This is a rather uncommon lateral cervical swelling which usually is seen in infants or young children. Typically, it is found in the lower third of the neck and enlarges as

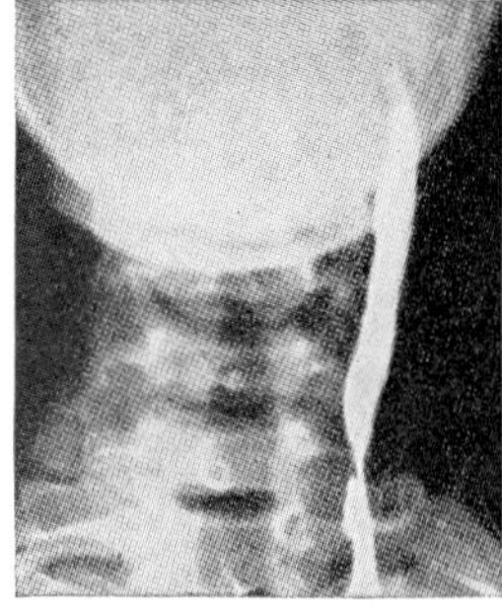

FIG. 30. Roentgenogram of an injected branchial fistula. The external opening is located at the *anterior* border of the sternocleidomastoid muscle, and the internal opening extends into the pharynx.

it extends upward toward the ear. If it extends downward, it can pass behind the clavicle to the dome of the pleura; it may extend into the axilla also. It feels soft and irregular and usually is located *behind* the sternocleidomastoid muscle. Pain or local discomfort usually are absent unless secondary infection has occurred. Since it lies in a superficial plane, it tends to bulge outward and rarely produces pressure symptoms upon the cervical viscera. If it is large, it may interfere with movements of the head. Occasionally, it ruptures spontaneously and disappears.

THYROID GLAND

The normal thyroid is palpable in slender individuals but cannot be felt in thicknecked or obese people. Each lobe normally extends from the middle of the thyroid cartilage to the 4th or the 5th tracheal ring. The isthmus, which is usually but not always present, connects both lobes and passes across the 3rd tracheal ring (Fig. 31).

The size of the gland is not related to its toxicity.

A useful *clinical classification of the thyroid state* is the following:

Toxic Goiter

A. Diffuse
B. Adenoma (nodose)

Nontoxic Goiter

A. Diffuse
B. Adenoma (nodose)

Hyperthyroidism

Hyperthyroidism resembles 2 other great masqueraders, namely, tuberculosis and syphilis, since they affect any or all of the major systems (Fig. 32). The 5 major systems are the cardiovascular, the respiratory, the gastrointestinal, the genitourinary and the nervous.

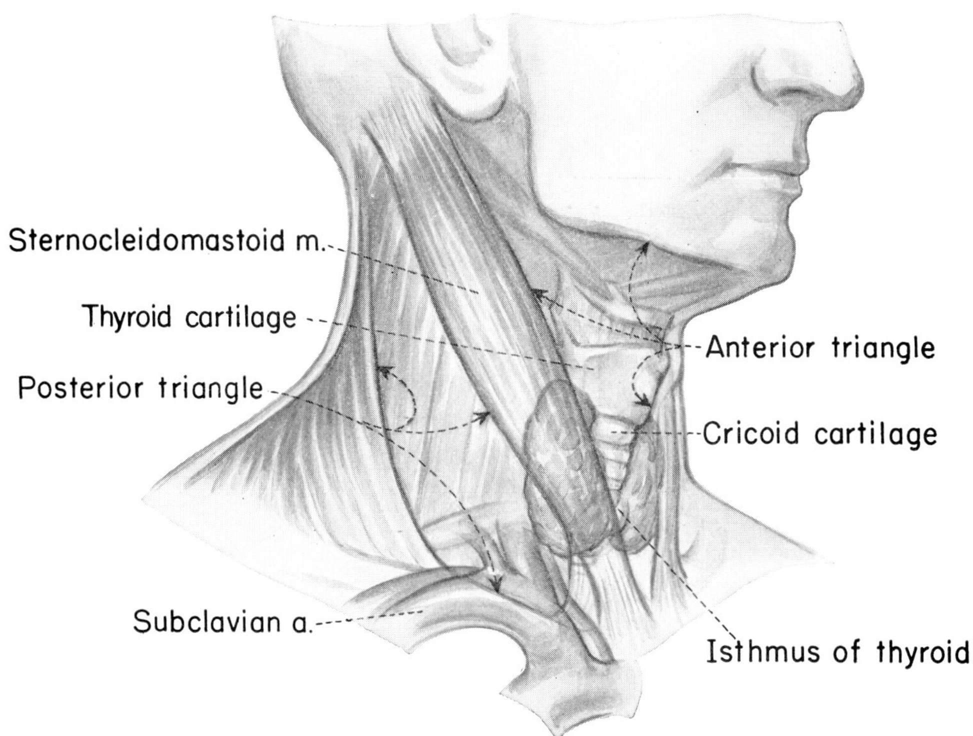

Fig. 31. The normal thyroid gland extends from the middle of the thyroid cartilage to the 4th or the 5th tracheal ring. The isthmus usually crosses the 3rd tracheal ring.

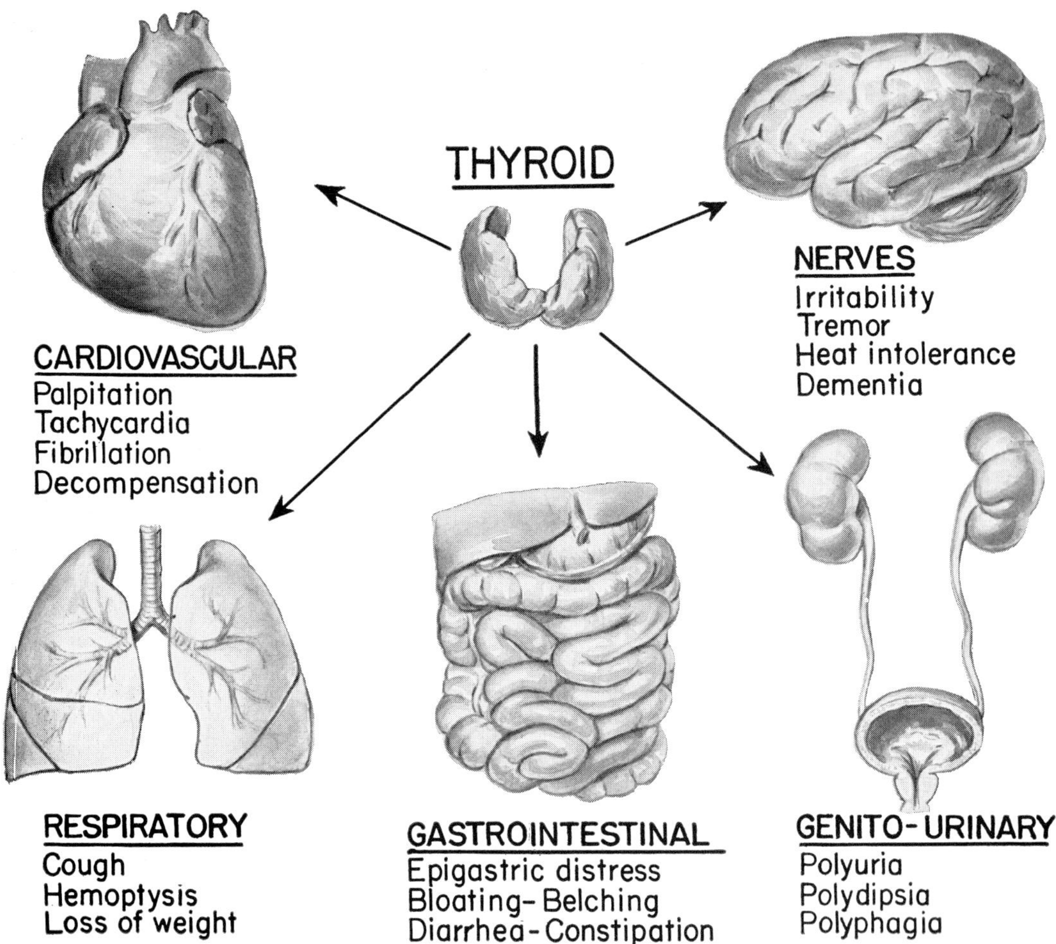

FIG. 32. Hyperthyroidism. This great masquerader can involve any of the 5 major systems. When cardiovascular complaints are foremost, the case may be mistaken for organic heart disease. Respiratory symptoms suggest tuberculosis. The gastrointestinal symptoms may lead to erroneous diagnosis which involve the gallbladder, the stomach or the bowel. Involvement of the nervous system focuses attention on psychiatric conditions. Unfortunately, the hyperthyroid patient may be mistaken for a diabetic when polydipsia, polyuria and polyphagia constitute the primary complaints.

The cardiovascular symptoms make the patient heart-conscious. He seeks medical aid because of his "heart trouble." This results from such symptoms as palpitation, tachycardia, dyspnea or decompensation. Lahey has aptly referred to these patients as "thyrocardiacs." Should decompensation take place, the unseasoned clinician is misled by the orthopnea, ascites and dependent edema. Paroxysmal auricular fibrillation, when present, should make one suspicious of a toxic thyroid.

The respiratory symptoms, such as cough, loss of weight and blood-streaked sputum, might suggest tuberculosis. It is well to remember that the patient with hyperthyroidism has a ravenous appetite, but the tuberculous individual is finicky about his food. Determination of the blood pressure is a simple and excellent way of differentiating tuberculosis from hyperthyroidism. The hyperthyroid patient has a somewhat elevated systolic and a normal or lowered diastolic pressure. This results in the almost pathog-

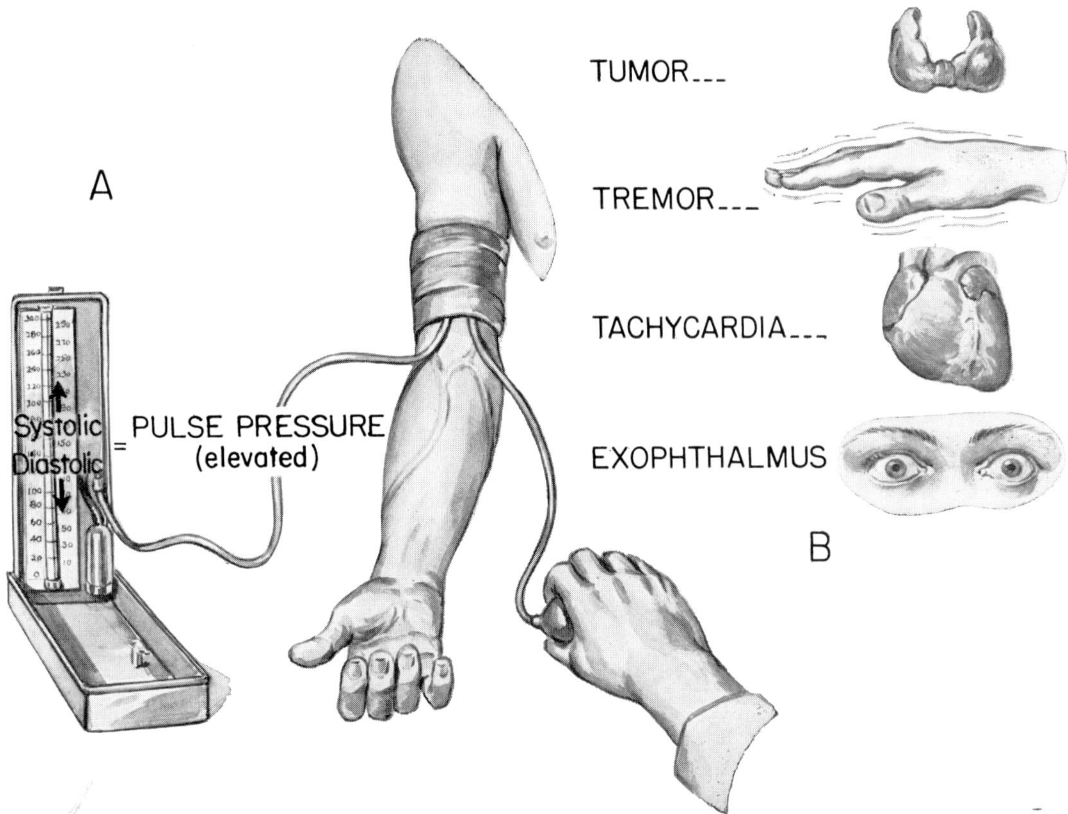

FIG. 33. Hyperthyroidism. (A) The blood pressure is characteristic, since the systolic is elevated, the diastolic somewhat lower, and the pulse pressure increased. (B) The cardinal signs of hyperthyroidism.

nomonic elevated pulse pressure of the toxic thyroid (Fig. 33 A). The tuberculous patient does not reveal this characteristic change.

The gastrointestinal symptoms of the hyperthyroid patients are numerous and bizarre. Among these are alternating diarrhea and constipation, bloating, distention and vague abdominal pains; usually these are associated with extreme weakness. The appetite is excellent, but with impending thyroid crises, anorexia, nausea or even vomiting may be present. With such gastrointestinal complaints, carcinoma, gallbladder disease, ulcer and enterocolitis must be ruled out.

The genitourinary system may be involved also, and diabetes mellitus may be diagnosed erroneously, because these patients present the diabetic triad, namely, polydipsia, polyphagia and polyuria. Since these patients consume large quantities of carbohydrates and sugars, they frequently have an alimentary glycosuria. This is differentiated readily if the fasting blood sugar is determined.

Nervous symptoms vary from irritability to dementia.

Heat intolerance is usually present; such individuals are the first to open the windows, to turn down the heat and to use few or no covers despite a very cool room. Most of them sweat excessively.

Physical examination should determine the size and the consistency of the thyroid gland. This gland moves with swallowing; hence, it should not be confused with other masses. The cardinal signs of hyperthyroidism have been listed as tumor, tremor, tachycardia and exophthalmus (Fig. 33 B).

TREMOR. A tremor is usually present; it may be quite fine and easily overlooked. To demonstrate such tremors, the patient

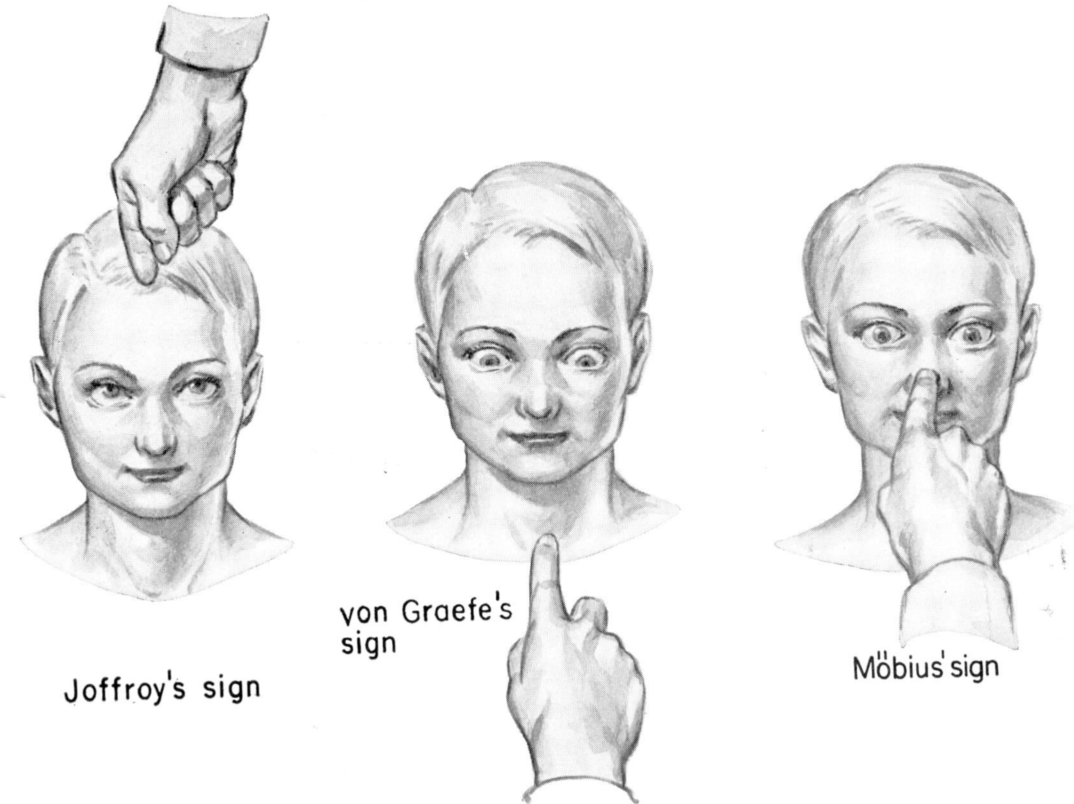

FIG. 34. Eye signs associated with hyperthyroidism.

should be asked to spread his fingers; as the physician places a piece of paper over them, the movements of the paper are readily seen.

EYE SIGNS. At times eye signs are present and helpful as diagnostic aids (Fig. 34).

Exophthalmos may or may not be present; it is usually bilateral.

Lid lag (von Graefe's sign) is positive when the upper lid lags behind the lower lid as the patient looks down; this exposes the white eyeball.

Failure of convergence (Möbius' sign) is positive when 1 eye or both eyes fail to converge on an object which is brought close to the midline of the face.

Retraction of the upper lid (Stellwag's sign) is often associated with spasmodic contractions of the lid as the patient looks upward.

Failure to wrinkle the forehead when the patient suddenly turns his eyes upward is Joffroy's sign.

THRILL AND BRUIT. A palpable thrill and an audible bruit are sometimes present in the more advanced cases.

DERMOGRAPHIA is readily demonstrable in hyperthyroidism; it is a manifestation of vasomotor instability.

The use of Lugol's solution as a therapeutic test is helpful; 10 drops 3 times a day should produce vast improvement and diminish most of the symptoms. Then the solution should be utilized only as a preparatory measure for surgery.

"TUMOR." Palpation gives valuable information in that the size and the consistency of a nodule can be detected readily. As was stated previously, all thyroid tissue and masses move with swallowing. The lower pole can be felt if the sternocleidomastoid muscle is pushed aside; if one fails to feel this lobe, a retrosternal thyroid should be suspected. Percussion over the manubrium reveals a specific dullness which is most sug-

TABLE 2. LABORATORY FINDINGS IN NORMAL, HYPOTHYROID AND HYPERTHYROID CONDITIONS

DETERMINATION	NORMAL	HYPOTHYROID	HYPERTHYROID
BMR	−10% to 15%	Below −10%	Above +15%
PBI	4 to 8 μg. %	Below 4 μg. %	Above 8 μg. %
I^{131}	20 −50% uptake	Below 20%	Above 50% uptake
PBI^{131} (24 hrs.)	0.010–0.086%	0.003–0.054%	0.085–1.45%
Cholesterol	110–300 mg. %	Above 300 mg. %	Below 110 mg. %

gestive of a retrosternal mass. It is important to detect solitary nodules in the thyroid gland, particularly the nontoxic variety. Statistical data suggest that malignancy is fairly common in such nodules; figures varying from 5 to 20 per cent have been reported.

As stated, the size of the gland is not related to the degree of toxicity. Marked enlargements encroach upon the trachea, displace it and produce dyspnea. Pressure on the esophagus produces dysphagia. Such displaced viscera can be demonstrated readily by the roentgenogram (Fig. 35).

Laboratory Tests. Some laboratory tests are helpful in the diagnosis of hyperthyroidism. The multiplicity of tests available for an evaluation of the thyroid function presents both a help and a headache to the clinician. We have the time-honored determinations of basal metabolic rate and blood cholesterol; the widely used serum protein-bound iodine levels and thyroid uptake of radioactive iodine have been joined by the serum level of butanol-extractable iodine, the I^{131} conversion ratio, the thyroid I^{131} clearance and the in-vitro erythrocyte uptake of I^{131}-labeled tri-iodothyronine, to mention only a few. Time will determine the efficacy of all of these; some of the more practical ones will be discussed (Table 2).

The *basal metabolic rate* is a most reliable test. In hyperthyroidism the rate is elevated; however, it must be recalled that no tests are foolproof, and other conditions might produce elevated basal metabolic readings. Leukemia, febrile states and pheochromocytoma, to mention only a few, produce increased readings.

The *blood cholesterol* is usually normal or below normal (140 to 200 mg. %) in hyperthyroid states.

The *serum protein-bound iodine* (*P.B.I.*)

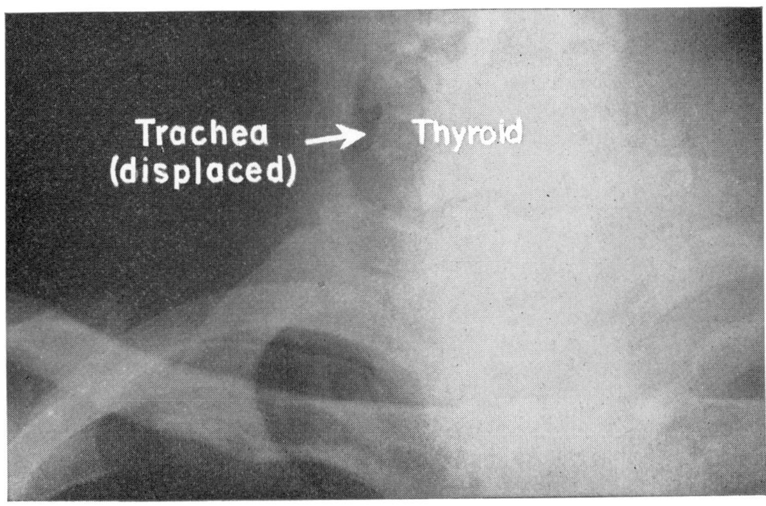

FIG. 35. Roentgenogram revealing displacement of the trachea and the esophagus by an enlarged thyroid.

is elevated in hyperthyroidism. In most clinics levels above 7.5 mcg. per 100 ml. are considered as diagnostic of this condition. Iodine containing medicaments or tests (cholecystography) make the test valueless.

ET-3 is a test which calls for special discussion; it deals with the erythrocyte uptake of iodine. The patient need not be in a fasting state or off iodine or thyroid therapy. This aspect of the test is particularly useful when such factors interfere with the diagnostic interpretation of other assays. There are some who believe that there is a slight variation in the range of normals between males and females. Hence, the following figures are given:

	Males	Females
Euthyroid	12-19%	11-17%
Hyperthyroid	19-38%	17-35%
Hypothyroid	6-12%	6-11%

Radioactive iodine tests seem to be a highly satisfactory method for determining thyroid function. Table 2 gives the normal and the abnormal values.

The *thyroid scan*, a graphic representation of the distribution of a radioactive tracer in the thyroid gland, is generally known as a *scintigram*. After the patient has ingested a given amount of radioactive iodine, the scintigram is interpreted by comparing an abnormal area in the gland with an adjacent normal one. In this way the normal area acts as a standard against which any abnormal regions can be measured.

Figure 36 reveals the uniform distribution of a radioactive substance in a patient with a normally functioning thyroid gland. "Hot nodules" are areas that concentrate more radioactive material than the surrounding normal tissues. Figure 37 demonstrates the pattern in such a nodule with increased thyroid activity. The "cold nodule" will do the reverse and indicates a nonfunctioning part of the thyroid gland. This scanning has become an important aid in the recognition and particularly the management of the so-called nontoxic goiter or the solitary thyroid nodule.

Nontoxic Nodular Goiter. There is little or no controversy concerning the treatment of large nodular goiters; thyroidectomy is advisable because of pressure symptoms (dysphagia and dyspnea) and/or cosmetic reasons. It is the smaller asymptomatic nodular goiter which presents problems. Astonishingly divergent views still exist regarding their management. Some authorities believe that practically never is thyroidectomy indicated, since carcinomas are rare. Equally experienced specialists state that thyroidectomy should be performed in practically all such patients because of the danger of malignancy. A study of statistics regarding this question is inconclusive. Obviously, neither position is entirely tenable. A "common-sense" approach has been suggested by some

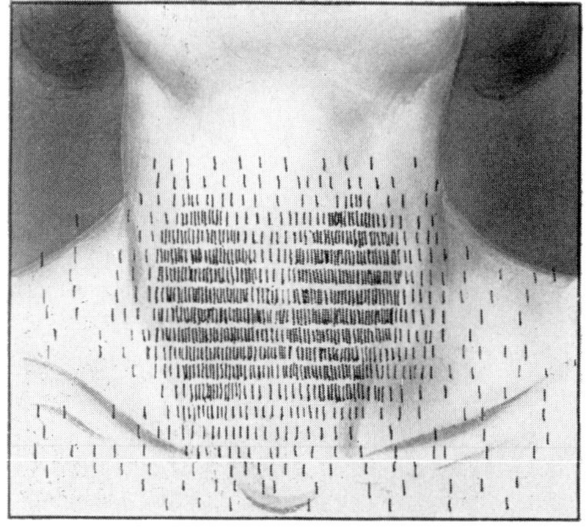

Fig. 36. A normal thyroid scan (scintigram).

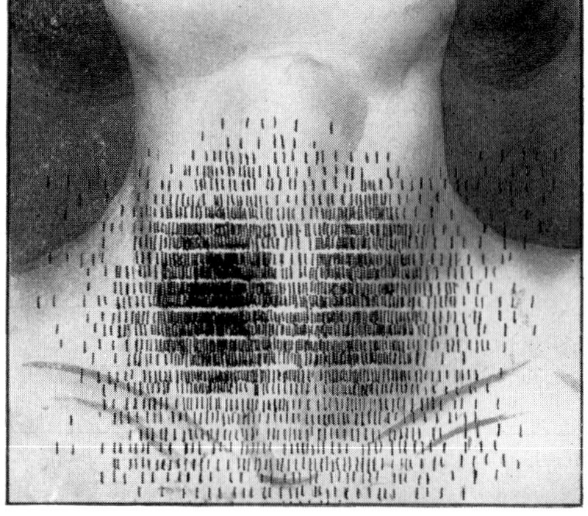

Fig. 37. A scintigram revealing a "hot" nodule (dark area).

clinicians regarding cancer and the "cold nodule." It can be stated as follows: Since hyperfunctioning nodules are almost always benign, they should be treated with antithyroid or radioactive drugs. Functioning or so-called "warm nodules" have an extremely low incidence of malignancy and should be given a therapeutic test with thyroid extract. If the size of the lesion does not diminish, or if it enlarges, surgical therapy is indicated.

Hypothyroidism

This condition produces a clinical picture that is the opposite of hyperthyroidism. Hypothyroidism is characterized by a diminution of practically all the vital processes; this results from an insufficiency or an absence of thyroid substance. Clinically, it is manifested by a slowing of the metabolism. No primary cause for the disease has been discovered except myxedema, which results from excessive removal of the thyroid gland. Nonoperative myxedema may be congenital (cretinism) or may occur in infancy or adulthood. Decreased thyroid function may be secondary to radiotherapy or certain drug ingestions.

Thyroiditis

The thyroid gland may be involved in inflammatory conditions. These are usually present in one of 3 types: acute thyroiditis, Hashimoto's thyroiditis or Riedel's chronic thyroiditis (Fig. 38).

Acute thyroiditis is a nonspecific condition usually caused by a staphylococcic or streptococcic infection. It is associated most frequently with an acute upper respiratory infection but may appear also as part of the clinical picture of a generalized septicemia. It is characterized by pain in the region of the thyroid gland which radiates to the neck, the head and particularly the ear. The gland is tender, and the patient complains of distress when swallowing or making movements of the head. The usual signs of inflammation, redness, swelling and induration are present; they are associated with spasm of the "strap" muscles, which forces the patient to hold the head in flexion. Dysphagia, dyspnea, hoarseness or aphonia may be present. A characteristic laboratory triad consists of an increased sedimentation rate, a high concentration of protein-bound plasma iodine, and a low uptake of radioiodine by the thyroid gland. The serious complications are abscess formation, perforation into the trachea and/or extension of the infection into the mediastinum. The disease may respond to chemotherapy, subside in its acute phase or become chronic.

Hashimoto's struma almost always occurs

Hyperthyroidism and Hypothyroidism Compared

Hyperthyroidism	Hypothyroidism
1. Accelerated metabolism	1. Low metabolism
2. Frequent accelerated pulse, often irregular	2. Slow, small, regular pulse
3. Anxious expression	3. Apathetic, quiet appearance
4. Vasomotor instability	4. Vasomotor stability
5. Wide lid slits	5. Puffiness around the eyes and lack of lateral half of eyebrows
6. Appetite usually ravenous	6. Normal appetite or anorexia
7. Vascular and moist skin	7. Thick, wrinkled, dry skin
8. Long, slender fingers	8. Short, thick fingers
9. Hypersensitiveness	9. Dulled sensation
10. Insomnia and restless sleep	10. Drowsiness and sound sleep
11. Mental excitations, mania or melancholia	11. Apathy
12. Feeling of heat	12. Feeling of cold
13. Loss of weight; emaciation	13. Increase of body weight; obesity
14. Laboratory tests	14. Laboratory tests

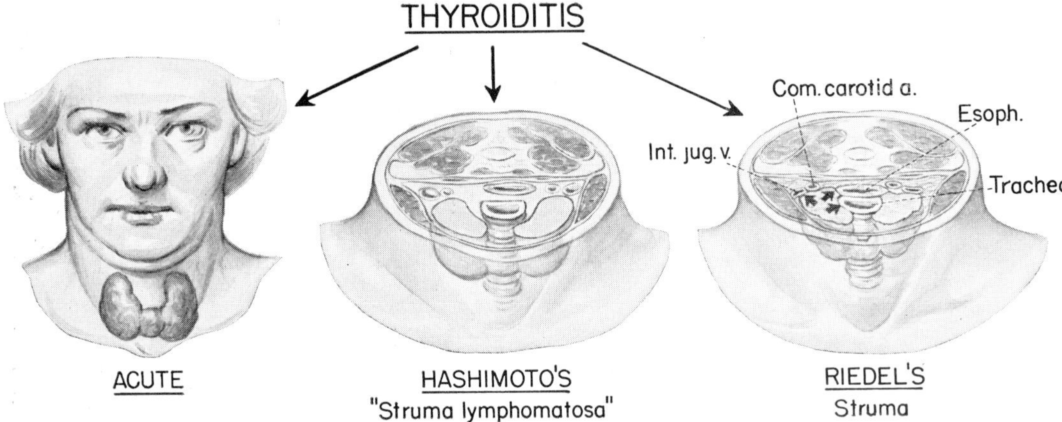

FIG. 38. Thyroiditis. Three types of inflammatory conditions which may involve the thyroid gland are: acute thyroiditis, Hashimoto's struma and Riedel's struma. Acute thyroiditis is a nonspecific condition caused by streptococci and/or staphylococci. Hashimoto's struma does not attach itself to surrounding structures, and the symptoms associated with it are mild. Riedel's struma extends into adjacent structures. These conditions must be differentiated from carcinoma.

in females. It is characterized microscopically by a marked lymphoid overgrowth and has been referred to as "struma lymphomatosa."

The first sign usually is the presence of a lump in the neck. Later the gland becomes uniformly enlarged and acquires a firm, rubbery consistency. It is characteristic of this disease that the contour of the gland can be clearly defined, but in some instances the hardness may suggest carcinoma. Occasionally, the enlargement becomes so severe that surgery becomes necessary to relieve obstructive symptoms. Desiccated thyroid therapy is fairly specific for this type of thyroiditis. The symptoms are usually mild; but if a subtotal thyroidectomy is performed, hypothyroidism may result.

Riedel's struma is characterized by excessive fibrosis. This usually starts in one lobe and eventually extends to the entire gland. Because of the characteristic woody hardness this type of chronic thyroiditis has been referred to as ligneous thyroiditis. As a rule the gland is not increased in size but feels extremely hard; the outlines of the gland may be lost because of direct extension into adjacent structures. Dyspnea and dysphagia may be present, and if the sclerosing process involves the jugular veins, an edema of the face and the neck occurs. In the early stages hyperthyroidism may be present, but as the condition progresses, a hypofunction of the gland becomes evident.

It is incumbent on the physician to keep these conditions in mind and to differentiate them from carcinoma of the thyroid. This can be done only by a microscopic examination.

Carcinoma of the thyroid has been the subject of much confusion and disagreement in clinical medicine. These carcinomas may appear at any age but are most common from the 5th to the 7th decades. Despite their greater frequency in later life, some patients with thyroidal cancer are discovered in the first 2 decades of life. Many of these younger patients were subjected to radiation therapy in and about the head and the neck in early life, a decade or so before the thyroid malignancy became clinically apparent. Radiation might have been given to these youngsters for the removal of tonsils, the treatment of enlarged thymus or acne. Even if the amount of radiation is seemingly small, the hazards must be kept in mind.

It is difficult to classify thyroid carcinoma; however the following is one of the accepted classifications. Three types have been described, namely, papillary, follicular and simplex. The *papillary* is the most common and comprises about 70 to 80 per cent of all thyroidal malignancies. At times the thyroid gland reveals nothing unusual on palpation except a lateral mass in the neck. Such masses usually are metastases from a cancer of the thyroid which is too small to be detected. The microscopic picture of these lateral cervical masses gives a deceptively benign appearance; hence, they have been erroneously referred to as *lateral aberrant thyroid rests*. These are very slow-growing carcinomas. Formerly, surgical resection was the treatment of choice. Presently, it is believed that such tumors are thoroughly dependent on thyroid-stimulating hormone, a characteristic which makes them vulnerable to medical treatment. Such tumors have been adequately controlled or even made to disappear with thyroid hormone treatment, which presumably depresses TSH levels (Crile). Even if left untreated, the life history of these tumors makes them compatible with survival of 15 to 25 years. Only rarely do they metastasize to distant organs.

Follicular carcinoma has been described according to various types. The classic picture reveals a lesion appearing insidiously as an enlarging thyroid mass. These carcinomas enlarge slowly, but their adherence to surrounding structures may produce pressure symptoms, such as dysphagia, dyspnea and recurrent laryngeal nerve paralysis. These lesions metastasize to regional nodes, bones, skull, lungs, and usually produce death in 3 to 5 years.

Carcinoma *simplex* is the highly malignant undifferentiated thyroid cancer which grows rapidly, invades the capsule and the blood vessels and results in death within 6 months to 1 year.

The more closely thyroid cancer resembles normal thyroid tissue, the greater is the uptake of radioactive iodine. The undifferentiated carcinomas do not take up significant amounts. Any firmness in the gland must be considered as cancer until proved to be otherwise; this can be accomplished only by biopsy. Advanced cancer is characterized by stony hardness, irregular nodularity and fixation to the underlying tissues. The obstruc-

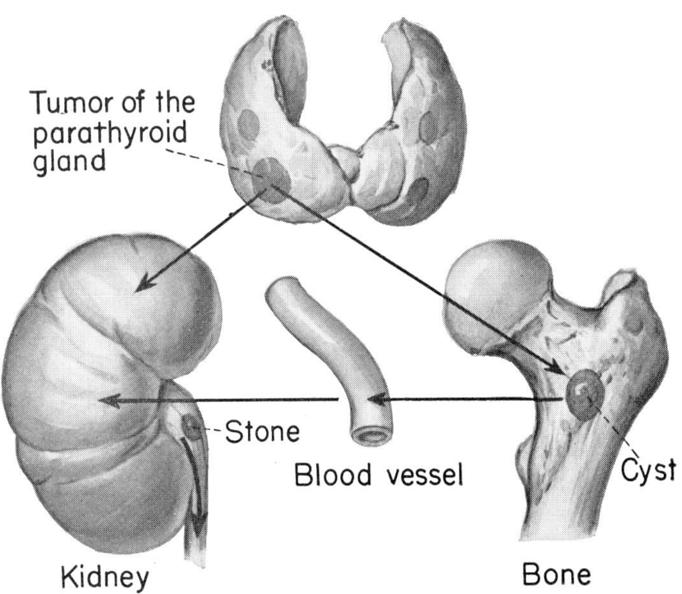

Fig. 39. Hyperparathyroidism. The overproduction of parathormone results in the formation of kidney stones (nephrocalcinosis) and the development of bone cysts—osteitis fibrosa cystica (von Recklinghausen's disease).

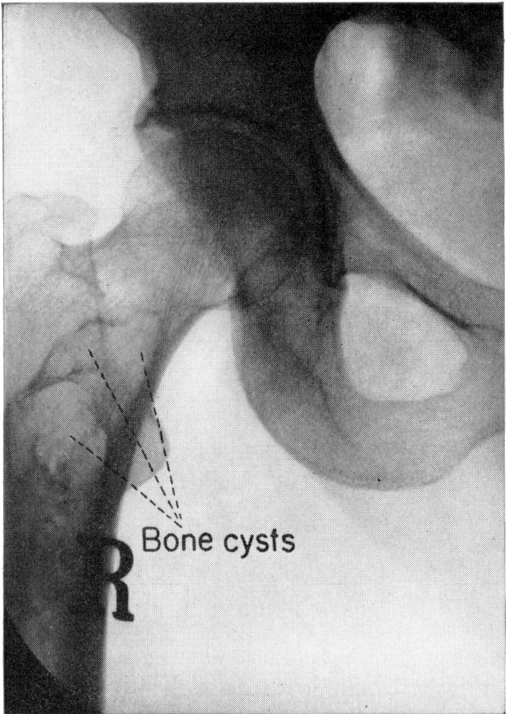

FIG. 40. Roentgenogram of bone cysts (osteitis fibrosa cystica) in a case of parathyroid adenoma.

tive symptoms and hoarseness associated with chronic thyroiditis may be present in carcinoma also.

PARATHYROID GLANDS

The parathyroid bodies or glands are small structures, usually 4 in number, which are located along the posterior aspect of the thyroid gland. Their most important function is associated with calcium metabolism. The two most common conditions to which they are related are hyperparathyroidism and hypoparathyroidism (tetany).

Hyperparathyroidism may be produced by a parathyroid tumor or a generalized hyperplasia. In either event the active principle of the gland, parathormone, is produced excessively. Such excess production of the hormone results in at least 2 major physiologic effects (Fig. 39). The first is that of decreasing the reabsorption of phosphate by the renal tubules, which results in phosphate

TABLE 3. NORMAL LEVELS OF LABORATORY TESTS FOR PARATHYROID DISEASES

TESTS	NORMAL LEVELS
Serum calcium	9.0–11.0 mg. % (4.5–5.5 mEq./L.)
Serum phosphorus	3.0–4.5 mg. % (1.0–2.3 mEq./L.)
Serum alkaline phosphatase	1.5–4.0 Bodansky units
Urine calcium	0.1–0.3 Gm./24 hrs.
Urine phosphorus	0.09–0.11 Gm./24 hrs.

diuresis. The second effect acts directly on the osteoclasts and brings about a demineralization of bone. The total effect is a marked increase in the amount of phosphate lost from the body through the kidneys and a lowering of the serum inorganic phosphorus level. In an attempt to compensate for this loss, calcium and phosphorus are mobilized from bone (decalcification). The excess calcium and phosphate precipitate in the kidney (nephrocalcinosis), form stones and damage the organ. This condition has been referred to as "the disease of bone and stone."

The diagnosis of hyperparathyroidism is simple when the condition is fully developed. Decalcification of the bony skeleton appears as severe cystic changes, a condition known as osteitis fibrosa cystica (von Recklinghausen's disease). Complete bony decalcification is demonstrated readily on the roentgenogram (Fig. 40). Sequelae include spontaneous fractures, collapse of vertebral bodies, rounding of the back, and nerve root pains. Such changes are usually irreversible. Any patient with a rounding of the back and/or evidence of decalcification of the skeleton should be suspected of having hyperparathyroidism. The same may be said for any patient with a history of kidney stones or renal or ureteral colic. The earlier cases are more difficult to diagnose, since they present such vague symptoms as muscular weakness, pains in the extremities and the back, polyuria and polydipsia. Lassitude, undue fatigue and constipation are symptoms which usually are overlooked.

Rarely is a parathyroid tumor palpable.

If one suspects parathyroid overactivity, the laboratory tests usually will reveal con-

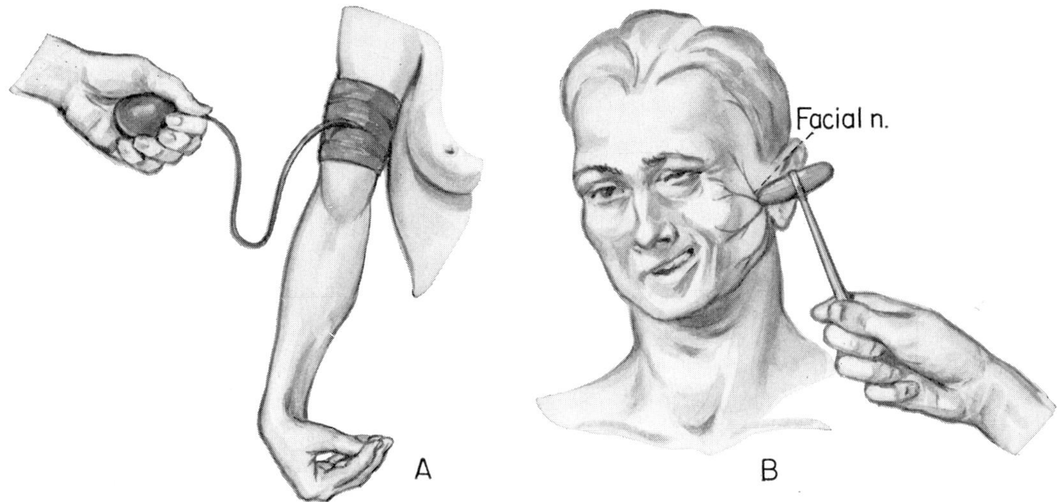

FIG. 41. Tetany. (A) Trousseau's sign: a blood pressure cuff is placed around the arm, and the pressure is raised to 200 mm. Hg. If tetany is present, the typical muscular spasm of the hand ("obstetrician's hand") appears within 5 minutes. (B) Chvostek's sign: tapping the facial nerve lightly produces spasms of the irritable facial muscles.

clusive evidence (Table 3). Typical findings consist of an elevation of serum calcium from the normal of 10 to a level varying from 12 to 20 or more milligrams per 100 ml. of serum and a depression of serum phosphorus. The serum alkaline phosphatase which is dependent largely on the amount of bone change may be elevated.

Localized bone defects noted on the roentgenogram are found usually in the long bones and/or the mandible. They appear in one of two forms, either as bone cysts or benign giant cell tumors (osteoclastomas).

Two further clinical forms of hyperparathyroidism recently have been considered, namely, peptic ulcer and a form of pancreatitis unassociated with alcoholic binges. The incidence of hyperparathyroidism and its relationship to these two conditions is not clearly understood, but because of current concepts and investigations they should be kept in mind.

Hypoparathyroidism (tetany) is observed most commonly following a thyroidectomy in which inadvertently the parathyroid glands have been removed or injured. The condition is manifested within 24 or 48 hours after operation; however, it might appear some weeks later. Headache, restlessness, tachycardia, irritability and twitching of the muscles, particularly those of the upper extremities, comprise the usual signs and symptoms. The serum calcium level is lowered. Most diagnostic are the typical carpopedal spasms, which consist of flexion at the metacarpophalangeal joints with adduction of the thumb and similar contractions of the feet. The muscular spasm of the hand can be induced by pressure which interferes with the blood supply to the nerves; this can be produced by a tourniquet (Trousseau's sign) (Fig. 41 A). Irritability of the muscles may be so pronounced that gentle tapping over a nerve may instigate a spasm; this is readily demonstrated when the facial nerve is tapped lightly (Chvostek's sign) (Fig. 41 B). Occasionally, spasm of the laryngeal muscles produces respiratory difficulty.

There are types of tetany which are not associated with the parathyroid glands. For example, the tetany from avitaminosis, particularly vitamin D, results in failure to absorb and retain adequate amounts of calcium. Another form of tetany results from alkalosis induced by overbreathing. So-called gastric tetany is caused by a depletion of hydrochloric acid produced by persistent vomiting; it is a manifestation of alkalosis.

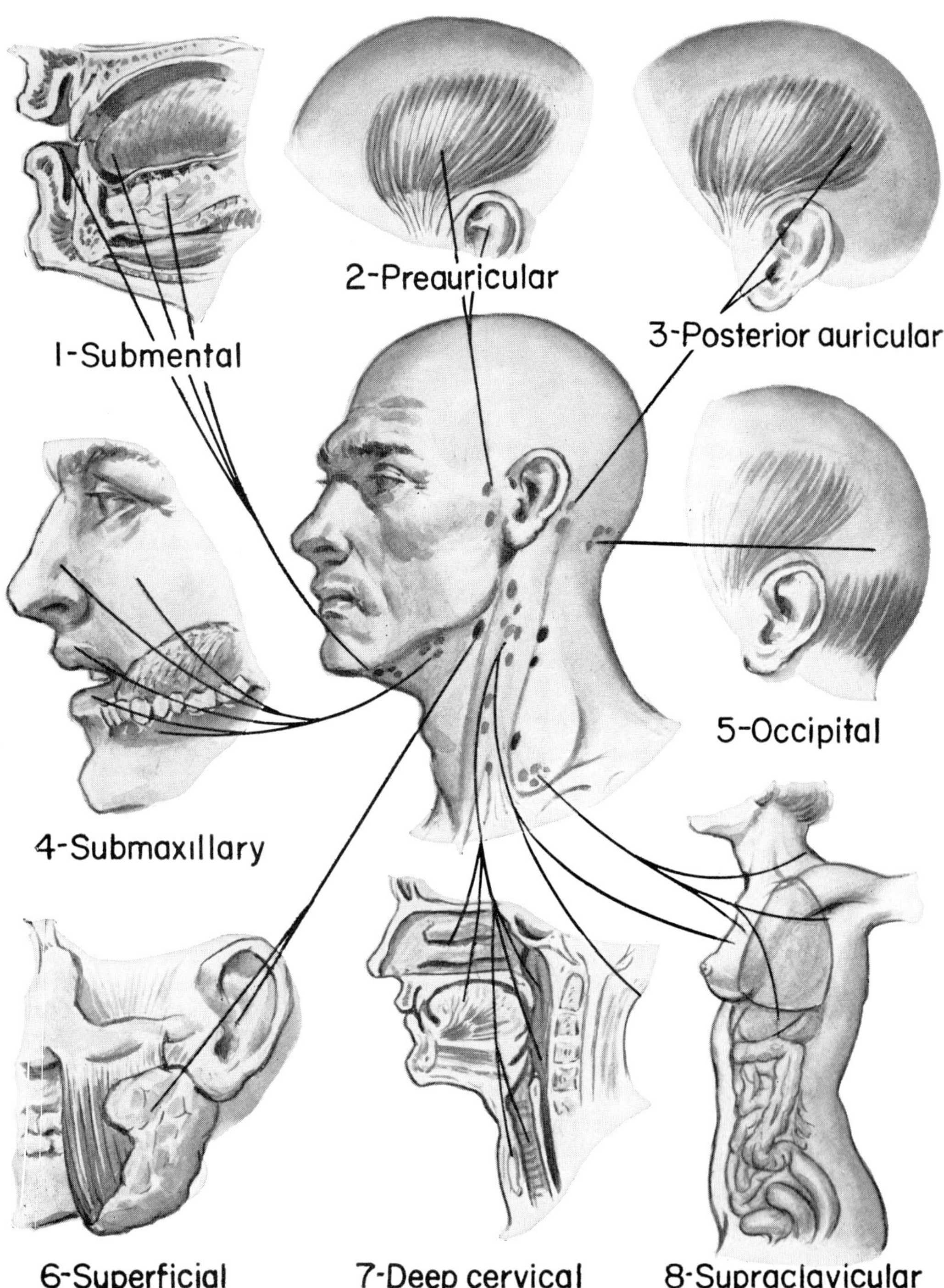

FIGURE 42 (*Caption on facing page*)

CERVICAL LYMPH NODE DISEASES

Cervical lymph node enlargements are evidence of some pathologic process, either past or present; this is particularly true in the adult. Investigation must be instituted when such enlargements are present (Fig. 42).

The enlargements can be discussed conveniently under the following headings: local inflammatory conditions, chronic infections, metastatic lesions and primary malignant lymphoid tumors.

Local Inflammatory Conditions

These conditions are responses to pyogenic infections. If the primary infection is a minor one, this leads to moderate enlargement and tenderness of the involved glands, but should the infection be grave, the glands may break down and form abscesses. The usual signs of inflammation, namely, tenderness, redness and heat, are found in the overlying skin. Systemic manifestations are also present.

Chronic Infections

Chronic lymphadenitis occurs frequently as a result of chronic or recurrent mild pyogenic infections of low-grade virulence. A common example is repeated chronic upper respiratory infections with cervical lymphadenopathy. Another example is pediculosis; hence, the scalp and the hair should be examined for nits in such cases. Chronic lymphadenitis may be associated with a specific granulomatous disease, such as tuberculosis, syphilis, actinomycosis and chronic brucellosis.

Hodgkin's disease produces large, discrete nontender lymph nodes of a firm consistency. Tuberculosis, on the other hand, results in a matting together and a conglomeration of these nodes, which may become soft, fluctuate, break down and produce draining sinuses. This inflammatory lesion is rarely tender and lacks the signs of acute pyogenic infections (redness, edema and local heat).

Fig. 42. Submental lymph nodes (1) drain the lower lip, the floor of the mouth and the apex of the tongue. Their efferents drain into the submaxillary and the deep cervical nodes.

2. The preauricular lymph nodes drain the lateral surface of the ear and the adjacent temporal region. Their efferents pass into the superficial deep cervical lymph nodes.

3. The posterior auricular nodes drain the posterior part of the temperoparietal region, the back of the ear and the external acoustic meatus. Their efferents communicate with the superficial deep cervical nodes.

4. The submaxillary lymph nodes drain the side of the nose, the cheek, the upper lip, the lateral lower lip, the gums and the anterior part of the margin of the tongue. Their efferents drain into the superior deep cervical nodes.

5. The occipital lymph nodes drain the occipital part of the scalp. Their efferents drain into the superior deep cervical nodes.

6. The superficial cervical lymph nodes are found along the sternocleidomastoid muscle. They drain the lower parts of the ear and the parotid region. Their efferents pass into the superior deep cervical node.

7. The deep cervical lymph nodes follow along the carotid sheath from the base of the skull to the root of the neck. For convenience they are divided into superior and inferior groups. The *superior* deep cervical lymph nodes are above the posterior edge of the sternocleidomastoid muscle. They drain most of the tongue, the thyroid, the larynx, the trachea, the nasopharynx, the tonsils, the nasal cavities, the palate and the esophagus. The *inferior* deep cervical nodes are found below the posterior margin of the sternocleidomastoid muscle. They drain the back of the scalp and the neck, the superficial pectoral region and the superior deep cervical nodes.

8. The superclavicular lymph nodes are part of the deep cervical chain. They drain the back of the neck, the superficial pectoral region, and receive efferents from the axillary nodes. These nodes receive metastases from involved abdominal and thoracic viscera.

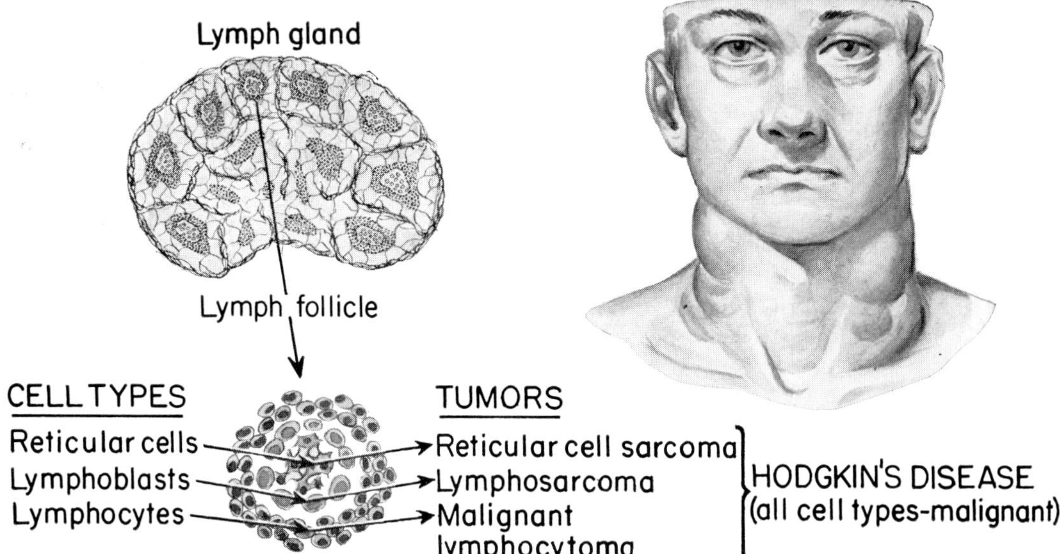

FIG. 43. The lymphoblastomas. This simple plan aids in understanding the terminology and the classification of these conditions. The predominant cell type determines the nature of a specific tumor and the name by which it is designated.

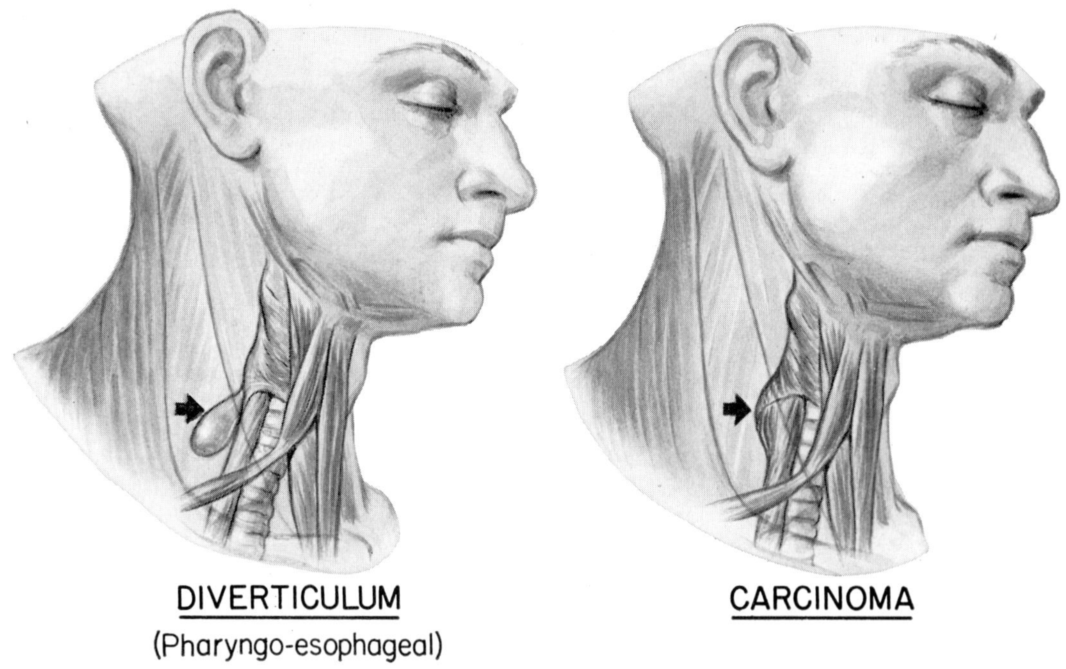

FIG. 44. The cervical portion of the esophagus. Pharyngo-esophageal diverticula and carcinoma affect this part of the organ. Frequently, a carefully elicited history can differentiate the two.

Metastatic Lesions

Metastatic tumor tissue, carcinoma and sarcoma, may involve the cervical lymph nodes when the primary source arises in the area drained by these glands. If the primary site is not evident, examinations must be directed particularly to the base of the tongue, the nasopharynx and the tonsils. The nasopharynx and the sinuses may be examined by means of the laryngeal mirror, endoscopy and roentgenograms. In these areas a small asymptomatic neoplasm may produce extensive cervical metastases. If an exhaustive search for the primary lesion proves to be fruitless, then biopsy of one of the cervical nodes becomes necessary. Occasionally, the histologic picture of the metastasis suggests the primary site. Superimposed inflammation may be present and obscure the underlying malignancy.

Primary Malignant Lymphoid Tumors of the Neck

These tumors constitute a most important group. There are many classifications of such tumors. It has been found advantageous to classify them according to the cells from which they are derived. These lymphoid tumors represent the neoplastic overgrowths of the various cells that make up a normal lymph node. When we recall the structural arrangement of a normal lymph follicle, we note the reticular cell in the center, a 2nd zone of lymphoblasts and a 3rd or outside zone of mature lymphocytes (Fig. 43).

Macrofollicular lymphoma (Brill-Symmers disease) is a manifestation of abnormal growth that originates in the lymphocyte layer. This is the most benign of all the lymphomas; it may take many years before the malignant nature of this disease is manifested. Terminally, it can change its histologic picture to any one of the other forms.

Malignant lymphocytoma has been referred to as small cell lymphosarcoma. This condition also originates from the layer which comprises the mature lymphocyte (the peripheral layer). The differentiation between this condition and chronic lymphatic leukemia is extremely difficult; some authorities are of the opinion that they are one and the same condition.

Lymphosarcoma, also called large cell lymphosarcoma, originates from the lymphoblast layer. Microscopically, there is a complete replacement of the architecture of the lymph nodes, and mitotic figures are numerous. *Reticulum cell sarcoma* has been called stem cell sarcoma, since it originates in the innermost layer where the reticular cells are found. Occasionally, an anaplastic carcinoma or melanoma may simulate reticulum cell sarcoma.

Hodgkin's disease (Hodgkin's sarcoma) is a malignant manifestation in which all of the cell types of the lymph node have undergone malignant changes.

Overlapping of the conditions is frequent, and one form blends with another. At times 2 different histologic pictures appear in the same node.

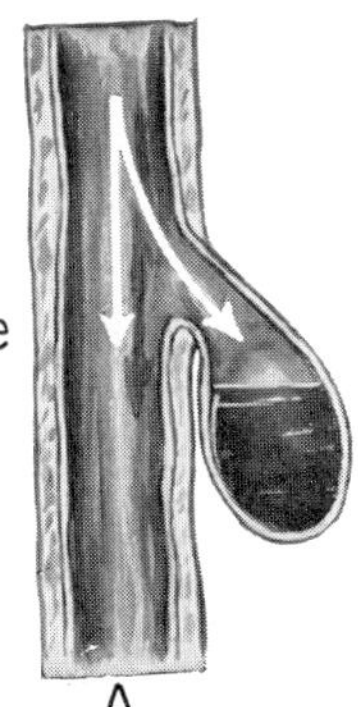

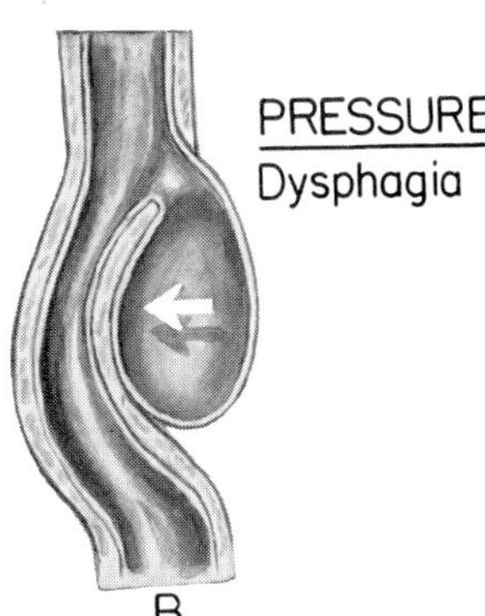

Fig. 45. Symptoms from esophageal diverticula are due to stasis or pressure. (A) Stasis results in the complications listed. (B) Pressure is associated with dysphagia.

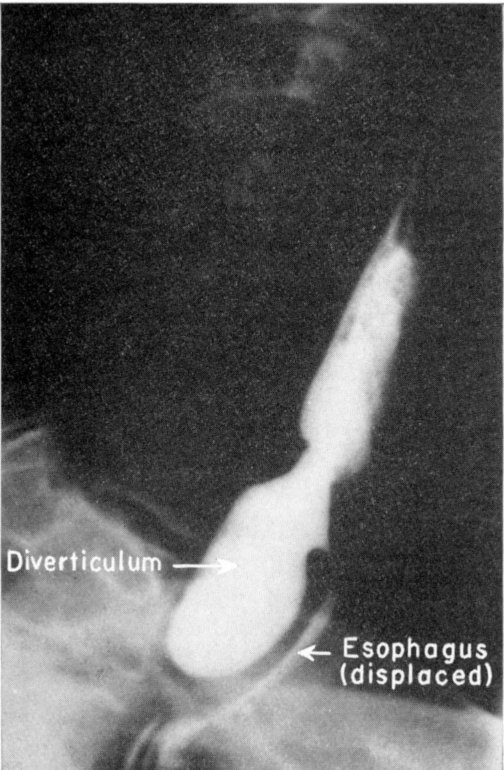

FIG. 46. Roentgenogram of a pharyngo-esophageal diverticulum. Note the pressure on and displacement of the esophagus.

Midline cervical lymphoid tumors are extremely rare, since the nodes are located in the lateral aspects of the neck.

Biopsy is essential, but it is well to remember that frozen sections are difficult to study. It is preferable to await a study of the permanent fixed sections.

PHARYNX, CERVICAL ESOPHAGUS AND LARYNX

Although the esophagus is heir to many diseases, the two which are found most frequently in the cervical portion are pharyngo-esophageal diverticula and carcinoma (Fig. 44).

PHARYNGO-ESOPHAGEAL DIVERTICULUM

This condition has also been referred to as Zenker's diverticulum. It occurs at the weakest point, which is located at the lower border of the inferior constrictor muscle (pharyngo-esophageal junction). These diverticula result from a herniation of mucosa through the muscularis (pulsion). The earliest symptom may be a mild dysphagia, or a choking or coughing spell which occurs during eating and may pass unnoticed at first. Repeated clearing of the throat, particularly when associated with increased salivation, is notably significant. Changing the position of the head may affect the ease or the difficulty of swallowing. Also of importance is the fact that difficulty in swallowing fluids is noticed first; this is the reverse of the story related by a patient with a tumor. As the pouch develops, retrosternal pain is experienced, and the patient complains of an actual sense of pressure in the neck, particularly during mealtime. Regurgitation of food usually is present and may be demonstrated by direct pressure upon the diverticulum. The regurgitated material contains food taken at an earlier meal. Should *stasis* develop, infection and its train of complication—ulceration, hemorrhage, perforation and mediastinitis—may result (Fig. 45 A). Other symptoms result from pressure (Fig. 45 B); marked dysphagia, dyspnea, and alteration in voice are common examples. Death may result from aspiration of retained material into the tracheobronchial tree. The physical examination is usually noncontributory unless the pouch is of tremendous size. The diagnosis is confirmed by the roentgenogram and at times by esophagoscopy (Fig. 46). The latter method may result in trauma and perforation.

CARCINOMA OF THE ESOPHAGUS

This lesion is usually epidermoid or squamous cell in nature. The onset and the progress of symptoms follow a definite pattern. Dysphagia is the first symptom and is associated with difficulty in swallowing solid foods. This becomes progressively worse; the patient finds it easier to swallow soft foods and finally liquids. There may be periods of intermittency during which time the patient may be misled and concludes that his difficulty has passed. In a short time, however, the dysphagia reappears and progresses. Relief from symptoms is explained by the fact that the central portion of the tumor may ulcerate; this partially restores the lumen. A feeling of vague discomfort rather than actual pain in the chest is usually present. This may be a substernal burning or a steady boring ache felt deep within the chest. Radiation of pain into the neck or the interscapular region is frequent. The patient usually points to the exact level at which the lesion is located. Signs of dehydration and loss of weight become apparent and suggest a far-advanced lesion. Physical signs are minimal or absent. The roentgen examination and the biopsy determine the exact nature of the lesion.

Differential diagnosis includes diverticula, stricture, coronary disease, foreign bodies, extrinsic pressure, benign tumors, thyroid enlargements, globus hystericus, esophagospasm, retropharyngeal abscess, Plummer-Vinson syndrome and specific granulomatous diseases. Although the disease predominates in males, it is interesting to note that cancer of the cervical esophagus occurs more frequently in females.

Laryngeal Cancer

This lesion is predominately a disease of the adult male, nearly all of the patients being over 40 years of age. Although it occasionally develops in the nonsmoker, 80 per cent of the cases occur in smokers. The first symptom of laryngeal carcinoma is hoarseness or alteration of the voice. A desire to clear the throat or a constant feeling of something in the throat are early complaints that cannot be overlooked. The author has stressed continually the importance of the phrase "change in habit"; a change in "voice habit" is usually the earliest symptom of laryngeal carcinoma. Other symptoms are pain in the throat or pain referred to the ear, hemoptysis, or the presence of a mass.

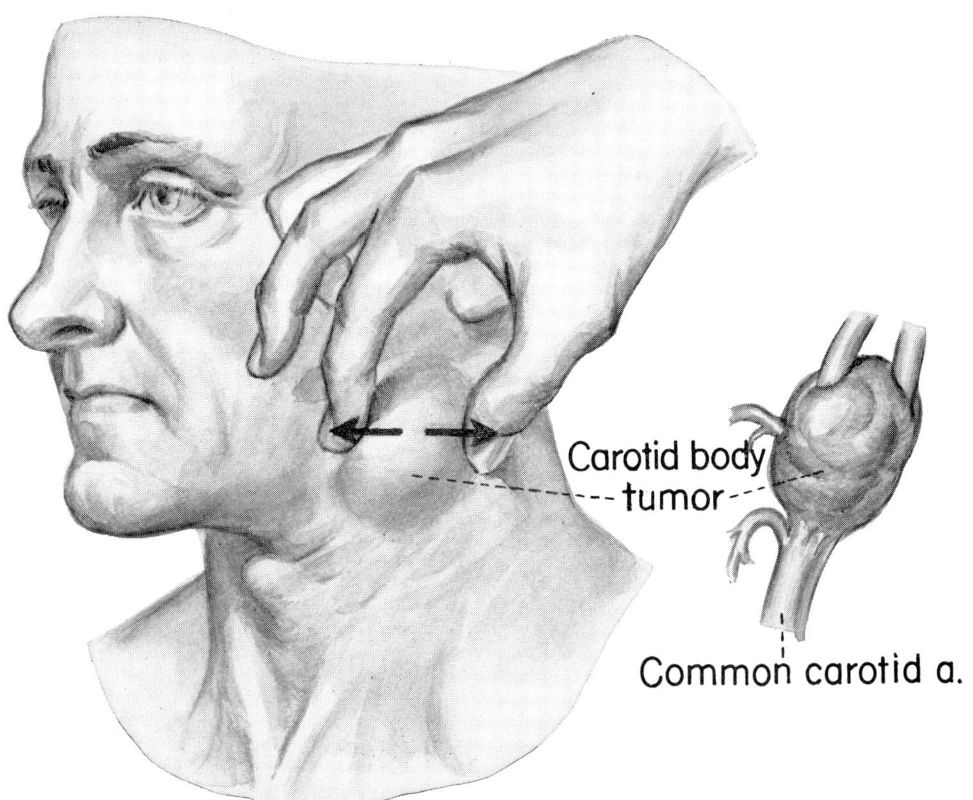

Fig. 47. A carotid body tumor can be moved in a horizontal but not in a vertical direction.

The visual examination of the larynx with the laryngeal mirror is quite satisfactory and can be conducted quickly and easily. A few cases require direct laryngoscopy and pharyngoscopy to visualize the postcricoid area. The diagnosis is established from microscopic study of the biopsy.

CAROTID BODY TUMORS

Tumors of the carotid body are relatively uncommon. They are serious, because they may encircle the carotid arteries or may become malignant. Their origin is still moot. Whether or not they are associated with the sympathetic nervous system is still a debatable point. Present consensus refers to these lesions as nonchromaffin paraganglioma which arises in the carotid bulb. As a result of the confused origin, the nomenclature also has become confused. The term "carotid body tumor" is probably the best.

The function of the carotid bodies is debatable—i.e., whether they are or are not chemoreceptors; it is believed that they are sensitive to changes in hydrogen ion concentration. Most authorities are of the opinion that they do not secrete epinephrine. They are paired structures which are situated near the bifurcation of the carotid artery. The average size is 5 mm. in diameter, and they have a reddish-brown or gray color.

Tumors of the carotid body are usually unilateral but may be bilateral; they may project into the pharynx. Essentially, they are asymptomatic slow-growing masses. Such symptoms as pain in the face and the neck, hoarseness and dysphagia may be present; however, it is the presence of the mass that is noticed first. Occasionally, a

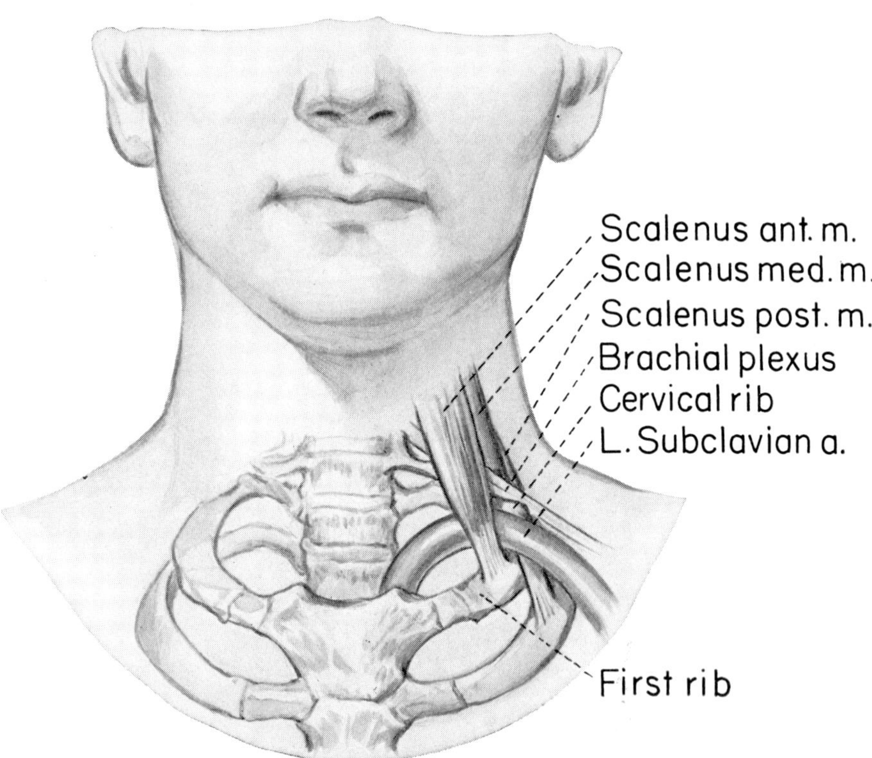

FIG. 48. The scalenus anticus syndrome. An anatomic vise is formed by the scalenus anticus muscle anteriorly and the scalenus medius posteriorly. A cervical rib, a vertebrocostal ligament or the scalenus minimus muscle may be present and add to the compression on the neurovascular bundle posteriorly.

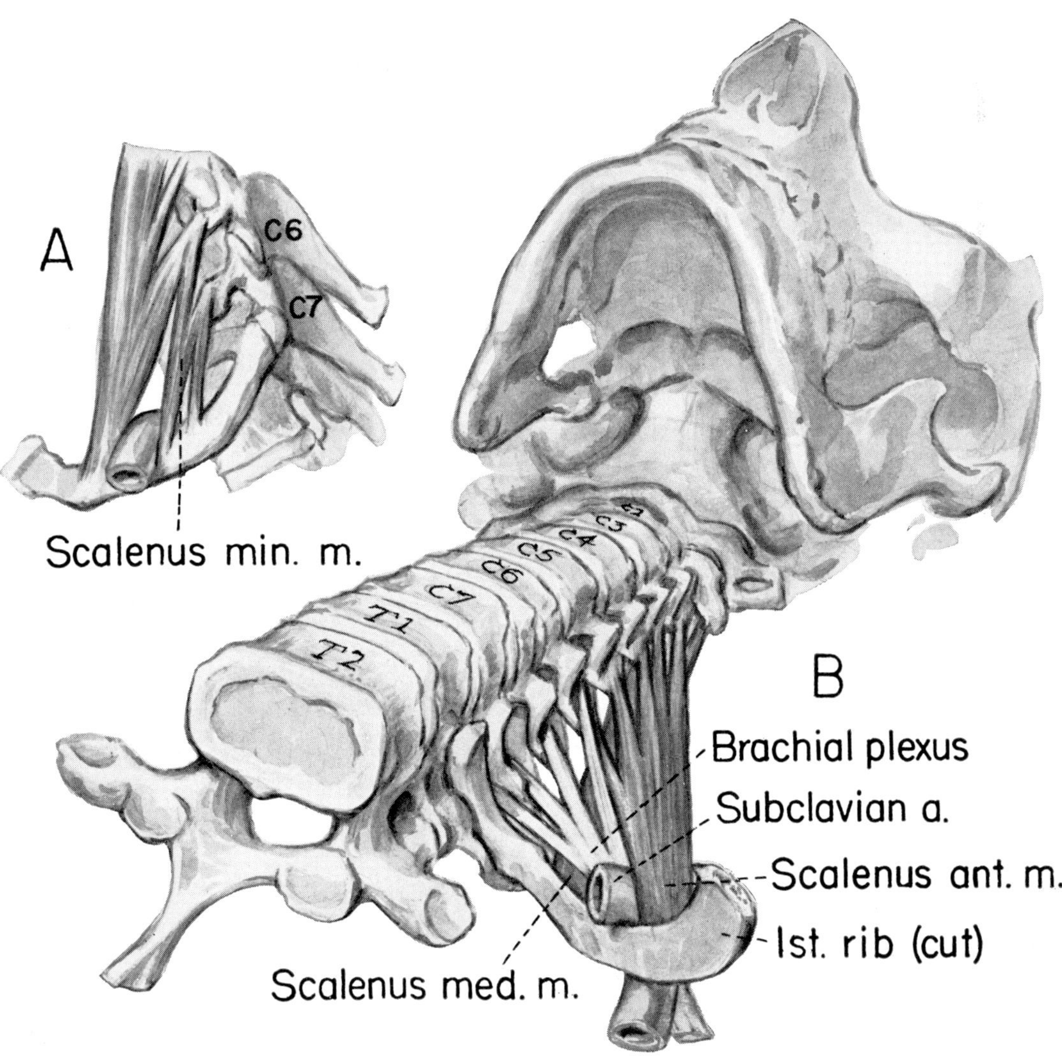

FIG. 49. The scalenus "vise" seen from below.

thrill and/or bruit are detected. At times the hypoglossal nerve and the recurrent laryngeal nerve may be involved.

Since they are located in the carotid notch and appear along the anterior border of the sternocleidomastoid muscle, they may be confused with branchial cysts. In differentiating this tumor from other masses in the neck, it should be recalled that because of its location in the fork of the carotid notch and its close association with the carotid vessels the mass may be moved from side to side but not in a vertical direction (Fig. 47). It can be differentiated from thyroid masses because it does not move when the patient swallows. Carotid angiography is the most valuable diagnostic aid. It has been stated that because of the increased vascularity the tumor "sparkles" with numerous areas of dye concentration. Displacement of involved carotid vessels will be demonstrated. It is interesting to note that regardless of the tumor's size the lumen of the artery rarely is compressed to obliteration.

It is the consensus that the incidence of malignancy is lower than is generally thought. Most authorities consider them as low-grade malignant lesions with potentialities toward invasion and metastases. Indiscriminate removal of such tumors, particu-

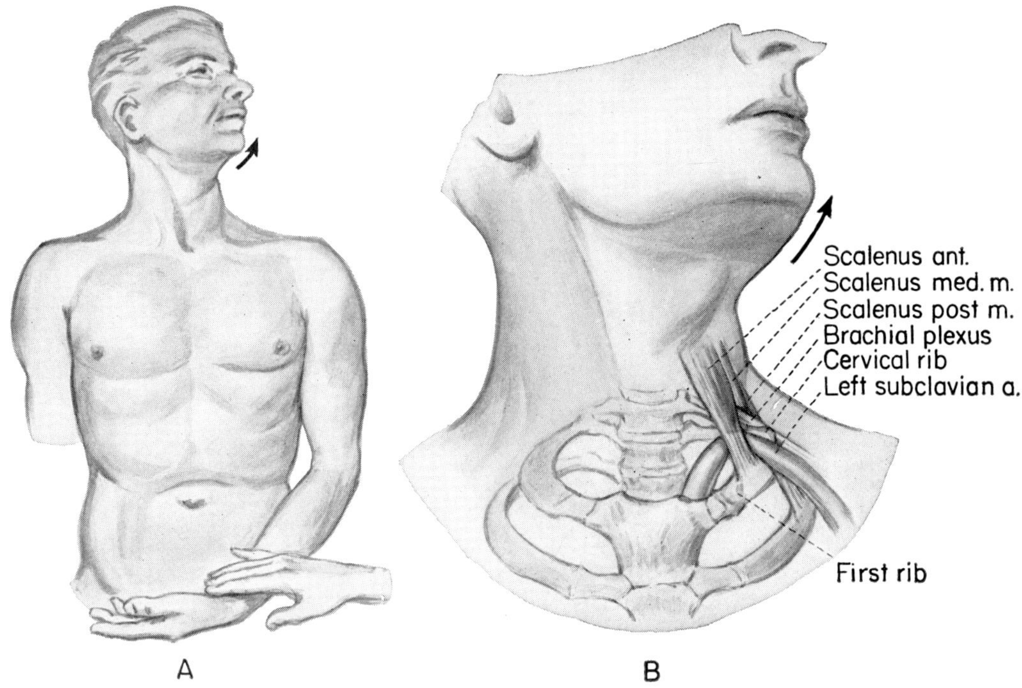

FIG. 50. Vascular compression test (Adson). Note that the patient's chin is elevated toward the *affected* side. If the radial pulse is altered or obliterated, the test is considered to be positive and indicates a scalenus anticus syndrome.

larly when this requires division of the carotid vessels, is not justifiable unless definite malignant degeneration has been suspected or is established.

SCALENUS ANTICUS SYNDROME

The so-called scalenus anticus syndrome is a brachial plexus neuritis caused by chronic pressure. The pain associated with the condition may be very disabling. Any movement which produces a downward pull on the arm or the shoulder may bring on the syndrome (pain, numbness, tingling and coldness of arm, forearm or hand). Equally important is pressure on the subclavian artery, which results in such circulatory changes as finger nail and local skin atrophy with destruction of the digits, particularly the 3rd and the 4th (Figs. 48, 49). The anatomic configuration and the relationship of the scalenus anticus muscle anteriorly to the 1st rib and the scalenus medius posteriorly explains the physiopathology. An anatomic vise is formed which compresses the neurovascular bundle. If a scalenus minimus muscle is present, it further adds to the compression effect. In some individuals fibrous bands replace the minimus muscle; such bands are referred to as the vertebrocostal ligament. A cervical rib may or may not be associated with the scalenus anticus syndrome.

The vascular compression test of Adson is significant when positive. The test is conducted in the following way (Fig. 50): The patient is seated, takes a deep breath, holds it and turns his chin up and to the *affected side*. An alteration or obliteration of the radial pulse on that side or a change in blood pressure indicates that the subclavian artery is compressed. The test is not pathognomonic, since it may be caused also by reflex sympathetic stimulation in the presence of a cervical arthritis. Digital pressure over the insertion of the scalenus anticus muscle will intensify the symptoms when the syndrome is present. Thorough roentgenographic study of the cervical spine should be made for the purpose of ascertaining the presence or the absence of cervical ribs or cervical arthritic spurs (Fig. 51). If a cervical rib is present, it may be necessary to excise it. In the absence of bony projections or cervical ribs, the procedure which produces most gratifying results is the surgical division of the scalenus anticus muscle at its insertion into the 1st rib.

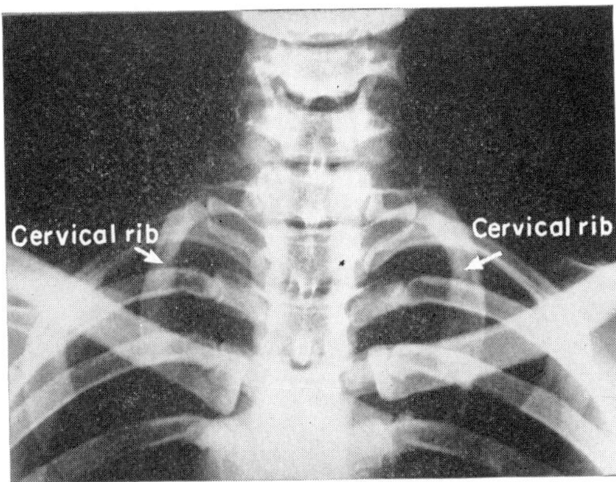

FIG. 51. Roentgenographic demonstration of bilateral cervical ribs.

Cervical lipomas are frequent; they may be above or below the deep cervical fascia. The so-called *hibernoma* is under the fascia and appears in the posterior cervical triangle. Supposedly, it is related to that fat which is found in hibernating animals. Other tumors that may appear are osteomas, neurogenic chondromas and hemangiomas. Aneurysms of the carotid artery and arteriovenous aneurysms that involve the carotid-jugular systems must be considered also in the differential diagnosis.

4

Chest

THORACIC CAGE

The thoracic cage may be involved in malformations, inflammations, neoplasms and traumatic conditions.

DEFORMITIES

The *congenital condition* known as *funnel chest* (pectus excavatum) presents a depression and concavity of the sternum; it may result from trauma (Fig. 52). In most cases it is asymptomatic, but serious pressure effects on the heart, the great vessels, the esophagus and the liver can occur. If pressure effects are present, it becomes necessary to remove the offending part of the chest wall. Another condition which results in a thoracic malformation is absence of the anterior thoracic wall (complete or partial). This may be associated with displacement of the heart outside of the thoracic cavity (ectopia cordis). The overlying skin may be absent. Fortunately, the condition is rare.

INFLAMMATIONS

Inflammations of the chest wall result from the ordinary pyogenic infections. Frequently, they manifest themselves as subpectoral or subscapular abscesses, both of which are worthy of special mention.

A subpectoral abscess arises from an infection which begins in the loose areolar tissue beneath the free border of the pectoralis major or the pectoralis minor. The constitutional symptoms can be severe. The swelling is apparent under the outer border of the pectoralis major muscle. Localized hyperemia may be absent. Any movement of the arm is painful, particularly adduction and outward rotation. If adequate drainage seems to have been instituted in infections of the superior extremity or the breast, and constitutional effects persist, a subpectoral abscess must be considered.

Subscapular abscess is rare. Frequently, it is mistaken for a tumor of the chest wall or the scapula. There may be an absence of local evidence of inflammation.

Osteomyelitis of the sternum and the ribs is rare. However, secondary osteomyelitis is more frequent, especially after surgical drainage of an empyema. Tuberculosis is the most common inflammatory disease of the ribs and the sternum except for those that follow compound injuries. Usually, a swelling is noticed by the patient; it is soft and not red. Signs of fluctuation are present. Aspiration reveals the characteristic curdy pus.

Nontuberculous costochondritis (Tietze's disease) is a frequently overlooked entity. In civilian life it is more frequent in women. They complain of a painful swelling of the chest wall. The patients consider it to be a "lump in the breast." It is the "lump" that causes them most concern. The usual costal cartilages that are affected are the 3rd, the 4th and the 5th. Palpation reveals that the swelling is caused by an expansion of the costal cartilage at its junction with the rib. When Tietze's disease is present in the male, it generally is associated with military men who carry heavy equipment strapped across the chest.

NEOPLASMS

Tumors of the chest wall usually arise from bone. So-called *osteomas* have been described, but practically all of these contain cartilage. Often *enchondromas* are malignant. This is particularly true of the cartilaginous tumors which arise from the costal cartilages. They are rarely found in the scapula. The most frequent malignant tumor arising in the chest wall is *sarcoma. Carcinoma* of the chest wall is secondary except those that arise in the mammary gland or the skin. The so-called *superior pulmonary sulcus tumor* has been described by Pancoast and is located at the thoracic inlet. It is believed to arise in the 5th pharyngeal pouch and presents some features of carcinoma. The present concept is that Pancoast tumors are bronchiogenic carcinomas that have arisen from a small bronchus in an upper lobe of the lung and have invaded the superior pulmonary sulcus (p. 65).

Injuries

These injuries are conveniently classified as nonpenetrating and penetrating.

Nonpenetrating Injuries. These are particularly important because vital intrathoracic structures and functions can be involved without external evidence of injury or fracture to the chest wall. Fractures of the bony cage without external evidence of injury are common. Numerous complications may result; however, 3 deserve particular attention: intrathoracic hemorrhage, tension pneumothorax and mediastinal emphysema.

Intrathoracic Hemorrhage. This complication may result from injury to lung vessels, intercostal vessels, or internal mammary vessels. Hemoptysis usually is present when the lung is lacerated. The early development of shock is suggestive of bleeding within the thoracic cavity. Pneumothorax may be associated with such an injury (hemopneumothorax). Lacerations of the great intrathoracic blood vessels are rapidly fatal. Bleeding from the lung parenchyma is more readily arrested spontaneously than bleeding from the internal mammary or the intercostal artery.

When the lung is injured, air escapes into the pleural cavity and adds pressure to the already increased pressure from blood. This is especially dangerous if the tear in the lung acts as a valve and produces the so-called tension hemopneumothorax (p. 49).

The symptoms of progressive bleeding are pallor, restlessness, thirst, increased pulse rate, and a reduction in the volume of the pulse. Periodic recording of the pulse rate and the blood pressure are mandatory. Pressure on the large thoracic veins is accompanied by a sense of tightness in the chest, increased pulse rate, shallowness of breathing, cyanosis, and engorgement of the veins of the neck. The outstanding sign is displacement of the apex beat toward the opposite side; hence the importance of marking frequently the position of the cardiac apex. Dullness to percussion is noted over the involved area.

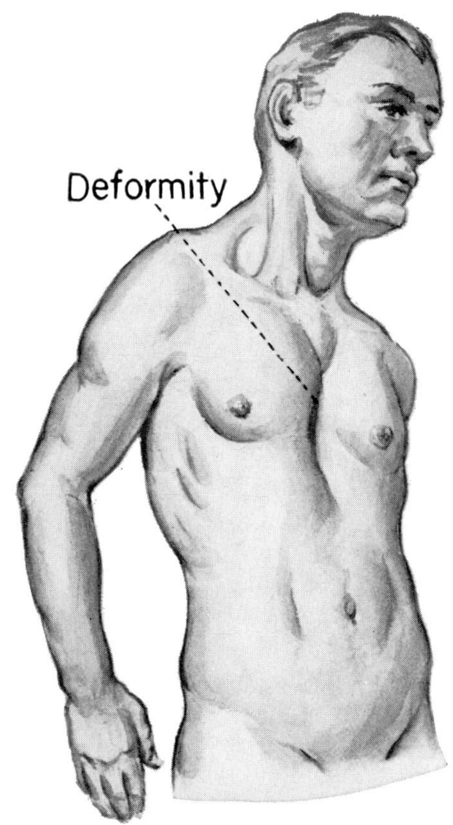

Fig. 52. The sternal deformity produced by funnel chest (pectus excavatum).

Since blood is irritating to the pleura, a secondary pleural effusion develops which may be massive within the first 24 hours. Such effusion added to the already present blood produces a rapid increase in intrapleural pressure which leads to dangerous compression symptoms.

Unless a foreign body or infection is present, blood in the pleural cavity does not

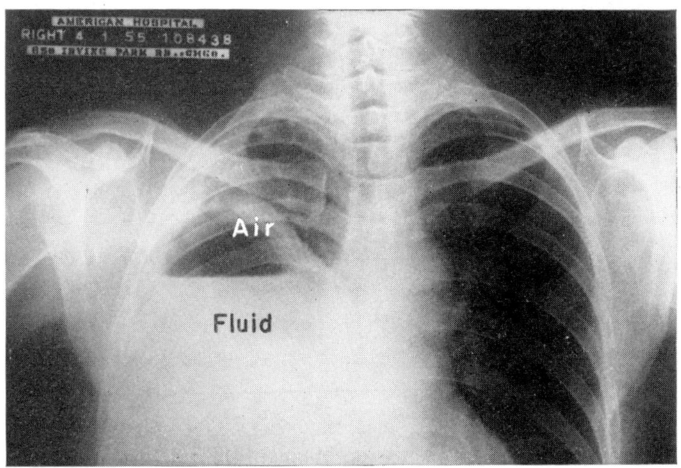

Fig. 53. Roentgenogram revealing fluid and air in the chest.

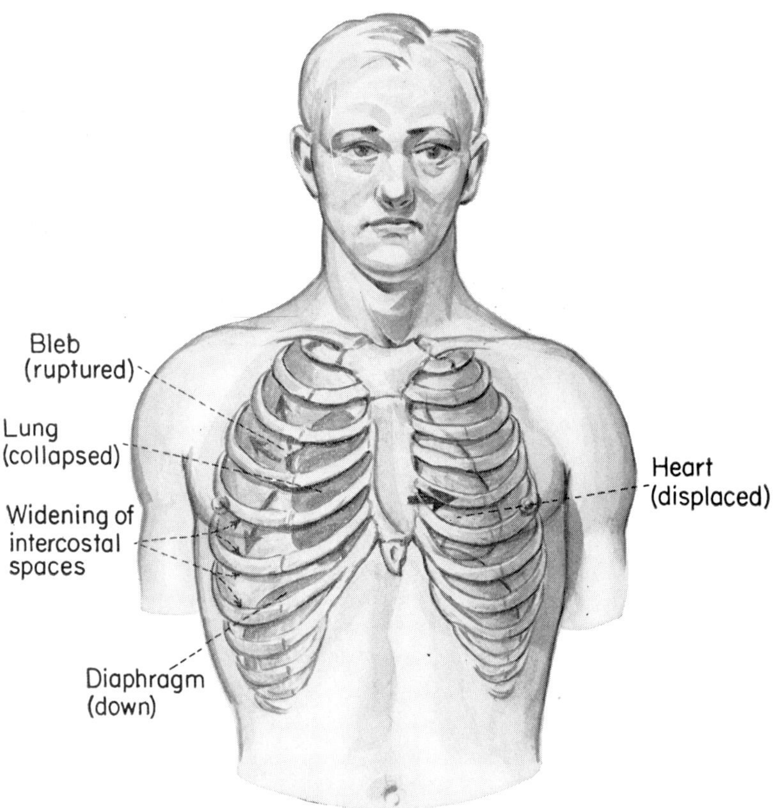

Fig. 54. Tension pneumothorax. This is produced by an injury to the tracheobronchial tree or lung which permits air to enter but not to leave the pleural cavity.

clot. There is a deposition of fibrin and endothelial cells which eventually becomes organized and forms a so-called "peel." The visceral and the parietal pleurae then become encased in a dense fibrous tissue and produce a "frozen chest." This prevents the lung from expanding and results in an immobile contracted chest which is accompanied by scoliosis and crowding of the ribs.

Roentgenograms are most helpful in ascertaining the diagnosis (Fig. 53). Aspiration is advocated by some for diagnostic purposes as well as being consistent with the safety and the comfort of the patient.

TENSION PNEUMOTHORAX. This condition results from a type of injury to the bronchial tree which permits the entrance of air into the pleural cavity but prevents its exit (Fig. 54). Alarming symptoms of respiratory embarrassment can occur which require prompt aspiration of the trapped air. Immediate diagnosis is mandatory. Owing to the positive intrapleural pressure, the intercostal spaces on the affected side are widened, and the normal intercostal depressions are obliterated. The thorax on the involved side is immobile and distended and looks smooth and bulging as compared with the other side. It is necessary to view the uncovered chest as a unit so that both sides may be compared. If the mediastinum is not fixed, the trachea and the apex beat will be displaced. The percussion note is hyperresonant, and vocal fremitus is absent over the affected side. The diaphragm may be displaced downward if the tension is marked. A flat roentgenogram confirms the diagnosis. (Fig. 55).

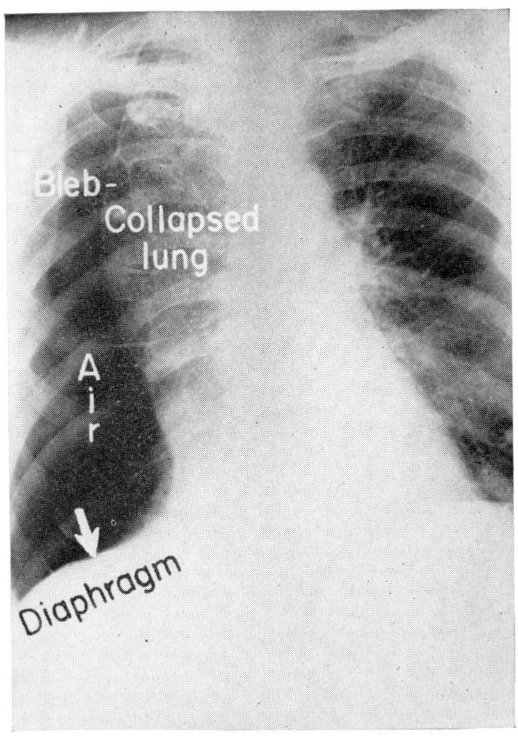

FIG. 55. Spontaneous pneumothorax which resulted from a ruptured emphysematous bulla. The right hemidiaphragm is displaced downward, and an unruptured bleb is shown in the collapsed lung.

MEDIASTINAL EMPHYSEMA. This condition usually occurs after laceration of the trachea or a main bronchus. Air may escape also into the mediastinum from a perforated esophagus, from a rupture of an overdistended alveolus, or from a pneumothorax accompanied by rupture of the mediastinal pleura (Fig. 56). The escaped air travels from the mediastinum throughout the body. The main symptom is pain, which may be anginal in type; dyspnea is marked if the accumulation of air is considerable. Subcutaneous emphysema is present in the neck, and a tympanitic note is elicited over the mediastinum; sometimes the latter is associated with obliteration of cardiac dullness. The subcutaneous tissue crackles (crepitation); this is most marked over the neck and the face but may be found as far down as the feet. The air apparently travels along the course of the blood vessels.

Penetrating Wounds. The complications associated with nonpenetrating injuries may be present also with penetration. Infection is due to the direct introduction of pathogenic bacteria and/or to the retention of a foreign body.

When there is an *opening in the chest wall,* normal respiration becomes disturbed (Fig. 57). In an open pneumothorax, air rushes to the area of lesser pressure within the pleural cavity. As the intact chest wall on the opposite side expands with inspira-

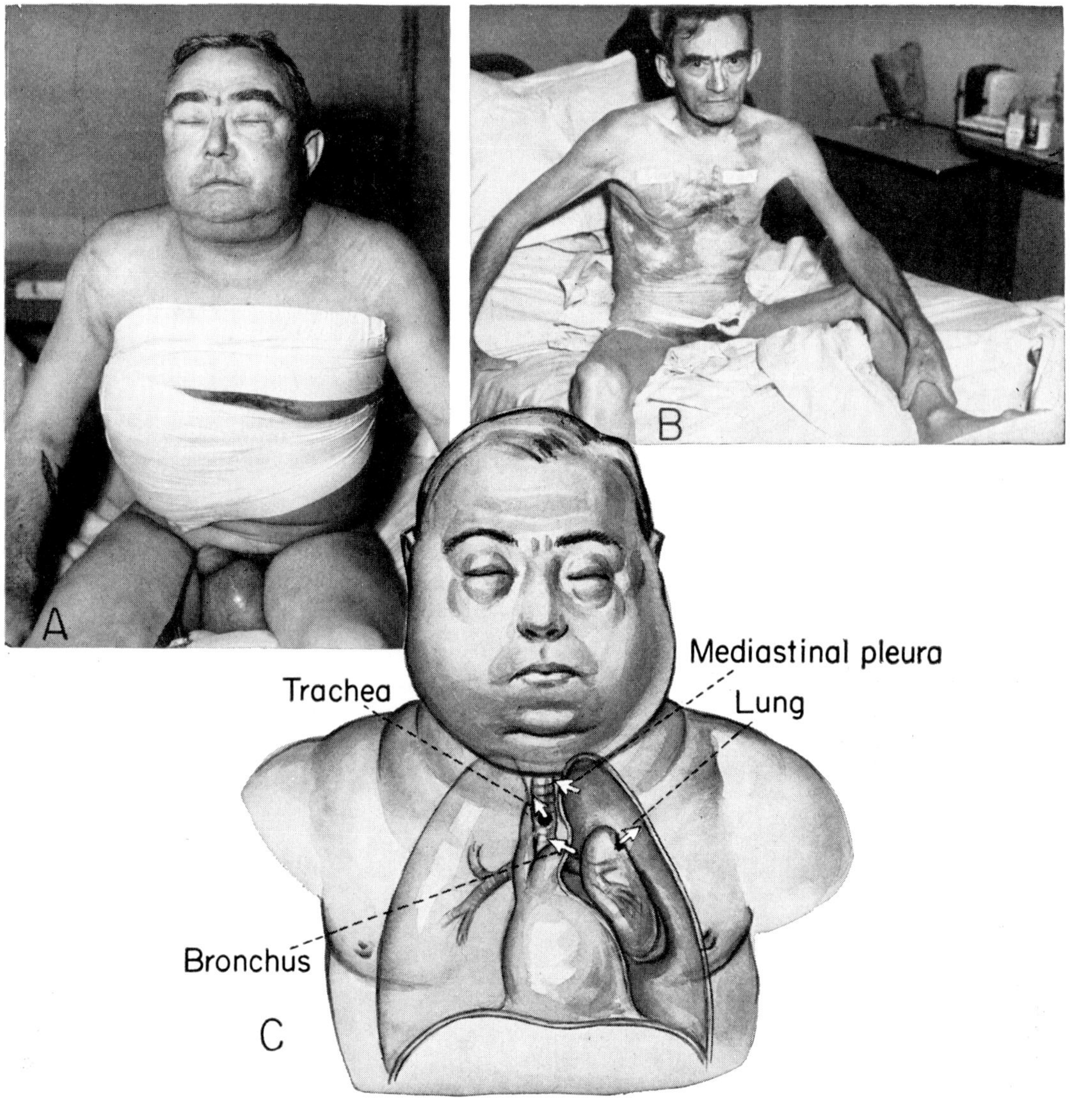

FIG. 56. Subcutaneous emphysema. This can result from a pneumothorax or a tear in the trachea, the bronchus, or the esophagus; frequently it is accompanied by a rent in the mediastinal pleura. (A) This patient had a chest injury and developed a crackling subcutaneous emphysema which extended from his head to his feet. A retention catheter was necessary because of the severe genital emphysema. (B) The same patient 10 days later. (C) Injuries which might produce mediastinal emphysema.

tion, the mediastinum is pulled to the sound side by increased negative pressure, and the contralateral lung fails to expand completely. During expiration more air passes out through the opening in the chest wound than through the glottis, and the mediastinum swings back to the midline or beyond it. This to-and-fro motion of the mediastinum is called *mediastinal flutter.* Pathologic alterations in circulatory dynamics result. The efficiency of the pumping action of the thorax in returning venous blood to the right heart is interfered with, and the venae cavae and other great vessels may become kinked. There is also a useless interchange of poorly oxygenated air between the

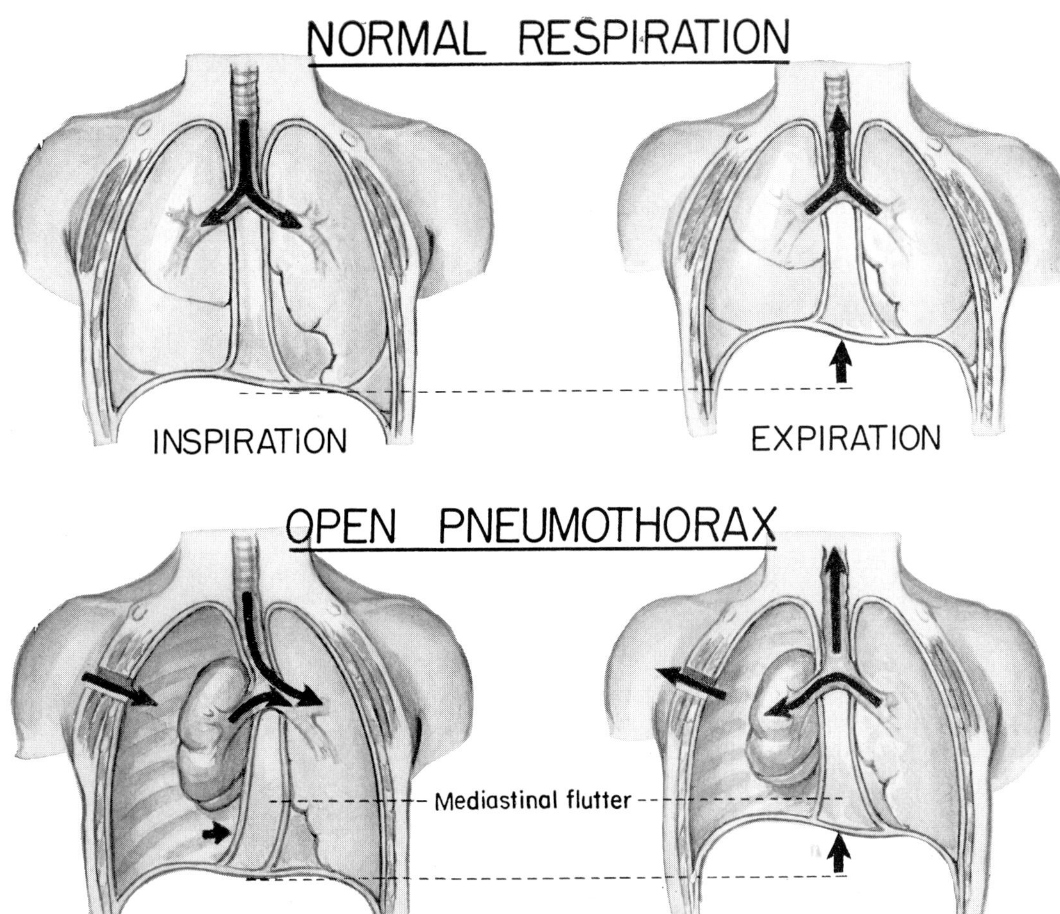

FIG. 57. Open pneumothorax and mediastinal flutter. Air rushes into an open chest wound during inspiration because of diminished pressure within the pleural cavity. Expansion (inspiration) pulls the mediastinal contents toward the sound side, and the contralateral lung fails to expand completely. During expiration a greater amount of air can pass out the chest wound than out the glottis, and the mediastinum swings to the midline or beyond it. This to-and-fro motion is called mediastinal flutter. Normal respiration has been shown for comparison.

2 lungs. These conditions must be corrected rapidly.

The diagnosis is not difficult, since an open sucking thoracic wound is apparent. The open pneumothorax must be closed. To be differentiated are compression of pulmonary parenchyma by blood or air (p. 49) and obstruction of the airway by blood or secretions. When partial obstruction of the airway is present, rales and rhonchi are audible. Frank hemoptysis also may be present. If a large amount of air is removed from the pleural cavity and re-accumulates rapidly, causing recurrent dyspnea, a tension pneumothorax must be suspected. With this a subcutaneous emphysema usually is found.

Paradoxical motion is caused by severe crushing injuries and often is associated with multiple rib fractures (Fig. 58). Normally, on inspiration all portions of the thoracic cage move outward, and the dia-

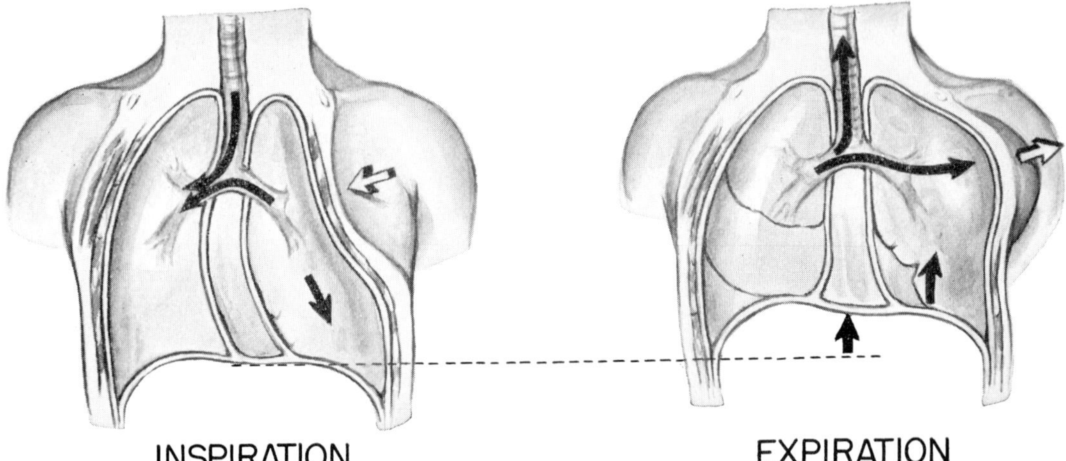

Fig. 58. Paradoxical motion. The flexible area is pulled inward on inspiration and pushed outward on expiration. A useless exchange of stagnant air within the lungs results. The mediastinum swings, and circulatory dynamics become seriously altered.

phragm moves downward; during expiration, motion is in the opposite direction. In paradoxical motion the flexible area is pulled inward on inspiration and pushed outward on expiration. Paradoxical motion is present sometimes following thoracoplasty and diaphragmatic paralysis. As a result of this, ventilatory efficiency is diminished, and there is also a useless exchange of stagnant air within the lungs. On inspiration, air is "pulled in" from the portion of the lung underlying the area of paradoxical motion into expanding portions of both lungs; during expiration part of the expiratory air is "pushed out" into the portion of the lung that balloons the flexible part of the chest wall (Fig. 58). Should this paradoxical motion involve a large area, there is a wide swing of the mediastinum, and the circulatory dynamics may be altered seriously. The venous pressure rises, filling of the right side of the heart becomes inadequate, and the arterial pressure eventually falls.

Recognition of these abnormalities should not require elaborate armamentarium. A stethoscope and a thoracentesis tray should be adequate. Early accurate diagnosis is mandatory, since the results of treatment are highly satisfactory.

DISEASES OF THE PLEURA

Pleurisy

The parietal layer of pleura lines the internal aspect of the chest wall; it is thicker than the visceral layer that invests the lung. The visceral pleura dips down into the interlobar fissure lining them. Whereas it is impossible to strip the visceral layer from the lung, it is quite easy to separate the parietal pleura from the parts that it covers except over the heads of the ribs, the vertebral column, the diaphragm and the pericardium. The two pleural layers are separated by a thin film of fluid which acts as a lubricant between these sliding surfaces. The normal pleura can rapidly absorb various solutions, toxins and dyes, by means of both the blood and the lymph vessels.

Inflammation of the pleura (pleuritis) may be caused by trauma or infection. The initial response is congestion of the pleural membranes. The inflamed membrane becomes thickened, and an inflammatory exudate pours into the pleural cavity. This may vary from a few ml. to several pints. At first it is straw-colored but may become turbid because of the presence of pus cells; the presence of blood gives it a red color which varies in the depth of its intensity. If the pleurisy is due to an acute infection, the causative organisms and the leukocytes may be found in the fluid. However, if it is due to tuberculosis, it may be impossible to detect the organisms without special tests. In the latter instance the predominant cells are likely to be lymphocytes. A purulent pleuritis (empyema) which presents many important problems will be discussed subsequently (p. 54). Any inflammation may result in pleural cicatrizations; these may vary from localized adhesions to a thickened solid shell covering both pleural membranes. If the diaphragmatic pleura is involved, pain can be referred along the sensory fibers of the lower intercostal nerves; this may be mistaken for an abdominal condition.

Pain is usually present on the involved side; this may be sharp, stabbing or tearing. It is aggravated by coughing, deep inspiration or pressure, and it is most intense at the end of inspiration. The pain disappears when the pleural fluid appears. Dyspnea, pyrexia and the presence of a pleura friction rub are usually present. The term "pleurisy with effusion" is a latter stage of so-called "dry pleurisy." The etiologic factors of pleurisy with effusion may be injury, in-

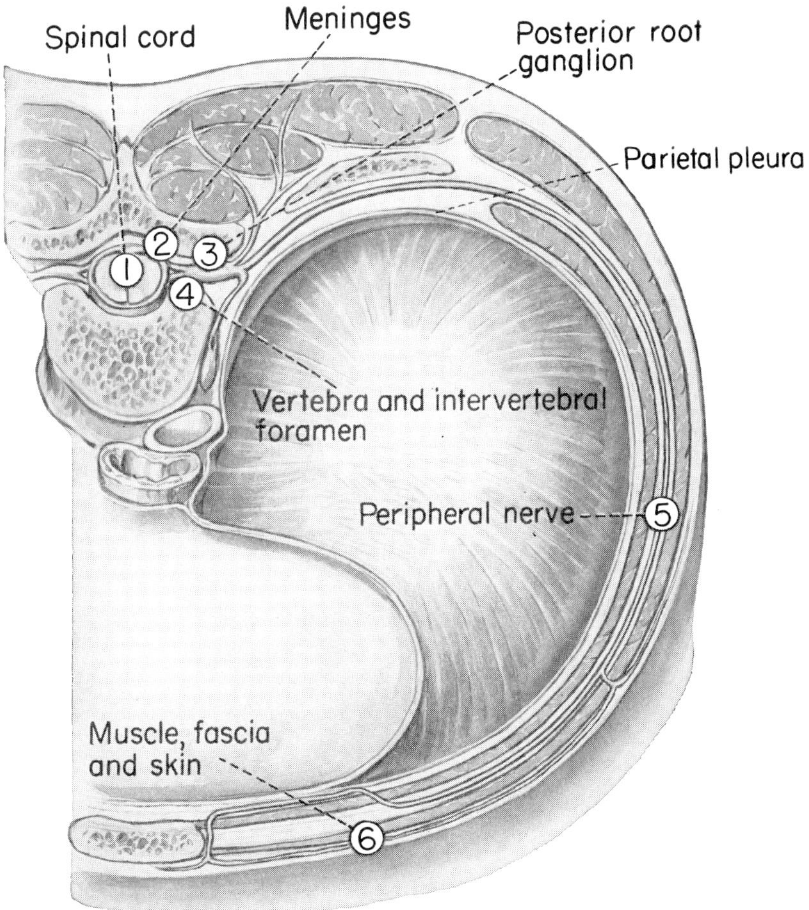

FIG. 59. Pleural pain. The pain associated with pleurisy may be confused with conditions involving the structures enumerated in the illustration.

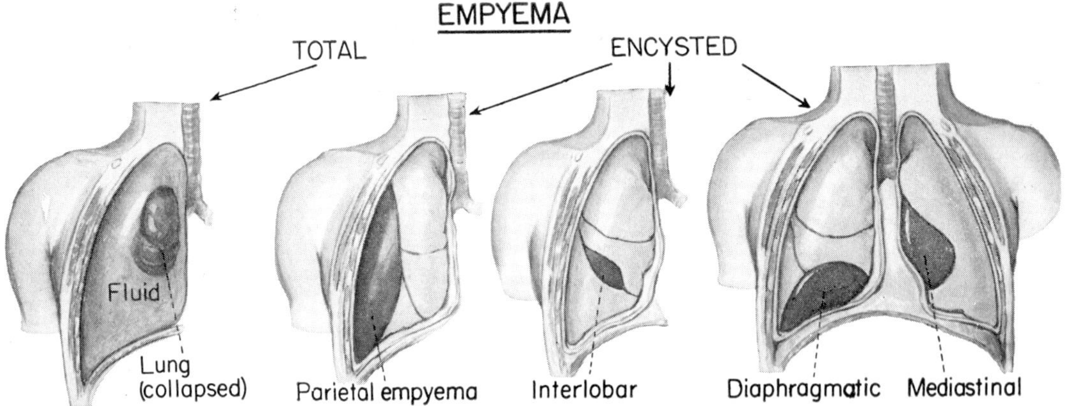

FIG. 60. Types of empyema thoracis. The total empyema has no limiting fibrinous adhesions.

flammation, neoplasm of the chest wall and parietal pleura, foreign material (especially blood), and lesions of the lungs and the visceral pleura.

A noninflammatory transudation of fluid may be present in the pleural cavities and occur as a complication of heart or kidney disease, ovarian fibroma (Meigs) or because of a tumor compressing the pulmonary veins.

Although pain in the chest may be the main feature of a diseased pleura, other conditions which may be associated with referred pain are caused by lesions of the spinal cord, the meninges, the posterior root ganglia, involvement of the foramina, peripheral nerve pathology, and diseases of the muscles, the fascia and the skin (Fig. 59).

Effusion affects the contents of the thorax, and it has been estimated that at least a half a pint of fluid in the pleural cavity of the average-sized chest is necessary to produce changes that can be detected clinically. Normally, the heart and the mediastinum maintain their median position by the elastic traction of both lungs. When an effusion collects in the pleural cavity, the corresponding lung is compressed, and traction of the lung on the sound side pulls the mediastinum toward it. This is possible only if the mediastinum is not fixed. Therefore, it is thought that the displacement of the heart is not a pushing to the opposite side by the pressure of the fluid. When fluid accumulates in a pleural cavity, the intrapleural pressure on that side becomes *less negative,* with the result that the now relatively larger negative pressure on the sound side pulls the mediastinal contents toward it.

The *physical signs* that are associated with pleural effusion are dullness on percussion, displacement of the apex beat, and an absence of normal vesicular breath sounds. The patient has a tendency to lie on the affected side, which permits him to get maximum expansion of the healthy lung. If the effusions are massive, the intercostal depressions are obliterated on the diseased side. Voice and breath sounds are absent over the area of effusion. The roentgenogram is most helpful in diagnosing effusions and associated lung lesions. It may become necessary to withdraw 5 or 10 ml. of fluid to arrive at a diagnosis through proper bacteriologic, cytologic and chemical investigations.

EMPYEMA

Acute empyema, more properly designated as **empyema thoracis,** is a condition in which pus is present in the pleural cavity (an abscess of the pleura). Purulent pleural effusions for practical purposes are always considered to be secondary. Although they may be due to any pathogenic organisms, the most frequent ones are the pneumococcus and the streptococcus. It is usually a complication of some type of pneumonia except when it occurs with a penetrating wound of the chest or by a spreading upward of an abscess beneath the diaphragm. When due to the pneumococcus, it is usually the sequel

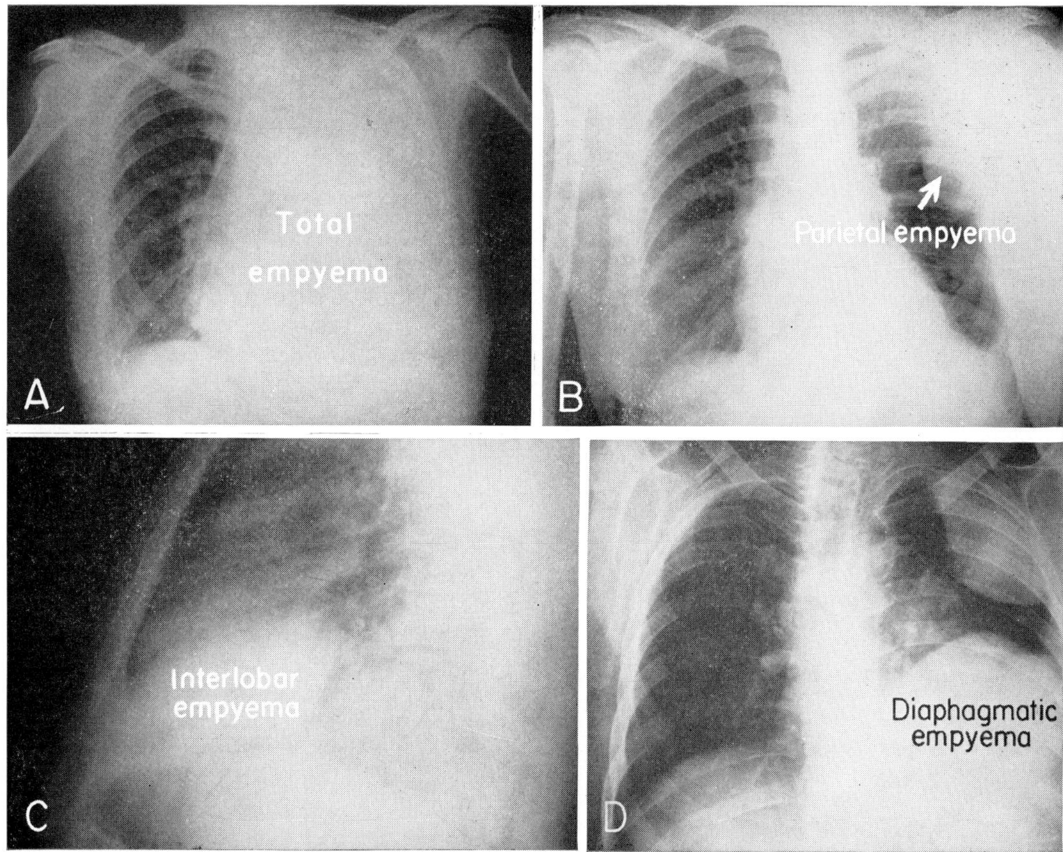

FIG. 61. Roentgenograms revealing types of empyemas.

of a lobar pneumonia; when streptococcus is the offending organism, it most often is a complication of bronchopneumonia; when other pyogenic organisms are present, it is usually a complication of some suppurative inflammation of the lung such as bronchiectasis or pulmonary abscess. Staphylococcal empyema, more frequent in infants, requires special mention, because this type of pneumonitis is associated with multiple small peripheral abscesses which may rupture into the pleural cavity with the development of a pyopneumothorax.

Empyema may be one of 2 types, namely, a *total empyema* with no localizing adhesions or an *encysted empyema,* in which localization is brought about by adhesions between the lung and the thoracic wall. Other types of encysted empyemas are interlobar, diaphragmatic and mediastinal (Figs. 60, 61).

It usually takes from 10 days to 2 weeks for the development of frank pus. Bilateral empyema is far less common than the unilateral variety. So-called *empyema necessitatis* is an unusual complication in which there is a spontaneous perforation through the chest wall. Fibrin is deposited on both pleural layers; in chronic cases the pleural membranes, particularly the parietal, may become tremendously thickened, measuring an inch or more.

The physical signs are those which are found in connection with any fluid in the pleural cavity (p. 54). In early cases the mediastinal contents are displaced to the healthy side, but chronic fibrotic changes result in displacement toward the affected side. A diagnosis of interlobar empyema is difficult; the condition may be confused with a lung abscess or a consolidated area of lung parenchyma. Clubbing of the fingers and the toes is present in subacute and chronic cases (Fig. 71). The roentgenogram reveals fluid in the chest or a combination of fluid and gas. The ultimate diagnosis depends on exploratory aspiration or operation. A high polymorphonuclear leukocytosis is nearly always present.

The complications most commonly associated with empyema are bronchial fistula, perforation through the thoracic wall, blood stream infection, suppurative pericarditis, peritonitis, mediastinal abscess, and a host of other complications which include meningitis, brain abscess and arthritic manifestations. Scoliosis is present in the chronic and neglected cases.

The creation of an open pneumothorax by the establishment of drainage of the pleural cavity should not be undertaken until frank pus has been demonstrated by aspiration. During the formative period of an empyema there is little or no stabilization of the mediastinum because of the lack of development of firm adhesions. Few patients will die of acute empyema per se, but many will die from an injudicious operation performed too early. The correct diagnosis as to type of fluid must be most exacting. If, on aspiration (thoracentesis), clear or turbid fluid is revealed, it is unwise to operate. Such aspiration can be repeated to relieve pressure effects or to determine the type of fluid.

Chronic empyema frequently is caused by a failure to provide adequate drainage of an acute empyema. Other causes of this condition are foreign bodies, communications with bronchial or lung fistulas, unobliterated fibrotic cavities, tuberculosis and other infections. Rare infections which involve the pleura are tuberculosis, syphilis, actinomycosis, blastomycosis and streptotrichosis. Injection of radiopaque material into a draining sinus may aid in determining the size of the empyema cavity. Study of the discharge and biopsies of pleura also are diagnostic aids.

Tumors

Tumors, both benign and malignant, attack the pleura; frequently these are associated with breast carcinoma. So-called endothelioma has caused much confusion in the literature. Whether it is primary in the pleura or metastatic from a bronchus carcinoma is still moot. Primary malignant tumors of the pleura are usually a type of sarcoma. Benign tumors such as lipoma, fibroma, angioma and leiomyoma have been reported. Regardless of whether the lesions are benign or malignant, almost all are associated with pleural effusions. If the tumor is malignant, the fluid appears to be bloody. Cytology, exploratory thoracotomy and biopsy are helpful methods in arriving at a final diagnosis. Occasionally, areas of calcification in the pleura may simulate a new growth. Congenital as well as echinococcal cysts must be differentiated also.

DISEASES OF THE TRACHEA

The conditions that involve the trachea are relatively few.

Foreign bodies are common, but with the advent of the bronchoscope most of these are diagnosed and treated readily.

Tumors of the trachea are rare. The benign neoplasms may be fibromas, lipomas, papillomas, chondromas, chondro-osteomas and lymphomas. Of the malignant tumors, carcinoma is found more frequently than sarcoma, although both are infrequent. The benign tumors occur more frequently in the upper third of the trachea, but the malignant lesions are found more commonly in the lower third. Symptoms suggestive of a malignant neoplasm are coughing, hemoptysis, dyspnea and pneumonitis. Metastases usually occur late. If the tumor arises in the posterior wall, early perforation might be expected.

Tracheo-esophageal fistulas are relatively infrequent and usually occur as a complication of carcinoma of the esophagus (p. 88).

DISEASES OF THE BRONCHI

Obstructive Lesions

An obstructive lesion of a bronchus (bronchostenosis) may be complete; if so, it is followed by an absorption of air in that portion of the lung to which the involved bronchus leads; this results in *atelectasis* (p. 64). Because of the straighter direction of the right bronchus the right lower lobe is involved most frequently. Foreign bodies are aspirated with greater ease into the right

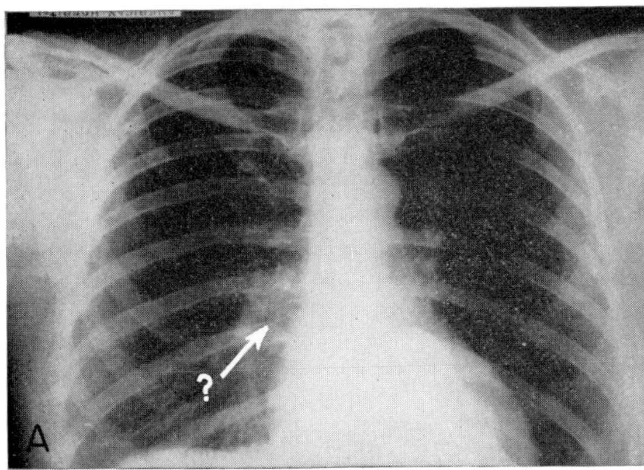

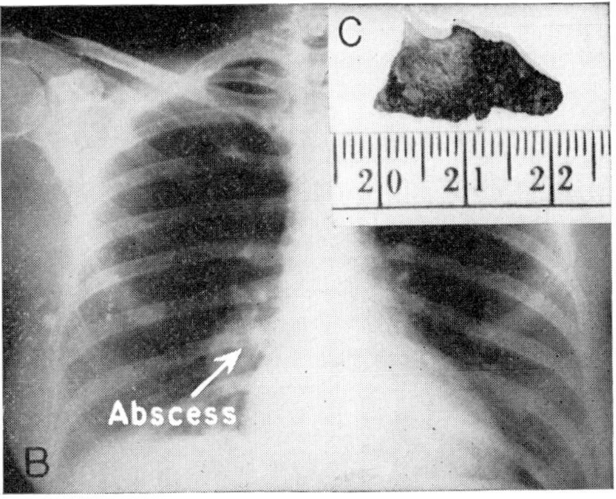

FIG. 62. Chicken bone in the right bronchus producing lung abscess. (A) Questionable lesion in the right lung. (B) Abscess demonstrated 3 months later. (C) Extracted chicken bone.

bronchus. Obstructive lesions are not always due to foreign bodies but may be caused by new growths, scars which result from severe inflammations or mucus plugs.

FOREIGN BODIES

Frequently, foreign bodies are aspirated by children or by inmates of mental institutions. If the aspirated object is nonopaque, it will not be seen on the roentgenogram; a typical example of this is peanuts. Immediately after such aspiration, the patient coughs violently, becomes cyanotic and usually complains of dyspnea. Cyanosis is less marked if the foreign body is located in the larynx or the trachea. Serious complications result from these foreign bodies if they are not removed. The inflammation which results produces destruction of the cartilaginous walls and bronchiectasis. Associated with this may be destruction of lung tissue with the formation of single or multiple lung abscesses and lung gangrene (Fig. 62).

Foreign bodies in the bronchus may cause either partial or complete obstruction. If partial, a diminished amount of air may pass in and out of the lung past the foreign body; however, the partial obstruction may be such that air is inspired but not expired (ball-valve action). Behind such an obstruction an obstructive emphysema may result.

TUMORS

Most tumors which are found in the bronchi are carcinomas; these will be discussed under the section dealing with tumors of the lung (p. 61). The benign tumors are usually adenomas or polyps which arise from the bronchial epithelium. The term *bronchial adenoma* is currently considered to be something of a misnomer. These adenomas are much less common than the frank epidermoid bronchiogenic carcinomas. They are slow-growing, but they are locally invasive and may metastasize. Although this will be discussed more thoroughly presently (p. 66), it must be emphasized that the differentiation between a benign and a malignant tumor of a bronchus is not always easy even with the aid of bronchoscopic and microscopic studies.

FISTULA

Bronchial fistula refers to a communication between a bronchus and another organ or surface. The most common bronchial fistulas are located between the bronchial tree and the pleural cavity. They may result from the surgical treatment of empyema or lung abscess; these usually communicate with the skin. They can occur with any type of lung inflammation in which there is destruction of pulmonary tissue. Hence, we find them associated with pulmonary suppuration as well as pulmonary tuberculosis. If a fistula communicates with a small bronchus, closure is spontaneous and rapid. Larger fistulas frequently become chronic and remain open. The fistula usually secretes mucus or mucopus; however, anything that

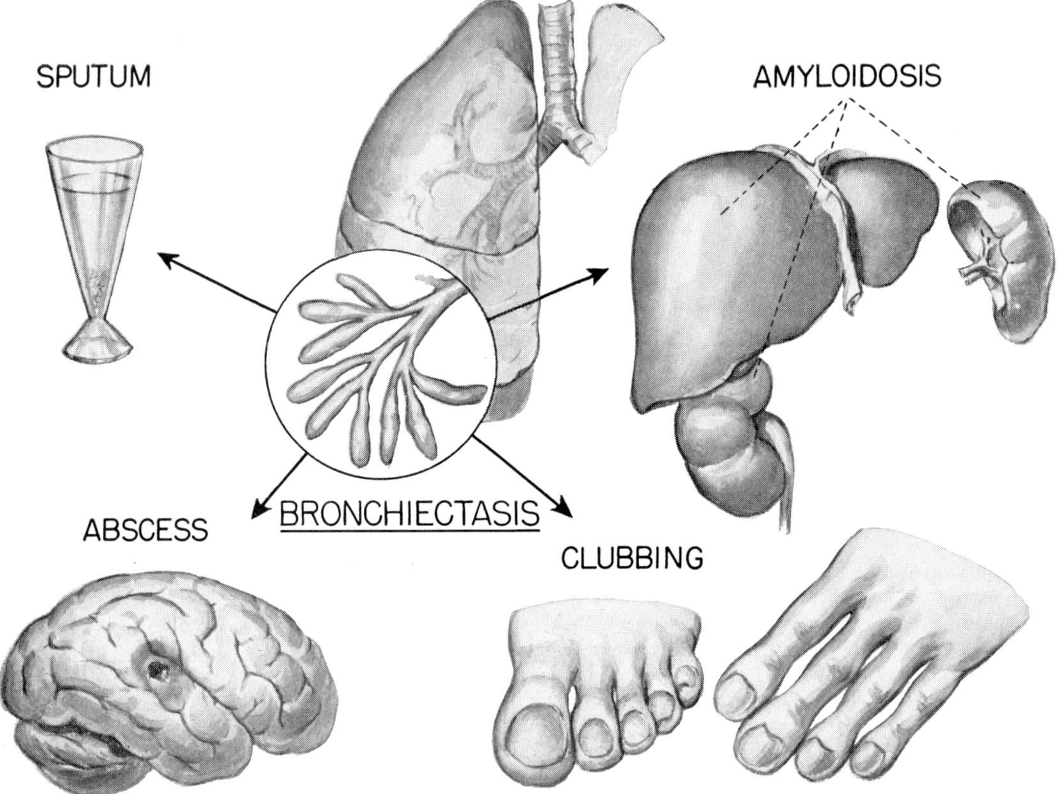

FIG. 63. Bronchiectasis and some of its manifestations and complications.

is secreted by the organ with which it communicates may appear; for example, bile in bronchobiliary fistula. Hemorrhage which can be serious is possible. When bronchial fistulas are present, there is always danger of drowning from the entrance of water into the lung through the external opening. These patients must be warned not to immerse the fistula below water.

Attempts always should be made to determine the size, the depth and the extent of the fistula as well as the presence or the absence of a foreign body. This can be done by roentgenography and the injection of radiopaque substances. Such information is important in determining the extent and the type of therapy indicated.

BRONCHIECTASIS

As its name indicates, bronchiectasis is a disease that is characterized by dilatation of the bronchi (Fig. 63). It may affect the tube uniformly (cylindric); it may occur as irregular pockets (sacculated); or the dilated tubes may have bulbous terminal enlargements (fusiform).

Etiology. Whether it is caused by one or a combination of factors is still unknown. The etiologic factors usually mentioned are chronic bronchial infection, bronchostenosis, pneumonitis and its sequel pulmonary fibrosis, and pulmonary atelectasis. The theory of congenital origin has not been accepted. An intriguing etiologic factor of septic bronchiectasis is that it is a penalty which modern man pays for assuming the erect posture of a biped. Normally, a bronchus prevents accumulation of secretions and stasis by ciliary action and peristalsis. Loss or diminution of these excretory actions in the dependent bronchi results in an accumulation of secretions which produces stasis and encourages bacterial growth.

The symptoms are by no means constant.

If marked, they are associated with spontaneous remissions and successive exacerbations. It is not uncommon for the disease to exist undiagnosed for 2 or 3 decades. In such instances the patient may be reduced to a state of chronic invalidism. Persistently dilated bronchi, unable to rid themselves of their secretions, tend to become obstructed and produce recurrent alveolar atelectasis. Ultimately, the mucus within these bronchi becomes infected, and an inflammation develops in the bronchial wall. The wall is weakened by destruction of its muscle and elastic fibers; such dilated bronchi cannot heal.

Recurrent respiratory infections may date back to early childhood, and the patient recalls frequent attacks of "colds." Each attack leaves the patient a little weaker. A chronic cough develops; this tends to be periodic and becomes worse in the winter. The cough is worse on arising and is associated with violent bouts of coughing which persist until the bronchi are emptied of their secretions. Then the patient is relieved for many hours. The *sputum* varies in amount but is usually copious. Acute infections increase its volume and alter its appearance. Sputum types vary from bland white or mucopurulent to a frankly deep-colored foul material. The odor is excessively offensive and becomes a socioeconomic problem. Because of the foul breath and coughing these people are likely to be shunned socially and have difficulty in securing steady work.

Hemoptysis occurs in about half of the cases and varies in amount from a tiny fleck of blood to several hundred ml. Many of these patients are diagnosed erroneously as tuberculous despite the fact that the tubercle bacilli are not demonstrated in their sputa.

Gastrointestinal symptoms include anorexia, nausea and vomiting. Frequently, nausea and vomiting are associated with paroxysms of coughing. Diarrhea may develop in chronic cases and suggests amyloidosis.

Pain in the chest is not severe but appears as a vague heaviness. *Fever* is associated with bronchial and pulmonary infection. Clubbing of the fingers and the toes is frequently present (Fig. 71). The clubbing is so gradual in its onset and progress that the patient is unaware of its presence. Joint pains are not infrequent.

The condition most commonly involves the lower lobes. The middle lobe on the right and the lingular segment of the left upper lobe may be involved also. The per-

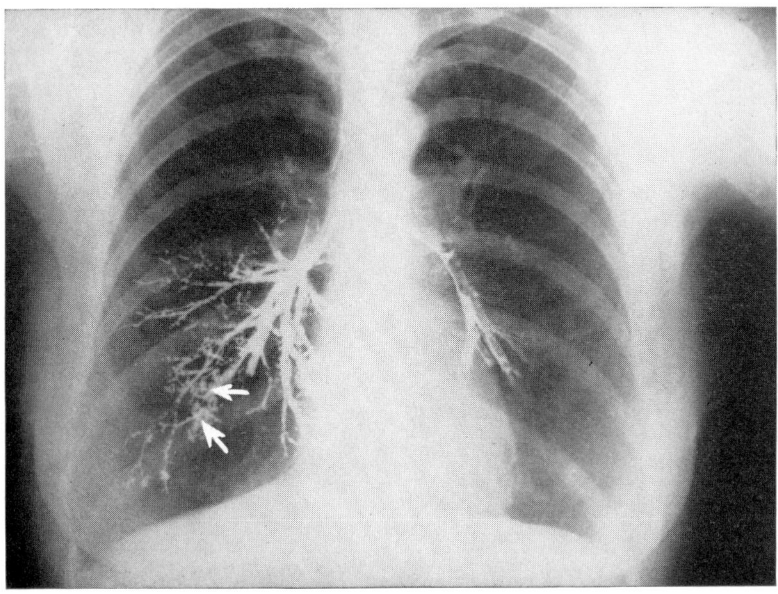

FIG. 64. Roentgenographic demonstration of bronchiectasis.

cussion note is dull over the involved areas. Rales, when present, are moist and medium to coarse in intensity. It is characteristic of bronchiectasis that the physical signs vary from time to time or even from hour to hour.

Complications. The more common complications are brain abscess and amyloidosis, which particularly involves the liver, the kidney and the spleen.

Diagnosis. A most important diagnostic adjunct is bronchography. This roentgenographic outlining of the bronchial tree with an opaque medium requires accurate positioning of the patient (Fig. 64). Bronchoscopic examination is helpful in determining from which side a purulent secretion or blood emanates. Exploratory thoracotomy should be performed if the diagnosis is doubtful and also for definitive therapy.

The physician must be aware continually of this common condition and realize its intractability. Its ultimately disastrous outcome makes early diagnosis and treatment imperative.

Broncholithiasis (Lung Stones)

This condition, although not too frequent, is found more often than a survey of the literature would indicate. The stones vary in size from mere granules to those weighing several grams and consist of calcium phosphate and calcium carbonate. They are seen in individuals who have healed pulmonary tuberculosis or other types of infections or granulomas. It has been suggested that they are concrements which have ulcerated into a bronchus from calcified tracheobronchial lymph nodes. Severe attacks of coughing and chest pain are frequently present. Following the expectoration of the stone there usually is blood in the sputum; the bleeding is due to trauma. If the stone is of sufficient size, it is seen on the roentgenogram. It is important to be aware of such stones to avoid confusion with such conditions as tuberculosis, bronchiectasis and carcinoma, particularly when hemoptysis is present.

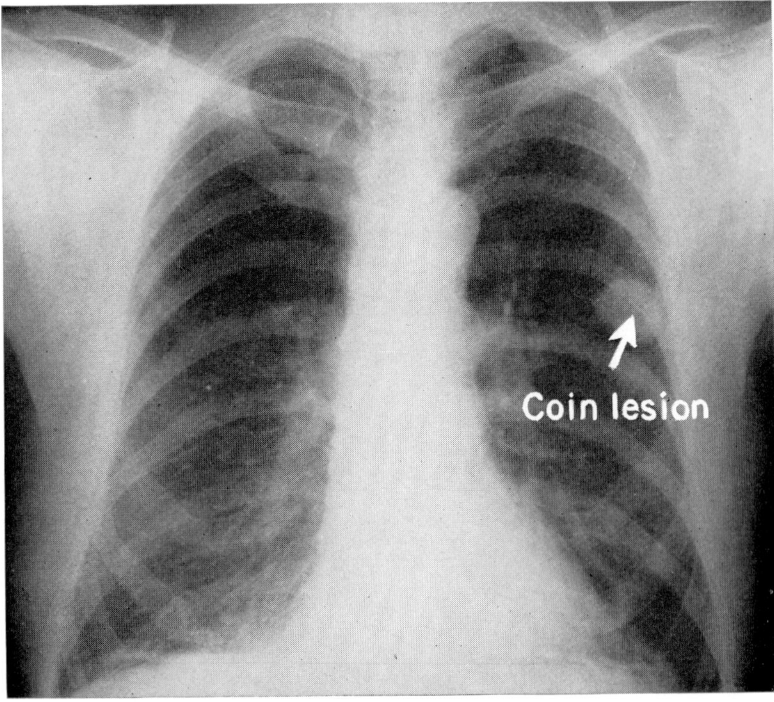

Fig. 65. Roentgenogram of a so-called coin lesion.

LUNGS

TUMORS

Tumors of the lung are benign, malignant or metastatic.

Benign tumors appear in a variety of forms as fibromas, lipomas, chondromas, osteomas, hemangiomas, polyps and cartilaginous hamartomas. The so-called bronchial adenoma is listed with the malignant tumors (p. 57). With the exception of hemangioma the benign tumors per se do not present unusual features. They are uncommon; and if symptoms are present, they usually result from obstruction to a bronchus. Chest roentgenograms have become a routine; hence, these tumors are frequently discovered when they are still asymptomatic and small.

A *hemangioma* differs because it may be associated with an arteriovenous fistula. Such a fistula permits a considerable volume of unsaturated blood to return to the left heart and the systemic circulation. This causes cyanosis, polycythemia, dyspnea, weakness and, as a rule, clubbing of the fingers (Fig. 71). The symptoms are relieved promptly by resection of the fistula-containing lung.

Also presenting some interesting features are the cartilaginous *hamartomas* of the lung. This tumor is usually small and firm and moves freely in the surrounding soft lung substance. It appears to be lobulated, and microscopically well-differentiated cartilaginous cells can be seen.

If a tumor is discovered on routine roentgenographic examination, a great responsibility is placed on the physician. Such a lesion may be a benign tumor, a tuberculoma, primary carcinoma, metastatic carcinoma, a cyst or an abscess. Tuberculomas should be suspected if signs of tuberculosis are present elsewhere in the lung, and if calcium deposits are noted in the spherical lesion. Chrondromas and cartilaginous hamartomas also may reveal areas of calcification.

The term *coin lesion* has been applied to a spherical well-circumscribed intrathoracic nodule which is demonstrated on the roentgenogram (Fig. 65). Any of the previously mentioned conditions may present the roentgenographic appearance of a coin lesion. If a diagnosis of a benign tumor of the lung could be established with certainty, one would be justified in withholding exploratory thoractomy. Since these lesions are discovered accidentally, and since they are usually asymptomatic, the proper course of therapy is difficult to outline; however, positive diagnosis is made with the greatest degree of certainty only when exploration and biopsy are performed. Other methods used to aid in the diagnosis are sputum examination, cytology, bronchoscopic study, specialized roentgenographic methods and intensive thorough study to search for a possible extrathoracic primary tumor.

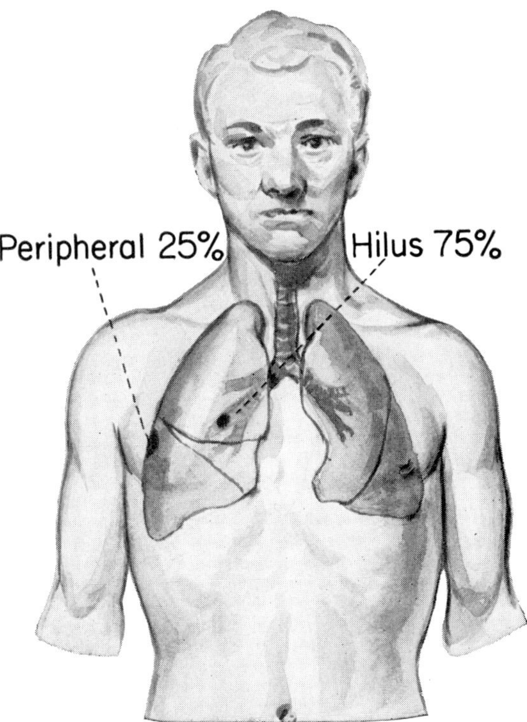

FIG. 66. Carcinoma of the lung can be classified according to location. Hilar lesions include those originating in a primary stem bronchus; peripheral lesions are at the lung surface.

Malignant tumors of the lung are unfortunately common; *carcinoma* is the most common type. It usually appears in the so-called "cancer age" groups, which constitute

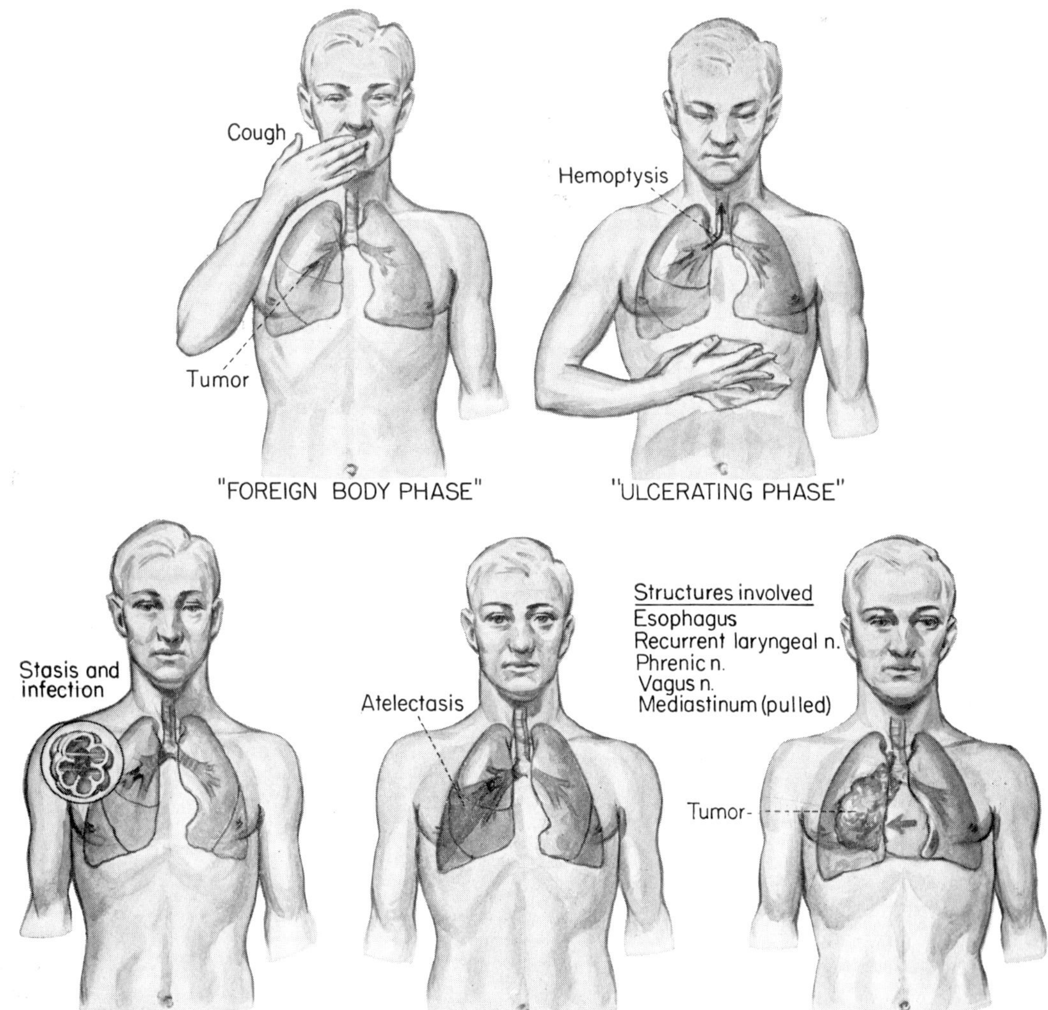

FIG. 67. The symptomatology as related to the growth of carcinoma of the lung. These phases must not be considered in a dogmatic fashion, since they can overlap or skip. The patient may be seen for the first time in any phase.

those in the 5th and 6th decades. It is 6 times more common in males. Little is known of the etiology. Those conditions that have a tendency to produce chronic irritations of the respiratory tract have been singled out as causative factors. Such irritative agents are those associated with smoking, exhaust gases, coal-tar products, lung abscess, silicosis, bronchiectasis, tuberculosis and chronic bronchitis.

A practical classification for these growths is based on their site of origin. Therefore, they are divided into 2 groups: *hilar* lesions, which include those arising in a primary stem bronchus (75%); and *peripheral* lesions, located toward the lung surface (25%). The latter are difficult, if at all possible, to see through the bronchoscope (Fig. 66). If the tumor is near the hilum, cough and hemoptysis may be early symptoms, and bronchoscopy usually reveals the neoplasm. If the tumor is peripheral, local symptoms may be lacking until either the pleura is involved or metastases occur.

SIGNS AND SYMPTOMS. The clinical picture is not stereotyped. It varies so tremendously from patient to patient that it is best to consider the symptomatology in the light of the growth of the tumor (Fig. 67).

An *early* neoplasm growing in the bronchial wall acts as a foreign body, and the patient attempts to expel it by *coughing*. As the tumor increases in size, it may ulcerate and bleed and produce hemoptysis. Such hemorrhage varies from a few specks of blood to copious hemorrhage; the latter is uncommon.

Later, as the growth increases, it may produce an incomplete blockage of the involved bronchus. This interferes with proper venti-

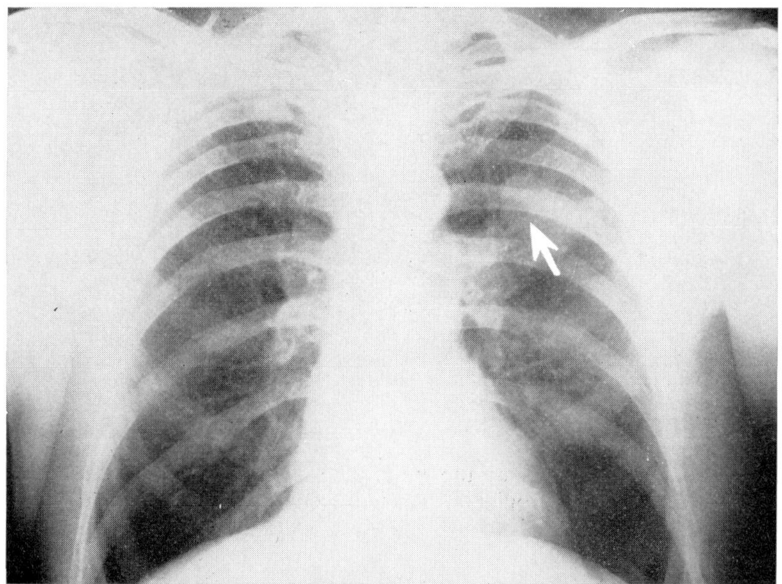

FIG. 68. Roentgen appearance of a proved bronchiogenic carcinoma as seen in the so-called "silent phase." Such lesions are discovered accidentally with routine roentgen screening of chests.

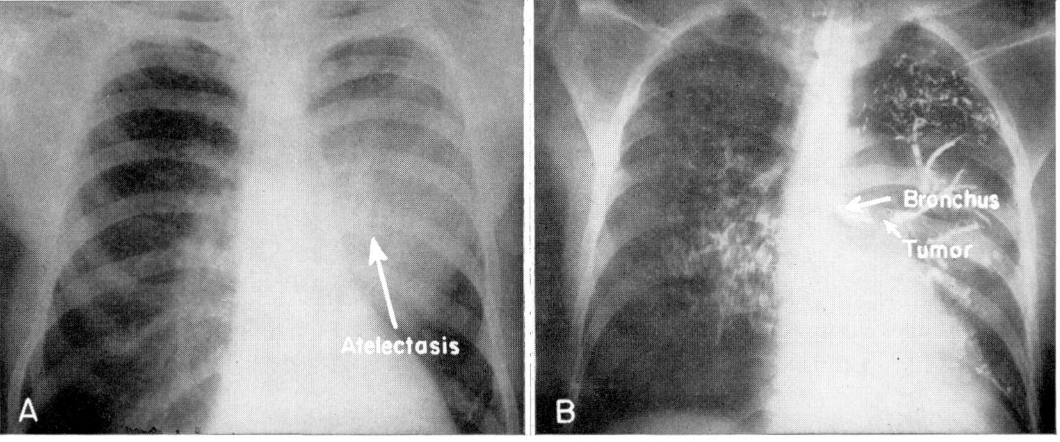

FIG. 69. Roentgenogram of pulmonary atelectasis caused by a lung carcinoma.

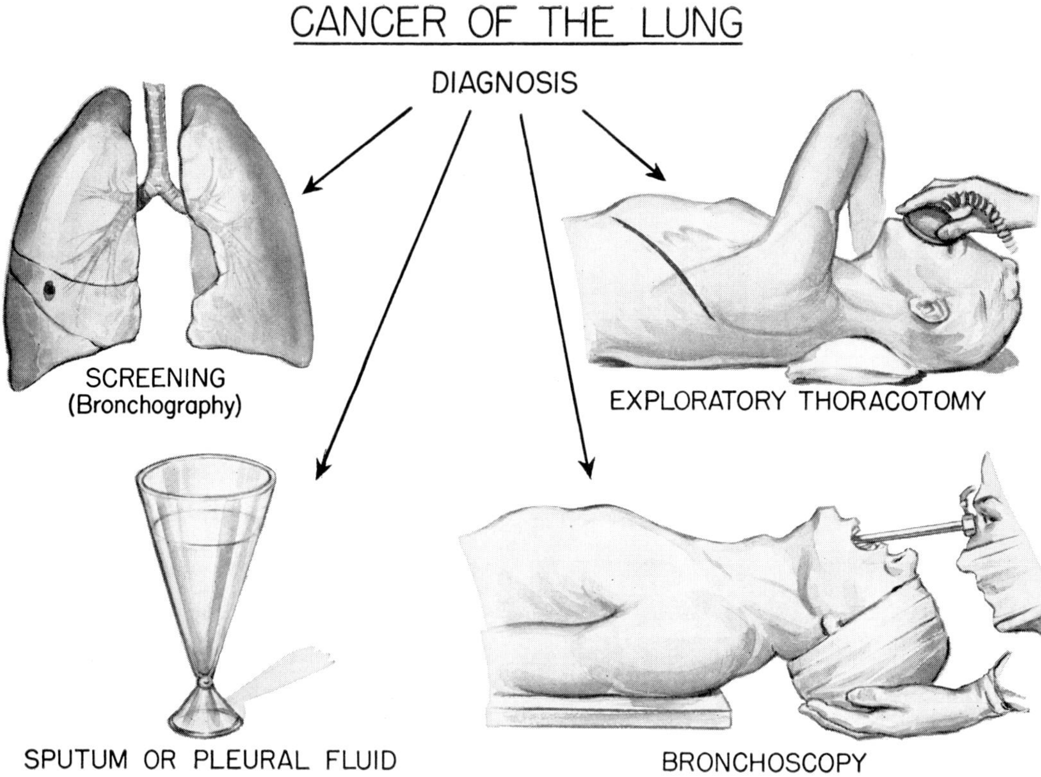

CANCER OF THE LUNG

DIAGNOSIS

SCREENING (Bronchography)

EXPLORATORY THORACOTOMY

SPUTUM OR PLEURAL FLUID

BRONCHOSCOPY

FIG. 70. Diagnosis of carcinoma of the lung. The cytologic study on sputum or pleural fluid is helpful only if the results reveal malignant cells.

lation of the corresponding lobe, and the patient becomes conscious of an inability to expand the lung fully, especially on exertion. At a comparative early stage some degree of *cyanosis* may be present. Wheezing may be heard over the narrowed bronchus; it is particularly significant when it is sharply localized and unilateral. Partial bronchial obstructions interfere with free drainage of secretions, and stasis results. This predisposes the patient to infection and bouts of fever. Such attacks are overlooked as "colds" or attacks of "flu." Pneumonia, abscess, or pleurisy are frequent complications (Fig. 67).

When the bronchus becomes completely *blocked*, the air in the alveolae distal to the lesion becomes absorbed (*atelectasis*). The mediastinum is displaced toward the affected side, and the ribs are pulled inward. Physical examination is helpful if the chest expands poorly on the involved side; this is accompanied by dullness and a complete absence of breath sounds. Toxemia, loss of weight and anemia are late signs.

As the growth progresses, it may involve such mediastinal structures as the phrenic nerve, the recurrent laryngeal nerve, the esophagus, the sympathetic nervous system, the superior vena cava and the vagus nerve (Fig. 67).

If the growth originates near the periphery of the lung, there is an early appearance of *pleural effusion;* this can be serofibrinous but more often is hemorrhagic. The study of such fluid may reveal tumor cells.

Carcinoma of the lung differs from other carcinomas in that it produces *pain relatively early*. Such pain is not pleuritic but is rather dull and situated deep in the chest. It is surprising how often the patient can localize this area of pain correctly.

Hemoptysis is present in about 50 per per cent of the cases. Any patient who complains of a bloody sputum must be examined immediately for "*the big three*": (1) carcinoma of the lung, (2) tuberculosis, (3) bronchiectasis. Although other conditions might produce hemoptysis, these 3 conditions must be ruled out first.

The so-called "silent phase" of carcinoma may be detected with a routine roentgen screening of the chest (Fig. 68). It has been stressed that the air within the expanded lung provides a good natural contrast medium for the early detection of density changes in the lung. Small tumors growing in the *periphery* usually cast a direct shadow. Small tumors that are *centrally located* cause segmental bronchial obstruction which may be seen as a corresponding thinned atelectatic segment (Fig. 69). Since an airless segment will cast a shadow many times the size of the tumor itself, these lesions should be demonstrable. Well-qualified roentgenologists stress that it is possible to demonstrate a lesion in the lung prior to the appearance of symptoms. They emphasize the importance of demonstrating the following roentgenographic findings: segmental emphysema, a difference in the size of the root of the 2 lungs, linear atelectasis, and a nodule in the periphery. Any or all of these should be considered as carcinoma until proved to be otherwise.

Routine screening of the entire population should be carried out. If any suspicious lesions appear, stereoscopic and tomographic studies should be made. Cytologic examination of the sputum and the pleural fluid should be done. Bronchoscopic examination may be most informative; if all of the tests are inconclusive, exploratory thoracotomy should be done (Fig. 70).

Clubbing of the fingernails may be the first indication of lung carcinoma (Fig. 71). It has been stressed that this osteoarthropathy may precede the usual signs and symptoms, including roentgenographic findings, by many months. When joint pain (arthralgia) is also present, it is due practically always to a pulmonary malignant lesion or a pleural mesothelioma, never to tuberculosis.

When a peripheral carcinoma is located in the lung apex, a so-called *Pancoast tumor*

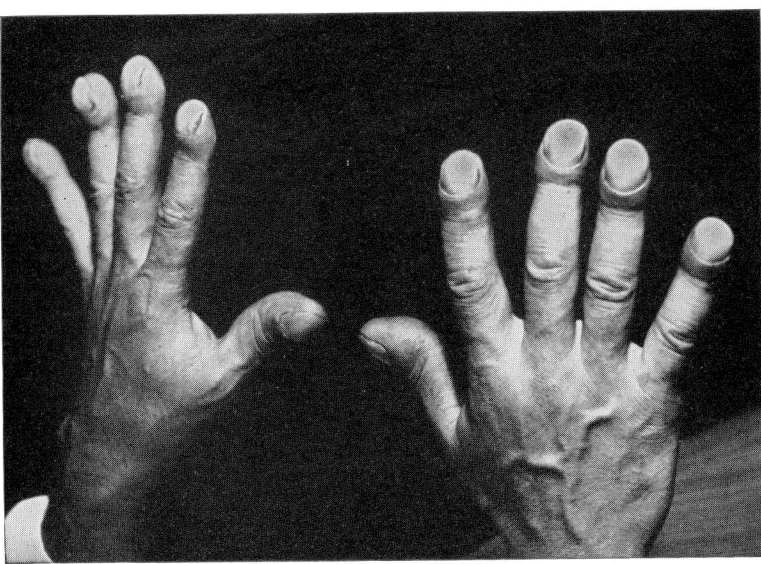

FIG. 71. Clubbed fingers. This is a condition characterized by enlargement of the terminal phalanges and curving of the nails. It is secondary to chronic conditions of the lungs and the heart. It may involve the toes. Other names have been applied to the condition, such as hippocratic nails, osteoarthropathy and pseudohypertrophic osteoarthropathy. This may be the earliest sign of lung cancer.

is diagnosed (p. 47). This is characterized by involvement of the ribs, the brachial plexus, the axillary vessels and the sympathetic nervous system. This results in pain in the shoulder, impairment of circulation of the upper extremity, and an ipsilateral Horner's syndrome (ptosis, miosis and enophthalmos). It is not unusual for the first symptoms of a peripherally located lung carcinoma to appear as remote metastases in the brain or the skeleton.

In the differential diagnosis of pulmonary carcinoma the 2 conditions which are also associated with hemoptysis, namely, tuberculosis and bronchiectasis, must be ruled out. Other lesions may simulate carcinoma. *Lipoid pneumonia* is associated with the instillation of oil into the nose and the throat or the oral intake of liquid petrolatum and allied preparations. *Chronic pneumonitis* and *pulmonary fibrosis* must be considered. Broncholithiasis was mentioned previously (p. 60). *Bronchial adenoma* is one of the most interesting, confusing and controversial tumors involving the bronchial tree. The majority of authorities are of the opinion that this lesion should be considered as a carcinoma with a slow rate of growth and with a tendency for the late development of metastases. Therefore, the term "bronchial adenoma" is a misnomer but probably will continue to be used because of habit or early teaching. This lesion is located characteristically either in a main bronchus or in a primary bronchial division. Grossly, it is distinguishable from carcinoma. It occurs with equal frequency in both sexes.

Metastatic Neoplasms. These pulmonary lesions are particularly important when one realizes that in recent years the resection of pulmonary tissue containing metastases has produced relief in some cases. The presence of such tumors does not always imply widespread dissemination; hence an overall pessimistic attitude is not justifiable.

The blood vascular spaces of the lungs represent the first major obstruction for tumor cells that arise in the somatic areas of the body. Malignant emboli that enter the portal vein and its tributaries are likely to be stopped by the sinusoids of the liver; later they may spread to the lungs via the hepatic veins and the vena cava. The lungs can be involved through the lymph channels and also by direct extension from adjacent structures. Primary tumors that spread to the

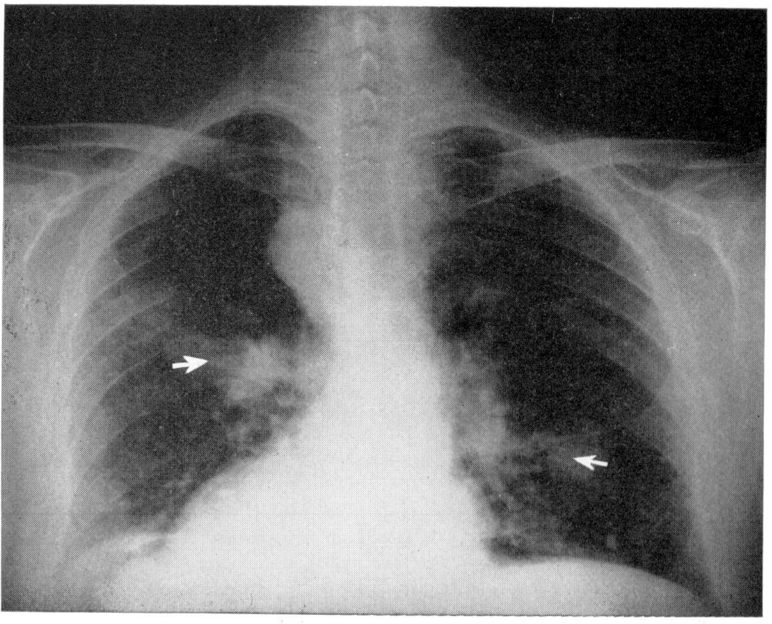

FIG. 72. Roentgenogram of metastatic tumors of the lung.

lungs by the blood vascular spaces include sarcomas, particularly Ewing's tumor and osteogenic sarcomas. Thyroid carcinoma, hypernephroma and chorio-epithelioma are the most common offenders in the carcinoma group. Metastatic tumors of the lungs often are spherical in shape and sharp in outline; if multiple, they are roughly uniform in size (Fig. 72). If the tumors are multiple and small, an early fatal prognosis is self-evident; however, the solitary metastatic lesion should be looked upon with some hope for survival. Such solitary lesions warrant removal.

Congenital Conditions

Various congenital abnormalities may affect the lungs. Occasionally, an entire lung may be absent. Another condition that has been described is one in which the fetal state has been maintained, so that the lung never has expanded. Variations involving the fissures and the lobes have been recorded frequently.

Congenital cystic disease of the lung has received great attention in the past few years. It has been known also as fibrocystic adenoma pulmonare. The cysts may be single or multiple, small or large; they have a tendency to be confined to a single lobe, although the condition may be bilateral. They are filled with either air or fluid. If asymptomatic, they are discovered accidently on routine roentgenographic examination of the chest. At times they give rise to alarming symptoms. If the cyst communicates with the bronchial tree through a narrow aperture, a valvelike action results in which air is drawn in during inspiration but prevented from escaping on expiration. Such an air-filled cyst rapidly increases in size, compresses the surrounding lung parenchyma and displaces the mediastinum to the opposite side. The clinical signs and symptoms resemble a tension pneumothorax (p. 49), including cyanosis, dyspnea, enlarged veins of the neck, and tachycardia. Death may occur if the condition is not diagnosed and treated rapidly. Needle aspiration to relieve the tension may be a lifesaving procedure. Cysts can become infected; the patient then presents the general signs and symptoms of sepsis plus localizing signs of a lung abscess (p. 67). The underlying condition is not suspected until bronchography is done. The demonstration of multiple cystic spaces may lead to an erroneous diagnosis of bronchiectasis. The differentiation between bronchiectasis and small multiple congenital cysts of the lung may be extremely difficult, particularly if the cysts are associated with chronic secondary infections.

Infections

The common surgical infections are pneumonitis, lung abscess, gangrene and tuberculosis.

Pneumonitis occurs in either acute or chronic forms. The *acute* type is important to the surgeon because of the frequency with which it follows surgical procedures (postoperative atelectasis). The *chronic* nontuberculous inflammatory lesions of the lung are of equal significance, because they must be differentiated from bronchiectasis, carcinoma, tuberculosis and lung abscess. The chronic form is a disease which occurs most frequently in middle-aged males. It is characterized by an insidious onset, a productive cough, pain in the chest, hemoptysis and a low-grade intermittent fever. The cough and the chest pain may be present for several years prior to the appearance of the hemoptysis. Of diagnostic importance is the fact that unlike many other chronic pulmonary diseases this condition does not have a noticeable effect upon the general condition of the patient. Bronchoscopic examination usually reveals an associated bronchitis; bronchography rules out bronchiectasis. The roentgenogram reveals an area of increased density lacking sharp demarcation from the surrounding lung tissue. Since conservative treatment usually suffices, a correct diagnosis is imperative. The right middle lobe is affected most commonly, but more than 1 lobe or bilateral involvement has been reported.

Pulmonary abscess and gangrene, which formerly were considered as separate lesions, should be considered together. An extensive gangrene of the lung can become an abscess, or an abscess may produce a gangrenous process. Although the condition is less frequent and less dangerous since the advent of improved technics of anesthesia and antibiotic therapy, it still is serious when present. About half the cases of lung abscess result

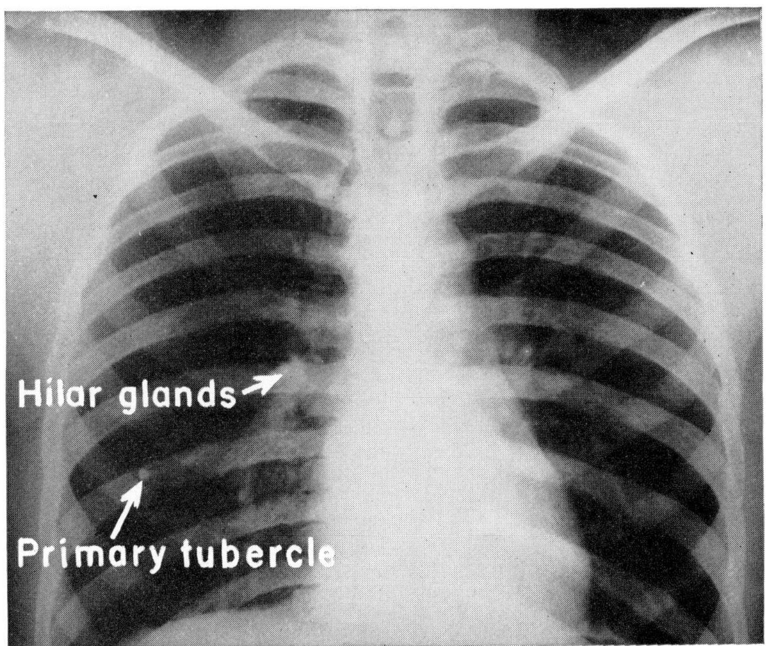

FIG. 73. Roentgenogram of the Ghon tubercle and primary pulmonary complex.

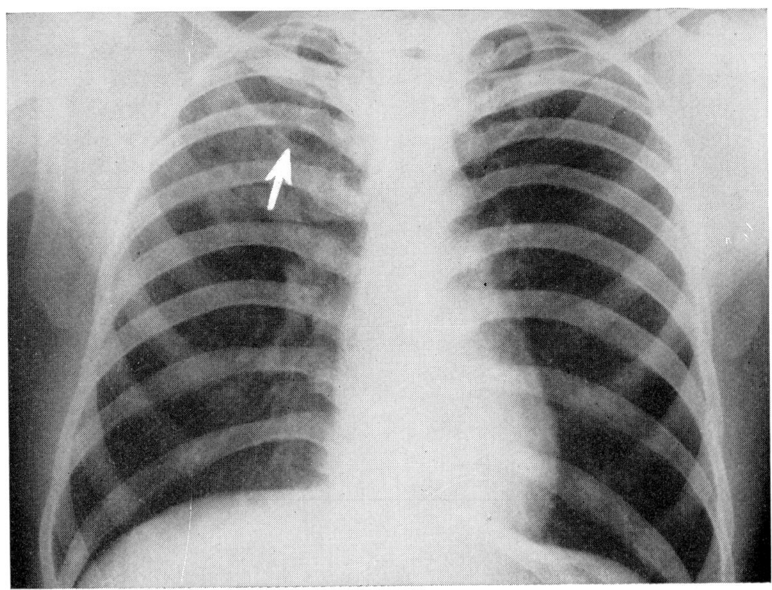

FIG. 74. Roentgenogram of tuberculosis involving the right upper lobe.

from pneumonia. The majority of the remaining cases reveal a history of aspiration of infected material. Tonsillectomy has been the greatest offender. In children, lung abscesses frequently result from the aspiration of foreign bodies. Other causes are infected chest wounds, congenital cystic disease and bronchiectasis. The putrid sputum contains spirochetes, fusiform bacilli, pneumococci, staphylococci and hemolytic streptococci. Cough is the most common symptom; also, hemoptysis may be present. Roentgenographic examination is of great value in the localization of the abscess. If the roentgenogram is taken early, an area of increased density is noted; later in the course of the disease and after bronchial communication has been established, the abscess cavity is seen, and a fluid level is present. Bronchoscopic examination is particularly helpful and also rules out or identifies an associated foreign body or tumor. Bronchoscopy also aids in aspiration of mucus and pus and provides a means of drainage. The abscess may perforate into the pleural space, giving rise to empyema; it may rupture into the pericardium and the mediastinum. *Brain abscess* as a complication of lung abscess is due to the passage of septic emboli from areas of thrombophlebitis in the intercostal and the bronchial veins by way of the azygos and the spinal veins upward to the brain.

Pulmonary Tuberculosis. The primary involvement of the lung by the tubercle bacillus results in the formation of the Ghon tubercle (Fig. 73). This is a small nodule usually located in the peripheral portion of the midzone of the lung. Secondary foci of tuberculosis in the hilar lymph glands are also present with the primary tubercle. This primary complex heals with scarring and calcification. A positive cutaneous reaction to tuberculin may be obtained later; this is the most obvious clinical manifestation. Occasionally, the primary form of the disease may be progressive and terminate fatally as a pneumonia or miliary tuberculosis.

The disease with which the surgeon is concerned is usually the result of a 2nd infection. Any portion of either lung may be involved. The most common sites are the apices, the right side being affected more often than the left (Fig. 74).

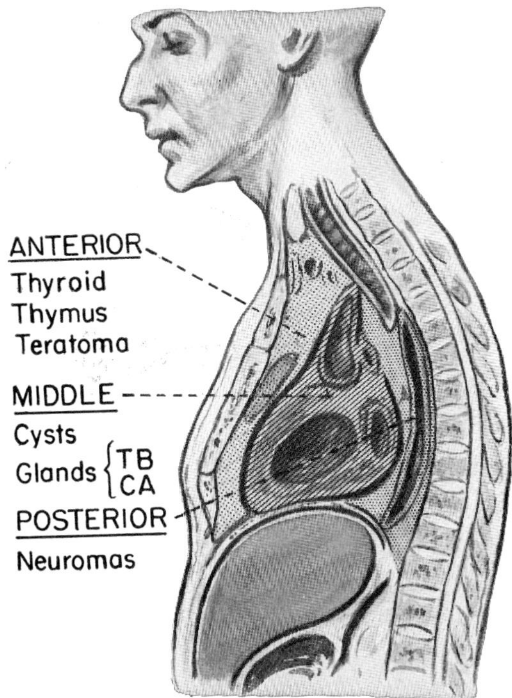

FIG. 75. Mediastinal enlargements. In the anterior mediastinum are masses associated with the thyroid, the thymus and teratomas; the middle mediastinal growths are related to bronchogenic cysts, lymphomas and metastatic and tuberculous lymph glands; the posterior mediastinal tumors are predominantly neurogenic.

Nature's process of healing a tuberculous cavity is by means of immobilization. This brings about some collapse of the affected side of the chest by drawing the ribs together, by pulling the diaphragm upward and the mediastinal contents toward the affected side. When these natural phenomena can occur satisfactorily, the cavity closes spontaneously and becomes obliterated. However, Nature's efforts may fail, because the structures to which the lung is attached by adhesions are unyielding and prevent spontaneous collapse. The basis of modern surgical methods assists Nature to overcome this resistance. These methods are referred to under the general terms of collapse procedures.

The medical aspect of tuberculosis and the signs and symptoms of the disease are well

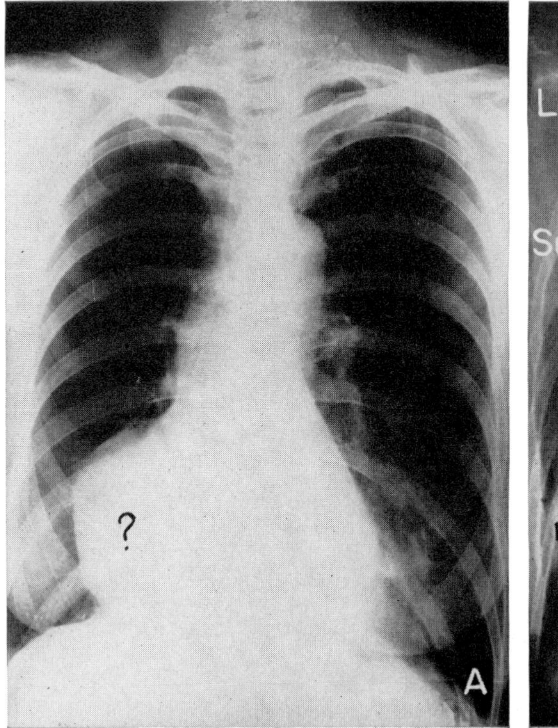

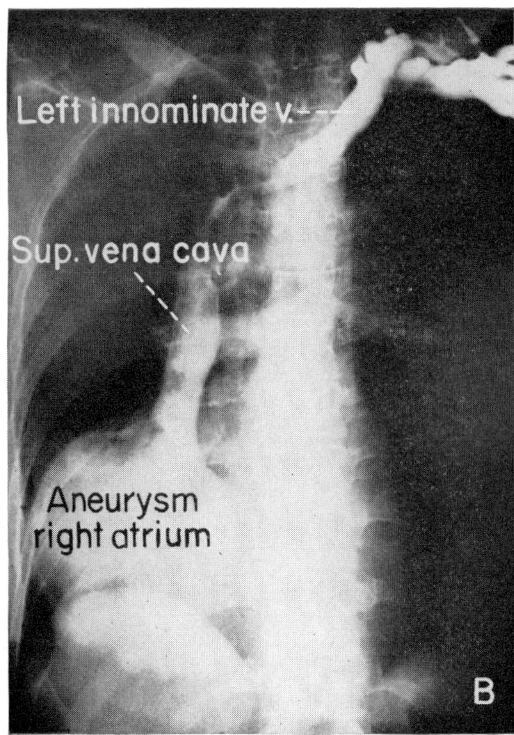

FIG. 76. (A) A mass is noted extending from the right border of the heart and involving the mediastinum. (B) An angiocardiogram showed this to be an aneurysm of the right atrium. Angiocardiography has become an outstanding adjunct in the diagnosis of lesions of this type.

known and described in appropriate texts. It might be well to emphasize, however, that unless the tubercle bacilli are demonstrated, one should hesitate to make a diagnosis of pulmonary tuberculosis, regardless of how suggestive the signs and the roentgenograms appear.

MEDIASTINUM

The mediastinum is that space which is situated between the lungs; it is divided into the superior, the anterior, the middle and the posterior mediastina. The tumors that involve this area have a tendency to be located in specific mediastina (Fig. 75). In the anterior mediastinum thyroid enlargements, thymomas and teratomas occur. The middle mediastinal masses are associated with bronchogenic cysts and esophageal conditions; this particular part of the mediastinum frequently harbors metastatic and tuberculous lymph nodes and lymphomas. The posterior mediastinal tumors are predominately neurogenic. It should not be forgotten that the heart is a mediastinal structure, and conditions involving this organ also must be considered (Fig. 76).

TUMORS

The subject of mediastinal tumors is complicated because of the large variety of lesions that may occur here. Almost any type of tumor can occur in this region. Dermoids and the neurogenic neoplasms usually are malignant. It is impossible to determine the exact nature of the growth without a microscopic study. Since the possibility of malignancy is high, and the morbidity and the mortality of exploratory thoracotomy is low, there is no justification for permitting mediastinal tumors to remain undiagnosed and untreated. The so-called "trial of irradiation" is inconclusive, and "punch" or needle biopsies are to be condemned. A biopsy of the scalenus anticus lymph nodes might be helpful. A group of cervical lymph nodes is situated on the scalenus anticus muscle; if one wishes to avoid an exploratory thoracotomy, exploration of these glands can be done easily (Fig. 77). Currently, some investigators advocate bilateral scalene lymph node excision associated with thoracic duct cannulation. In some cases of lung cancer they are able to demonstrate both positive nodes and positive cytologic findings in thoracic duct lymph and chyle. Fluoroscopy and roentgenography may be helpful. Barium studies of the esophagus may reveal an intrinsic lesion or esophageal displacement (Fig. 78). Tumors of the mediastinum are primary or secondary; hence, a complete examination and investigation must be conducted.

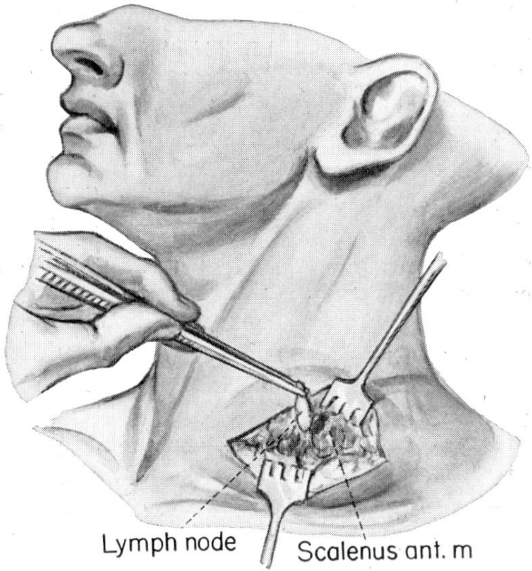

FIG. 77. The scalenus biopsy. A telltale lymph node may be situated on the scalenus anticus muscle.

The most common symptom caused by increased mediastinal pressure is *dyspnea.*

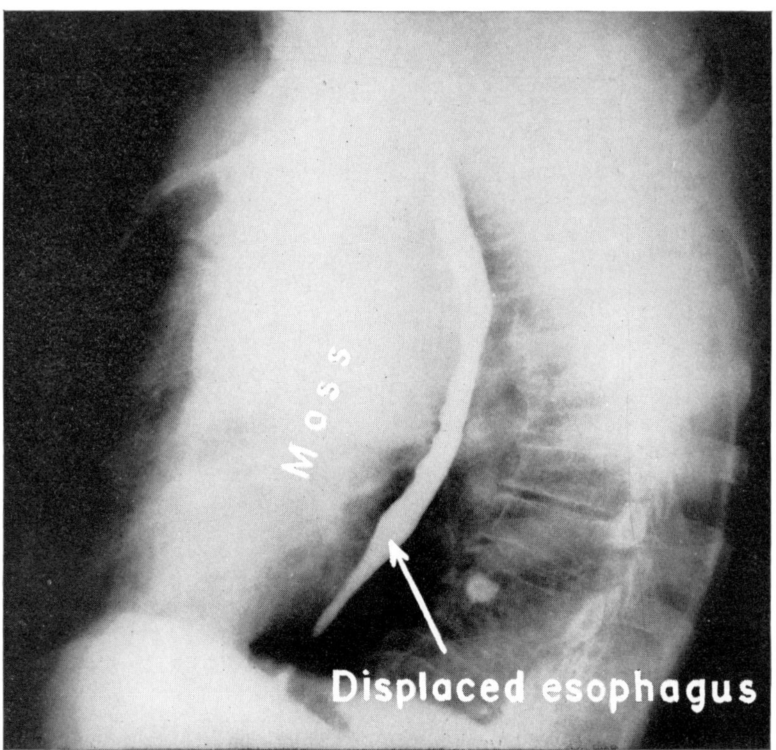

FIG. 78. Roentgenogram revealing displacement of the esophagus by a mediastinal lymphoma.

This is probably due to compression on the large veins and the air passages. The vein that is affected most commonly is the superior vena cava. Obstruction of this vessel results in cyanosis, orthopnea, dilatation of the superficial veins of the thorax and the neck, and later pleural and pericardial effusions. In severe cases of superior caval obstruction there may be headache, dizziness, epistaxis and tinnitus; subcutaneous edema of the head, the neck and the upper part of the thorax may occur also. If the obstruction is above the azygos vein orifice, the symptoms are less severe.

Modern thoracic surgery has made possible the removal of mediastinal tumors that have not infiltrated. However, mediastinal tumors of thyroid origin still can be removed through the usual thyroidectomy approach. Median sternotomy gives the best exposure for the removal of thymus tumors. A neurogenic tumor may have an extension into the spinal canal which necessitates the addition of a laminectomy.

Mediastinitis

Infections of the mediastinum comprise a wide range of conditions which vary from mild degrees of inflammation to suppurative mediastinitis and gangrene. These infections can arise from inflammatory or traumatic conditions which involve the thorax, the abdomen or the cervical region. Many acute mediastinal infections occur from lesions of the esophagus (p. 82).

Perforations of the esophagus result from trauma (instrumentation), tumors or inflammatory processes. Chronic infections of the mediastinum often are tuberculous in nature; they may originate from a tuberculous spine. Roentgenography and fluoroscopy are valuable aids.

Mediastinal Emphysema

This condition has been described elsewhere (p. 49). It produces increased mediastinal pressure.

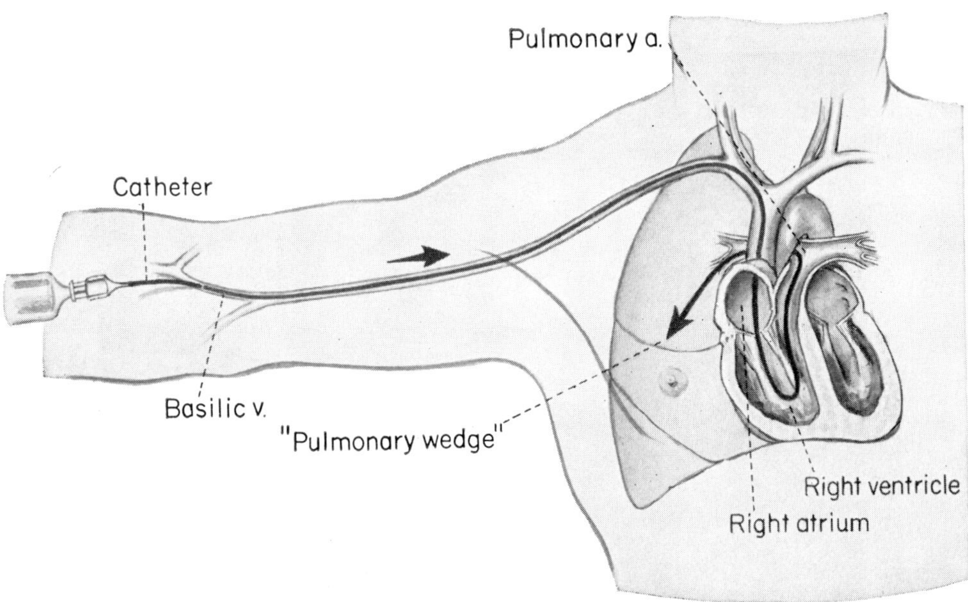

Fig. 79. Right-heart catheterization. The catheter has been passed through the basilic vein into the vena cava, the right auricle, the right ventricle, the pulmonary artery and into the "pulmonary capillary" position in the right lung. In infants it may become necessary to perform this procedure through the external jugular or the saphenous vein.

CONGENITAL HEART DISEASE

History and Physical Examination

In spite of the many new diagnostic methods, a carefully taken history and an accurate physical examination still are of the utmost importance. In eliciting the history one should attempt to date the appearance of the symptoms (cyanosis and exertional dyspnea) and their crippling effects. *Fatigability* is an important symptom unfortunately too often overlooked; it suggests inadequate cardiac output. Frequently, it is mistaken for a "feeding problem." Left-sided heart failure is characterized by dyspnea on exertion or even at rest. If this becomes severe, marked respiratory distress ensues with tachypnea (60 to 100 per minute), flaring alae nasi and retractions at the supersternal notch. A mother may accidently discover the orthopnea by observing that the baby is more restful on her shoulder in an upright position. It is peculiar to infants with left-sided heart failure that rales are rare. In right-sided heart failure also the symptoms may differ from those of older patients. Dependent edema is rare, and venous distention of the jugular veins is difficult to detect. With right-sided failure the enlarged liver loses its sharp edge and is particularly tender.

In the course of the physical examination one should record the presence of any cyanosis, clubbing of the fingers and the toenails, cardiac murmurs and the character of the pulses in all 4 extremities. Since polycythemia accompanies most lesions associated with cyanosis, a study of the peripheral blood becomes important.

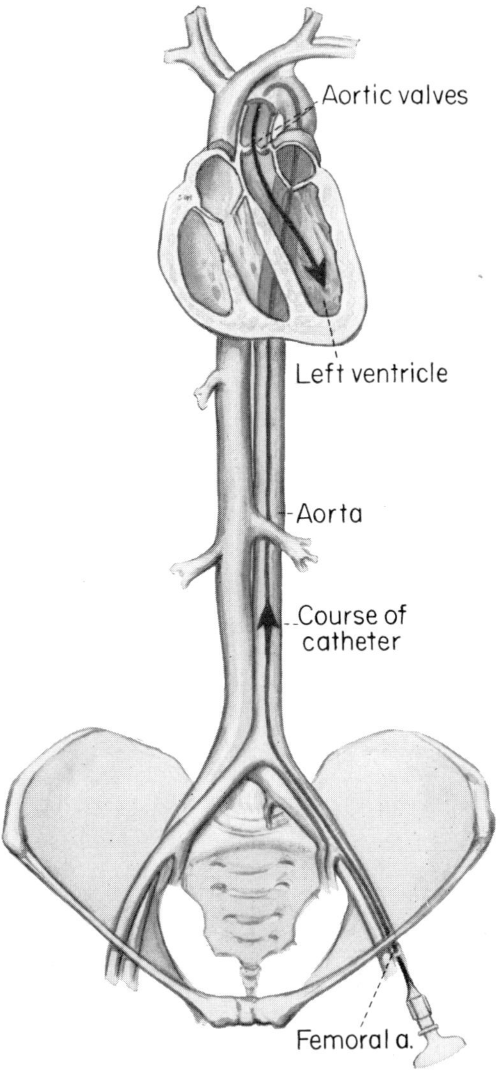

Fig. 80. Left-heart catheterization. In this instance the catheter has been passed retrograde up the femoral artery through the abdominal and the thoracic aorta past the aortic valve and into the left ventricle. Other methods of left-heart catheterization have been accomplished via the left atrium or the left ventricle by direct punctures.

Special Diagnostic Procedures

These aid immeasurably in the diagnosis and the treatment of cardiac lesions. Among those diagnostic procedures which are most helpful are fluoroscopy, roentgenography, vectorcardiography, electrocardiography, cardiac catheterization, angiography and aortography. Progress in the field of cardiac surgery has been so rapid and so breathtaking that it would be presumptuous to attempt to portray in this volume a semblance of the material available. The material here presented is given only as a suggested basis for some of the diagnostic procedures available.

Cardiac catheterization is probably the most important recently developed diagnostic

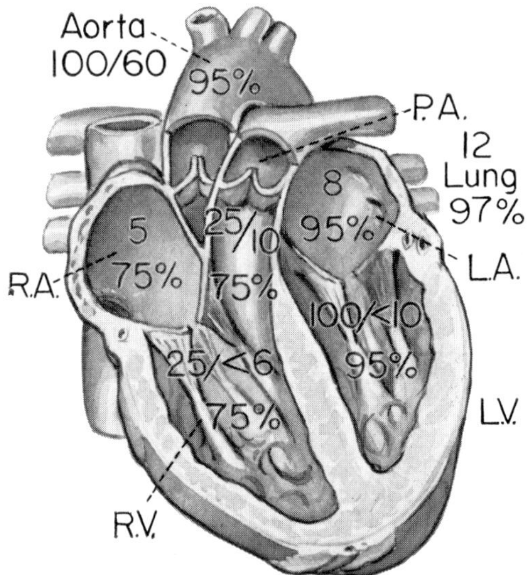

FIG. 81. Pressures and oxygen saturations of the blood in a normal heart. (After Warren)

procedure. By this method one frequently may obtain precise diagnosis of the anatomic abnormality. Furthermore, it permits evaluation of the degree of disability, and often it predicts impending cardiac decompensation.

RIGHT-HEART CATHETERIZATION is performed through a cutdown in the basilic vein (Fig. 79). The catheter is advanced into the right atrium, the right ventricle, the pulmonary artery and into the so-called "wedge or pulmonary capillary" region. During this procedure the position of the catheter must be checked repeatedly under the fluoroscopic screen or by means of an electrode-tipped catheter connected to the electrocardiograph. The presence of oxygenated blood in the right heart suggests a left-to-right shunt. The oximeter is an extremely valuable adjunct, since a determination of oxygen can be made continuously while the catheter is being withdrawn from the pulmonary artery to the vena cava. In this way amounts of oxygen can be determined and the localizations of various saturations; thus the location of the shunt can be diagnosed accurately.

LEFT-HEART CATHETERIZATION can be accomplished by passing a catheter from the femoral artery through the aorta and into the left ventricle (Fig. 80). Two other routes for left-heart catheterization have been utilized: into the left atrium by direct puncture or into the left ventricle via a similar direct puncture. By these methods pressure recording and oxygen sampling on the left side of the heart are possible. This information has resulted in increased diagnostic accuracy by detecting localized right-to-left shunts because of the low oxygen saturation of blood on the left side of the heart.

Angiography is accomplished by means of rapid injection of a radiopaque substance into the circulatory system, thereby providing a roentgenographic means of visualizing the chambers of the heart and the great vessels. With proper equipment the course of the solution throughout the heart, the lungs and the aorta can be followed, and repetitive films can be taken.

Aortography is another method of diag-

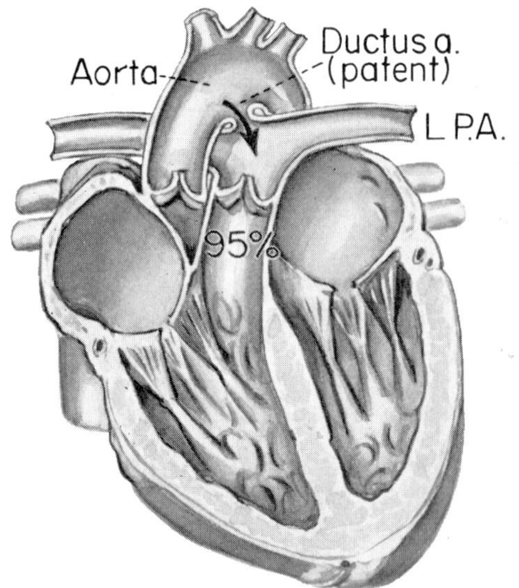

FIG. 82. Patent ductus arteriosus. The fetal communication between the pulmonary artery and the aorta remains open. The direction of the blood flow in the ductus is reversed, and the oxygen content in the pulmonary artery has a higher than normal saturation—in this instance, 95 per cent (normal is 75%). This takes place in the absence of pulmonary arterial hypertension.

nostic importance. The dye is injected into the left branchial artery, and the entire aortic arch can be visualized.

The oxygen saturations and the pressures in the various heart chambers and the great vessels are shown in Figure 81.

Classification

Earlier classifications were based on the presence or the absence of cyanosis, but recent knowledge relating to the hemodynamics and the physiopathology of these lesions have resulted in newer classifications. *A right-to-left shunt will produce a cyanosis, whereas a left-to-right shunt will not.* There are malformations which are not associated with shunts. These have been classified as *distal to* and *proximal to* the mitral valves.

Whereas one classification lists truncus arteriosus under large left-to-right shunts (aorticoid-pulmonary), equally qualified authorities list the same condition under the heading of malformations with combined shunts predominately left-to-right. For those interested in detailed discussions of the subject, numerous excellent texts and articles are available. A few examples will be discussed in this text.

Patent Ductus Arteriosus. This ductus is a vascular connection which directs blood from the pulmonary artery to the aorta during fetal life (Fig. 82). If the ductus remains open after birth, the direction of blood flow is reversed owing to the higher pressure in the aorta. The hemodynamics in this lesion result from a shunt of saturated arterial blood from the aorta into the pulmonary artery. Therefore, this produces an acyanotic lesion. The decrease of the pulmonary arterial resistance and the increase of the systemic pressure explain the direction of the shunt. The symptoms, the signs and the laboratory data are dependent on the size of the shunt. A small ductus with small volume produces minimal signs, whereas a large ductus can produce startling findings.

The two outstanding symptoms are dyspnea and fatigue. The finding of a persistent murmur heard over the pulmonic area, both systolic and diastolic, is characteristic. This murmur has been described as a "machine-like" constant, to-and-fro hum. Cardiac catheterization reveals a demonstrable left-to-right shunt at the level of the pulmonary artery; the oxygen tension of the blood in the pulmonary artery is above normal. At times the tip of the catheter may pass through the ductus and appear in the descending aorta. If there is associated pulmonary hypertension, the shunt becomes reversed to a right-to-left shunt. Cardiomegaly is directly associated with the diameter of the patent ductus. It has been stated that patients with typical clinical findings do not require cardiac catheterization. The procedure is not without danger and should be utilized only when definitely indicated.

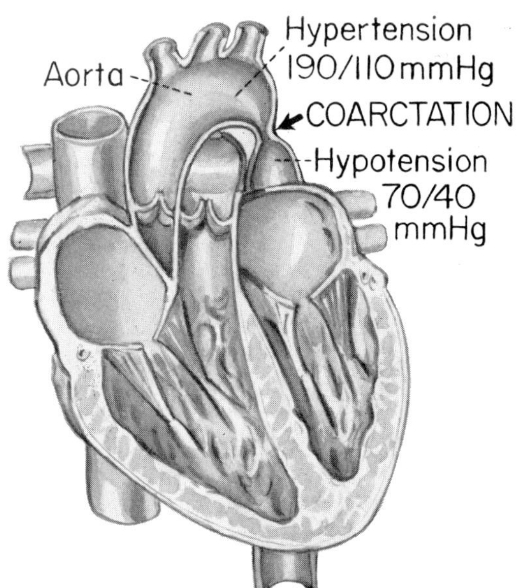

Fig. 83. Coarctation of the aorta. As a result of a narrowing in the coarctated aortic area, there are hypertension in the upper extremities and hypotension in the lower extremities. The aortic pressure, which normally is 100 to 120 over 60 or 70, now is elevated to 190 over 110. The pressure distal to the coarctated area is diminished, frequently to 70 over 40 or less.

Coarctation of the Aorta. This disease is characterized by narrowing or complete obstruction of the aortic lumen, usually involving the distal segment of the aortic arch (Fig. 83). The descending thoracic and even the abdominal aorta may be involved. The usual location is just distal to the left subclavian artery. The decrease in the size of the lumen prevents an adequate amount of blood from reaching the lower part of the body. A number of different classifications have been proposed for aortic coarctation because of the wide variations in its anatomic forms. The type most frequently encountered is located just distal to the aortic insertion of the ligamentum arteriosum.

The chief clinical findings are upper extremity hypertension and decreased to absent pressure in the lower extremities. Faint or absent femoral pulsations should arouse suspicion. Normally, the pressure in the legs is as high or higher than that in the arms. Cardiac murmurs may or may not be present, and the classic roentgenographic findings of the so-called "notching of the ribs" usually appears after the age of 14. Aortography is an aid in confirming the diagnosis; frequently, it will identify the extent of the coarctated area and the state of collateral circulation. Cardiac catheterization is not useful as a diagnostic aid. Without surgical intervention many of these patients succumb from the complications (cardiac failure, cerebral

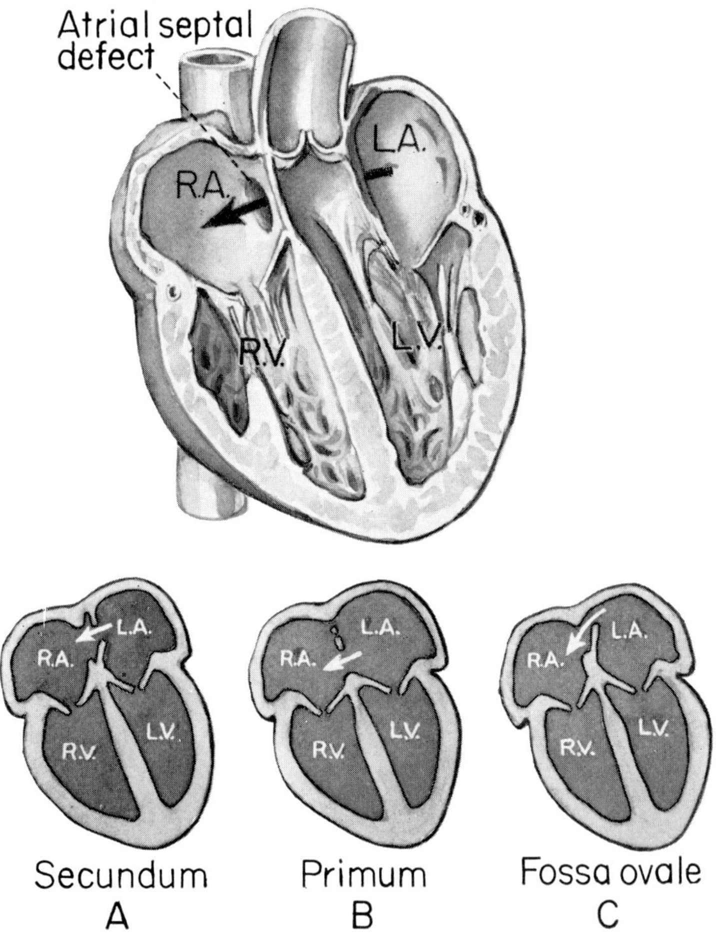

FIG. 84. Atrial septal defects. This defect is characterized by an abnormal opening in the atrial septum. It permits a shunt of blood from left to right. (A) The osteum secundum defect, which is situated high in the atrial septum. (B) The osteum primum defect, which is situated low in the septum. (C) A patent foramen ovale.

hemorrhage and subacute bacterial endarteritis). Mild cases are asymptomatic and are discovered only at necropsy.

Atrial Septal Defects. This defect presents an abnormal opening in the atrial septum (Fig. 84). A left-to-right shunt results, because the pressure in the left atrium exceeds that on the right side, and the flow is reversed. In the typical case no cyanosis is present. With increased pressure on the right side of the heart, as can occur with crying or straining, venous blood may be shunted from right to left, and the patient then develops a *transient cyanosis*. With the typical left-to-right shunt the pulmonary flow becomes greater than the systemic; consequently, there is an increased burden on the right ventricle. A potential secondary pulmonary hypertension is possible.

The symptoms depend on the size of the shunt. If the defect is small, the patient may be totally asymptomatic. With a larger defect the patient tires easily and becomes dyspneic. A systolic murmur usually is heard over the base of the heart. The degree of cardiac enlargement is in direct relation to the size of the defect. The electrocardiogram reveals right axis deviation and incomplete right bundle branch block.

The two types of atrial septal defects have been described as a persistent osteum secundum, in which the defect is high in the septum, and a persistent osteum primum, in which the defect is low in the septum. The patency of the foramen ovale also must be considered in these defects. The persistent osteum primum is the more serious of these. Usually, the diagnosis is clinched following cardiac catheterization. If such a defect is present, there is an increased oxygen content in the right atrium, and at times an easy passage of the catheter from the right atrium to the left atrium becomes possible.

Ventricular Septal Defects. These defects vary in size and may occur either in the membranous or the muscular portion of the ventricular septum (Fig. 85). Due to the higher pressure in the left ventricle, a shunting of blood from left to right occurs during systole; in these typical cases there is no cyanosis. The small ventricular septal defect (maladie de Roger) is a very noisy lesion but is of little physiologic moment. Usually, it is found in the muscular portion of the septum and rarely requires surgery. When the defect occurs in the upper or membranous portion, the symptoms will be dependent on the size of the defect. Cardiac catheterization usually reveals a greater oxygen saturation in the right ventricle than in the right atrium; at times the catheter may be seen passing from the right into the left ventricle.

Tetralogy of Fallot. This condition accounts for the most common type of "blue baby." The 4 parts which constitute the tetralogy are pulmonary stenosis, ventricular septal defect, right ventricular hypertrophy and dextroposition of the aorta (Fig. 86). The course of blood in such a heart takes the following paths: From the right atrium the blood passes into the right ventricle, and from here a small portion of the venous (unoxygenated) blood enters the stenosed pulmonary artery. This portion will undergo oxygenation in the pulmonary circulation. The major portion of blood in the right ventricle is shunted from right to left through the interventricular defect. The shunt is ex-

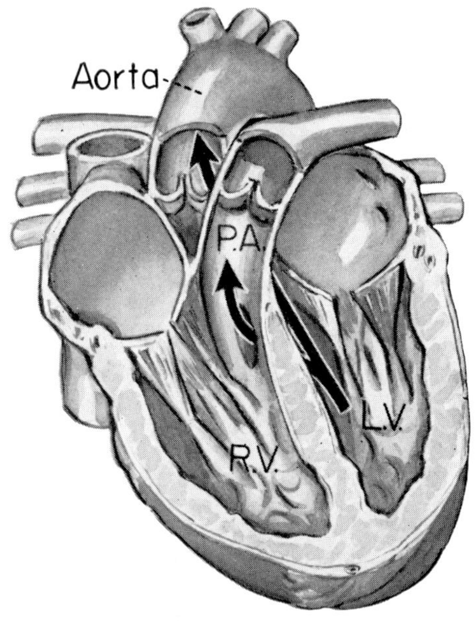

FIG. 85. Ventricular septal defect. This is a composite drawing showing the possibility of the bidirectional shunt.

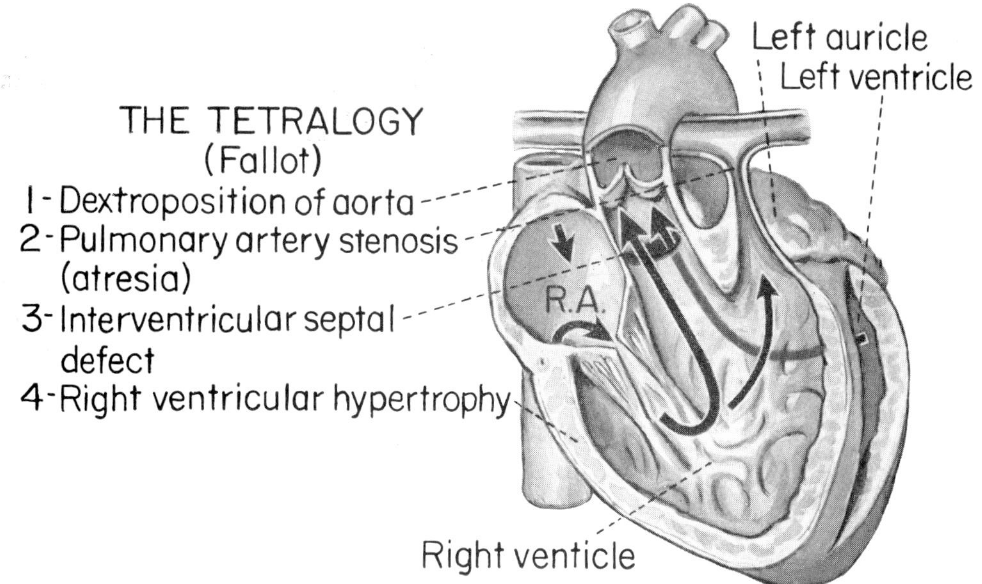

FIG. 86. Tetralogy of Fallot. The 4 parts which characterize this most common cause of the "blue baby" are (1) dextroposition of the aorta, (2) pulmonary artery stenosis, (3) ventricular septal defect and (4) right ventricular hypertrophy. The arrows indicate the possible courses of blood flow.

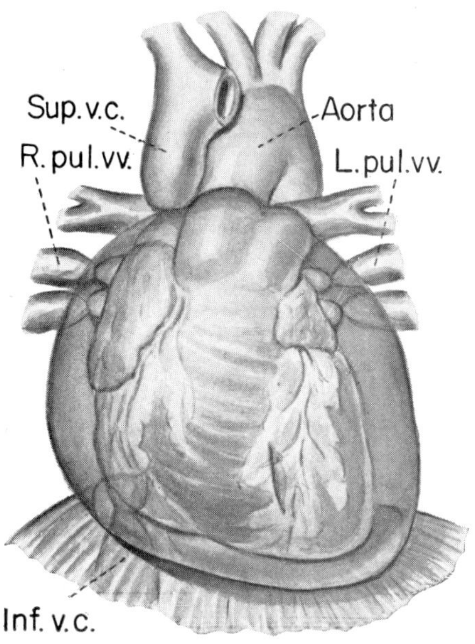

FIG. 87. A schematic drawing of the heart and the pericardium, showing the effect of acute cardiac tamponade on the venae cavae and the pulmonary veins. The compression interferes also with the diastolic filling of the ventricles.

aggerated by the stenosis in the pulmonary artery. Mixing of the oxygenated blood (from the pulmonary system) occurs in the left ventricle. From the left ventricle this mixed blood enters the aorta and thence passes into the systemic circulation.

The severity of the symptoms depends on the degree of pulmonary stenosis, the size of the ventricular septal defect and the degree to which the aorta overrides the septal defect. Cyanosis during the early months of life, increasing with exertion, is characteristic. Also predominant is clubbing of the fingers and the toes, a systolic murmur along the left sternal border, paroxysmal attacks of dyspnea and loss of consciousness. The squatting position is particularly characteristic. Cardiac catheterization demonstrates an elevated right ventricular pressure due to the right-to-left shunt. The arterial oxygen tension is below normal. Frequently, the catheter may be directed through the defect into the aorta.

Numerous other congenital heart lesions, such as subaortic stenosis, complete transposition of the great vessels, truncus arteriosus, tricuspid atresias and anomalous venous return, to mention only a few, are described in texts dealing with this subject.

PERICARDIUM

The common disorders of the pericardium which are of particular interest to the diagnostician and the surgeon are wounds, acute pericarditis and chronic constrictive pericarditis.

WOUNDS

Morgagni in 1761 stressed the dangers of cardiac compression due to hemorrhage into

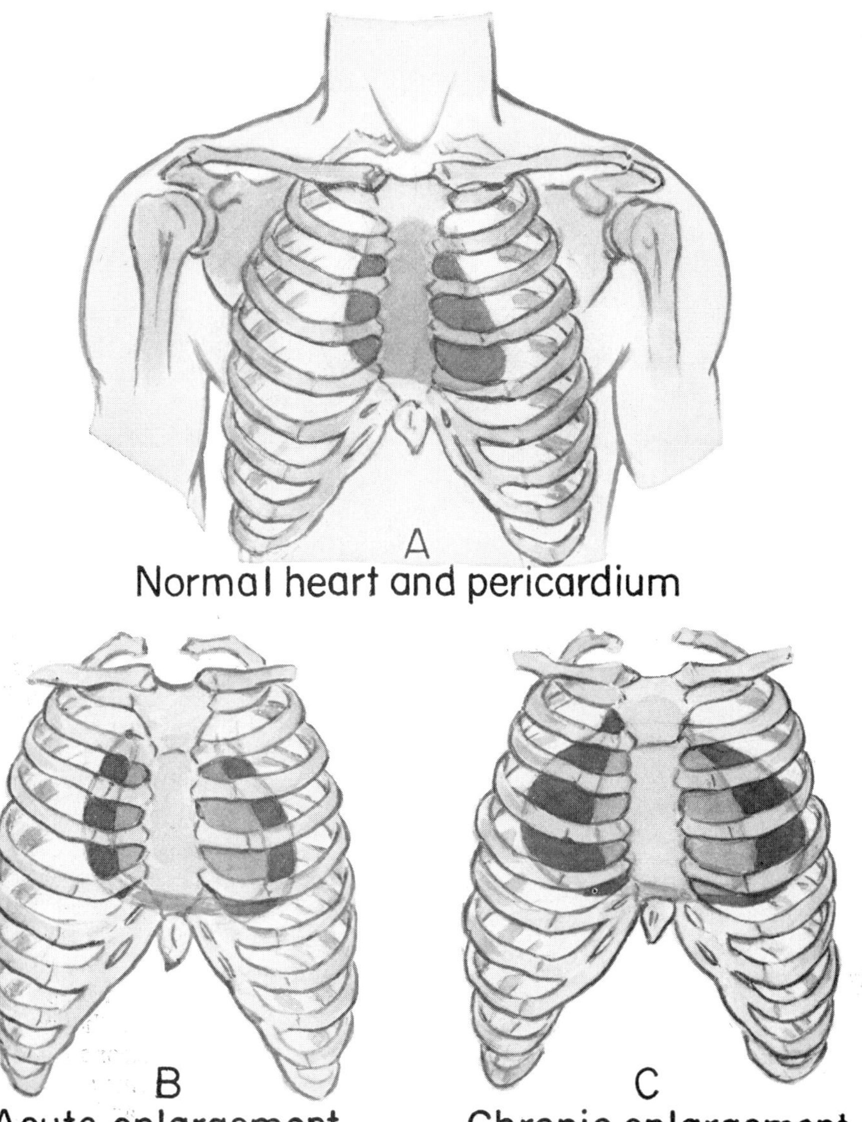

FIG. 88. Schematic drawing of cardiac silhouettes in (A) the normal heart and pericardium, (B) acute cardiac tamponade and (C) chronic enlargement. Because the fibrous pericardium is inelastic, it does not allow the massive pericardial enlargement in the acute tamponade that it does in the chronic or delayed form.

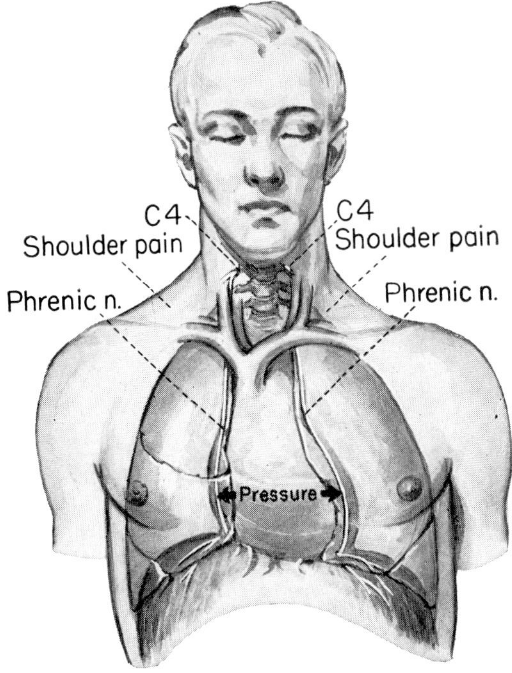

FIG. 89. Pericarditis and shoulder pain. When the pericardial sac distends, pressure on the phrenic nerve results; this in turn produces pain in the shoulder region.

the pericardium and thus originated the concept of pericardial tamponade. It was Napoleon's surgeon, Larrey, who is credited with performing the first successful pericardicentesis in 1829.

Wounds which involve the pericardium almost always involve the heart; hence, this is the most common cause of *cardiac tamponade*. Because of its vulnerable anterior position, the right ventricle is the chamber most frequently injured. Oozing of blood from a heart chamber into the pericardial space may occur when the heart is injured directly or by compression injuries of the chest. An accumulation of blood within the pericardium produces a progressive compression of the heart and obstruction of the great veins (Fig. 87). The compressed veins are the venae cavae and the pulmonary veins. When venous pressure and pericardial pressure become equalized, arterial pressure rapidly falls, and cardiac action ceases. Beck has described a diagnostic triad for cardiac tamponade which can be remembered by using the letter *H*:

1. *H*igh venous pressure
2. *H*ypotension
3. *H*eart sounds distant and difficult to hear

The high venous pressure is manifested by distention of the neck veins. Since the systolic pressure is low, and the diastolic level rises, it is diagnostic when one can demonstrate the presence of a diminished pulse pressure. Pulsus paradoxicus is present and is best demonstrated with the use of a sphygmomanometer. The systolic pressure falls with each inspiration. This decline can be demonstrated by maintaining the blood pressure cuff at a level at which the systolic sounds are first heard. With each inspiratory phase the sounds will disappear. Fluoroscopy, if available, will demonstrate diminished cardiac pulsation. Roentgenograms are not as useful in acute tamponade as they are in the chronic form, since the relatively inelastic pericardium does not immediately become greatly distended. In the chronic or delayed forms of tamponade an enormous cardiac silhouette may be demonstrated (Fig. 88).

The recognition of this condition is vital, since aspiration of a small amount of blood from the pericardial sac can be lifesaving. In many wounds of the heart and the pericardium death results from cardiac tamponade rather than exsanguinating hemorrhage.

Fibrinous and Purulent Pericarditis

These acute conditions are encountered most commonly as complications of lung infections. During epidemics of streptococcal bronchopneumonia, purulent pericarditis is not uncommon. The serious aspects of this condition are not only those associated with the infection but also the pressure effects caused by the fluid in the pericardial sac; these produce a tamponade of the heart. The signs and symptoms are associated with precordial discomfort and pain, dyspnea and a sense of sternal oppression. The pain usually extends to the left shoulder region (phrenic nerve) (Fig. 89). Anxiety, cyanosis and weakened pulse are present often.

There are observed frequently an increase in precordial dullness, a pericardial friction rub and a palpable liver. The roentgenogram may be a valuable diagnostic aid. The normal adult pericardial sac holds between 150 and 250 ml. of fluid. When this amount increases, the effects of tamponade become evident. The heart sounds are distant, muffled or even lost. The veins in the neck become full and distended, and the upper abdomen is tense. If aspiration reveals pus, surgical drainage of the pericardium is indicated.

Chronic Constrictive Pericarditis

This condition has been referred to as the "compressed heart." It results from a conversion of adhesions and/or fibrinous deposits into dense, mature fibrous tissue which may go on to calcification. As the pericardium and the epicardium thicken and contract, the pericardial space becomes obliterated; this results in an imprisoned and restricted heart, which in turn alters hemodynamics. Some of the more common etiologic factors are tuberculosis, rheumatic fever and trauma with resulting hemopericardium. Some of the rarer causes are cholesterol pericarditis and specific infections such as actinomycosis (bovis) and staphylococcic infections (Fig. 90).

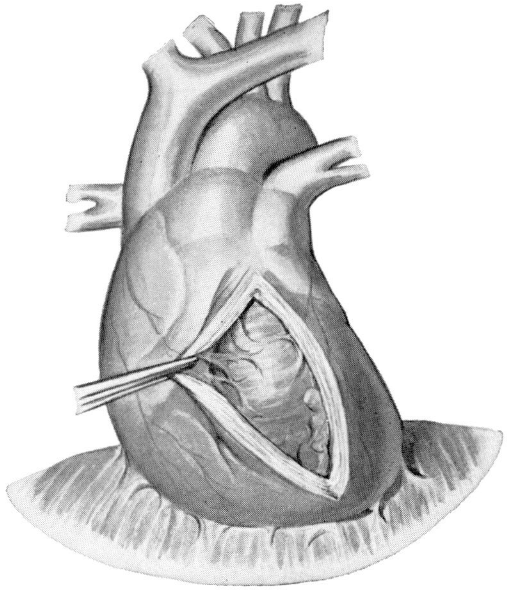

Fig. 90. Chronic constrictive pericarditis. The thick, dense fibrous tissue fills the pericardial sac and imprisons the heart.

The diagnosis of chronic constrictive pericarditis should be suspected whenever a patient presents a clinical picture suggestive but not typical of congestive heart failure. One of the most characteristic symptoms is ascites. The name "pseudocirrhosis" was given to this condition by Pick in 1896. The two conditions still may be confused when the patient is first seen, but the signs of increased venous pressure will differentiate the two conditions. The signs, the symptoms and the sequelae are due to inadequate diastolic filling of the heart, inadequate systolic ejection and a diminution in stroke volume. The venous pressure usually is elevated above 300 mm. of saline, and clinically one notices a marked distention of the neck veins as well as venous distention of the forehead, the arms and the chest. Beck's triad (p. 80) also is present. The blood pressure is low, and the pulse pressure is narrow. *Pulsus paradoxus* sometimes is present, namely, a marked decrease of pulse amplitude rather than a mild one on inspiration. Congestive cardiac failure may be excluded by the findings of dry pulmonary fields and a small, quiet heart without murmurs.

As the disease progresses, the abdomen becomes more prominent (ascites), and the liver becomes markedly enlarged. The vascular stigmata of hepatic cirrhosis (spider angioma and erythema of the palms) are not present. Although dyspnea is present, orthopnea is conspicuously absent. Probably, tachycardia is a compensatory mechanism. Peripheral edema frequently is seen. Roentgenographic examination reveals a small, quiet heart, and about one third of the patients have calcifications in the region of the pericardium. Cardiac catheterization (p. 73) rarely is necessary to make the diagnosis. Liver function tests may be somewhat affected by constrictive pericarditis but not to the extent that would be consistent with the size of the liver if this condition were due to cirrhosis. Pericardiectomy (removal of the constricting scar of pericardium) frequently produces dramatic surgical cures.

DISEASES OF THE ESOPHAGUS

It is incumbent on every physician to be "esophagus-minded." The esophagus is not a mysterious organ and has not received the attention that it warrants. The more common conditions to which this organ is heir include congenital defects, diverticula, achalasia, hiatus hernia, varices, inflammatory diseases, spontaneous rupture, strictures and tumors.

Congenital Defects

Although numerous congenital defects occur, the most common combination is that of esophageal atresia with tracheo-esophageal fistula. The most common type of this defect is depicted in Figure 91. These anomalies occur with the same frequency as harelip and cleft palate, which is approximately 1 in every 2,500 births.

The clinical manifestations are usually so distinct and uniform that the diganosis should or can be made within the first few hours after birth. The importance of early diagnosis cannot be overemphasized, since these children die early from aspiration pneumonia. The condition should be suspected if the child is "born with a cold," because it would be most unusual for a newborn to present such signs. If the child has spells of *C*hoking, *C*oughing and *C*yanosis following feedings, a diagnosis of tracheo-esophag-

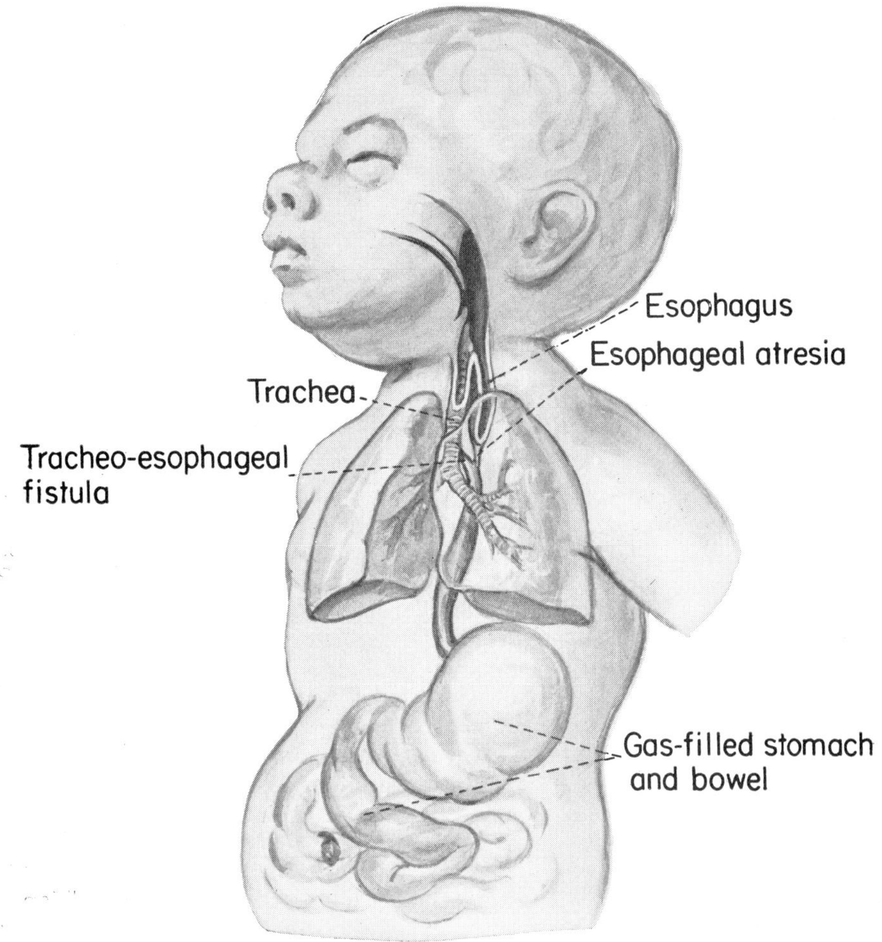

Fig. 91. Tracheo-esophageal fistula with esophageal atresia. This is the most common type and combination of congenital defect of the esophagus.

eal fistula and esophageal atresia can be made with considerable certainty. The diagnosis is verified readily by passing a No. 8 F or 10 F soft rubber catheter into the esophagus; if an obstruction is encountered, the diagnosis of atresia is practically confirmed (Fig. 92). Lipiodol (never barium) injected through this catheter can be seen on the roentgenogram as it is arrested in the blind end of the proximal esophageal segment. If a tracheo-esophageal fistula also is present, air is noted in the stomach and the intestine. This air is not swallowed but inhaled. If no air is demonstrated in the gastrointestinal tract, then esophageal atresia without tracheo-esophageal fistula is diagnosed. When the diagnosis is made, immediate preparation for surgery is initiated; many of these children can be saved. It should be emphasized that every "blue baby" is not a congenital heart lesion.

Diverticula

Sites. Diverticula of the esophagus usually occur at 3 sites: at the pharyngo-esophageal junction, on a level with the bifurcation of the trachea and above the diaphragm (epiphrenic) (Fig. 93).

The symptoms of diverticula, regardless of their locations, are similar. If the diverticulum can empty itself, inflammatory changes

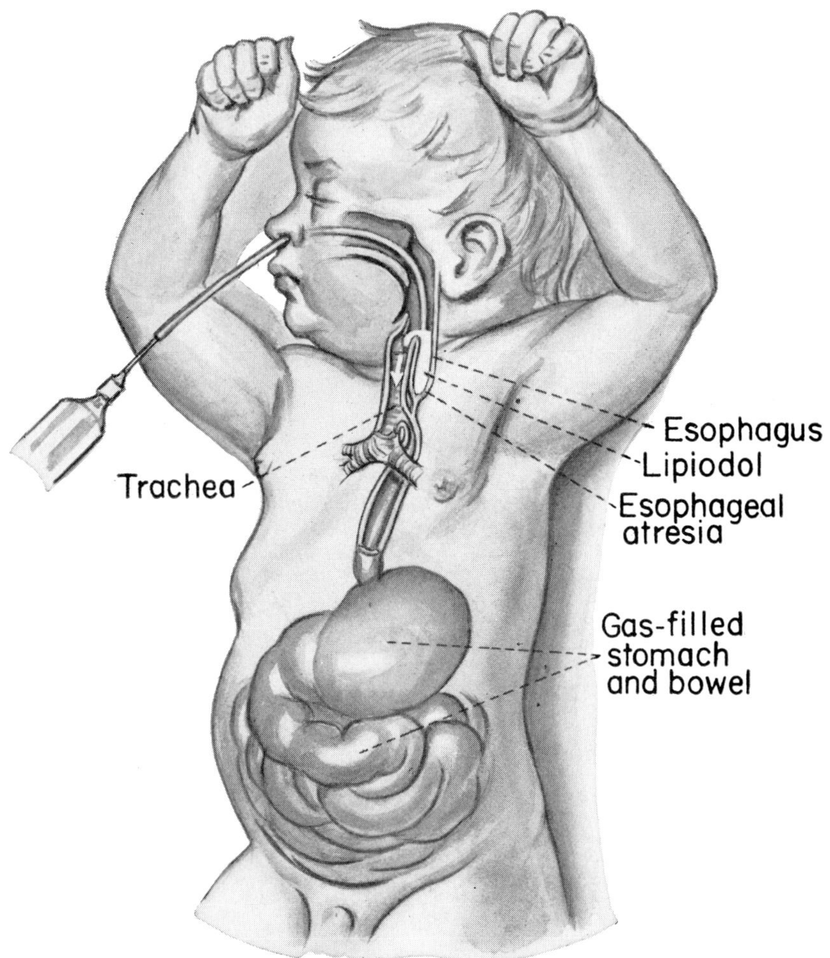

Fig. 92. Esophageal atresia with tracheo-esophageal fistula. The diagnosis is made by the radiologist, who injects a dye (never barium) into the esophagus. The dye is arrested at the point of the atresia. A gas-filled stomach and small bowel also are seen on the roentgenogram as a result of "inspired" air.

do not take place. If stasis develops, inflammation and the associated sequelae appear. One of the earliest symptoms is difficulty in swallowing or spells of coughing. The expulsion of thick mucus or continual clearing of the throat and salivation are particularly significant in the early stage. Dysphagia is a later symptom and is caused by pressure of the diverticulum on the esophagus. These patients first have difficulty in swallowing fluids, whereas solid foods pass with comparative ease. This is in contrast with the patients suffering from tumors, who first notice difficulty in swallowing solids. Retrosternal pain and a sense of pressure in the neck frequently are present and aggravated by eating. Food can be forced back into the mouth by direct pressure on the affected side of the neck. This regurgitated material usually contains food taken at an earlier meal. These pouches also may be emptied by postural methods. If stasis is present, infection, ulceration, hemorrhage perforation and mediastinitis may occur. Toxic absorption appears in the late cases and is accompanied by wasting. Unusual manifestations are pressure on vessels of the neck, pressure on local nerves, alteration in voice, and dyspnea. Aspiration of retained material has resulted in pulmonary complications and even death from aspiration pneumonia. The physical examination is noncontributory unless the pouch is of immense size. The diagnosis is made with certainty by means of roentgenography and esophagoscopy. Small diverticula frequently occur in the middle of the esophagus and are discovered in the course of routine roentgenographic examinations (Fig. 94). They do not require treatment as long as they empty satisfactorily and do not produce pressure.

Cardiospasm (Achalasia)

Numerous synonyms have been applied to this condition. It is characterized by dilatation, hypertrophy and tortuosity of the esophagus, and a nonorganic obstruction which involves the lower 3 to 6 cm. of the esophagus. The etiology is unknown. This condition accounts for 20 per cent of all cases of dysphagia and is twice as common in females as in males. Although more commonly seen in the 3rd and the 4th decades, no ages are exempt.

Symptoms. The cardinal symptoms are dysphagia, retrosternal pain and regurgitation. The pain usually is epigastric and may be referred to the xiphoid, the precordium, the neck, the lower jaw, behind the ears, or between the scapulae (Fig. 95). Because of these pain patterns, the cardiospasm may be overlooked and mistaken for coronary disease, gastrointestinal conditions or gallbladder infections. The pain may be mild or so severe that it requires repeated doses of morphine; addiction is not an infrequent sequela. Nitrites usually provide relief; this is another reason why the condition has been confused with coronary disease and angina

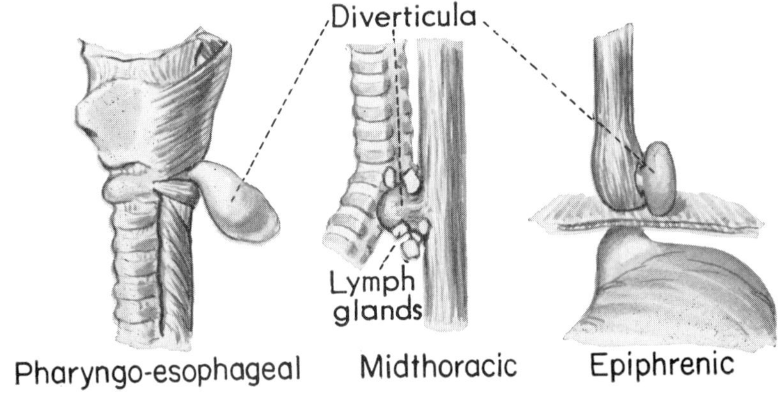

Fig. 93. The 3 types of esophageal diverticula. Their anatomic relation to the pharyngo-esophageal junction, the bifurcation of the trachea and the diaphragm are shown.

pectoris. The dysphagia differs sharply from the typical progressive dysphagia of organic stenosis, since in cardiospasm liquids are more difficult to swallow in the early phase than solids. Erroneously, the condition has been called globus hystericus, because patients complain of a discomfort or "ball" in the throat. Characteristic is the fact that solid foods usually must be washed down with large amounts of liquids. Because of the difficulty in swallowing and bouts of choking, the patient is embarrassed to eat in public or even with relatives and begins to lead a cloistered life. The weight may be maintained if he partakes of nourishing liquids and semisolids. The fact that dysphagia is present with little or no loss of weight speaks against an organic stenosis. Nocturnal regurgitation is particularly dangerous, since it can produce aspiration pneumonitis, bronchiectasis and lung abscess. The physical examination is noncontributory. The roentgenogram reveals the typical defect (Fig. 96). Esophagoscopy is indicated particularly to rule out carcinoma. Ninety per cent of these patients respond to medical treatment; the remaining 10 per cent can be cured by a simple surgical procedure which entails the severing of the muscle fibers at the esophagogastric junction.

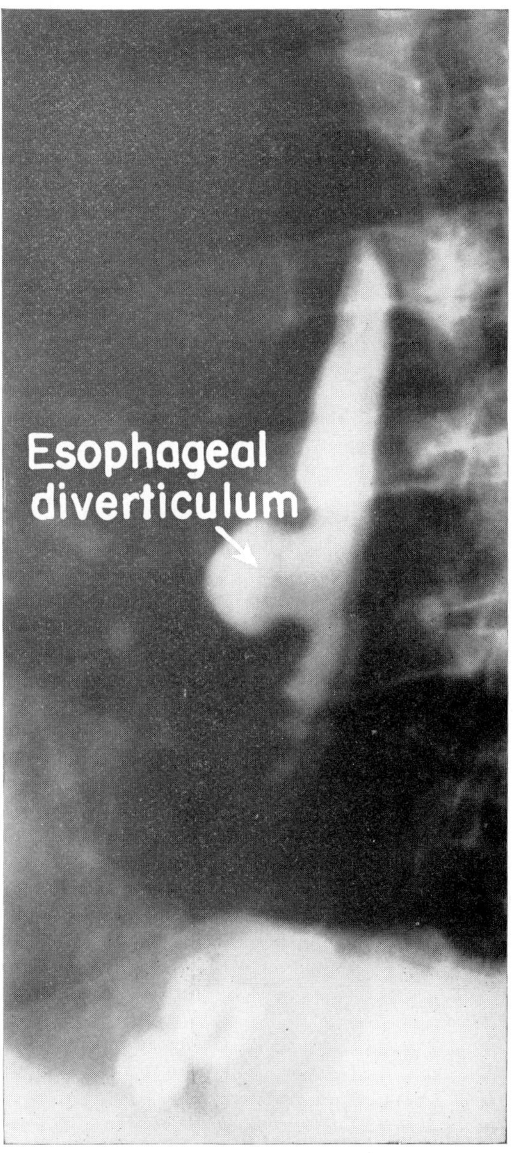

Fig. 94. Asymptomatic traction diverticulum of the middle of the esophagus discovered in the course of a routine roentgenologic examination.

Esophageal Hiatus Hernia

This is a type of diaphragmatic hernia which is present more frequently than is suspected (Fig. 97). The condition is properly referred to as the "great masquerader" of the upper abdomen, since it is readily confused with and must be differentiated from gallbladder disease, peptic ulcer, coronary disease and so-called idiopathic secondary anemia. The chief symptoms are epigastric distress, gaseous eructations, vomiting, anemia, hemorrhage, dyspnea, weakness and cardiac manifestations. The *anemia* calls for special comment. That part of the stomach which is herniated above the diaphragm contains dilated gastric veins that bleed either slowly or massively. The reason for the dilated veins is the constriction brought about by the surrounding and contracting diaphragm. It should be a general rule that any patient with an unexplained secondary anemia should have a careful roentgenographic evaluation; this must be done in the Trendelenburg position, since this reveals an otherwise reduced hiatus hernia (Fig. 98). The treatment is surgical and is quite satisfactory. Other types of diaphragmatic herniae will be discussed subsequently (p. 90).

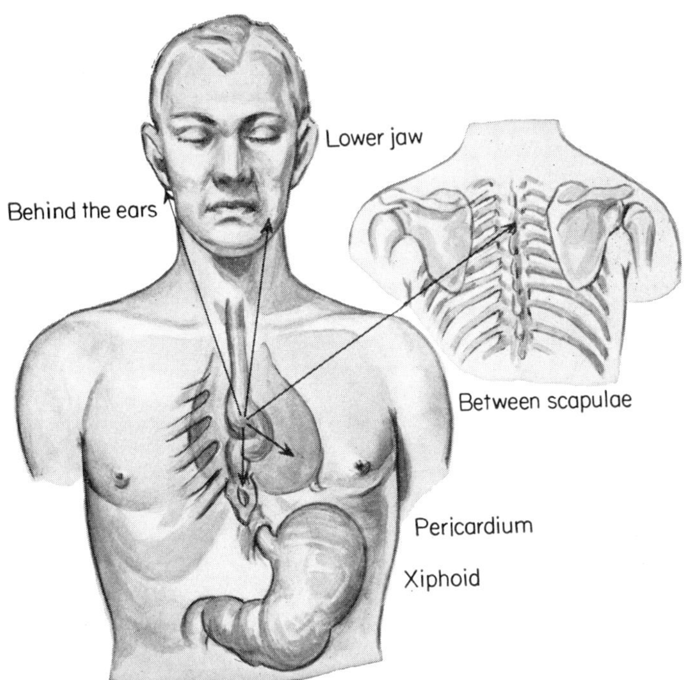

FIG. 95. Esophageal pain may be referred to the xiphoid, the pericardium, the neck, the lower jaw, behind the ears or between the scapulae.

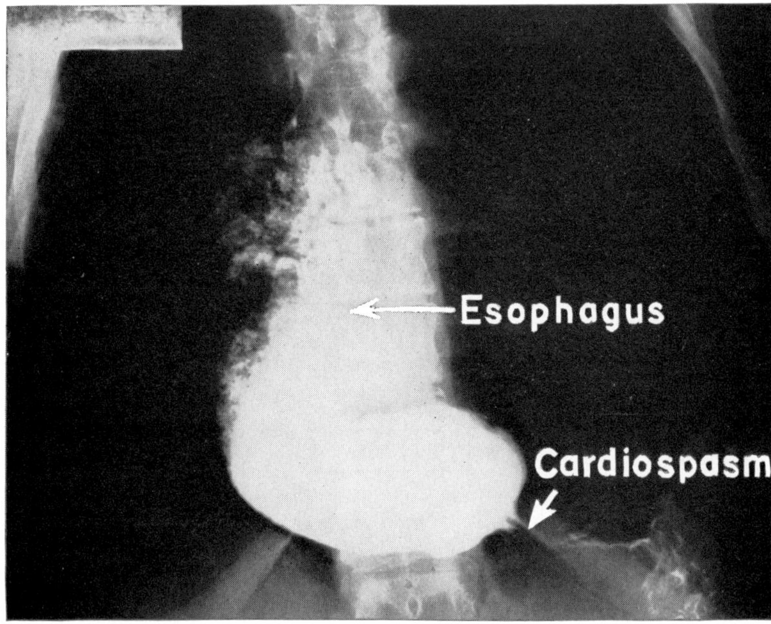

FIG. 96. Roentgenogram revealing a typical cardiospasm (achalasia). The nonorganic obstructed area is located at the distal end of the esophagus, and proximal to this is the dilated and tortuous esophagus.

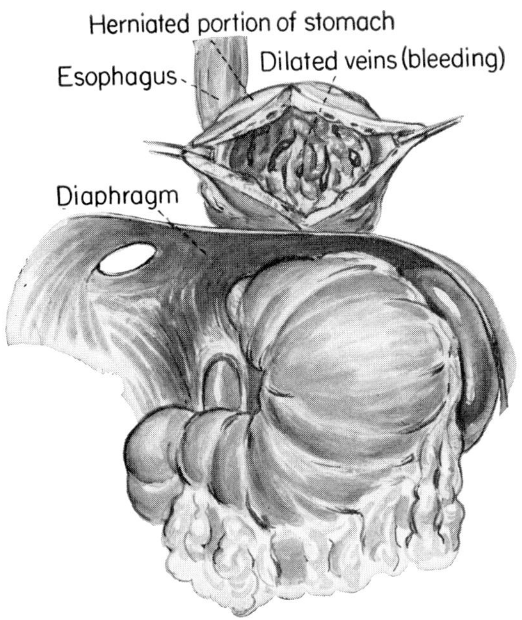

FIG. 97. Esophageal hiatus hernia. The veins in the intrathoracic part of the stomach dilate and may cause hemorrhage (acute or chronic).

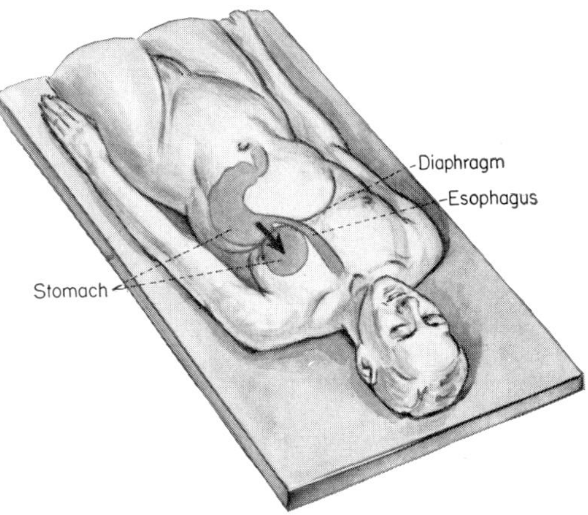

FIG. 98. Trendelenburg position will aid in the roentgenographic detection of a hiatus hernia. In the erect position the hernia may be reduced and overlooked.

ESOPHAGEAL VARICES

Esophageal varices usually result from a portal hypertension (p. 196). Although these veins develop silently and insidiously, they may rupture and produce an uncontrollable and fatal hemorrhage. Banti first called attention to this condition in 1883; it has been referred to as "Banti's disease." Portal hypertension results from intrinsic liver disease or extrinsic portal disease. These 2 types of portal hypertension can be differentiated by the various liver function tests (p. 191). If the liver is at fault, the tests are positive. Esophageal varices are found almost always at the lower end of the esophagus (Fig. 99); those that are located at the upper end are usually congenital. The most common causes are cirrhosis of the liver or thrombosis of the portal vein. There are few, if any, early symptoms of esophageal varices; most patients seek medical advice following a sudden massive hematemesis. Physical examination may reveal an enlarged spleen (congestive splenomegaly). I have been impressed by the so-called cirrhotic habitus (Fig. 189). This is characterized by a male who has little or no hair on his chest. The roentgenogram reveals the varices assuming a so-called "pearl necklace" appearance (Fig. 100). Esophagoscopy, if done, must be performed with great caution; it is rarely indicated in this condition. Blood examination may reveal a secondary anemia, leukopenia and thrombocytopenia.

TUMORS

Benign tumors are not rare; they occur more frequently in males (10 to 1). A wide variety have been encountered, the most frequent of which are myomas, fibromas, lipomas and polyps. Some benign tumors of the esophagus are extramucosal and are covered by normal epithelium. These usually arise from the muscle wall.

SYMPTOMS. The early symptoms are so slight that the patient rarely seeks relief. Mild retrosternal pain or an odd sensation in the "throat" may be so slight that it is overlooked. Erroneously, such cases may be called globus hystericus. As the tumor grows, dysphagia appears and becomes progressively worse. If the tumor is pedunculated—and they often are—they may be regurgitated into the mouth and reswallowed (a terrifying experience). In some instances pedunculated tumors have been aspirated and cause laryngeal obstruction. Roentgenographic and esophagoscopic examinations confirm the diagnosis. The results with surgical treatment are most gratifying.

Malignant Tumors. Carcinoma of the esophagus unfortunately is a common disease. The mucosa of the esophagus is squamous in type; hence, the lesion is of the squamous (epidermoid) variety. Adenocarcinoma is extremely rare and when found usually represents an extension upward from a gastric carcinoma. Secondary involvement of the esophagus is uncommon but must be kept in mind in any case of dysphagia; it can be embarrassing to resect such a lesion under the impression that it is the primary tumor. Secondary involvement arising from the hypopharynx, bronchus, larynx, stomach, breast, testis, pancreas, mediastinum and prostate have been reported. The history and the symptoms usually are stereotyped, with dysphagia being the first complaint (Fig. 101). If a history is taken carefully, frequently it reveals either increased salivation and/or definite bouts of choking. The choking usually occurs when the patient attempts to swallow semisolids. Retrosternal pain, loss of weight, signs of dehydration and toxic manifestations appear as the obstruction progresses.

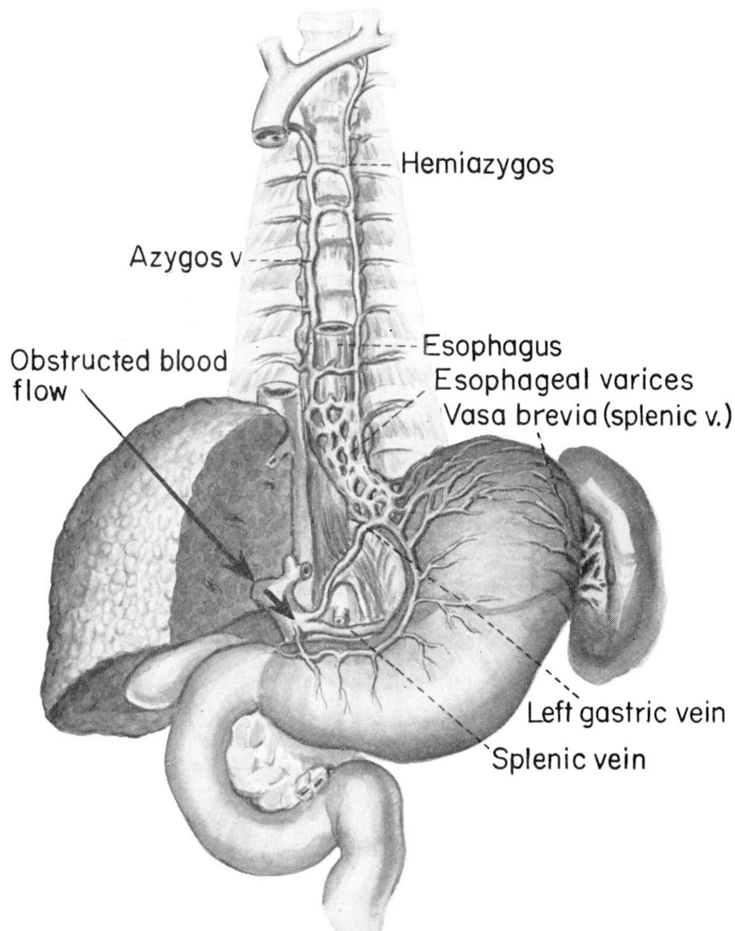

Fig. 99. Esophageal varices. The physiopathology associated with portal hypertension suggests a backflow of blood which cannot pass through the cirrhotic liver. It should be noted that the veins over the upper aspect of the stomach also are dilated.

The differential diagnosis includes a long list of conditions, the most important of which are diverticula, stricture, cardiospasm, esophagitis, foreign bodies, extrinsic pressure, benign tumors, perforating carcinoma from a bronchus, thyroid enlargements, retropharyngeal abscess, granulomatous diseases, Plummer-Vinson syndrome, mediastinal lymphadenopathy, esophageal cysts and polyps. The roentgenographic examination is a valuable aid; however, a definite diagnosis is made by esophagoscopy and biopsy. With modern surgical methods palliation and occasional "cures" can be expected.

Spontaneous Rupture of the Esophagus

This condition, which formerly was always fatal, has lost some of its horror since an accurate diagnosis, chemotherapy and modern surgical methods can save many of these patients. This is particularly true if the diagnosis is made early. The esophagus is closely related to the mediastinal pleura immediately above the diaphragm. This portion of the esophagus is weakest, and it is here that the increased pressure caused by vomiting or coughing produces the perforation. The mediastinal pleura is usually torn. The diagnosis should be suspected when the history reveals a sudden onset of severe pain in the chest or the abdomen which usually *follows* vomiting, coughing or trauma. (In perforated peptic ulcers the pain *precedes* the vomiting.) Shock develops rapidly. Finding crepitation and emphysema in the supraclavicular regions is particularly suggestive. The roentgenogram reveals a hydropneumothorax if the mediastinal pleura is torn. The abdominal rigidity which is often present unfortunately calls attention to the abdomen rather than the chest. If necessary, it is safe to allow a swallow of a nonirritant opaque material to determine the presence of the rupture.

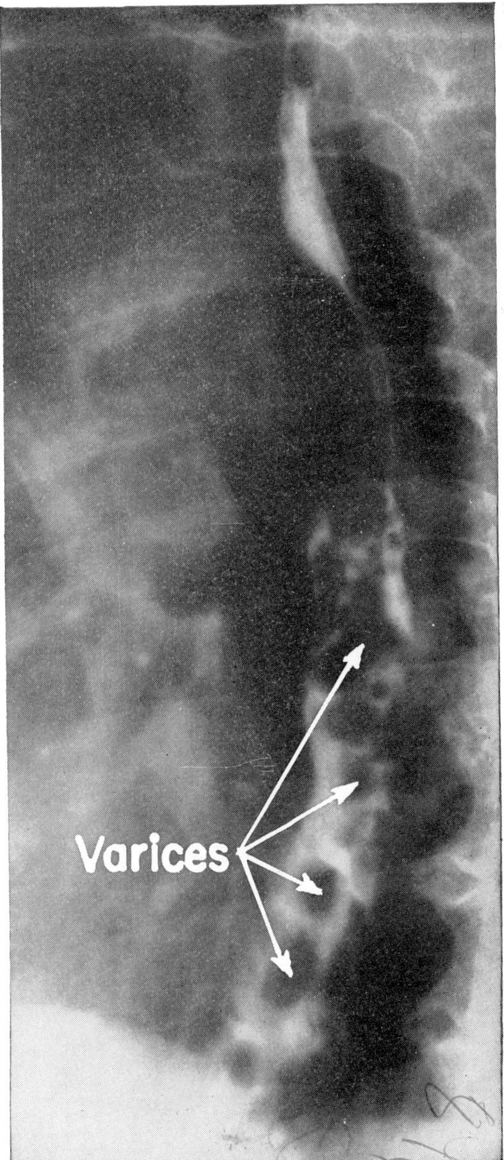

Fig. 100. Roentgenogram of esophageal varices revealing the so-called "pearl necklace" appearance.

Esophagitis and Peptic Ulcer

Esophagitis is probably the most frequent disease of the esophagus (Fig. 102). It is almost always a complication and not a primary disease. Among the etiologic factors are included reflux of gastric secretion, hiatus hernia, repeated vomiting, prolonged use of the nasogastric tube, and brain tumors. The end-result of prolonged esophagitis is stricture formation with shortening. Dyspepsia is present in about 75 per cent of these patients, and the vast majority of them complain of "heartburn." Dysphagia appears later. Medical treatment, diet and bougienage usually produce excellent relief.

Surgery is indicated for the complications of esophagitis.

Foreign Bodies

Foreign bodies usually are arrested at the 3 physiologic constrictions: immediately below the cricopharyngeus muscle, in the regions of the arch of the aorta, or immediately above the diaphragm. Sharp bodies may perforate and produce periesophagitis, mediastinitis and mediastinal abscesses. The symptoms are choking, coughing, gagging and dysphagia. The patient identifies a painful point which corresponds to the site where the foreign body has perforated or lodged. Radiopaque substances are demonstrable on the roentgenogram; however, should these be nonopaque, esophagoscopy is the only definite method of determining their presence and location.

DIAPHRAGM

Embryology

The embryology of the diaphragm is complicated. It can be simplified somewhat if one recalls the 4 sources from which it is derived (Fig. 103): (1) The septum transversum becomes the ventral portion; (2) the pleuroperitoneum membrane provides the dorsal portion; (3) parts of the body wall give rise to the lateral diaphragmatic portions; and (4) the dorsal mesentery becomes the dorsal median portion.

Hernias

All but traumatic diaphragmatic hernias have their inception in a developmental defect; hence, it is helpful to classify them in the following way:

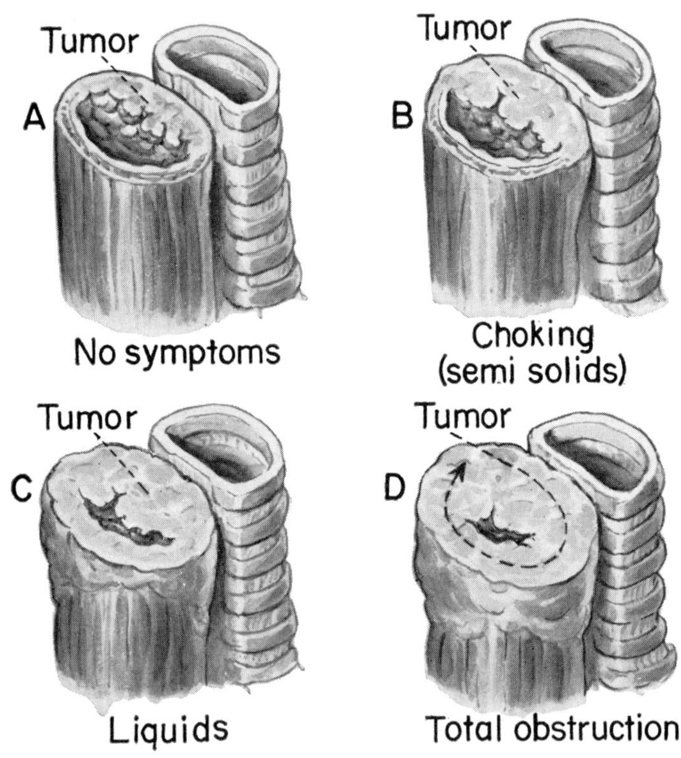

Fig. 101. Carcinoma of the esophagus. The size of the lesion in relation to the symptoms is shown.

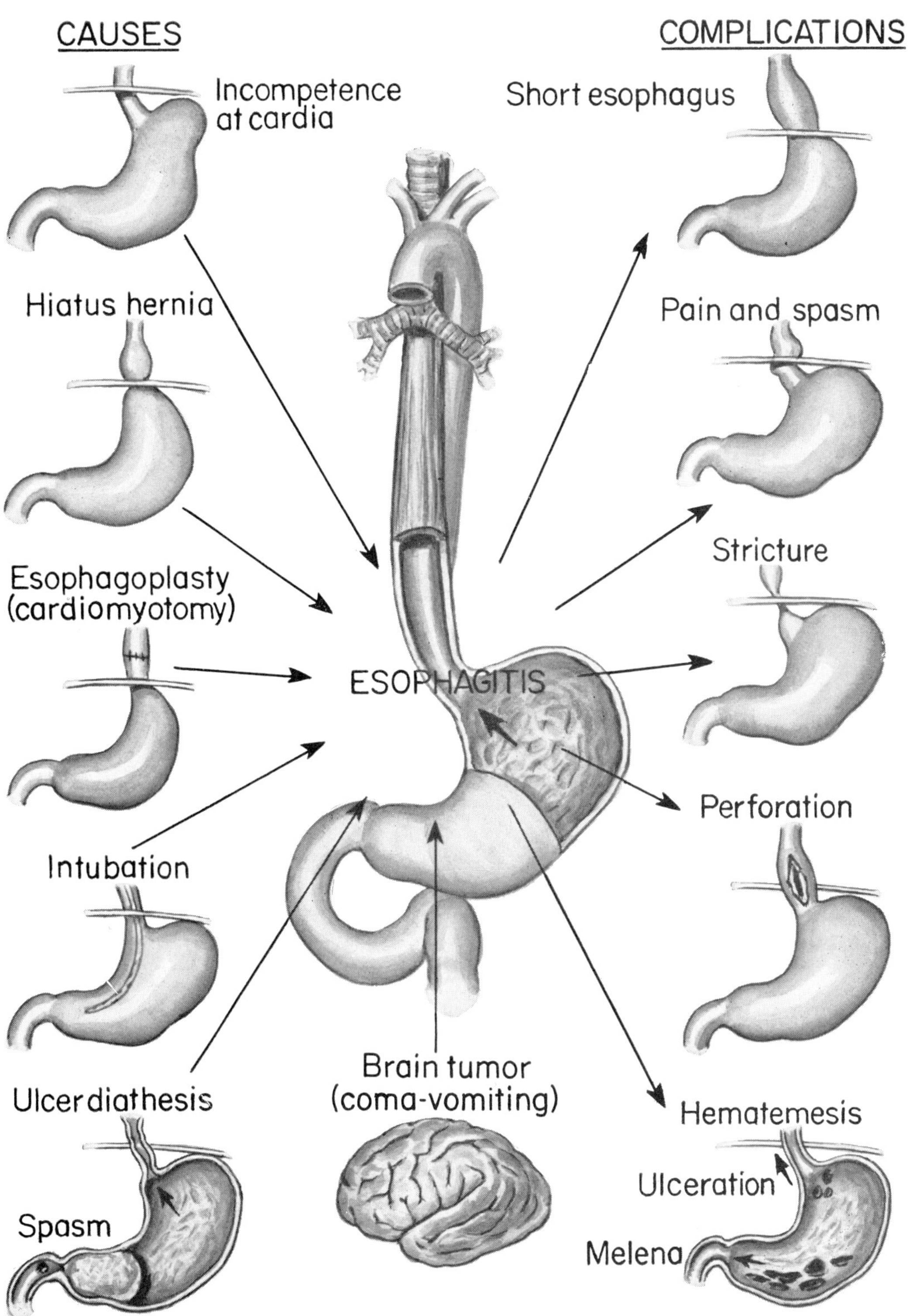

FIG. 102. Esophagitis and gastroesophageal reflux. Esophagogastric reflux, initiated by the conditions shown in the left-hand column, results in esophagitis (*center*), which may proceed to the complication depicted in the right-hand column. (After Benedict and Nardi)

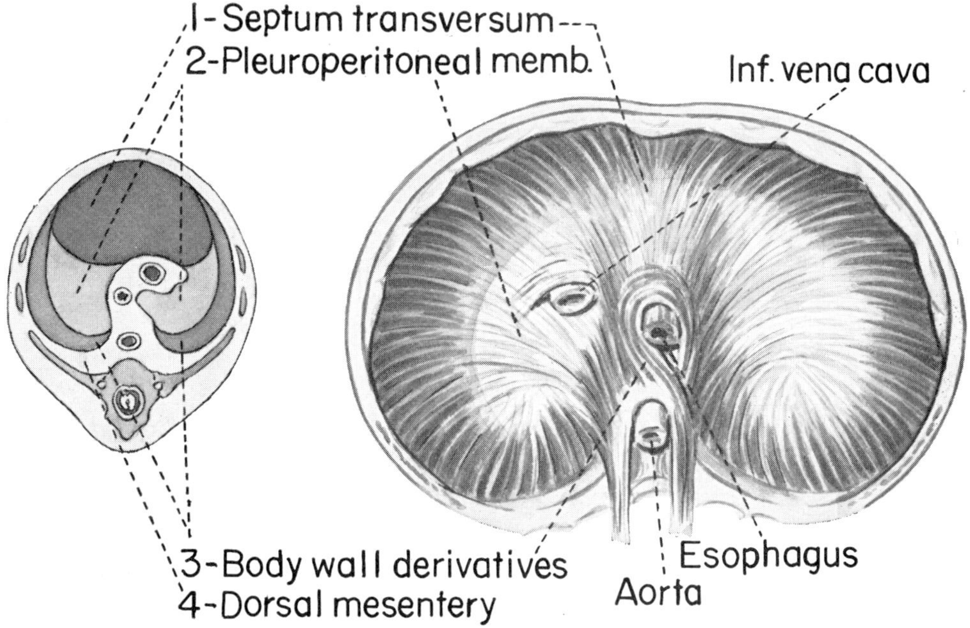

FIG. 103. Embryology of the diaphragm. The 4 embryologic sources from which the diaphragm is developed and the fully developed diaphragm are shown.

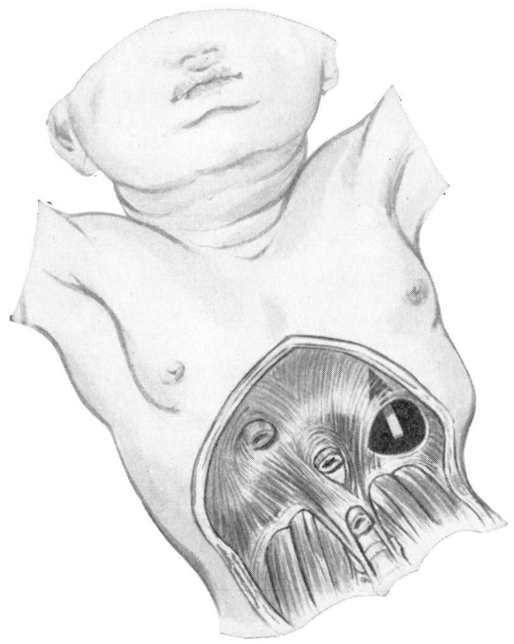

FIG. 104. Pleuroperitoneal foramen of Bochdalek. Arrow shows path of the hernia.

1. Congenital segmental absence of a portion of the diaphragm
2. Congenital weakness or imperfect fusion of diaphragmatic segments
3. Traumatic hernias

Congenital Segmental Absence of the Diaphragm. This is best illustrated as a hernia through the pleuroperitoneal foramen of Bochdalek (Fig. 104). This segment may be absent partially or completely. Occasionally, the corresponding part of the septum transversum also is deficient, so that the entire hemidiaphragm is lacking. The most common variety is a defect somewhat triangular in shape with its apex pointing medially. Since the pleuroperitoneal membrane is missing, there is no hernial sac, and there is a free communication between the abdominal and the thoracic cavities. The involved hemithorax usually is completely filled with abdominal viscera, the homolateral lung is collapsed, and there is a shift of the heart and the mediastinal structures to the opposite side, with compression of the opposite lung (Fig. 105). Since this condition is not compatible with life, early diagnosis and immediate surgical intervention are imperative. This is the only way in which strangulation and cardiorespiratory embarrassment can be prevented.

Congenital Weakness or Imperfect Fusion of Diaphragmatic Segments. The second group, which includes those hernias due to imperfect fusion of embryologic seg-

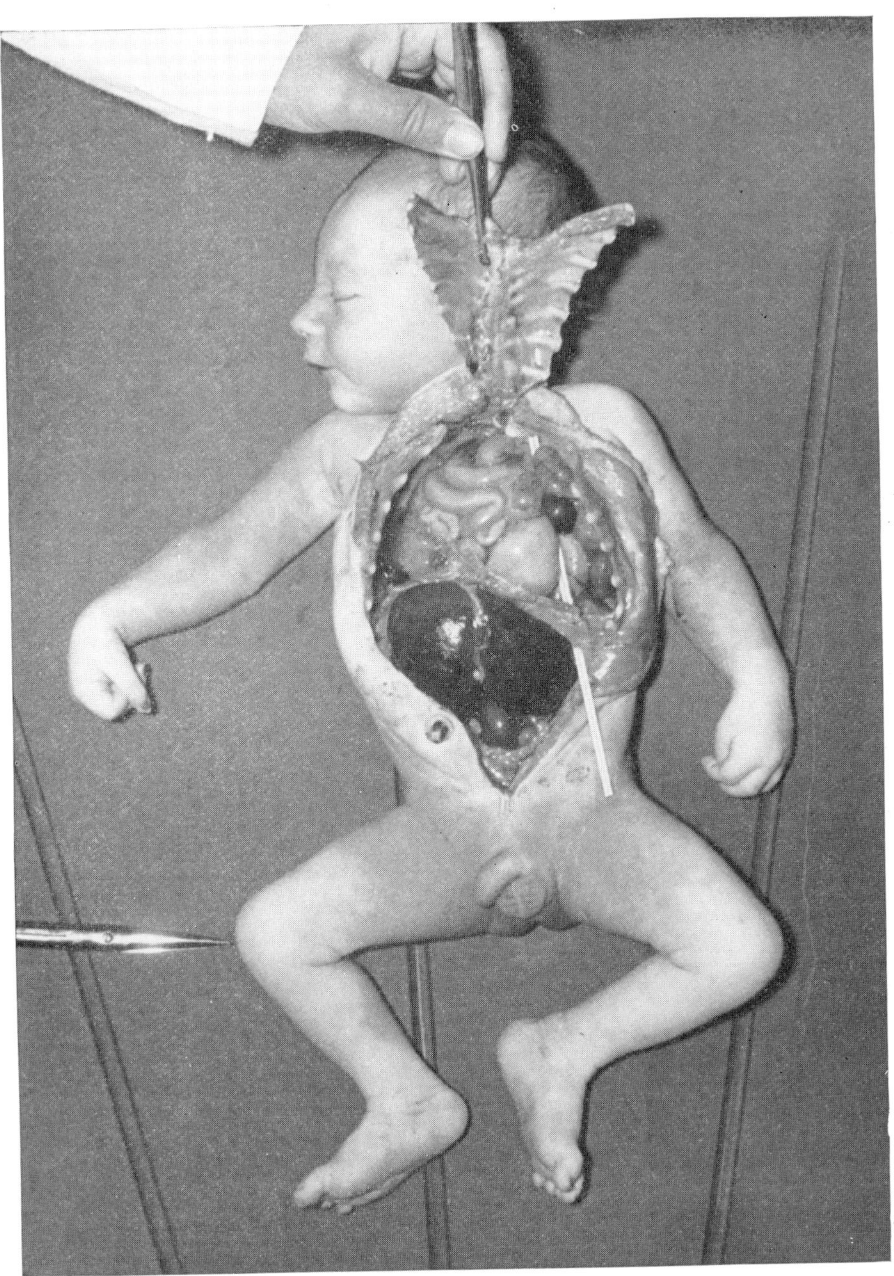

FIG. 105. Untreated herniation through the pleuroperitoneal hiatus. Death occurs early in these infants. (Thorek, P.: Diseases of the Esophagus, Philadelphia, Lippincott, p. 72, Fig. 65)

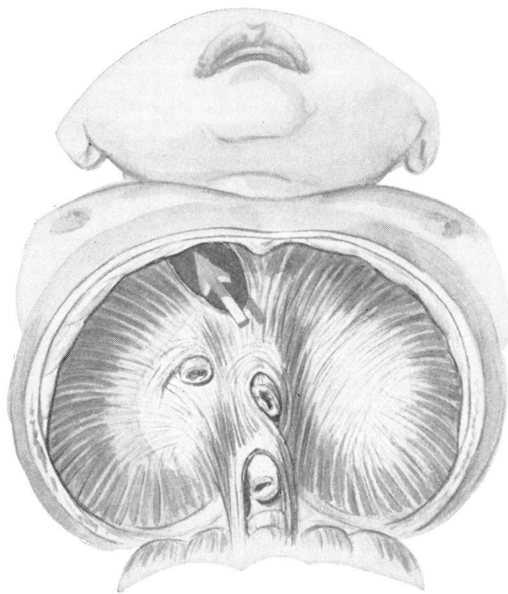

FIG. 106. Parasternal hernia (Morgagni). These may be bilateral. Arrow shows the hernial defect.

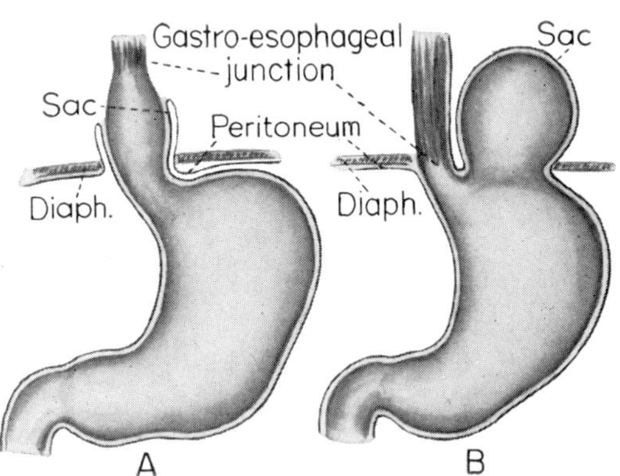

FIG. 107. Hiatus hernia. (A) A sliding hernia showing the gastroesophageal junction lying above the diaphragm and the stomach forming part of the sac. Because of the interference with the sphincteric function at this junction, acid reflux is present and accounts for the symptoms (esophagitis). (B) A para-esophageal hernia revealing the normally placed gastroesophageal junction; hence, no acid reflux symptoms—only those associated with pressure. Some believe that in this type the stomach always lies to the right of the esophagus.

ments, are best illustrated by the parasternal and esophageal hiatus hernias. Herniation through this cleft has been referred to also as a hernia of Morgagni (Fig. 106). The constant presence of a sac attests to the fact that the peritoneal membrane has divided the abdominal from the pleural cavity before the herniation has occurred. This type of hernia is quite uncommon; it may be unilateral or bilateral.

Hiatus hernias constitute the vast majority of all diaphragmatic herniations. They have been divided mainly into 2 types (Fig. 107).

SLIDING HIATUS HERNIA. In this hernia a portion of the peritoneal sac is made up of visceral peritoneum. In this type the cardio-esophageal junction precedes the stomach into the thoracic cavity and is therefore superior to the diaphragm.

PARA-ESOPHAGEAL HIATUS HERNIA. This hernia is distinguished from the sliding variety by the fact that the gastroesophageal orifice is maintained in its normal position beneath the diaphragm. In this instance the hernial sac is formed by the diaphragmatic covering of parietal peritoneum on its undersurfaces. The fundus of the stomach usually is found in the sac, and as the sac enlarges, most of the stomach may find its way into the thoracic cavity.

SYMPTOMS. Pain, dyspnea, bleeding, obstruction and bronchospasm are the symptoms of hiatus hernia. The pain is believed to be due to pinching of the peritoneal sac. Characteristically, it is located directly over the hiatus or the epigastrium. However, at times it may present the typical esophageal pattern of referred pain and appear in the upper abdominal quadrants, the scapular region, the dorsal spine, the top of the shoulders, the left side of the neck and the ear, or the inner aspect of the left arm down to the wrist. Pain is often relieved by gravitational reduction of the hernial sac when the patient is in the erect position. The "dyspeptic symptoms" are bloating, heartburn, or actual eructation of food. Bleeding is due to a diffuse hyperemia of the gastric mucosa within the hernial sac or associated esophagitis. Bronchospasm supposedly is due to a trigger point in the lower esophageal region close to the hernia. Actual asthmatic attacks have been precipitated by such hernias; these are completely relieved following hernial repair. Final diagnosis is dependent on roentgen and, at times, esophagoscopic examinations.

Traumatic Diaphragmatic Hernias. Most of these hernias involve the tendinous dome of the left diaphragm (Fig. 108). The right lobe of the liver can seal small perforated wounds; hence, fewer traumatic hernias occur on this side. This type of hernia does not have a peritoneal sac; at times adhesions prevent open communication between the abdominal and the pleural cavities. The correct diagnosis of diaphragmatic hernia is directly proportional to the index of suspicion of the examining physician. If the hernia is small, the symptoms usually are vague; but if the hernia is large, or if strangulation occurs, the symptoms become hyperacute and involve the heart, the lungs, and/or the gastrointestinal tract. The roentgenogram supplies the final evidence for diagnosis.

Eventration

In eventration the diaphragm is thin and membranous rather than muscular. It assumes an unusually high position, sometimes reaching the level of the 2nd rib. The left hemidiaphragm is involved more frequently. The symptoms, if present, are dyspnea, flatulence, indigestion and constipation. This condition is confused with diaphragmatic hernia, but in eventration the abdominal

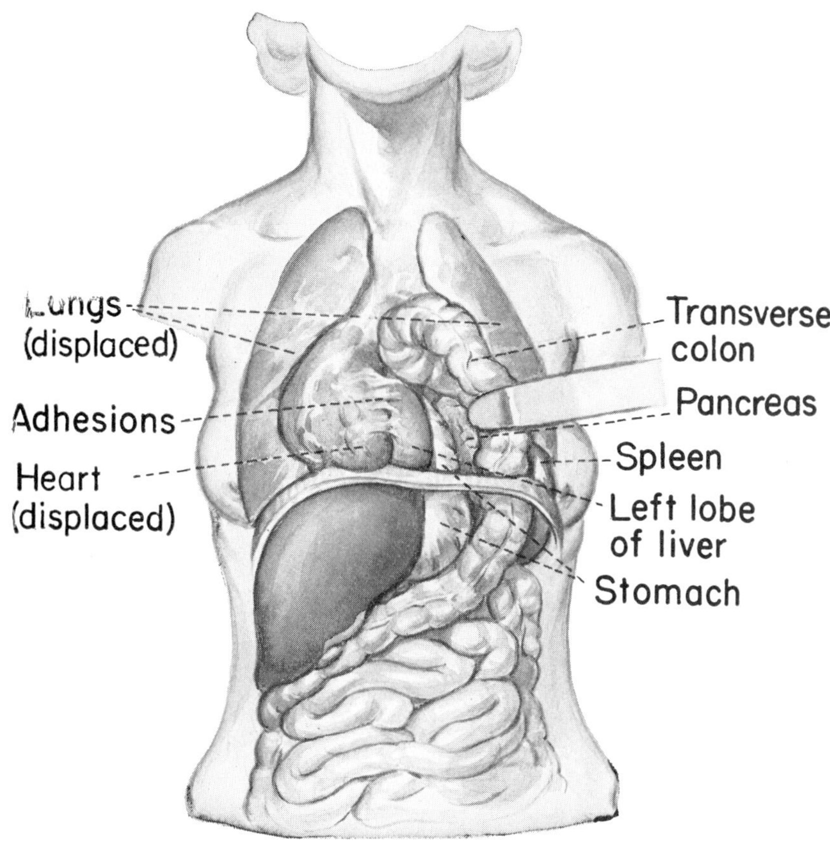

Fig. 108. Traumatic diaphragmatic hernia. The unusual feature in this case is the presence of the body and the tail of the pancreas in the thoracic cavity. The hernia had been present for 2 years, which accounted for the firm adhesions between the left lobe of the liver and the heart.

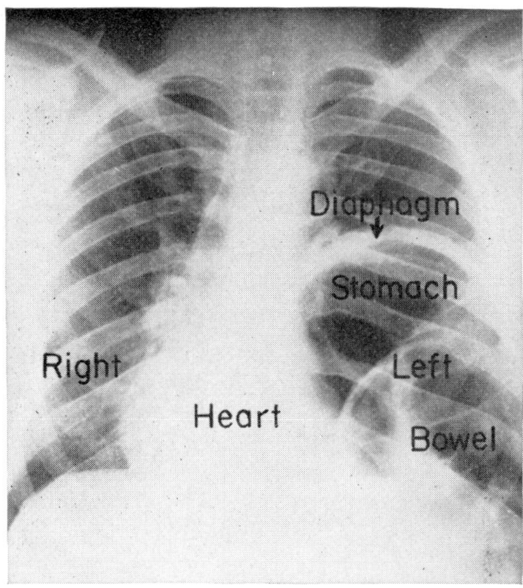

FIG. 109. A roentgenogram of an eventration of the left hemidiaphragm. The abdominal viscera are *below* the diaphragm.

viscera are *below* the diaphragm. Pneumothorax or pneumoperitoneum may be necessary if the diagnosis is obscure. This is important, because eventration rarely demands treatment (Fig. 109).

TUMORS

Primary tumors of the diaphragm are exceedingly rare. The benign tumors are frequently asymptomatic and are discovered accidentally. However, bulky tumors interfere with normal diaphragmatic function and cause dyspnea, cough, chest pain and shoulder pain. Pleural effusion may be present.

INFECTION

Infection in the subdiaphragmatic spaces may necessitate surgical drainage. The author has described 6 subphrenic spaces, each having a specific surgical approach.

FUNCTIONAL DISTURBANCES

The 2 most important functional disturbances that affect the diaphragm are hiccough and diaphragmatic flutter.

Hiccough (singultus) is paroxysmal clonic contraction of the diaphragm. It is usually mild and innocuous but may be so severe and persistent as to threaten life. It is associated with stimulation of the phrenic nerve; aneurysm, pleurisy, pericarditis and mediastinal lymphadenitis may be the source of such stimulation. Also, it can be related to perinephric or subdiaphragmatic abscess, trauma and hemoperitoneum. It may complicate such diseases as meningitis, encephalitis, cerebral hemorrhage, brain tumor and toxemias. Epidemics of singultus have been reported; probably these are viral in origin.

Diaphragmatic flutter is a rare condition that is poorly understood. It is characterized by a paroxysmal or sustained diaphragmatic contraction with a rate of 60 to 300 per minute. It usually affects both hemidiaphragms. There may be an antecedent history of encephalitis or some other nerve condition. It closely resembles coronary disease or angina pectoris, since it is associated with precordial and arm pain. The pain with diaphragmatic flutter is not aggravated by physical exertion. Physical examination reveals fibrillary or rapid tremors in the epigastrium. A characteristic to-and-fro shuffling sound, which may be confused with a pleuropericardial friction rub, is heard over the chest. However, this sound is not synchronous with the cardiac cycle but with the diaphragmatic contractions. There may be an associated hyperventilation and respiratory alkalosis.

5

The Breast

EMBRYOLOGY

The milk lines extend from the axillary regions to the pubis and the inner aspects of the thighs (Fig. 110). They represent an atavistic throwback. Supernumerary nipples and areolae occur frequently on this line. Occasionally ectopic nipples and breast tissue occur in such areas as the face and the gluteal regions.

The so-called axillary tail of Spence is a prolongation of breast tissue which is situated at the upper end of the milk line and extends into the axilla. Frequently it is mistaken for a lymph gland when it is enlarged and painful (Fig. 111). This differentiation can be made since the axillary breast tissue enlarges and becomes painful with each menstrual period.

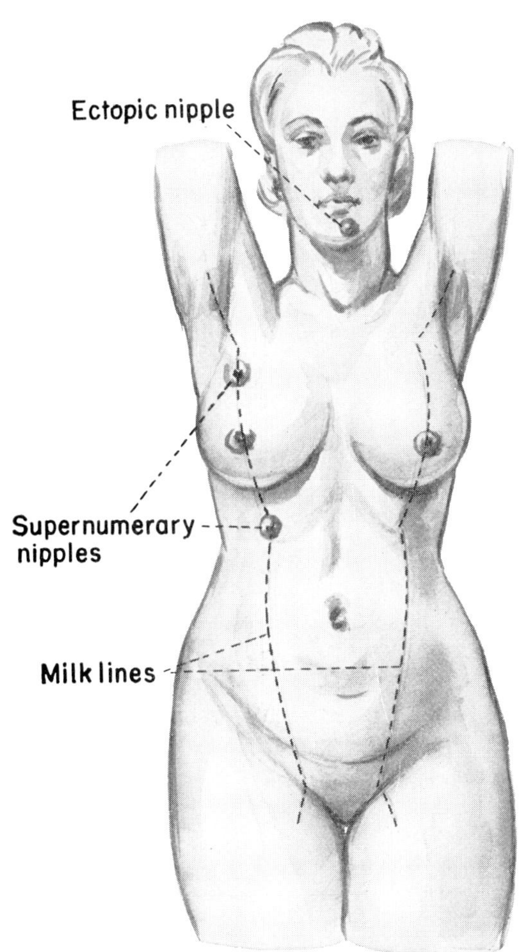

FIG. 110. The milk lines. These extend from the axillae to the hips. The ectopic nipple on the chin should be noted.

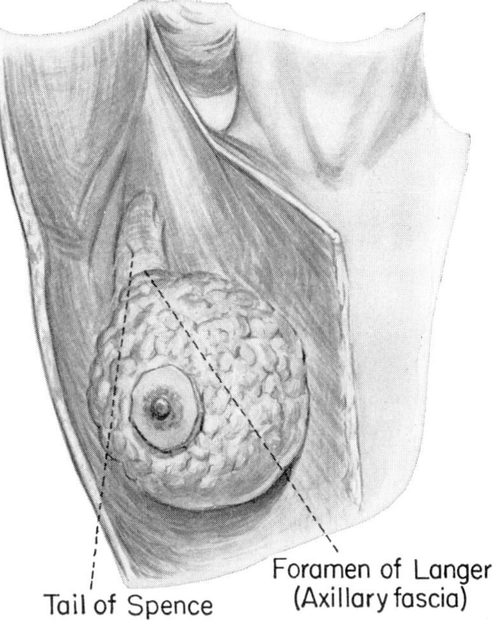

FIG. 111. The axillary tail of Spence. A prolongation of breast tissue which extends through the axillary fascia (foramen of Langer). Frequently it is mistaken for an axillary lymph gland.

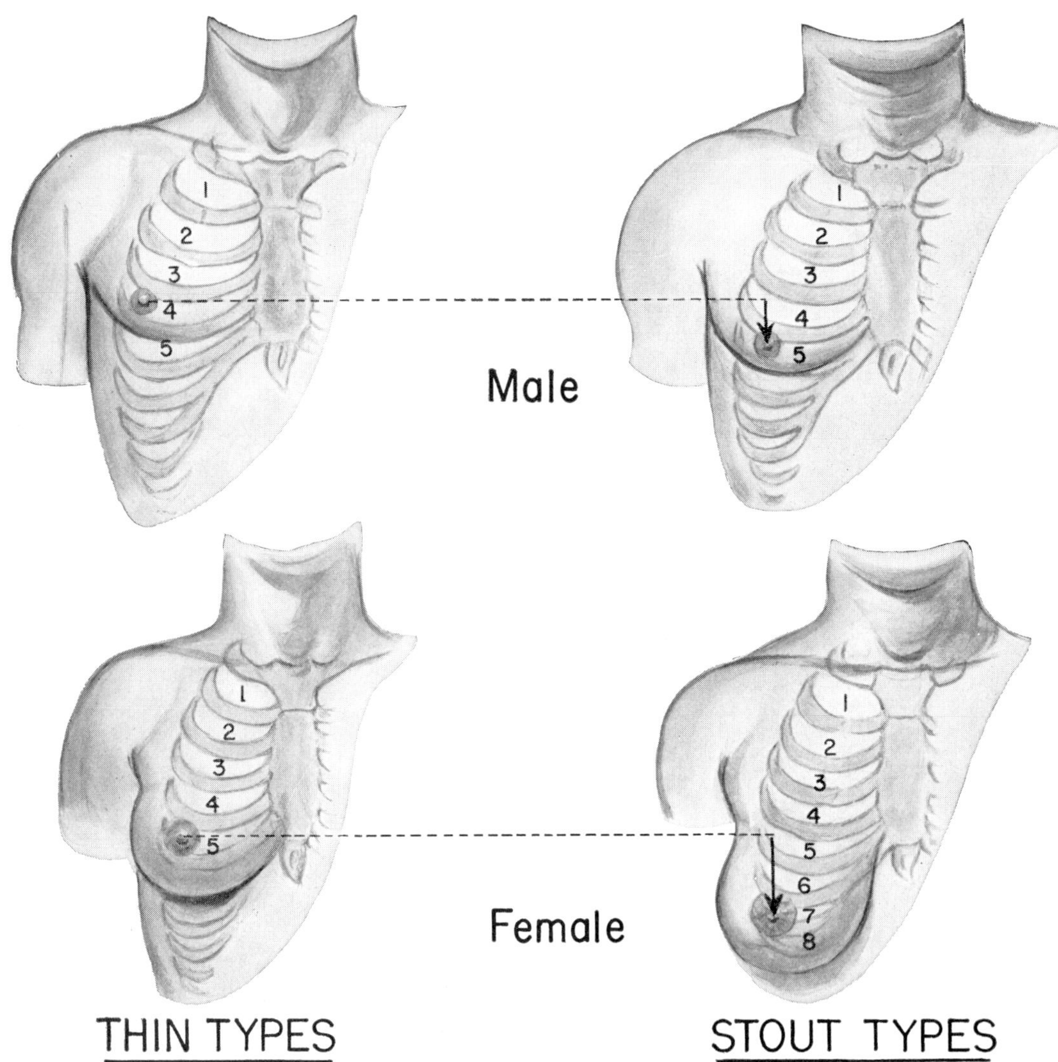

Fig. 112. Normal anatomic positions of the nipples in thin and stout individuals.

EXAMINATION

In the examination of the breast 2 methods, inspection and palpation, are particularly helpful.

Inspection

The physician should record the size and the position of the breasts and the nipples. Also, he should note any changes in contour, symmetry and redness. The usual *anatomic position* of the nipple is between the 4th and the 5th intercostal spaces and approximately in the midclavicular line; this applies to both young males and young thin females (Fig. 112). In these types, the nipple is an accurate anatomic landmark. With an increase of fat—and at times age—the nipple sags, and its position becomes extremely variable. In the pendulous breast (Fig. 124), the glandular tissue is at the lowest portion of the nipple, and the remainder of tissue consists of fat and fibrous tissue.

Palpation

The breasts should be palpated in both the sitting and the supine positions. In the supine position, the shoulder is elevated

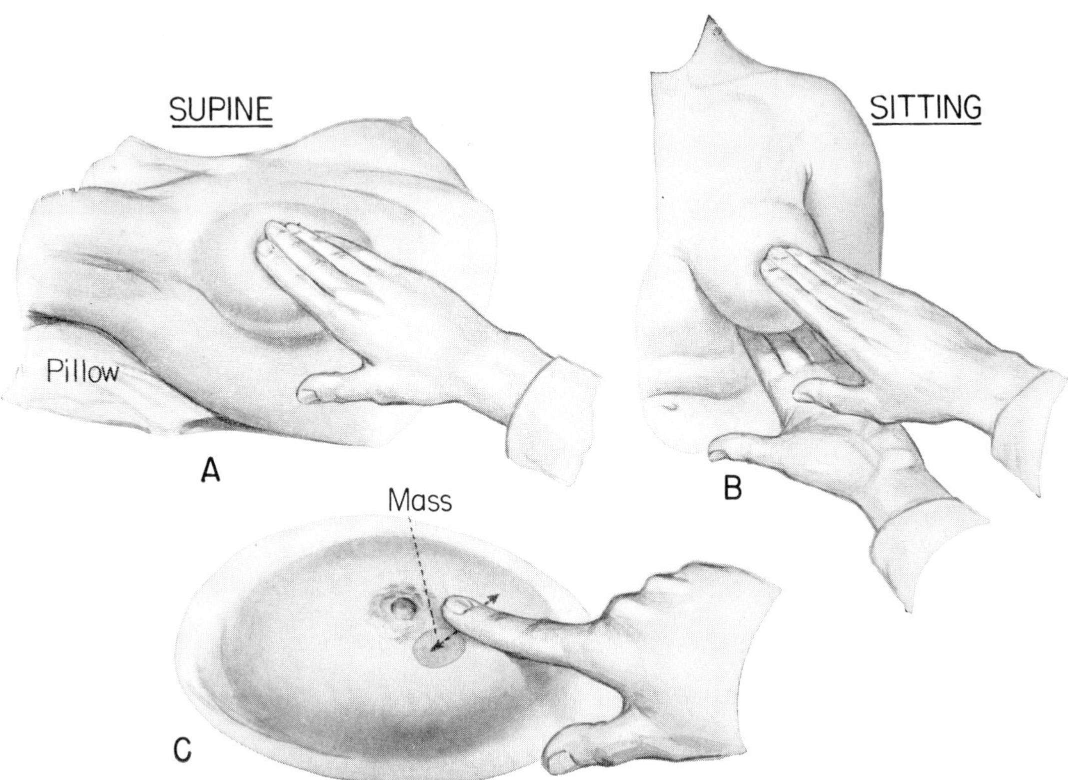

FIG. 113. Methods employed in examining the breast.

slightly by a pillow, and the breast is examined *gently* with the flat of the fingers of 1 hand (Fig. 113). It might be helpful while examining the medial portion of the breast to raise the patient's arm above the head, but while examining the lateral portion the arms should rest at the side. In the sitting position, the breast is palpated between the fingers of both hands (Fig. 113). This method is particularly helpful in detecting a lesion in the subareolar and nipple regions. In this central area the lactiferous ducts converge upon the nipple. A tumor situated in the soft subareolar tissue may be impalpable in the supine position; but when it is examined with the dependent breast between the examiner's fingers, it becomes readily palpable. Also of value in palpation is the method whereby 1 finger is used to determine fixation and movability of a mass (Fig. 113). Pressure against the mass is increased gently, and if the lesion is movable or encapsulated, it will slip away suddenly and appear to be lost; with release of the 1-finger pressure it reappears.

The *axillary* and the *supraclavicular regions* must be examined individually (Fig. 114). The patient should be sitting. In examining the axilla it is essential that the axillary fascia be relaxed. To achieve this the examiner supports the patient's arm on one of his own; this will permit palpation along the upper lateral chest wall and well into the apex of the axilla in a search for axillary and apical glands. The more gently this palpation is carried out, the more rewarding will be the information obtained. In obese patients, axillary palpation is particularly unreliable. The supraclavicular regions are conveniently palpated if the examiner stands behind the patient. The approximate number of glands, the consistency and the movability should be noted. One must remember that palpation cannot determine whether an enlarged lymph gland is inflammatory or metastatic.

RETRACTION PHENOMENA

Retraction phenomena, when present, may be demonstrated easily; they are par-

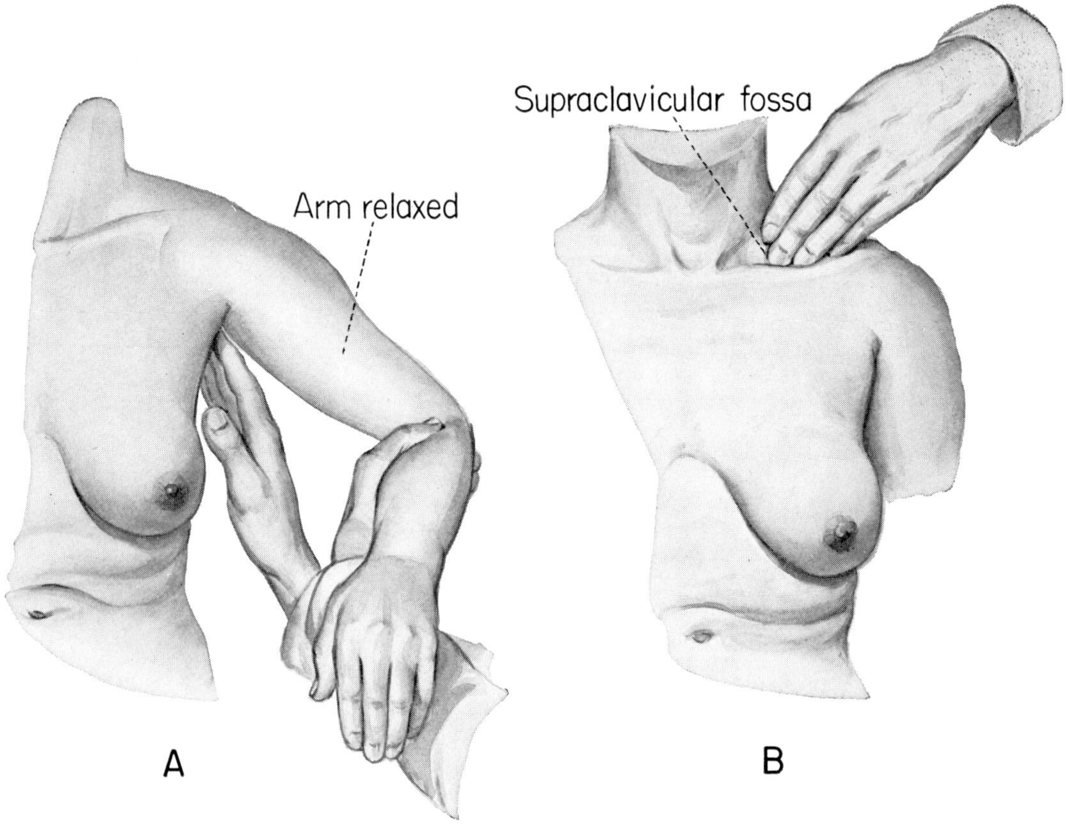

Supraclavicular fossa

Arm relaxed

A

B

FIG. 114. Examination of the axilla and the supraclavicular fossa. (A) The patient's arm is lowered and rests in the surgeon's hand. This relaxes the axillary fascia. (B) the surgeon stands behind the patient as he palpates the supraclavicular fossa.

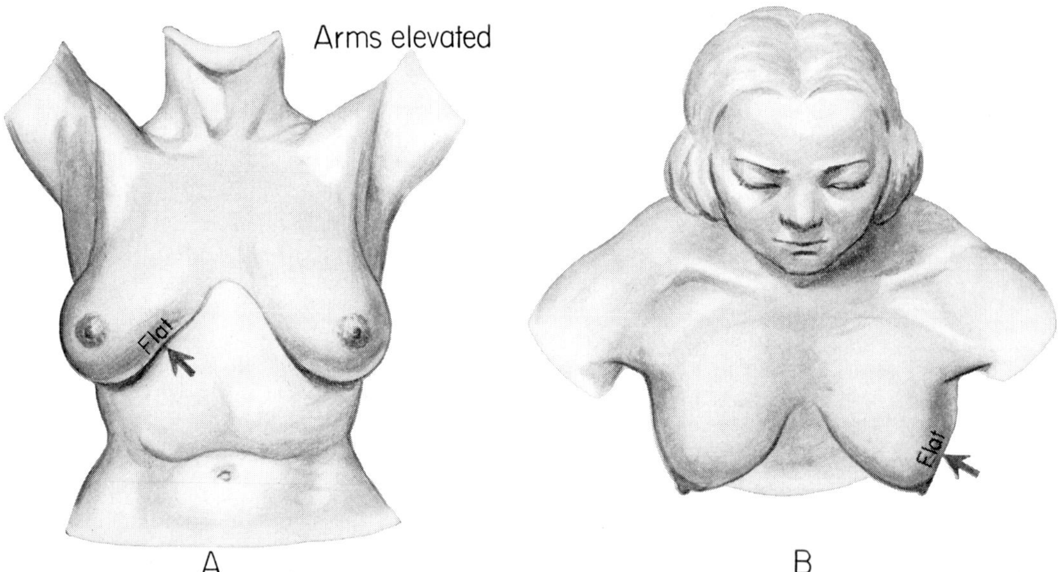

FIG. 115. Two simple methods of demonstrating retraction of the skin.

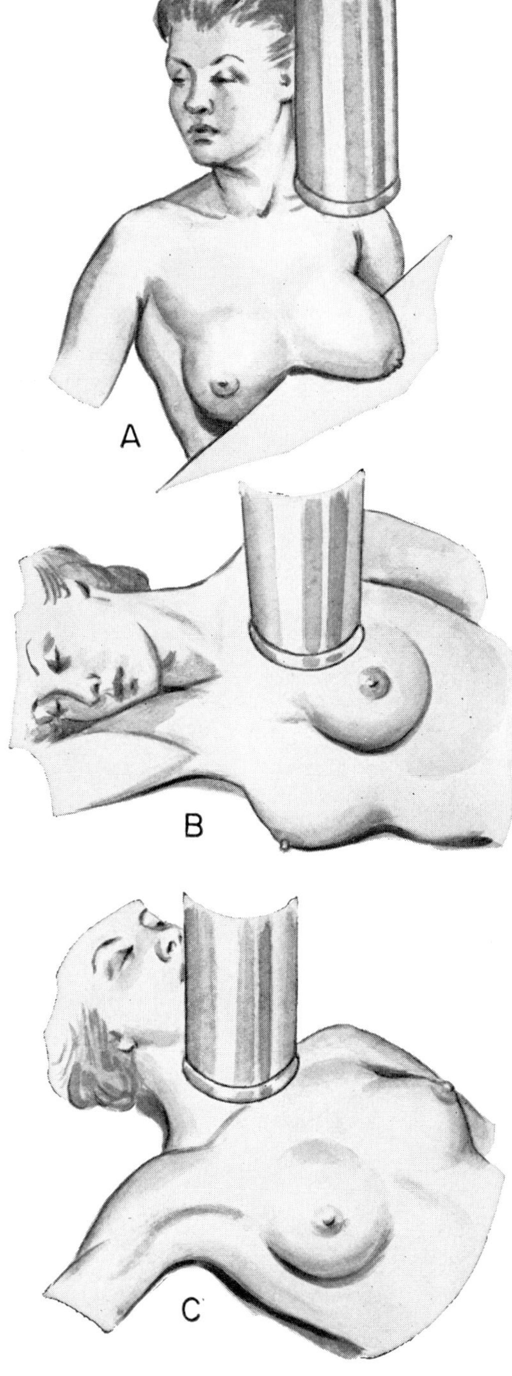

FIG. 116. The 3 views recommended in mammography. (A) The craniocaudal view, (B) the mediolateral view and (C) the axillary (oblique) view.

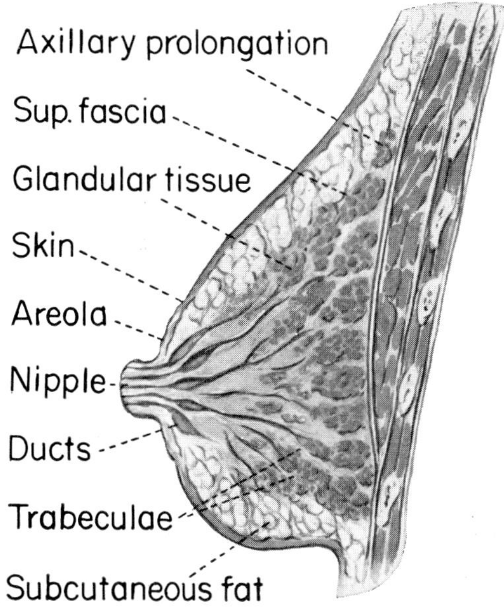

FIG. 117. A schematic representation of the anatomic breast structures which can be identified on the mammogram.

ticularly diagnostic, since they are suggestive of a malignancy. Such findings may be demonstrated when the arms are raised above the patient's head (Fig. 115 A). Another way in which retraction can be demonstrated is to have the patient bend forward from the hips, with the chin extended upward, and the superior extremity extended forward. Indentations and flattenings of the otherwise normal spherical contour of the breast immediately becomes apparent. (Fig. 115 B). Additional retraction phenomena are considered on page 113, where carcinoma of the breast is discussed.

MAMMOGRAPHY

Mammography is soft-tissue roentgenography of the breast. This type of mammogram does not utilize any opaque media injected into the ducts, and no air or gas is introduced into the retromammary space. Mammography is not a new procedure; it was first used in 1913 by a German surgeon named Salomon. He studied 3,000 amputated breast specimens and found that by this method tumors and various distortions

TABLE 4. DIFFERENTIAL DIAGNOSIS BASED ON MAMMOGRAPHY

MASS	BENIGN	MALIGNANT
Number	Often numerous	Usually single
Shape	Round or oval	Variable, ragged, tentacled
Border	Regular, well-circumscribed	Irregular, poorly circumscribed
Size	Same as palpable mass	Smaller than palpable mass
Density	Homogeneous	Nonhomogeneous
Surrounding tissue	Compressed, not invaded	Infiltrated
Calcification	Few coarse, isolated or widely scattered	Numerous, uncountable, confined to the lesion

of normal structures could be detected. Later contributions appeared in South American and European literature. Leborgne of Uruguay in 1951 improved the technic and was the first to reveal the significance of calcifications seen in malignant lesions of the breast. Others who have contributed largely to this method are Warren, Gershon-Cohen and Robert L. Egan. Egan performed prebiopsy mammograms on 240 breast cancers in a series of 1,000 cases and diagnosed cancer in 238—missing only 2 malignancies.

Three views usually are utilized (Fig. 116). The craniocaudal and the medio-

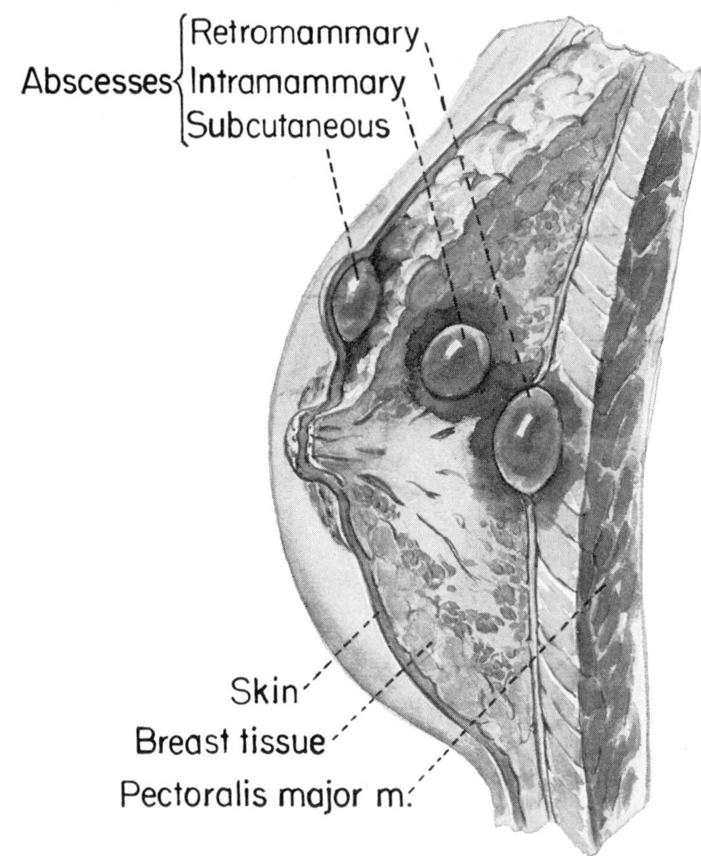

FIG. 118. Classification of breast abscesses according to location.

lateral are the ones used most frequently. The so-called axillary or oblique view is suggested to demonstrate the tail of the breast and/or the axillary nodes.

There are wide variations in the roentgenographic appearance of the "normal" breast, because the shadows transmitted are influenced by puberty, menstrual cycle, pregnancy, menopause, lactation and the state of nutrition. Much practice and perfection of technic are required to interpret mammograms properly. However, the time expended on this diagnostic method is most rewarding. Anatomic structures that should be identified on the mammogram are dependent on the anatomy (Fig. 117). On the roentgenogram the mammary gland projects as a triangle with the nipple at its apex and the base at the chest wall. The glandular portion is a denser triangle within the breast triangle, separated from the skin by the more radiolucent subcutaneous fat. The gland consists of 15 to 20 irregular lobes radiating from the nipple and separated by poorly defined fibrous septa. The virginal breast with its abundance of glandular and periductal tissue and its paucity of fat produces some contrast. A menopausal breast with its generous fat content produces the greatest contrast.

The mammogram *suggests* whether the lesion is benign or malignant (Table 4). Benign masses are rounded, homogeneously dense and surrounded by a thin radiolucent layer of fat which is pushed aside by the noninvading tumor. If calcium is present, it appears as a dense white mass or masses. Malignant tumors, on the other hand, are tentacled (with spiculated borders), denser in the center, invasive, and the calcification appears as faint stippled or "salted" small dots. Frequently, malignant lesions are associated with secondary changes, such as nipple or skin retraction, skin thickening, venous engorgement and enlarged axillary nodes.

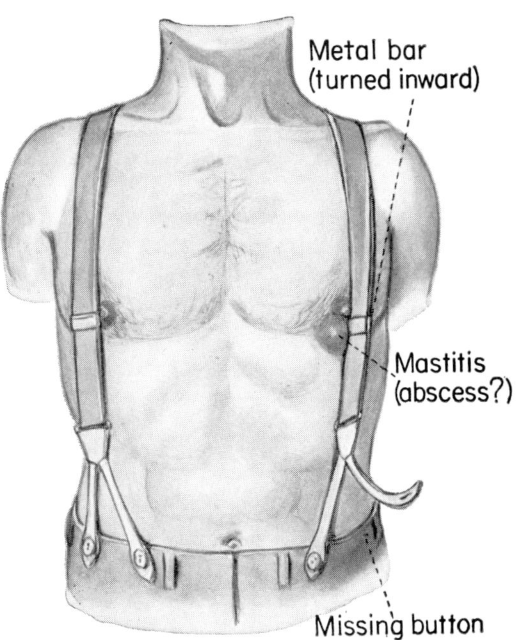

FIG. 119. Mastitis (breast abscess?) in the male. Frequently, this is caused by repeated trauma, such as constant rubbing from the metal bar on a pair of suspenders.

INFLAMMATION OF THE BREAST

ACUTE MASTITIS

This common form of breast inflammation almost always occurs during lactation and suckling. It is thought that organisms enter through fissures or openings in the nipple and pass into the breast tissue along the milk ducts. The offending organisms are usually streptococci and staphylococci which may come from the infant's mouth. The affected breast becomes enlarged, firm, tender, hot and painful; if unrelieved, systemic signs appear. With conservative treatment, the inflammatory process may subside completely; however, this may fail; in such instances necrosis and abscesses develop.

Breast abscesses may be single or multiple and may be located in 1 of 3 places: (1) subcutaneous, (2) intramammary or (3) retromammary (Fig. 118). The clinical signs depend on the location. If the abscess is subcutaneous, the inflammatory signs are visible early; they appear later if the abscess is intramammary and may be lacking entirely if the abscess is retromammary. A septic syndrome is usually present; this is characterized by spiking fever, true chills, marked sweats and a leukocyte count usually over 20,000. It is important to differentiate between acute mastitis and a suppurative process, since the former usually responds to conservative

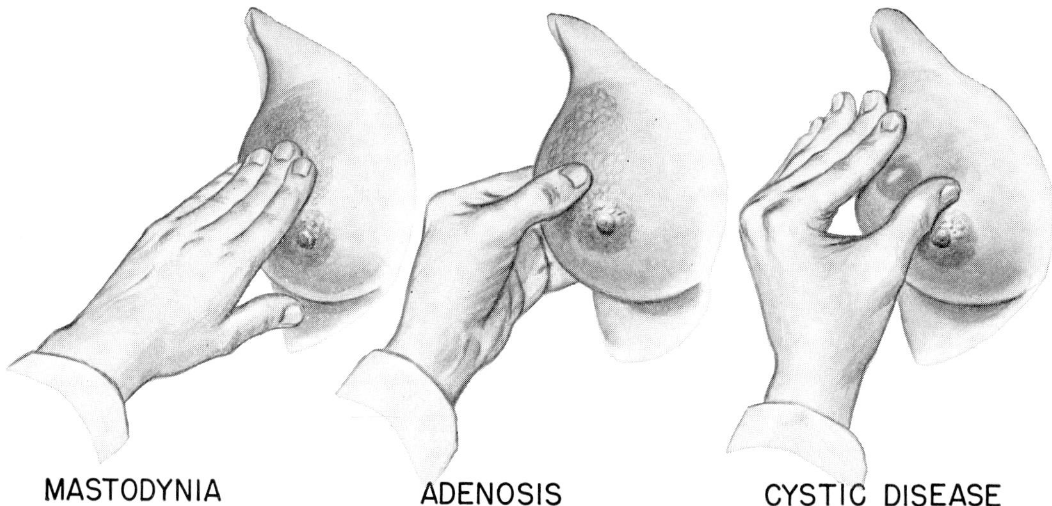

FIG. 120. Mammary dysplasia is a more appropriate term than the misnomer "chronic cystic mastitis." Three types of this dysplasia are recognized: mastodynia, adenosis and cystic disease. These are endocrine disturbances which must be differentiated from carcinoma. The saucerlike edge of adenosis is characteristic.

treatment, but an abscess requires drainage.

This condition may also affect the male breast. If so, it usually is associated with constant mild trauma such as rubbing. Those cases seen by the author are produced almost always by the rubbing of the metal part of a pair of suspenders against the hairy areola. This can be greatly exaggerated if one of the suspender pants buttons is missing, thereby turning the metal bar inward (Fig. 119).

So-called nonbacterial "mastitis" may occur during the first few days of life as a result of breast stimulation from the high circulating titer of maternal estrogens. This results in palpable tender breast tissue, particularly beneath the areola. No treatment is necessary, but the *parents* will require reassurance that this "mastitis" will subside as soon as the mother's hormones disappear from her newborn baby's blood. At puberty the hormonal level again becomes altered and may give rise to tender breasts; this may occur in either sex. The treatment is reassurance.

Chronic mastitis usually is manifested by a chronic draining sinus or sinuses; it frequently results from an inadequately drained breast abscess. A history of an acute process suggests the correct diagnosis. The possibility of tuberculosis should be kept in mind in all chronic mastitis cases. Although smears and guinea pig inoculations may be helpful, the definite diagnosis rests on a biopsy.

MAMMARY DYSPLASIA
(Chronic Cystic Mastitis)

This is the most common involvement of the female breast. Supposedly, it is due to an exaggeration and a distortion of the cyclic breast changes that normally occur in the menstrual cycle. Since 6 pituitary and 2 ovarian hormones have been shown to affect mammary tissue, mammary dysplasia becomes an extremely complex endocrinologic puzzle. The names applied to this condition are legion. Fibrocystic disease, cystic hyperplasia, mastopathy, fibroadenosis, Reclus' disease, Bloodgood's blue domed cyst, adenosis, mazoplasia, microcystic and macrocystic disease of the breast are only a few such appellations. The most persistent and widely used term, although totally inappropriate, is chronic cystic mastitis. The disease is not invariably chronic, nor is it always cystic, and it surely is not an inflammation. I have chosen to use the term "mammary dysplasia" as being the most inclusive and the least offensive.

Mammary dysplasia is intimately related

to the function of the ovaries and the pituitary as they pertain to *lobule formation*. Such dysplasia does not occur during normal puberty (lobule formation lacking); nor is it encountered frequently after the menopause, when the lobule structure has disappeared (senile involution). Lobule formation is not seen in the normal human male breast.

The estrogen secretion of the ovarian follicle brings about adolescent development of the breast and sexual maturity; when the corpus luteum hormone is added, development of the lobule system results. Estrogen is responsible for stimulating the growth of the duct tree, the lobular buds and proliferation of the supporting stroma. Without the previous action of estrogen, corpus luteal hormones cannot bring about lobule formation. An understanding of the normal physiology of the breast is essential if one is to comprehend the endocrine imbalances which result in breast pathology.

Mammary dysplasia can be divided into 3 types (Fig. 120): (1) mastodynia, (2) adenosis and (3) cystic disease. Despite variable behaviors it is possible to distinguish these 3 patterns according to their morphologic changes. They also conform fairly well as to age and distinctive clinical manifestations of a malignant transformation. It must be emphasized that there may be some overlapping; therefore, it becomes difficult to categorize every case dogmatically.

Mastodynia. This is the most common of the 3 forms of mammary dysplasia. It has been referred to as fibrosis of the breast, because the microscopic picture of this variant reveals a fibrous tissue overgrowth unaccompanied by epithelial hyperplasia. It is found most frequently in women between the ages of 25 and 35. In mastodynia lobule formation is partially suppressed.

This condition is characterized by breast pain and tenderness which is most marked in the premenstruum. The upper outer quadrant of the breast is involved most frequently; it may be unilateral or bilateral. The pain is mild in character in the early stages but ultimately becomes more severe and prolonged. In the chronic cases it may persist throughout the greater part of the menstrual cycle. Weight of excessively heavy and pendulous breasts increases the discomfort. Physical examination reveals a tender, firm and somewhat granular area of breast tissue which the patient refers to as a "lump." The fear of carcinoma brings her to the physician. The swelling is usually larger and more painful before each menstrual period. This cyclic association with the menses cannot be overemphasized as a diagnostic aid for all types of mammary dysplasia. Demarcation from surrounding breast tissue is usually indistinct.

When such breast tissue is seen on cut surface, the area is usually white, fibrous, not encapsulated, and at times associated with

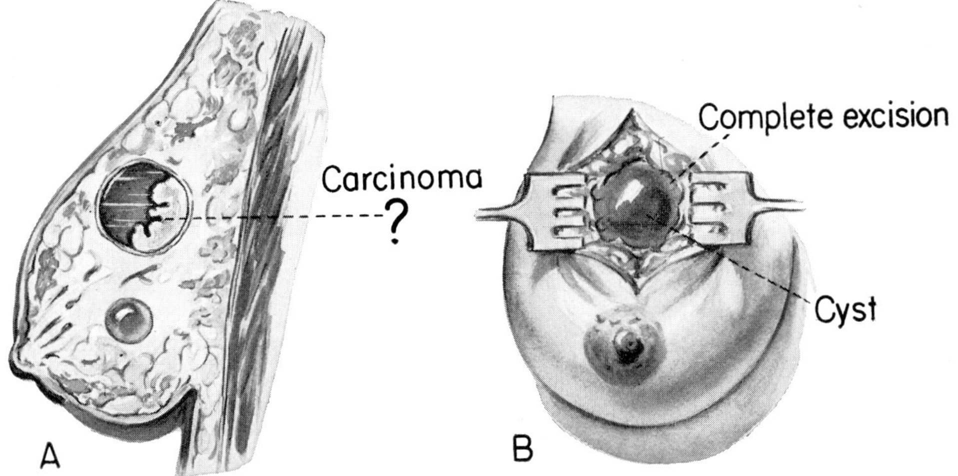

FIG. 121. Cystic disease of the breast (dysplasia). Because of the possible association of carcinoma these cysts should be excised and not aspirated.

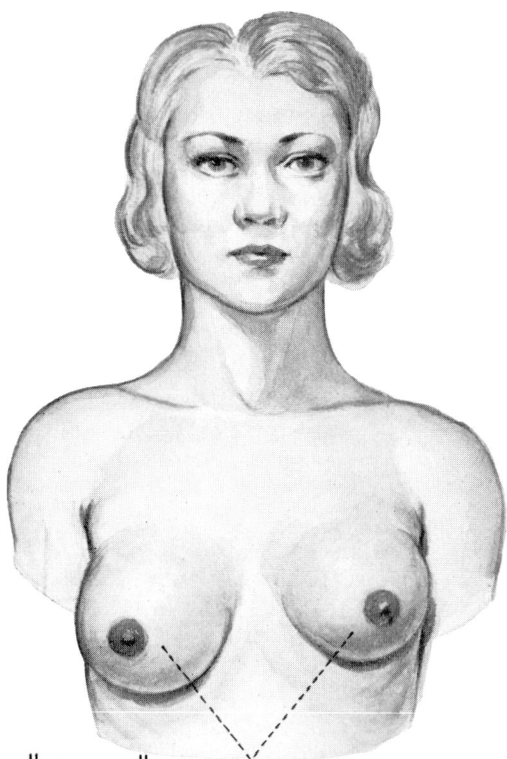

FIG. 122. Prepubertal enlargement in the developing female breasts. The resulting asymmetry should cause no alarm, since the condition almost always rectifies itself.

tiny cysts. The indurated areas tend to disappear after pregnancy and the menopause. If the cases persist, they are prone to develop adenosis. Therapy consists of mental as well as breast support.

Adenosis. This has been referred to as microcystic disease, Schimmelbusch's disease and ductal papillomatosis. It is characterized by epithelial proliferation beyond the ends of the tubules which replaces normal lobule formation. The age of incidence falls between the peak incidence of mastodynia, which affects younger women, and cystic disease, which tends to affect older women.

This form of dysplasia is fortunately the least common, since it is the most serious type. It is seen most frequently in women between the ages of 35 to 45 and is characterized by the presence of nodules in one or both breasts. In most instances the patient is aware of a distinct nodule which usually occurs in the upper outer quadrant of the breast. The majority of patients are childless, seem to be of a nervous type and frequently have irregular menses. Exacerbation of pain and enlargement of the nodule are commonly found during the premenstrual period. These nodules reveal a definite edge which is readily felt at the periphery. The induration suggests malignancy. The condition usually persists for years. About 4 per cent of these cases are associated with intraductal papillomas and bleeding from the nipples.

The differential diagnosis between adenosis and carcinoma may be very difficult. Statistical data show an incidence of carcinoma in patients with adenosis of approximately 4 per cent. The particular reason for the extreme difficulty in the differentiation is that the gradations of the 2 diseases dovetail. Biopsy is the only certain method of determining the nature of the lesion. In those patients who become pregnant, disappearance of the nodularity and tenderness usually occurs after midpregnancy, and the breasts become normal during lactation. It is interesting to note that some breasts in which previously adenosis has been present appear to be normal a year or more after childbirth.

Cystic Disease of the Breast. This condition has been referred to as the cystic disease of Reclus or the blue dome cyst of Bloodgood. This type of dysplasia is characterized by the presence of 1 or more cysts which occur during or near the menopause. The peak of the age incidence is between 40 and 45 years; it is unusual to find macrocystic breast disease under the age of 25. Authorities have found evidence to support the probability that an intense and unopposed estrogenic stimulus results in cyst formation.

The patient consults a physician when she discovers a "lump"; about one half of these are associated with pain and/or soreness. The cysts may change in size or disappear abruptly. The mass feels smooth, rounded, tense and freely movable (Fig. 113). Transillumination may be helpful at times. If the cyst is situated deep in the breast and lies close to the chest wall, its nature and extent will be difficult to appraise. Multiple cysts are found in one or both breasts in approximately 25 per cent. This tendency toward multiplicity and bilateral involvement suggests an endocrine imbalance. At times there is a serous discharge from the nipple.

During surgical exploration the cyst is found to have a tense, thin wall with a distinctive bluish tint, the latter being lost when the cyst is opened. The fluid is usually serous or cloudy, and the wall is smooth and glistening. Intracystic papilloma and carcinoma cysts must be considered first in the differential diagnosis. It is true that these latter conditions occur after the menopause as a rule and frequently affect the large ducts in the areolar area, whereas the cysts in the macrocystic disease per se usually occur during the menopause and affect the smaller ducts. Nevertheless, such differentiations are too difficult to make; hence, no time should be lost in excising these masses for thorough microscopic study (Fig. 121). If the pathologist has the slightest doubt regarding a frozen section, he should not be pressed for a snapshot diagnosis. It is better and safer for everyone concerned to await the study of the paraffin sections. Aspiration of cysts of the breast should be condemned (p. 116).

Two groups of cysts that are not associated with mammary dysplasia are galactoceles and sebaceous cysts. The former results from an obstructed duct (usually during lactation), and the latter resemble sebaceous cysts seen elsewhere in the body.

ABNORMAL BREAST ENLARGEMENTS

These may be prepubertal or postpubertal.

Prepubertal Enlargements

Between the ages of 10 and 12 years it is not unusual to discover a rather marked asymmetry of the developing breasts (Fig. 122). This should cause no alarm, since in almost each instance the condition rectifies itself.

In boys, there may be an enlargement beneath the areolae of the developing breasts (Fig. 123). The firm mass feels like a disk, about the size of a quarter, and is often tender. It has been referred to as *discoid hyperplasia*. These should be left alone, since they regress spontaneously.

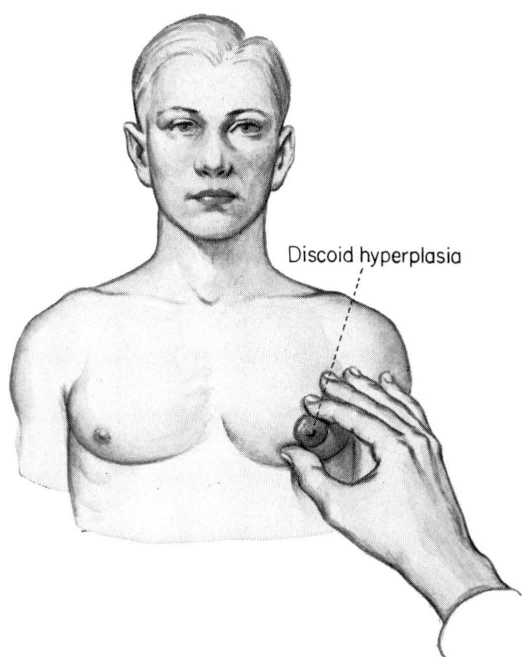

Fig. 123. Prepubertal enlargement in the developing male breast. This is known as discoid hyperplasia; it requires no treatment and disappears spontaneously.

Postpubertal Enlargements

The normal adult female breasts are slightly asymmetrical. In some instances both breasts become massively enlarged, producing the condition known as *virginal hypertrophy*. The cause of this condition is unknown. These patients complain of excessive weight and pain, particularly during the premenstruum. The author has seen the skin of the shoulders grooved so deeply by the weight of the breasts that the brassière straps caused severe dermatitis and even bleeding. Such breasts can be corrected by plastic surgery (Fig. 124).

In men, between the ages of 45 and 65, abnormal enlargement of one or both breasts may develop (Fig. 125). The lesion resembles those seen in boys at puberty, namely, a firm discoid mass beneath the areola which at times is tender. *Gynecomastia* may be related to diseases of the liver, the adrenal, the testicle or the pituitary. Of particular interest is the enlarged male breast seen in liver cirrhosis with its increased susceptibility to carcinoma. This condition is a response to an excess of estrogen. Hyperplasia of the male breast or breasts is encountered under a variety of circumstances. The most important cause for hyperestronism in the male is cirrhosis of the liver, since the liver is responsible for destroying estrogens. In very aged males presumably it is due to a relative increase in adrenal estrogens as the androgenic function of the testes fails. *Carcinoma of the male breast* forms a painless hard irregular mass which is abnormally fixed to surrounding structures and associated with signs of retraction. If the slightest doubt exists as to the nature of the lesion, excision and microscopic study should be done.

BENIGN TUMORS OF THE BREAST

Although not all-inclusive, a practical classification based on the type of tissue from which the tumor arises includes the following (Fig. 126): (1) fibroadenoma, (2) intraductal papilloma and (3) miscellaneous tumors: lipoma, angioma, etc.

Fibroadenoma

This is the most common benign tumor of the female breast. Though it may be encountered in all age groups, it is found most commonly during the 3rd and the 4th decades. It has a tendency to enlarge during pregnancy. The symptoms are usually insignificant, although slight pain may be present.

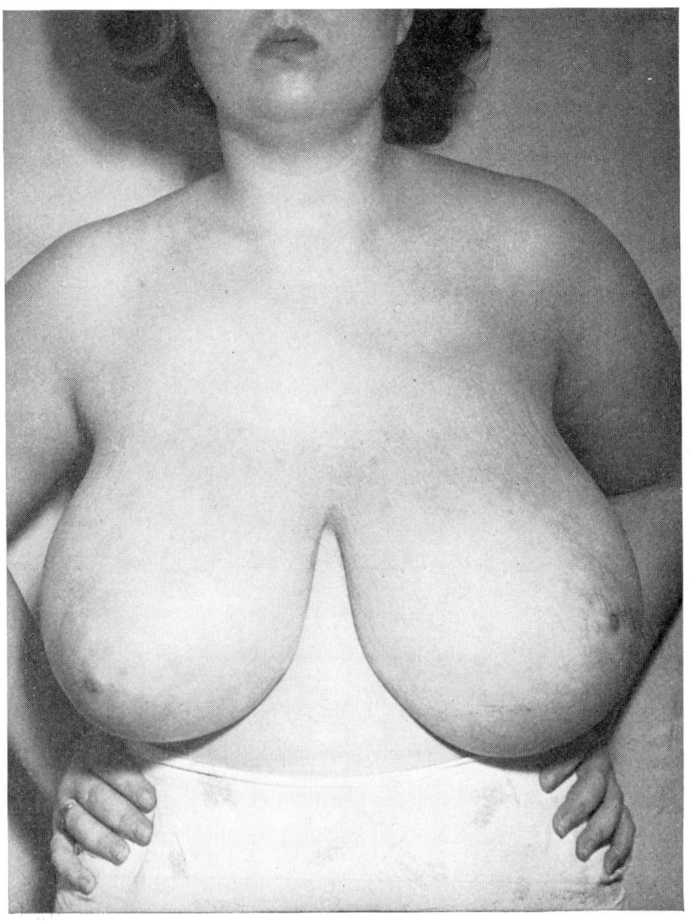

Fig. 124. Virginal hypertrophy is a postpubertal enlargement.

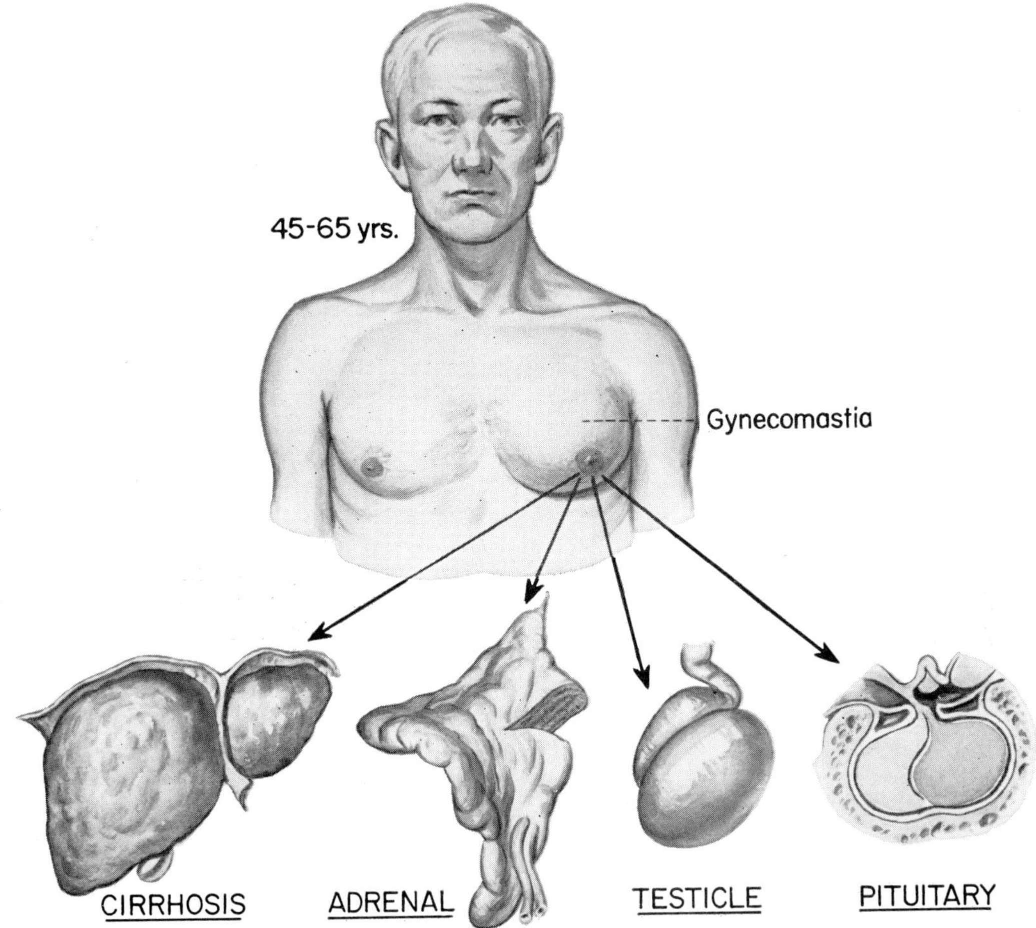

FIG. 125. Postpubertal gynecomastia. A thorough study of the liver must be conducted because of the frequency with which the gynecomastia is related to cirrhosis and other liver diseases. This condition may be associated also with diseases of the testicle, the adrenal or the pituitary.

Usually, the mass is discovered accidentally by the patient while bathing or dressing. Of diagnostic importance is the observation that the size remains stationary. The average fibroadenoma ceases to grow after attaining a size of 2 to 4 cm. in diameter.

Physical examination reveals a palpable smooth, firm nodule which slips about readily beneath the examining fingers (Fig. 113). This extreme mobility is an important point in differentiating it from malignant tumors.

Pathologists divide them into 2 types: intracanalicular and pericanalicular.

Since one can arrive at a correct diagnosis only by microscopy, these lesions should be excised and studied.

Intraductal Papilloma

As the name implies, this is a papillomatous growth of epithelium into the lumen of a duct. They usually occur singly and are located in the ampulla or close to it; they have been known to form in a pre-existing cyst.

In contrast with other tumors, they are frequently so small that they are not palpable. Occasionally, however, a thickened duct or tiny nodule can be felt immediately beneath the nipple. Almost always pressure *directly over the papilloma* will result in extrusion of a small drop of serous or bloody fluid (Fig. 127). They are the most frequent cause of bleeding from the nipple. When these papillomas are large enough to be palpable, they are apt to be undergoing malignant transformations. It is well to remember that whereas these tumors are located beneath the nipple, the fibroadenomas are rarely seen in this location.

Other Forms

Other benign tumors (lipoma, angioma, etc.) which may affect the breast resemble tumors found elsewhere in the body; they are mentioned for the sake of completion.

CARCINOMA OF THE BREAST

This is the most common form of malignancy in the female and is responsible for approximately 25,000 deaths per year in the United States. Some authorities believe that this form of cancer is increasing. Randall and his co-workers have estimated that slightly more that 5 women per 100 will develop breast carcinoma. The disease rarely occurs under the age of 25 but shows a steadily rising incidence with each advancing decade of life.

The etiology of carcinoma of the breast is unknown; there appears to be some relationship to the female sex hormones. Direct trauma, stagnation and heredity as etiologic factors also have their proponents. It is more common in nulliparous women and appears to be less frequent in women who have suckled their young. The term "precancerous" lesion is a misleading one. In this respect all breast lesions may be considered as precancerous; to quote Stewart, "the female breast is a precancerous organ."

Classification

Frequently, classification of tumor results in clinical dilemmas (Fig. 128). When the weary clinician reads such term as "encephaloid," "medullary," "carcinoma simplex," "scirrhus" or "adenocarcinoma," he may be left in a quandary. Encephaloid merely means resembling brain. Medullary suggests resembling marrow. Carcinoma simplex implies "simple" carcinoma. But who would consider carcinoma to be simple? Scirrhus means hard. Adenocarcinoma is a rather futile term, since the breast is a gland, and every carcinoma derived therefrom is funda-

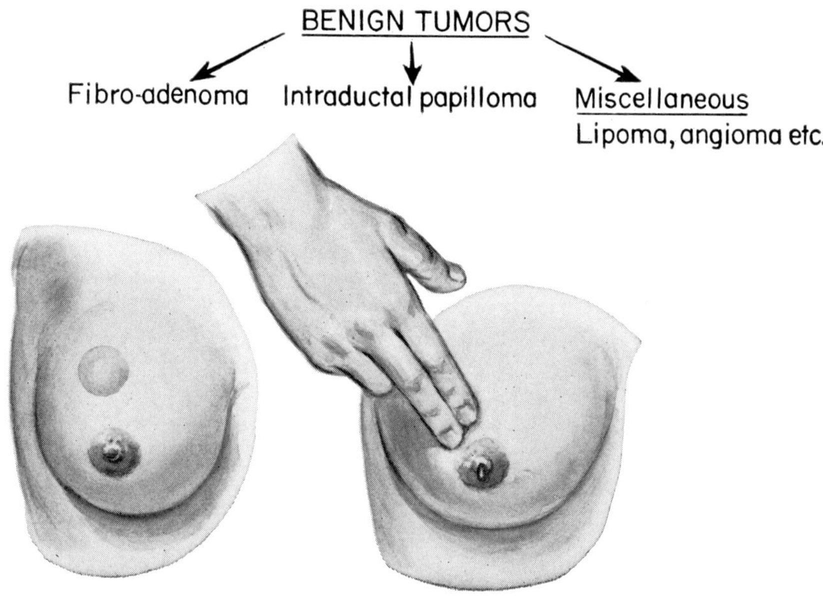

Fig. 126. A practical classification of benign breast tumors.

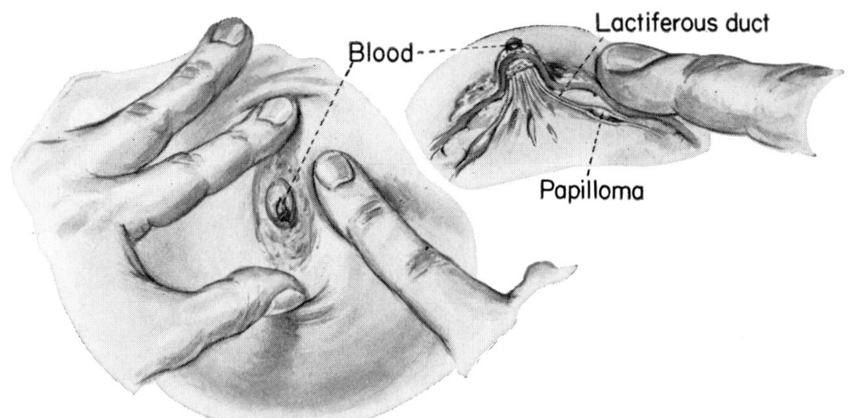

FIG. 127. Intraductal papilloma. The location of the papilloma can be determined if the surface of the breast is spread out, and if pressure is exerted in the direction of the nipple with the index finger placed at the periphery of the areola. This is repeated around the areola. A drop of blood will appear at a duct opening on the nipple when the papilloma is pressed.

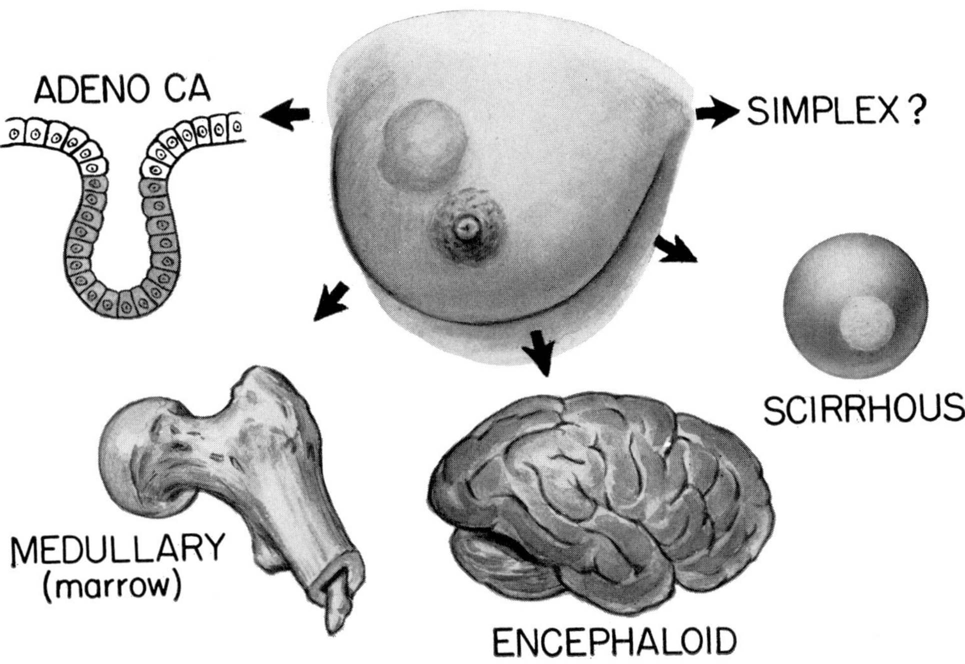

FIG. 128. Clinically, it is better to classify carcinoma of the breast as infiltrating or noninfiltrating. The descriptive terms applied to carcinoma are legion and are more confusing than helpful.

mentally an adenocarcinoma. Qualified pathologists have taught us that different parts of a given tumor may show different structural arrangements.

Numerous classifications can be found and consulted in any standard textbook of surgery or pathology. Of greater clinical and prognostic importance, however, is the simple classification of (1) infiltrating and (2) noninfiltrating.

If a tumor has broken through the normal anatomic boundaries and has invaded the surrounding lymph and blood vessels, the prognosis is worse. One might find some clinical value in classifying these tumors as being intraductal or extraductal. Some pathologists are of the opinion that "grading" carcinoma is of little or no value when it pertains to the breast, in contradistinction to "gradings" which appear to have prognostic value when pertaining to the skin and the cervix uteri. It is well to recall that those tumors that attain large sizes usually remain confined to the breast for longer periods of time.

Lymph Drainage

Numerous descriptions have been presented of the lymph nodes and drainage that are associated with the mammary gland.

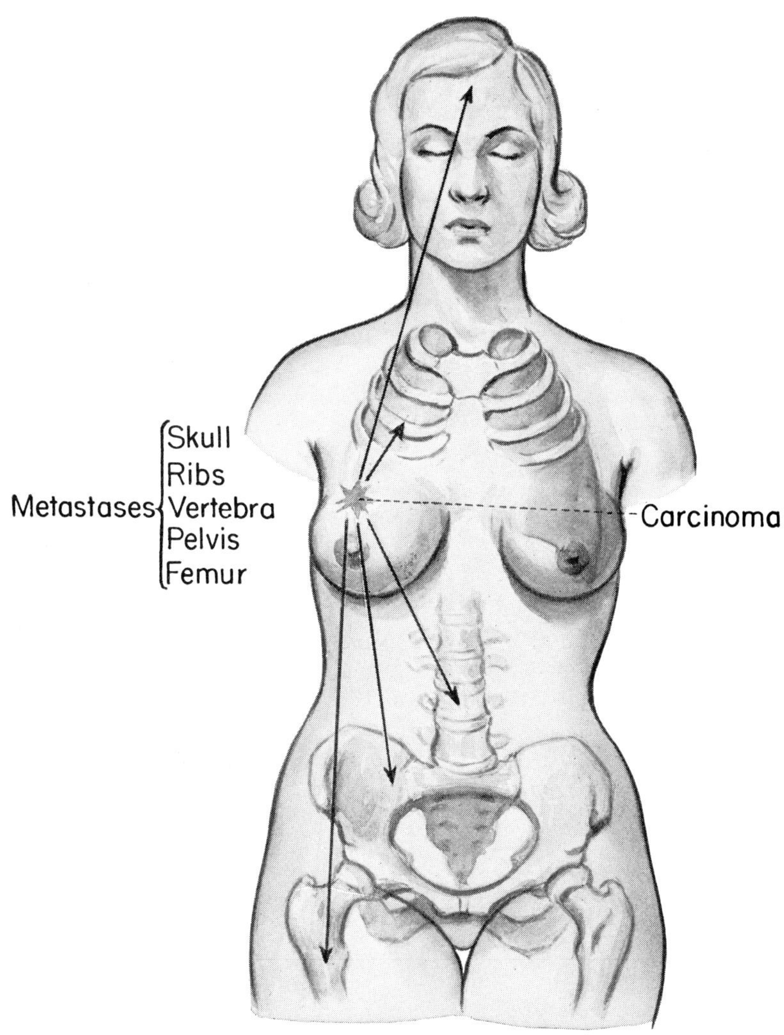

Fig. 129. The bones which most frequently reveal metastasis in carcinoma of the breast.

These may be found in any standard text.

After studying lymph drainage and the paths that spreading carcinoma may take, one is reminded of the terse statement of the late Dr. Richard Jaffe, who said, "Who am I to tell carcinoma where to go?" Metastases may appear in most bizarre and remote locations.

Breast carcinomas vary widely in their clinical courses; in younger individuals they usually spread more rapidly. Masses in the medial portion of the brest are particularly prone to spread to the opposite breast and the lymph nodes associated with it. Extension may take place via peritoneal lymph channels and thence to the liver. Frequently, the lungs and the bones are affected; the bones that usually are attacked are those which contain red marrow, namely, ribs, skull, vertebra, pelvis and proximal ends of the femurs (Fig. 129).

Clinical Manifestations

These can be remembered if one recalls the letters and the spelling of the word BREAST:

Breast mass
Retraction signs
Edema
Axillary involvement
Sanguineous nipple discharge
Tenderness

The mass may be located in any portion of the breast; however, it is found most frequently in the upper outer quadrant (Fig. 130). Usually, it is discovered accidentally by the patient while bathing or dressing. Its consistency is firm to hard, and its margin is ill-defined. It does not have the free mobility of benign tumors or cysts. The greatest of gentleness must be exercised in palpating these lesions.

Retraction signs can be demonstrated by dimpling of the skin and/or retraction of the nipple (Fig. 115).

Dimpling of the skin is a most valuable sign (Fig. 131). It is produced by invasion of the ligaments of Cooper by cancer cells. These ligaments are bands of fibrous tissue which anchor the breast to the overlying skin and the pectoral fascia. Following invasion, the ligaments contract and account for the

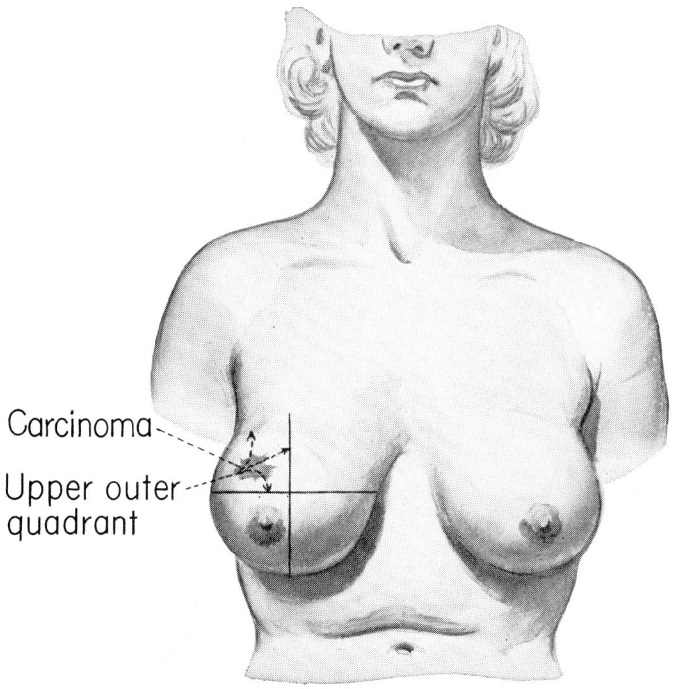

Fig. 130. The upper outer quadrant of the breast is involved most frequently by carcinoma.

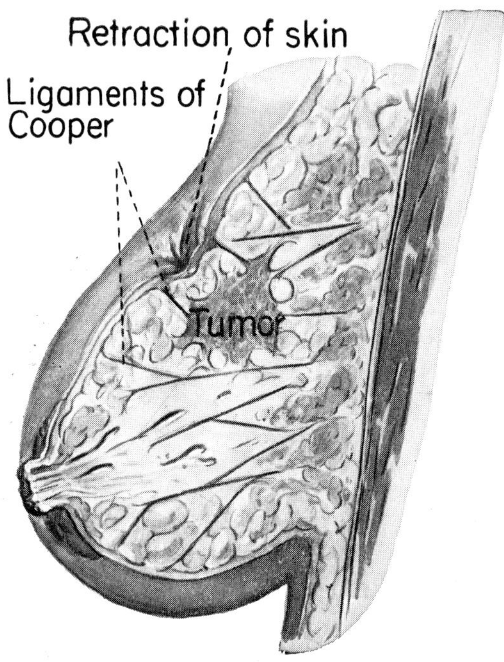

FIG. 131. Retraction of the skin is caused by invasion and contraction of the ligaments of Cooper.

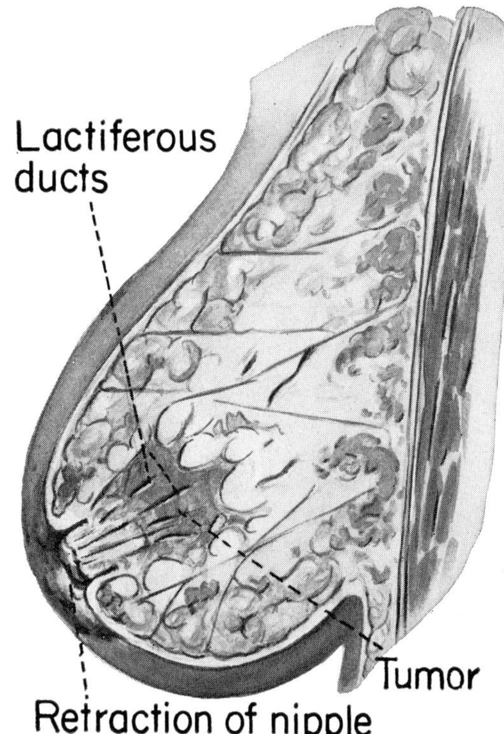

FIG. 132. Retraction of the nipple is caused by invasion, fibrosis and contractions of the lactiferous ducts. The tumor is located directly beneath the nipple.

dimpling and the fixation either to the skin above or the pectoral fascia below. The sign, although very helpful, is not pathognomonic, since it may be found in other conditions, particularly those associated with previous breast operations, acute mastitis, fat necrosis and plasma cell mastitis. In the first 2 conditions, the differentiation is easy, since the history is so informative; however, the differential diagnosis between carcinoma and fat necrosis taxes the experience and the ability of the most seasoned physicians and is frequently impossible until the tissue is excised and examined.

Retraction of the nipple is present when the tumor is located beneath the nipple (Fig. 132). It is due to extension of the growth along the lactiferous ducts with subsequent retraction and fibrosis. It must be recalled that retraction of the nipple may be congenital and may be bilateral.

Edema accounts for the "orange peel" or "pigskin" appearance of the breast. It results from obstruction of the lymphatics by the neoplasm (Fig. 133). The hair follicles and the sebaceous glands are more firmly fixed to the subcutaneous tissue than the rest of the skin. The skin around these openings bulges forward when the lymphatic drainage is interfered with, and the hair follicles appear as depressions in the edematous area. Since this sign may be produced by acute inflammatory conditions, it cannot be considered as pathognomonic of carcinoma.

Axillary metastases (p. 100). It is difficult to determine whether enlarged glands are inflammatory or neoplastic. These glands should be examined microscopically, as they may be of some value prognostically.

Bloody discharge from the nipple is a frightening discovery for the average woman (Fig. 134). Nipple discharge occurs in less than 5 per cent of the cases of carcinoma of the breast and in about half of these, the discharge is serous and not bloody. Benign lesions produce a nipple discharge. It is not pathognomonic for carcinoma. Ductal papillomas and some of the mammary dysplasias

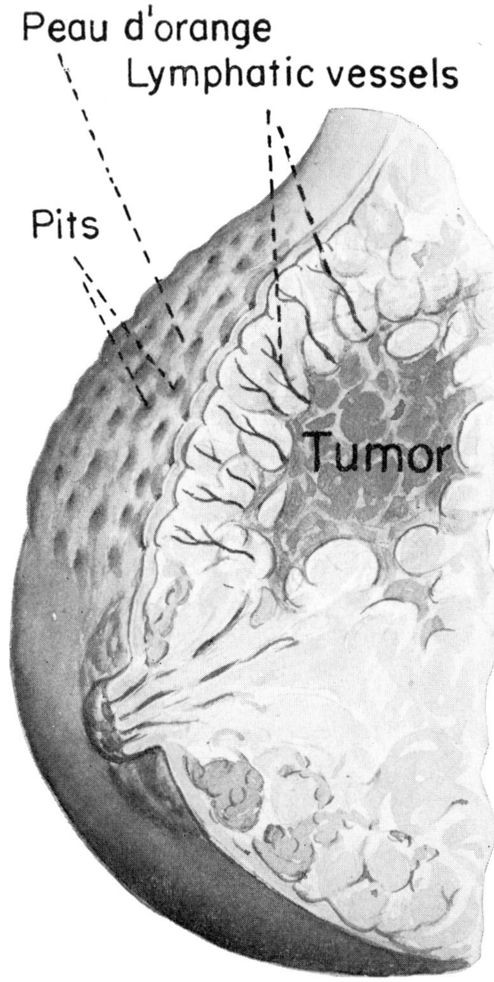

FIG. 133. Edema of the breast gives a characteristic "pitting." The fixation of the hair follicles and the sebaceous glands accounts for this.

may also produce bleeding from the nipple. Occasionally, it will be noted that the bleeding arises from more than one duct. If this is found in the absence of a palpable or a demonstrable lesion, it is unlikely that carcinoma is the cause.

Tenderness is more common than pain. In a fairly high percentage of patients the tenderness of the carcinoma leads to the discovery of the mass. Pain, uncommon in carcinoma of the breast, is associated with the late phase of the disease. Pain in the back and the extremities should make one suspect

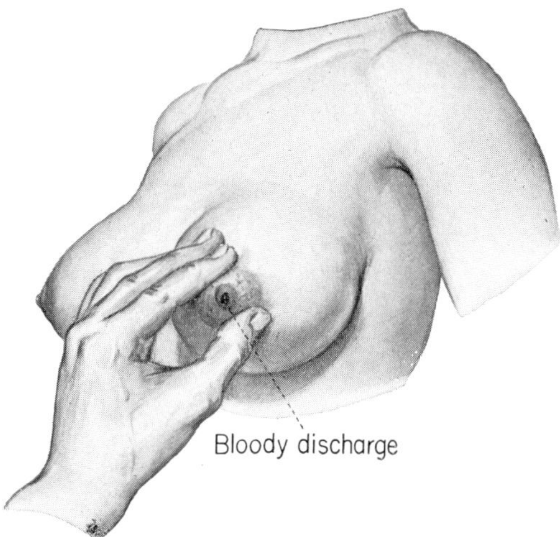

FIG. 134. Bloody discharge from the nipple is suggestive but not pathognomonic of breast carcinoma.

bone metastases. *Cough* suggests pulmonary metastases.

Cancer of the breast during *pregnancy* and *lactation* grows more rapidly and has a grave prognosis. *Carcinoma en cuirasse* is observed when the skin involvement is more rapid than that of deeper structures. The surface then presents a nodularity that is diagnostic. So-called "*inflammatory*" cancer of the breast is a rapid-growing neoplasm that is associated with infection. The hyperemia and the skin thickening may be so marked that it is mistaken for erysipelas. These cases usually take a rapidly fatal course.

DIAGNOSTIC EXAMINATIONS

Mammography has been discussed on page 101. This more recent method of examination has become an important part of the clinician's armamentarium.

Biopsy suggests the removal of a small amount of tissue for study. Such a piece of tissue should *not* be removed when it is possible to excise the entire mass. Although in most instances a frozen section will reveal the diagnosis, there are cases that cannot be diagnosed by this method. In such instances one must await a more thorough microscopic study made from paraffin sections.

Needle and *punch biopsies* are mentioned

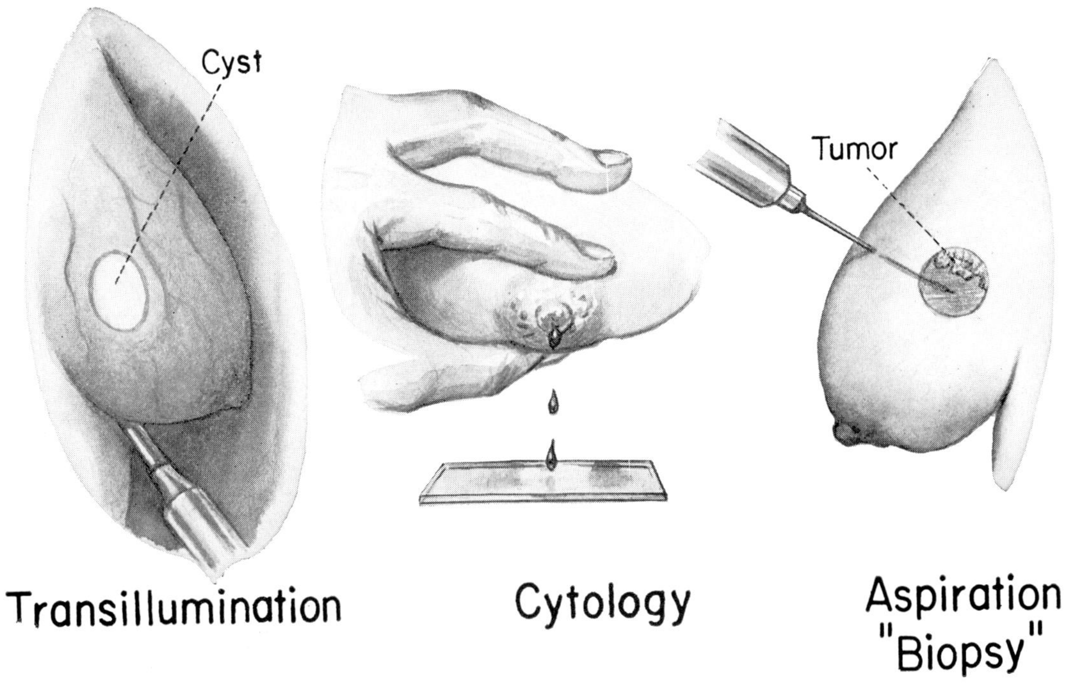

FIG. 135. Some methods used as diagnostic aids in diseases of the breast. These are mentioned only to emphasize their extreme limitations (see text).

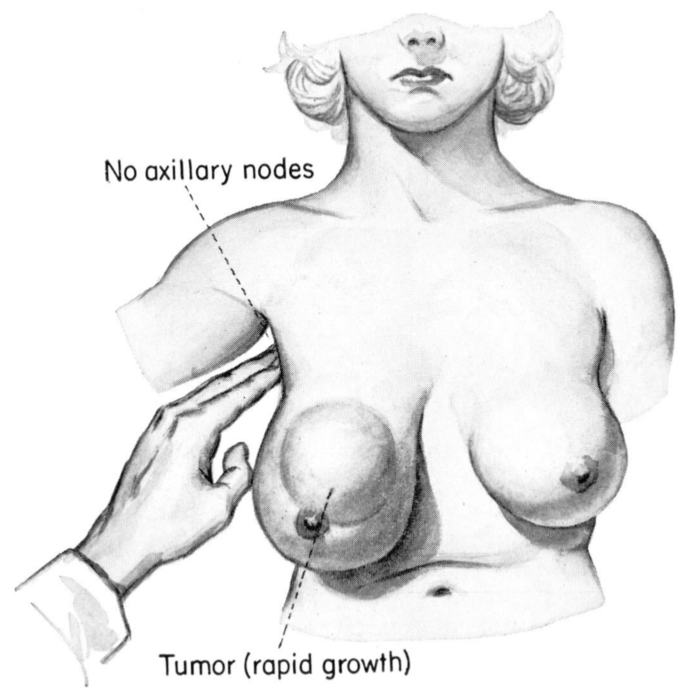

FIG. 136. Sarcoma of the breast grows rapidly and rarely involves the axillary lymph nodes early.

only to be condemned (Fig. 135). They traumatize and may miss or disseminate the tumor. A cyst associated with a tumor might reveal the fluid but miss the neoplasm.

Cytologic examinations are not as useful in studies of nipple discharges as in vaginal and cervical smears or material taken from the respiratory tract.

Transillumination is limited in its usefulness.

SARCOMA OF THE BREAST

This is a rare disease, its incidence being placed at 0.5 per cent. Numerous types have been described, the most common being fibrosarcoma and spindle cell sarcoma. At times the condition develops from a pre-existing fibroadenoma.

The 2 important features in the diagnosis are the rapid rate of growth (the tumor may reach the size of a grapefruit within a few months) and the absence of involved axillary lymph nodes (Fig. 136). There is a tendency toward ulceration. The prognosis is variable because of the great variety of sarcomas. The angiosarcomas are highly malignant.

Cystosarcoma phyllodes is an unfortunate designation because it is essentially benign. These tumors frequently are considered to be giant fibroadenomas. It is a relatively rare tumor, and any malignant degeneration is exceedingly unusual. It appears as a large bulky tumor which may distort the breast, producing bulging and even pressure necrosis of the overlying skin. When ulceration occurs, the tumor may rupture; the clinician's first impression is that this is a far-advanced fungating malignancy. Even in those excessively rare instances in which malignant transformation takes place, the tumors tend to remain localized for long periods of time. It is because of the excellent prognosis that stress must be placed on accurate diagnosis and removal of such breasts. When malignant, these tumors tend to spread hematogenously. Up to the present time only one case of lymph node metastases has been reported.

PLASMA CELL MASTITIS

The etiology of this condition is unknown. The disease presents 2 phases. (1) The *acute phase* consists of a mild inflammatory reaction that is associated with local heat, redness and tenderness. This phase is a transient one; the symptoms subside spontaneously, following a rather mild course for which the patient rarely seeks medical advice. (2) After some weeks or months the *residual phase* appears (Fig. 137). Examination now reveals a firm mass usually not tender and possessing an irregular ill-defined border. The importance of plasma cell mastitis lies in the fact that it is confused with carcinoma, because it may present "orange peel" skin, retraction of the nipple, discharge from the nipple and enlarged axillary lymph nodes. The signs of local inflammation are entirely lacking in this stage, so that the eliciting of a history that reveals a previous mild acute phase is extremely important in the differential diagnosis. The final diagnosis rests with a histologic examination.

Plasma cell mastitis has been referred to also as mammary duct ectasia and comedomastitis. Whether these are one and the same condition, whether they are entirely different conditions, or whether they represent different stages of chronicity of a given condition is still moot.

TRAUMATIC FAT NECROSIS

This condition is characterized by a lump in the breast which originates from the destruction and the necrosis of fat with subsequent inflammation and fibrosis. A history of trauma cannot always be elicited, but when present is of such severity as to produce a painful tender mass that is accompanied by ecchymosis (Fig. 137).

The disease is found most commonly in obese women between the ages of 30 and 60, since in the latter decades of life fat has a tendency to increase in the mammary glands. Although it is not common, it is important, because it is difficult to differentiate from carcinoma.

The necrosis results from a response of the body to the chemical irritation of fat and its decomposition products (fatty acids and glycerol). These products set up an inflammatory reaction ultimately followed by the deposition of dense, firm, scar tissue.

Only a small percentage of contusions of the breast result in fat necrosis, since the

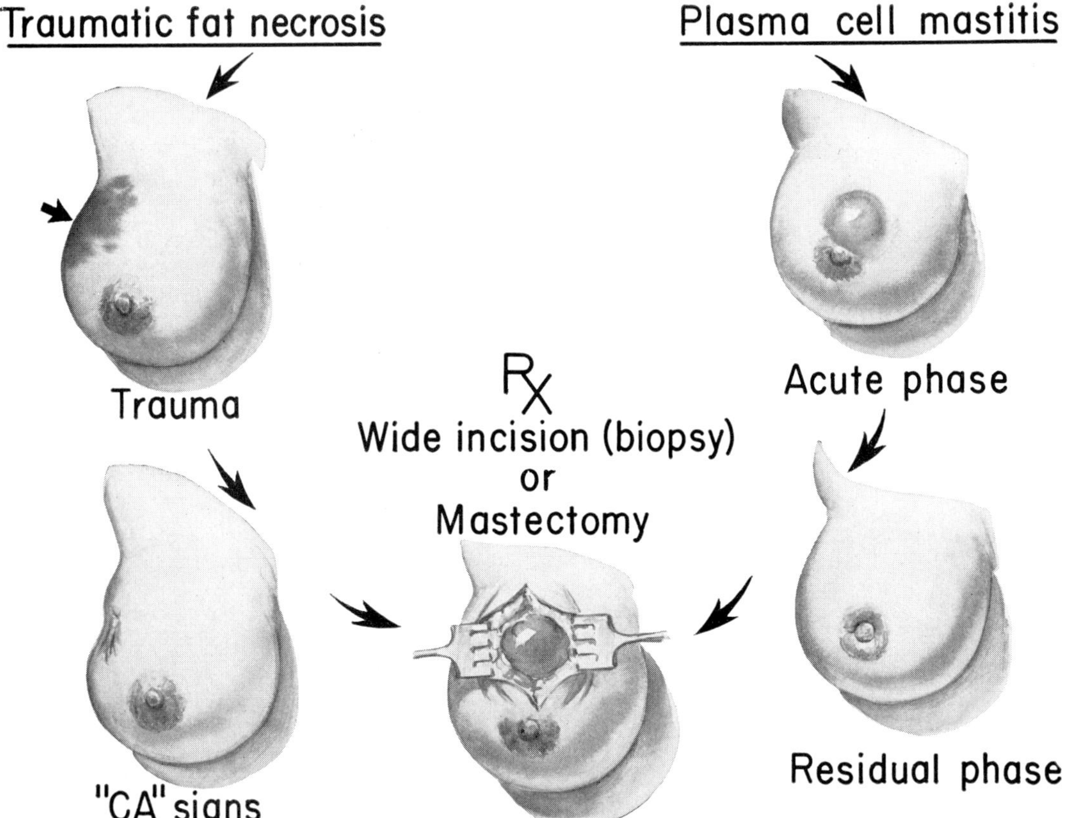

FIG. 137. Differential diagnosis of carcinoma of the breast. Two conditions—traumatic fat necrosis and plasma cell mastitis—may resemble a malignant neoplasm of the breast. The relationship of the lesion in plasma cell mastitis to the nipple should be noted.

majority heal without sequelae. In those cases that develop fat necrosis, the original pain, tenderness and discoloration disappear within 2 or 3 weeks, and the mass decreases in size. Rarely does the mass disappear entirely. It may take several months or years for the development of the dense fibrous tissue. When this latter stage appears, it is practically impossible to differentiate it from carcinoma. There is usually definite fixation of the mass to the skin, which gives rise to retraction of the skin as seen with malignancies. "Orange peel" skin rarely appears in fat necrosis, and retraction of the nipple is extremely uncommon. Enlarged axillary lymph nodes may be present.

Wide excision of the mass with thorough microscopic study is the only way in which a definite diagnosis can be made.

TUBERCULOSIS OF THE BREAST

This condition is quite rare and usually affects young women. Active lesions elsewhere in the body may or may not be demonstrable. The condition develops slowly with relatively little pain. It appears as a nodular mass fairly well localized at first but later involving the entire breast. The diagnosis is suspected if sinuses develop. Culture material from these may be helpful. Microscopic examination of tissue usually reveals tuberculosis. It may resemble carcinoma in many respects, and the differential diagnosis can be quite difficult.

SYPHILIS OF THE BREAST

This condition may be encountered in its primary, secondary or tertiary stage. The primary stage manifests itself as a chancre of the nipple; the secondary stage consists of skin reactions; tertiary stage gummas are rare. It is the tertiary lesion that must be differentiated from a neoplasm.

ACTINOMYCOSIS OF THE BREAST

This also is a rare condition. When found it is usually secondary to pulmonary actinomycosis which has broken through the thoracic wall and extended to the breast. At first firm nodules appear which become fixed to the skin; these finally form sinuses. It is prior to the sinus formation that these nodules simulate carcinoma. The diagnosis is confirmed by the finding of sulfur granules and the ray fungus.

PAGET'S DISEASE OF THE BREAST

It is currently thought that this disease represents a specialized form of intraductal carcinoma which arises in the main excretory ducts of the gland and extends upward to involve the skin of the nipple and the areola (Fig. 138). It was because of this malignant invasion of the skin and the resulting eczematoid changes that Paget believed the condition to be an inflammatory involvement of the skin. Careful morphologic study demonstrated that the intraductal carcinoma invariably antedates the skin changes. Therefore, any eczematoid lesion of the nipple must be considered as a sign of an underlying ductal carcinoma until proved to be otherwise.

Clinical Manifestations

The patient usually complains of itching and burning over an eczematous patch; this is accompanied by a constant weeping surface. The exudate is usually serous but may be bloody. Scabbing and crusting result in the formation of fissures. Ulceration develops, and retraction signs appear late. It is notoriously true that in a large percentage of cases no underlying mass is felt. However, when a mass is palpable, it has all the characteristics of a carcinomatous growth. A mass directly under the nipple may appear on the mammogram. Although such lesions

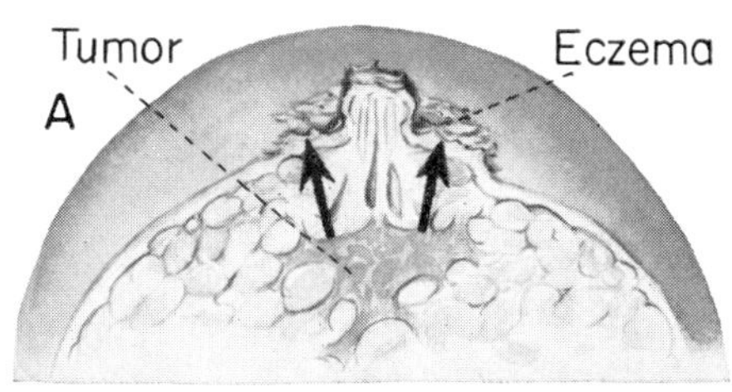

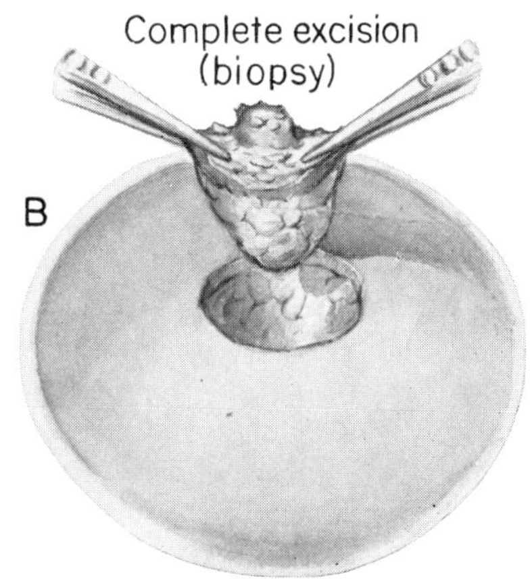

Fig. 138. Paget's disease is now thought to be a subareolar intraductal carcinoma frequently associated with an eczematoid lesion involving the overlying skin and the areola.

seem to be benign fibrosis, experience has taught that *every lesion under the nipple* must be considered to be malignant until proved to be otherwise. Microscopic study will determine the nature of the disease, particularly since the pathologist's landmark of this entity is the so-called pathognomonic Paget's cell. Since Paget's disease implies extension from an underlying carcinoma to the skin, the prognosis is somewhat unfavorable.

Treatment

It is agreed by most authorities that the nipple, the areola and the subareolar breast tissue should be removed en bloc (Fig. 138). This removes the entire involved area and affords adequate tissue for biopsy study. In the event that the lesion is benign, no future therapy is indicated; however, if a malignancy is discovered, mastectomy is indicated. How radical such mastectomies should be is still debated by experts.

6

Esophagogastrointestinal Tract

ESOPHAGUS

It is advantageous to consider an esophagogastrointestinal tract rather than an gastrointestinal tract. Many conditions that involve the lower end of the esophagus are frequently confused with lesions of the stomach and the bowel. These include cardiospasm, carcinoma, ruptured esophagus, diverticula, varices, esophagitis, and esophageal ulcers. They have been discussed elsewhere (pp. 82-89).

STOMACH

The more common conditions which affect the stomach are gastritis, peptic ulcer and its complications, tumor, acute dilatation, foreign bodies, specific granulomas, and infantile pyloric stenosis.

Mallory-Weiss Syndrome

In 1929 Mallory and Weiss described bleeding which resulted from lacerations of the cardiac end of the stomach. They noted this was associated with prolonged and/or forceful vomiting which usually *preceded* the appearance of blood (Fig. 139). Although uncommon, it is important, because it is one of those obscure sources of upper gastrointestinal hemorrhage that can be diagnosed preoperatively. Surgeons are reluctant to operate for gastrointestinal hemorrhage without a specific diagnosis. Some cases occur in

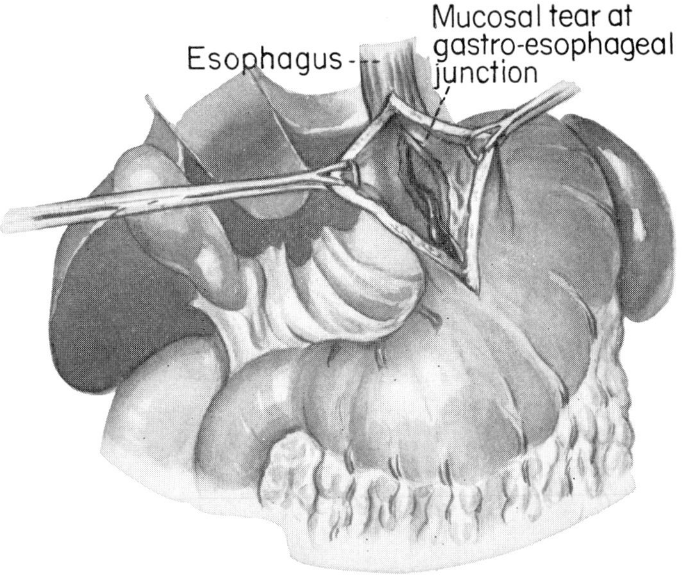

Fig. 139. Laceration of the esophagogastric area (Mallory-Weiss syndrome) with resultant massive gastric bleeding.

patients who retch and/or vomit repeatedly as a result of heavy drinking. Recent studies have related these tears to underlying and at times undemonstrable hiatal hernias. Atrophic gastritis may play a part in the production of such bleeding. Roentgenograms of the gastric cardia and the esophagogastric junction have failed to reveal the lesion. The flexible gastroscope may play a part in the diagnosing of this condition.

Gastritis

Gastritis or inflammation of the gastric mucosa occurs frequently. If it is present in a subclinical state, it is not a surgical problem. However, *2 forms* of gastritis are of surgical importance; these are chronic atrophic gastritis and chronic hypertrophic gastritis.

Chronic atrophic gastritis is of importance because of the possible relationship between it and gastric carcinoma. Fortunately, it presents certain pathologic characteristics which make it a recognizable entity. The involved area of mucosa is gray and flat and is covered with an excessive amount of mucus. Although it might affect any part of the stomach, the antrum usually is involved. Its symptomatology varies greatly. The patient may have few or no complaints, and the disease may be found coincidentally. Mild dyspepsia or epigastric distress might lead to an erroneous diagnosis of gallbladder disease, ulcer or carcinoma. At the operating table, the surgeon may demonstrate a mucosa that is difficult to diagnose; however, microscopic study reveals an atrophy of the mucous membrane.

Chronic hypertrophic gastritis usually presents more severe symptoms. In its focal form it is often confused with benign polyps; in its diffuse form it must be differentiated from multiple polyposis, infiltrating carcinoma and lymphosarcoma. The rugal folds may become so enlarged that they resemble the convolutions of the brain (Fig. 140). The epigastric distress can be severe; curtailment of food results in weakness and loss of weight.

Hemorrhage is particularly common; this fact has not been stressed sufficiently. The hemorrhage may be small in amount and chronic; this type is associated with severe secondary anemia. At times the hemorrhage may be acute and alarmingly massive. This type must be differentiated from hemorrhage associated with ulcers and varices.

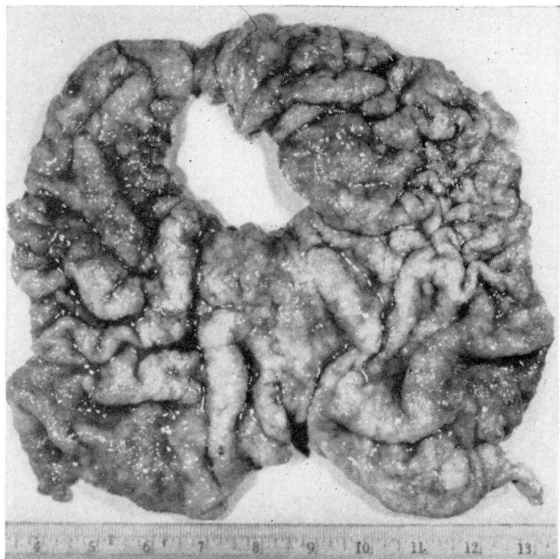

FIG. 140. Giant hypertrophic gastritis (Menetrier's disease). The stomach following partial gastrectomy has been opened along the greater curvature. The giant rugae resembling convolutions are noted.

Fluoroscopy and possible gastroscopy are of great value in diagnosing chronic hypertrophic gastritis. The symptoms may be so severe as to require gastric resection. The milder forms of the disease respond favorably to appropriate medical therapy. If the condition cannot definitely be differentiated from infiltrating carcinoma and lymphosarcoma, exploratory laparotomy becomes mandatory. The author has been particularly impressed with the value and the ease of gastrotomy. This permits careful inspection of the interior of the stomach and the removal of sections for microscopic study.

Gastric Ulcer

Most gastric ulcers are located in the pyloric region or along the lesser curvature (Fig. 141). Ulcers on the greater curvature are almost always malignant. Statistical data regarding malignant degeneration of these ulcers give a sense of false security. If every gastric ulcer is considered as a malignancy until proved to be otherwise, many lives will be salvaged.

Gastric and duodenal ulcers differ in many respects:

Gastric Ulcer	Duodenal Ulcer
1. Etiology apparently associated with a hormone secreted in the antrum of the stomach	1. Etiology apparently associated with the neurogenic (vagus) phase of secretion
2. Not related to hypersecretion and hyperacidity	2. Closely related to hypersecretion and hyperacidity
3. Potentially malignant	3. Rarely, if ever, malignant
4. Recurrence rate following adequate surgical therapy is low	4. Recurrence rate following adequate surgical therapy is relatively high
5. Treatment is preferably surgical	5. The treatment is preferably medical

To treat a gastric ulcer medically places a tremendous responsibility on the attending physician.

The typical ulcer story is described elsewhere (p. 127). In brief, it may be stated here that these patients complain of a burning or gnawing epigastric distress which ap-

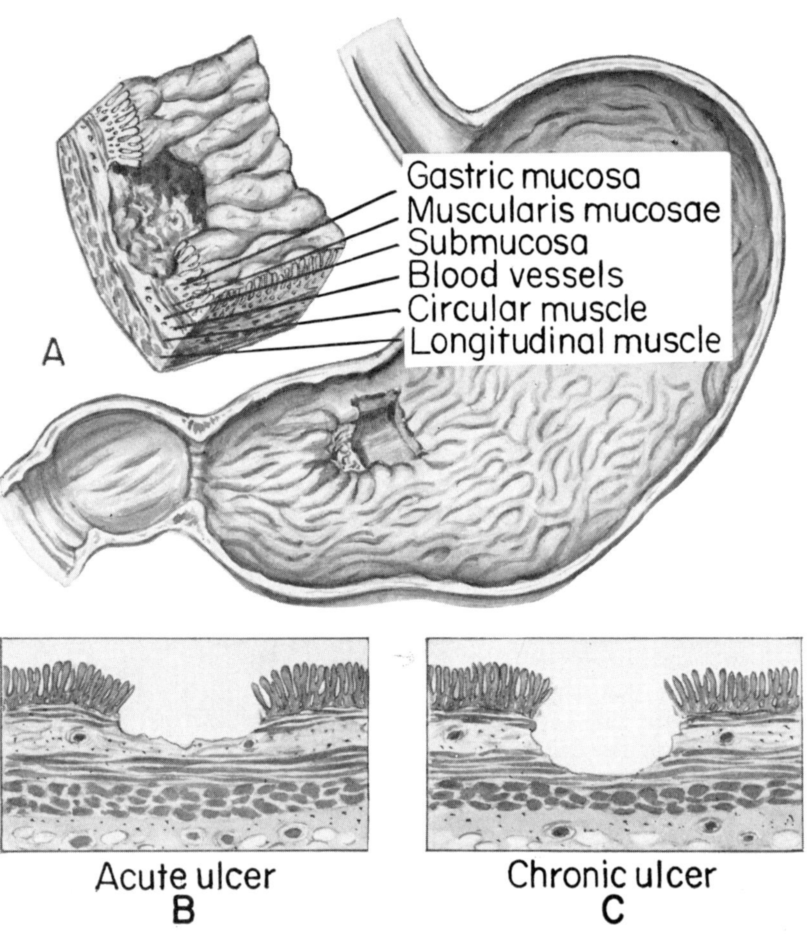

Fig. 141. (A) Gastric ulcers must be considered as carcinoma until proved to be otherwise. (B) The acute ulcer has a relatively small crater involving only the mucosa and possibly the superficial layers of submucosa. (C) The chronic ulcer is round or oval and presents a punched-out appearance with relatively straight walls. As it progresses downward, it incorporates the deeper layers.

pears a few hours after meals and is relieved by vomiting, alkalies or the intake of food. The symptom pattern of the gastric ulcer patient is a little less definite than that of the duodenal ulcer. The complaint of "dyspepsia" (heartburn, gas, eructations) is probably the most common one. Diagnosis is aided by means of fluoroscopic, roentgenographic and at times gastroscopic examinations. Studies of gastric acidity are of limited value and are not pathognomonic.

Various isotopic and radioactive principles are now being applied to the diagnosis of gastric lesions. It has been suggested that cancerous tissue has a greater appetite for phosphorus than normal tissue. Radioactive phosphorus (P^{32}) is used in the hope that beta particle emissions will indicate whether the lesion is malignant or not. Time will tell whether methods such as these will prove to be beneficial. Let us hope that this newer approach will lead us to earlier diagnoses of gastric carcinoma, since the surgical results for this condition are anything but gratifying. One must be particularly mindful of those gastric "ulcers" which respond, both clinically and radiologically, to medical management and return some months later with a far-advanced malignant lesion at the site of that "ulcer."

The complications of gastric ulcer which are similar to those of duodenal ulcer are discussed on page 129.

Benign Tumors of the Stomach

These tumors produce clinical manifestations sufficient to warrant surgery in only 1 to 2 per cent of cases. Most frequently they are polyps or leiomyomas.

The polyp is usually a well-formed rounded mass which varies in size; it may be sessile but usually presents a clearly differentiated head and stalk. It is definitely movable. The common secondary changes are inflammation, ulceration and hemorrhage. Diagnosis usually is made by roentgenologic or gastroscopic examinations or surgery. In patients with multiple polyps the exact number or locations can be determined only by gastrotomy. Since they might undergo malignant degeneration, their identification is important.

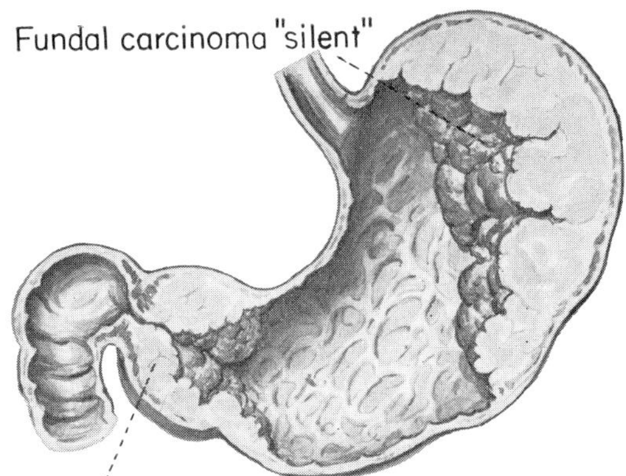

FIG. 142. Carcinoma of the stomach. The tumor manifests itself earlier when it involves the pyloric end, because it causes obstruction. A tumor at the fundal end of the stomach may reach huge proportions before producing clinical manifestations.

Carcinoma of the Stomach

Over 30,000 lives are lost annually in this country as a result of gastric carcinoma. It is the most common malignant tumor in males and is nearly as prevalent in females as carcinoma of the uterus or the breast. Although it is encountered most frequently in the 5th and the 6th decades of life, it is seen all too frequently in the 4th and the 3rd decades. Cases have been reported under 20 years of age. It is clinically "silent" for a considerable length of time; metastases are present in at least 50 per cent of patients by the time their first symptoms appear.

When a *change of habit* occurs in any organ or system in the body, carcinoma must be considered until proved to be otherwise. The stomach is no exception to this rule; these patients become aware of a change in their eating or digesting habits. Such a patient becomes "stomach-conscious." Although gastritis, peptic ulcer, gallbladder disease—to mention only a few—may produce this "change of habit," carcinoma must be the first condition to be ruled out. Epigastric distress, anorexia, nausea or vague abdominal complaints, if unexplainable and persistent beyond a period of a few weeks, require exhaustive study. A tumor at the pyloric end

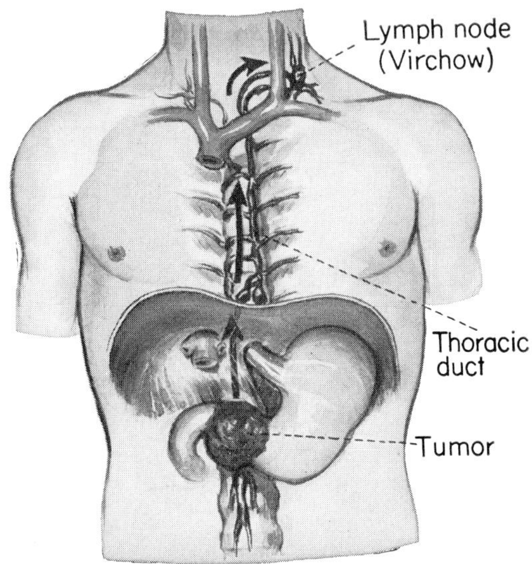

FIG. 143. Virchow's node. This is an involvement of the lymph glands in the left supraclavicular space frequently associated with carcinoma of the stomach.

will produce earlier symptoms because it obstructs; however, in the fundus the neoplasm may become very large before it manifests itself (Fig. 142). The fundal carcinoma is fortunately the rarer type; because of its chronicity, anemia may be the outstanding and only feature. The presence of "coffee-ground" vomitus is evidence of ulceration and bleeding associated with gastric retention. When the mass is palpable in gastric carcinoma, the lesion is usually far-advanced and often inoperable. Anemia and loss of weight are *late* manifestations.

A filling defect is the significant roentgenographic finding. Of limited value is the examination of the gastric contents, which may show blood, lactic acid, anacidity and sarcinae. People with apparently normal stomachs may have little or no gastric acid, and patients with gastric carcinoma have been known to have hyperacidity.

The tumor may spread by direct contiguity into surrounding structures, or it may spread by lymph vessels, blood vessels, or gravity. It is unfortunate that carcinoma of the stomach is notorious for the frequency with which metastases are present at the time of surgical exploration. Of particular serious prognostic importance is the finding of a left supraclavicular lymph node known as Virchow's sentinel node (Fig. 143). This node is no longer considered to be pathognomonic of gastric cancer, since it is found also in carcinoma of the lung or of the esophagus, or it may represent a primary lymphoma. In some clinics it is standard practice to take a biopsy of so-called *scalene nodes* when occult gastric carcinoma is suspected. As the carcinoma spreads through the muscularis and involves the serosa of the stomach, widespread secondary peritoneal implants may develop. The ovaries are particularly receptive to such cells. Such "gravity" or dropped metastases may form pelvic masses which are detectable on rectal and vaginal examinations. Blood-born metastases may appear in remote parts of the body.

When a peptic ulcer becomes malignant, the transformation occurs at the mucosal margins. If the lesion is not too far advanced, the base remains free of tumor infiltration. When a frozen section biopsy is taken, the mucosal margins must be included. It is sad to relate that many gastric carcinomas are inoperable at the time of discovery, and that the survival rate following gastrectomy is only 12 to 18 months in the vast majority of cases.

Sarcoma of the Stomach

This tumor constitutes about 1 per cent of all gastric malignancies; like carcinoma, it is observed more frequently in males. *Lymphosarcoma* is the most common type of gastric sarcoma. The clinical picture is similar to that of carcinoma. Microscopic examination reveals the true nature of the lesion. The differentiation between carcinoma and sarcoma of the stomach is important, since the prognosis in a well-localized sarcoma is much more favorable than that in carcinoma. The usual appearance of these mesenchymal malignancies as large bulky, soft tumors makes them quite distinctive macroscopically from carcinoma.

Syphilis of the Stomach

This disease may produce symptoms and roentgenologic findings similar to those of cancer or peptic ulcer. The differentiation becomes particularly difficult when a patient

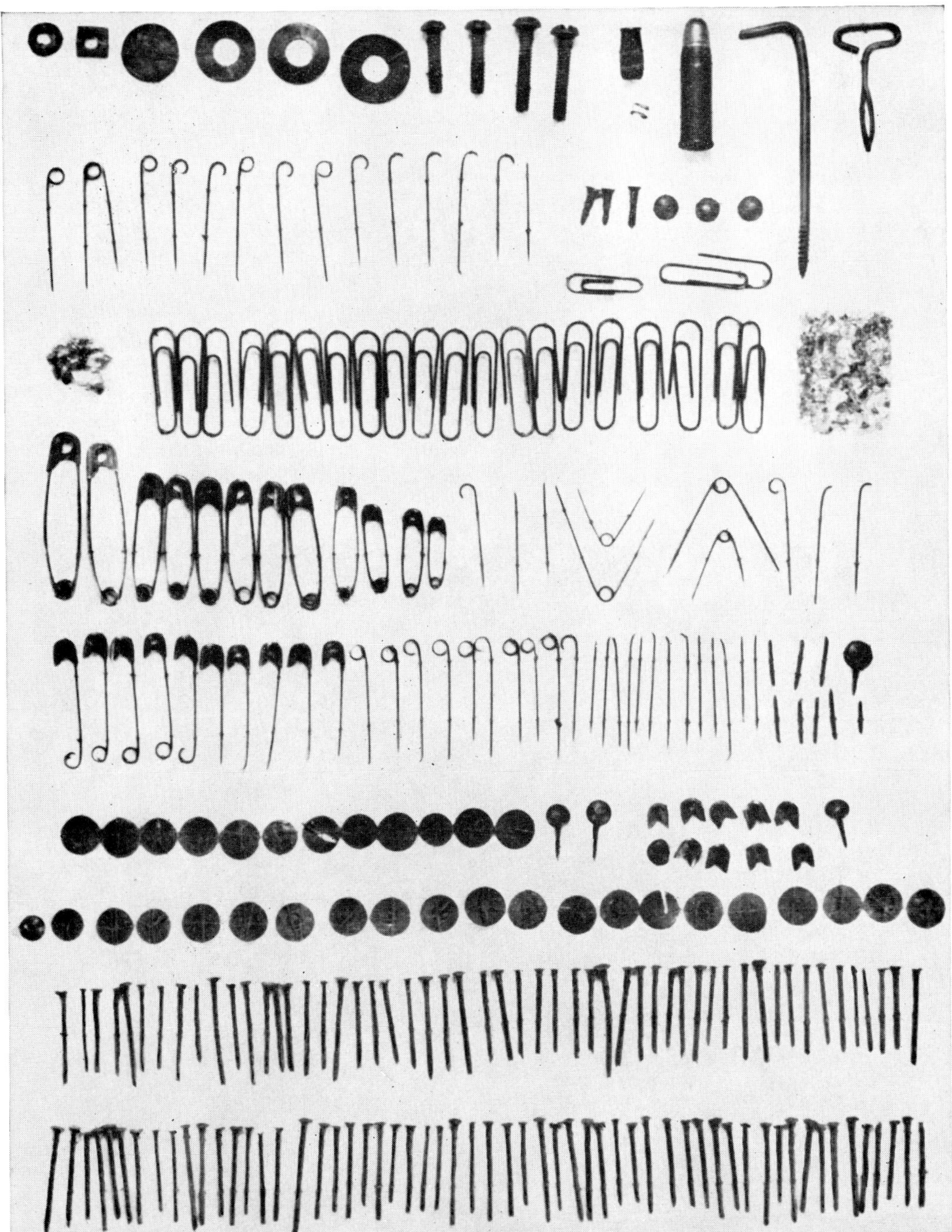

FIG. 144. It is surprising what can pass through the esophagogastrointestinal tract. This figure shows only a small number of objects removed from the stomach of a professional swallower. He performed his feats for many years, experiencing no difficulties whatsoever. One of the safety pins opened and perforated the stomach.

with a gastric ulcer has a positive serologic response.

Foreign Bodies in the Stomach

This condition is encountered frequently. Most objects that pass the mouth can be passed per rectum; however, they require constant observation with serial fluoroscopic and roentgenologic examinations. If the object is sharp, and periodic roentgenologic examinations reveal that it has become stationary, exploratory laparotomy is indicated (Fig. 144). *Food balls* represent a type of foreign body; they develop from tough vegetable fibers, particularly persimmons. They are referred to by the general term of "bezoars." Bezoars of vegetable origin are called phytobezoars, and those of animal origin (hair) are known as trichobezoars. Roentgen examinations after ingestion of barium reveal their presence.

Acute Dilatation of the Stomach

This change occurs as a postoperative or post-traumatic complication, particularly when peritonitis is present. The entire stomach becomes dilated with liquid and gas and produces upper abdominal distention (Fig. 145); if marked, such distention results in cardiorespiratory embarrassment. Pain is not a predominant symptom, but continuous vomiting produces rapid deterioration. Hiccough is a frequent symptom. Diagnosis is simple if the condition is kept in mind. Nasogastric siphonage results in deflation and immediate relief. If the condition remains un-

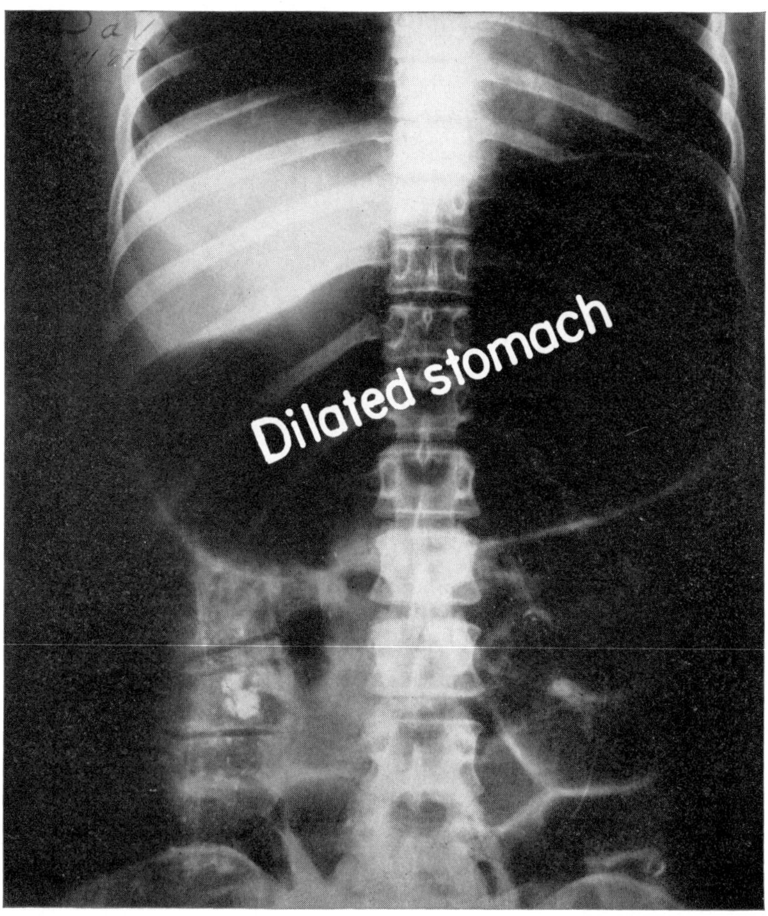

Fig. 145. Roentgenogram of acute gastric dilatation. The subdiaphragmatic air is postoperative.

diagnosed and untreated, death results quite rapidly.

Infantile Pyloric Stenosis

This condition is encountered in well-developed firstborn male infants (Fig. 146). The first 2 or 3 weeks of life are usually uneventful, and then without warning or apparent cause the child begins to vomit. This condition becomes progressively worse until little or nothing is retained. Emaciation, oliguria, obstipation and alkalosis result. If untreated, death occurs before 3 months of age as a result of starvation or complicating pneumonia.

Physical examination usually reveals vigorous gastric peristaltic waves which pass from left to right across the upper abdomen and terminate under the right costal margin (Fig. 146). In this latter area one can frequently palpate a firm olive-shaped (pyloric) mass. The vomitus does not contain bile, since the obstruction is complete and proximal to the ampulla of Vater (Fig. 146 B). A roentgenogram reveals a large dilated stomach (Fig. 147); fluoroscopy indicates pyloric obstruction.

Heredity plays an important role in the etiology of this condition, but its exact nature is unknown.

Microscopically, the mass consists of hypertrophied muscle involving the circular coat. The longitudinal muscle contributes little to the mass, and there is no significant increase in fibrous tissue. The muscle mass reaches its maximum firmness between the 4th and the 9th weeks of life, and then with gradual stretching of the serosa it becomes progressively softer. This coincides with the clinical observation that if a child can be maintained in good general health with medical treatment beyond 3 months of age, he is likely to recover without having to resort to surgical intervention.

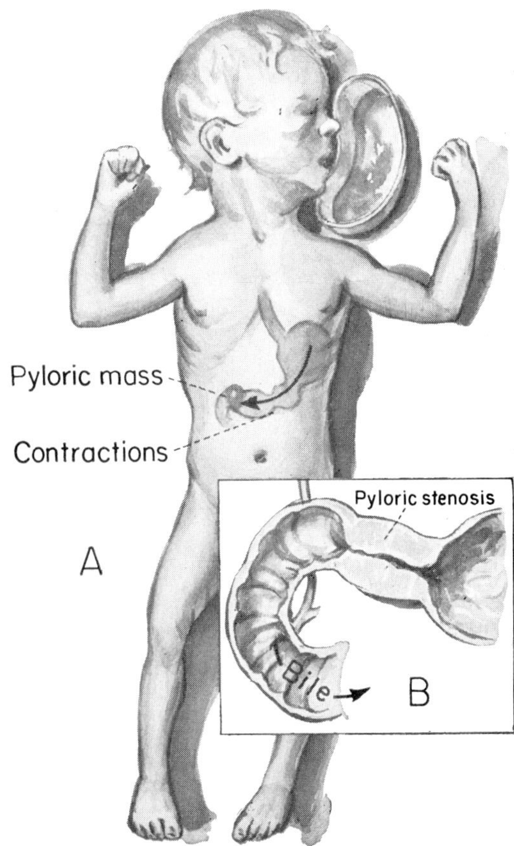

Fig. 146. Infantile pyloric stenosis. (A) Hyperperistaltic contractions passing from left to right and a palpable pyloric mass are characteristic. (B) The emesis is not bile-stained, since the obstruction is complete and proximal to the ampulla of Vater.

DUODENUM

Duodenal Ulcer

Incidence. This is a common disease. It has been estimated that from 5 to 10 per cent of our population is affected with this lesion. Some authorities are of the opinion that it is related to the increased tension of modern life. Men are afflicted more frequently than women; peptic ulceration occurs more frequently in the duodenum than in the stomach (5 to 1). It usually appears in the 3rd or the 4th decades, is worse in the spring and the fall, at times of great mental stress, and following infections. It is associated with remissions and exacerbations, so that in the symptom-free period the patient believes that he is cured.

Symptoms. A typical story is usually elicited. When the patient awakes following some hours of sleep, his pain is not present; this is believed to be due to the fact that his secretion, acidity and gastrointestinal activity are diminished. The pain appears between breakfast and lunch. Rarely is it unbearable and has been described as burning, gnawing or a "hunger pain." It is relieved by one of 3 things: food, alkalies or vomiting. It recurs some hours after lunch, usually between lunch and dinner, and appears again between dinner and bedtime. Frequently, these patients are awakened by the pain after a short sleep; they retire with milk or food at their bedside to relieve such distress. Heartburn and eructations, although present, are not characteristic, since they occur in many other conditions. If vomiting is present early in the course of the disease, it probably is due to edema or pylorospasm; if it occurs later, it is due to scar tissue (organic obstruction).

Examination. Physical examination may reveal tenderness deep in the epigastrium, presumably over the lesion. Superficial tenderness or hyperasthesia is due to referred pain. A study of gastric contents is of some value, because with duodenal ulcer there is usually a hyperacidity and hypersecretion. The roentgenographic examination usually reveals the ulcer, which is located most frequently in the first part of the duodenum.

Types. A *simple* peptic ulcer is one that has eroded or involved only the mucosa and has not involved the deeper layers (Fig. 148). A *penetrating* ulcer is one which involves the deeper layers and penetrates into an adjacent organ. These usually are located at the posterior aspect of the first part of the duodenum; they attack the pancreas. Because the pancreas seals these ulcers, they rarely perforate. A *perforating* ulcer is one which is not protected by an adjacent viscus and is perforating into the peritoneal cavity. These ulcers are usually on the anterior gastric or duodenal wall; if untreated, they will perforate into the peritoneal cavity. Clinically, penetrating and perforating ulcers differ from simple ulcers in 3 ways, in that the

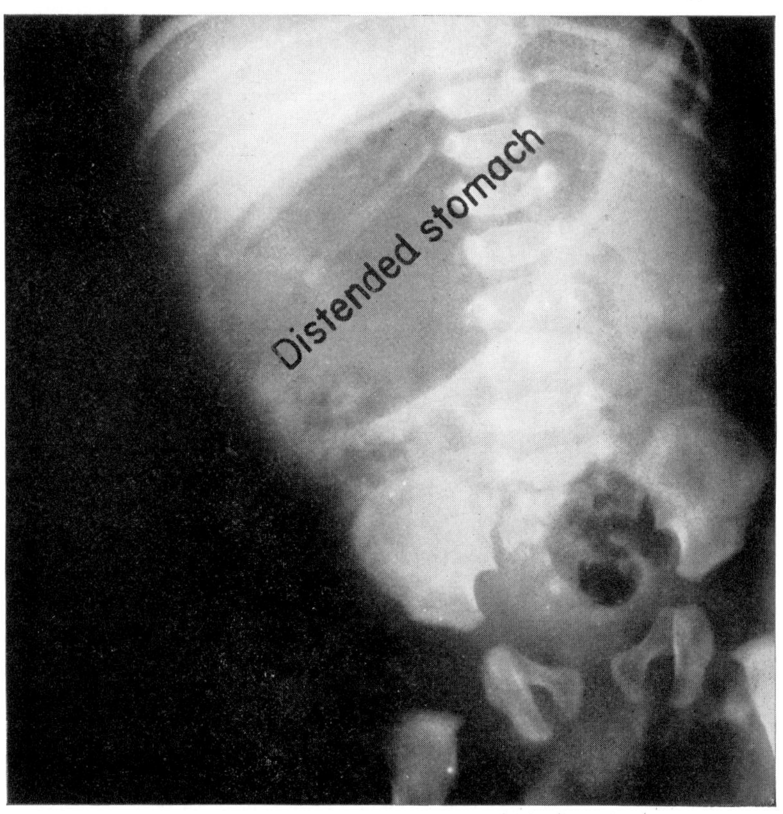

FIG. 147. Roentgenogram of an infantile pyloric stenosis.

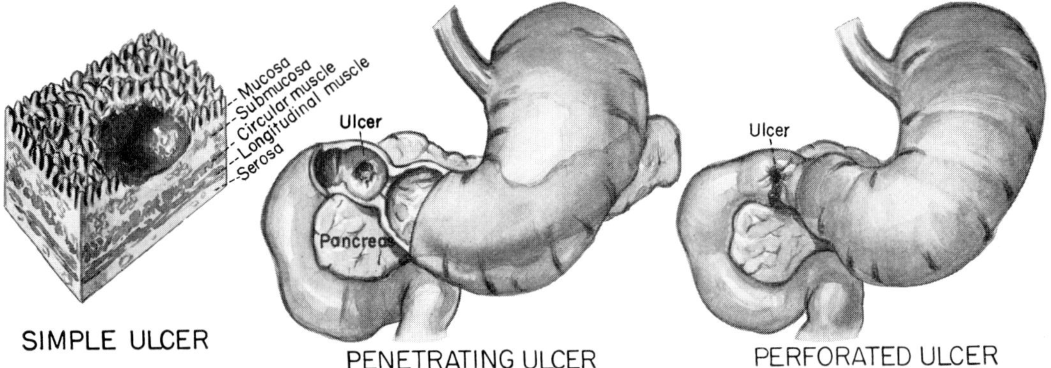

FIG. 148. Peptic ulcers may be simple, penetrating or perforated (see text).

pain becomes continuous, is far more severe and is difficult to relieve. Those ulcers which penetrate posteriorly into the pancreas usually are associated with pain in the region of the 9th to the 11th dorsal vertebrae. Tenderness is most marked in the perforating variety. Roentgenologic examination reveals the lesion. Such lesions have been known to perforate while under the fluoroscopic screen; hence, caution is the keynote.

Complications of Peptic Ulcers

The 3 most important complications are hemorrhage, obstruction and perforation (Fig. 149). Combined, they appear in serious forms in about 5 to 10 per cent of all peptic ulcer patients. They are present in both gastric and duodenal ulcers. Carcinoma is a 4th complication but applies almost entirely to gastric lesions (p. 123).

Hemorrhage. Bleeding from peptic ulcers may be mild, moderate or massive. The term "massive" is applied to those cases that present a sudden loss of at least 1 liter of blood; clinical manifestations of shock, and anemia associated with a red blood cell count below 2.5 million per cu. mm. are usually present. These patients vomit bright red blood or pass tarry black blood per rectum. The vessel that is usually involved is the gastroduodenal artery. Abdominal auscultation is helpful, since the bowel sounds are increased with intraintestinal hemorrhage. However, in intraperitoneal hemorrhage the abdominal sounds are diminished or absent (Fig. 150).

If the patients are in a younger age group (under 45 years), atheromatosis is usually not advanced; the elastic blood vessels contract and control the hemorrhage. If the patient is older, the sclerotic vessels are unable

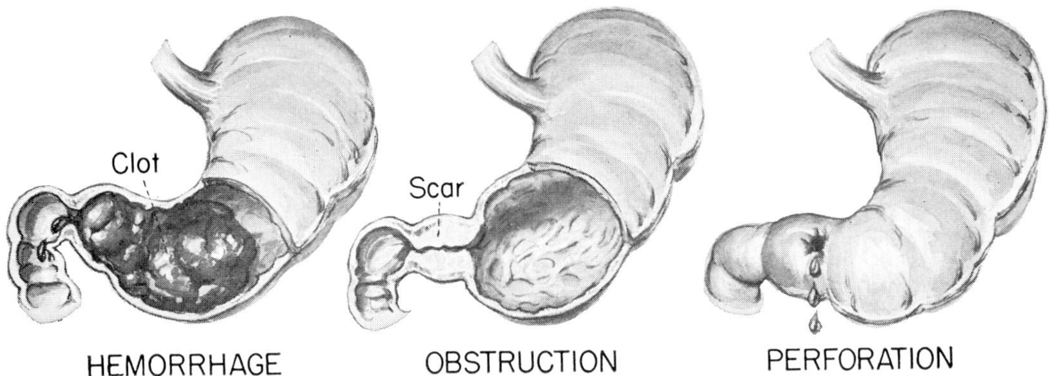

FIG. 149. Complications of peptic ulcers. Malignant degeneration, a 4th complication, applies almost entirely to gastric ulcers.

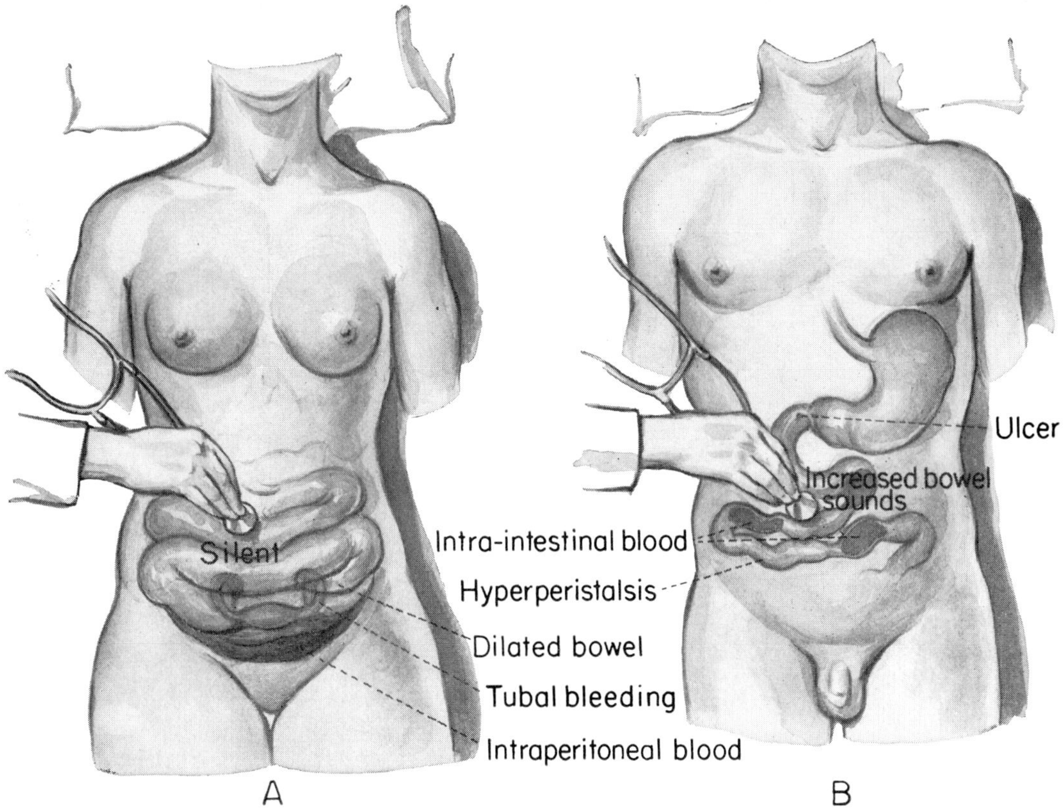

Silent
Intra-intestinal blood
Hyperperistalsis
Dilated bowel
Tubal bleeding
Intraperitoneal blood
Ulcer
Increased bowel sounds
A
B

FIG. 150. Intra-intestinal or intraperitoneal hemorrhage? (A) In intraperitoneal bleeding (regardless of cause) the bowel sounds are diminished because of the dilated bowel which results from the chemical peritonitis. (B) In intra-intestinal bleeding the bowel sounds are hyperactive because of the blood-filled gut.

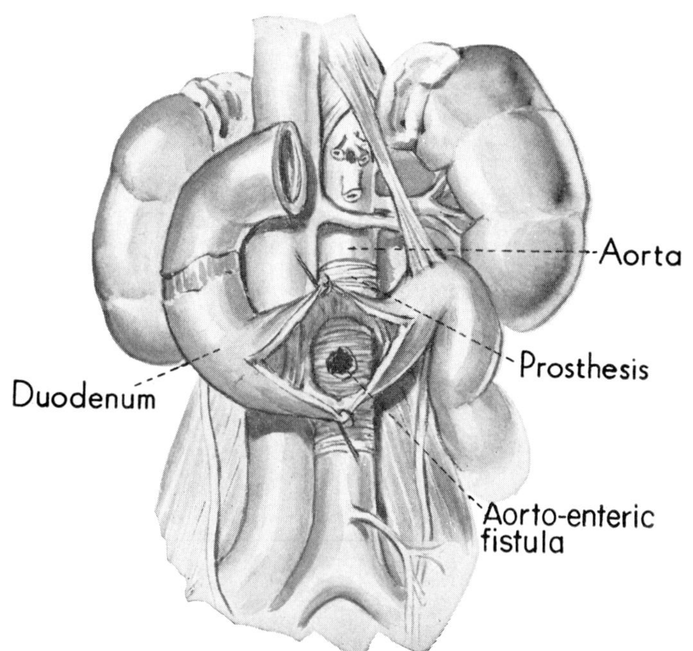

FIG. 151. Aorto-enteric fistula resulting from erosion of an abdominal aortic graft. This must be considered in the differential diagnosis of gastrointestinal bleeding.

to contract, and the bleeding usually continues. Massive bleeding from gastroduodenal ulcers must be differentiated from bleeding anywhere in the esophagogastrointestinal tract.

Since the advent of vascular surgery and the placement of aortic prosthesis, a new condition must be considered in the differential diagnosis of gastrointestinal bleeding. An abdominal aortic graft may give rise to an aorto-enteric communication as a result of erosion or the formation of a false aneurysm (Fig. 151). Successful treatment depends on prompt and accurate diagnosis. Although bright-red blood passed per rectum usually means lower (colon) intestinal bleeding, peptic ulcer bleeding also may produce bright-red blood in the stool because of the associated hyperperistalsis. This is the exception and not the rule.

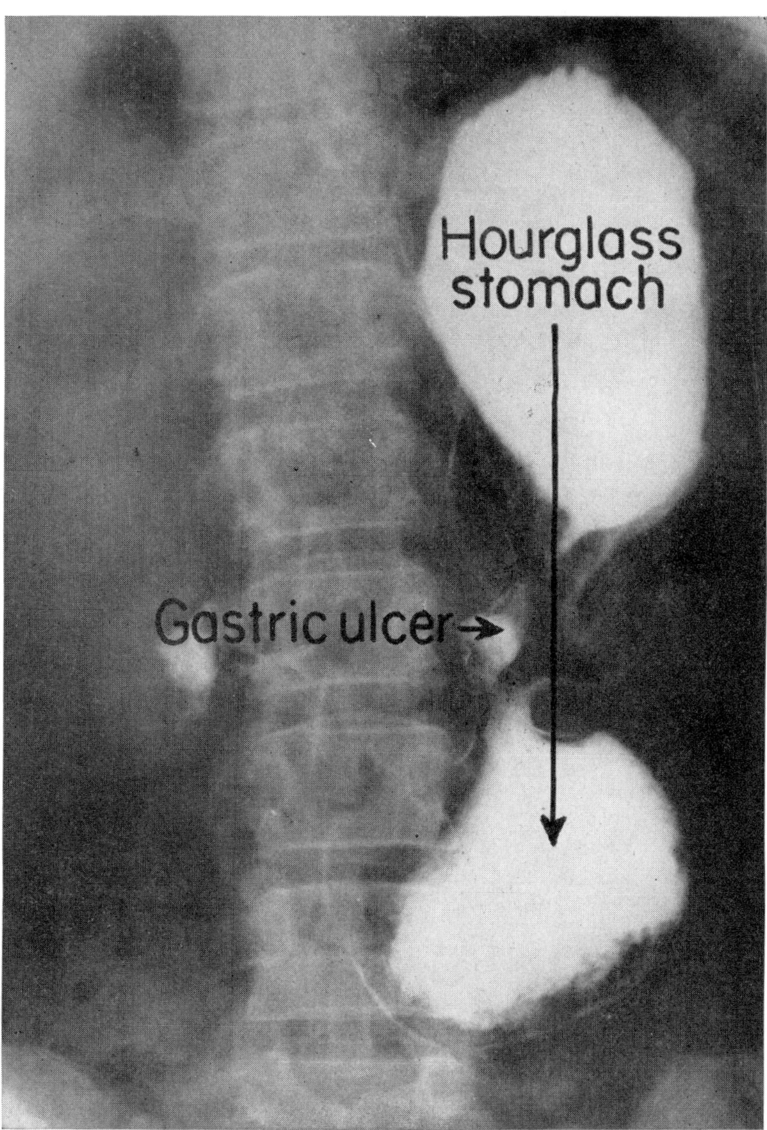

Fig. 152. Roentgenogram of an hourglass contracture of the stomach resulting from a gastric ulcer.

Inspection reveals marked pallor. Pain is almost always absent, and there are no signs of peritoneal irritation. Blood counts, hematocrit, blood volume, and hemoglobin determinations are helpful but are not as significant, particularly regarding the progress of the case, as are the blood pressure and the pulse.

Obstruction. As pyloric obstruction develops, vomiting increases and becomes the outstanding symptom. Little or no relief is obtained, and eating usually aggravates the distress. Gastric ulcers located in the pars media produce an hourglass contracture and obstruction (Fig. 152). Dehydration, emaciation and electrolyte imbalance develop rapidly. The vomitus contains undigested food; if bile is absent after repeated bouts of vomiting, the obstruction is complete. It may be difficult to determine how much of the obstruction is due to scar tissue, spasm or edema. A therapeutic test of conservative therapy may be tried. This consists of frequent feedings, alkalies, antispasmodics and nasogastric siphonage. If retention diminishes after such treatment, part of the obstruction was due to edema and spasm.

Perforation. This usually appears with dramatic suddenness. It occurs more frequently in males. A previous ulcer history is usually present. Following the ingestion of a meal, the patient experiences a pain so severe that he "doubles up" or "falls to the floor." At no time in his life has he experienced a pain of such severity. *Prostration* is present. This should not be confused with shock, which is unusual in these cases. Although the patient is bathed in a cold sweat, and the extremities are cold and clammy, the pulse and the blood pressure remain normal. The

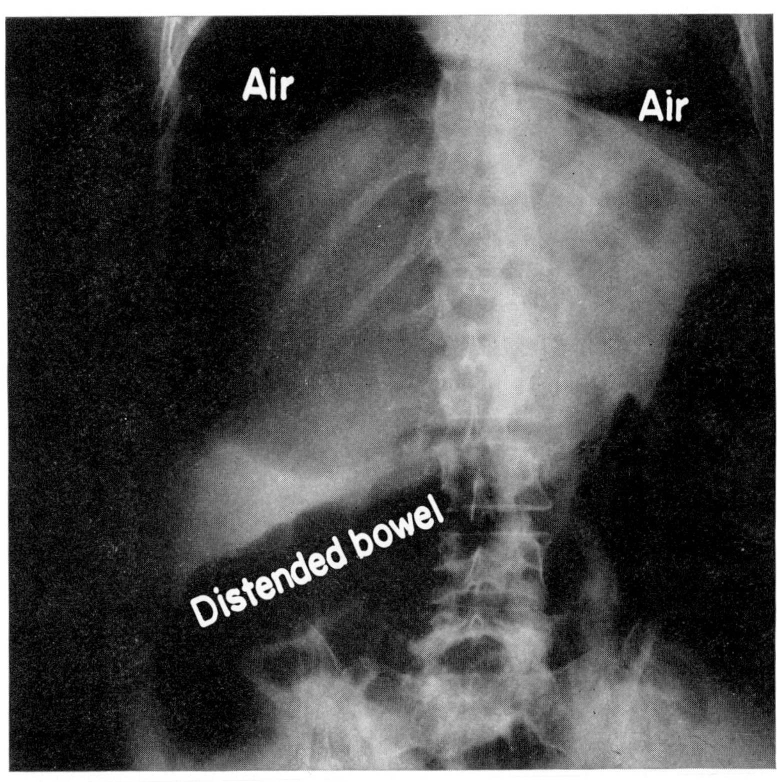

FIG. 153. Roentgenogram revealing a spontaneous pneumoperitoneum in a case of perforated peptic ulcer. These pictures must be taken with the patient upright or on his left side to permit the air bubble to "float up" and separate the right hemidiaphragm from the right lobe of the liver.

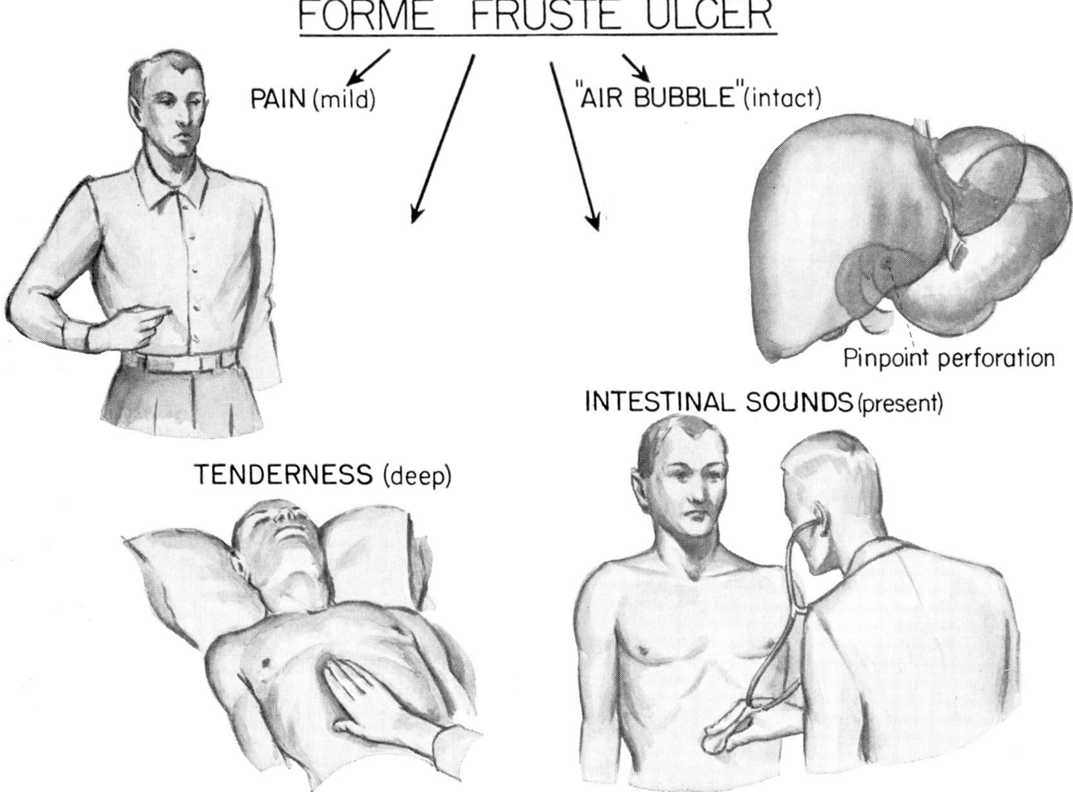

FIG. 154. The forme fruste ulcer. This pinpoint perforation seals off rapidly and produces minimal peritoneal signs. Therefore, it is easily overlooked. The patient has mild pain and is not prostrate but ambulatory; the tenderness is absent or deep, the bowel sounds are present, and a spontaneous pneumoperitoneum is not demonstrated on the roentgenogram.

patient has an anxious, pale expression, and the respirations are shallow and rapid. The reason for this type of breathing is that it is almost entirely thoracic without an abdominal component.

When a patient states that he does not wish to move or to be moved, one must suspect *peritonitis*. If the patient requests the driver of the auto or ambulance to "drive slowly" and "take the bumps easily," he has peritonitis. The patient with *colic* is usually restless and seeks relief by moving about; this is diametrically opposed to the patient with peritonitis, who wishes to be perfectly quiet (Fig. 294).

Abdominal rigidity in all 4 quadrants is present and is "boardlike." Tenderness is intense, particularly over the ulcer site. Abdominal auscultation is very helpful, since almost every patient with a perforated peptic ulcer has a *silent abdomen*.

A *spontaneous pneumoperitoneum* is present in about 75 per cent of these patients (Fig. 153). The presence and the visualization of free air in the peritoneal cavity indicates a perforation of a hollow viscus, not necessarily a perforated peptic ulcer. However, if there is an antecedent peptic ulcer history, the diagnosis of a perforated peptic ulcer is almost a certainty. The "air bubble" will be seen as a translucent area on the right side, as it separates the diaphragm and the right lobe of the liver. In the upright position, air may be seen under the left hemidiaphragm; this may be confused with the normal intragastric "air bubble." If the air

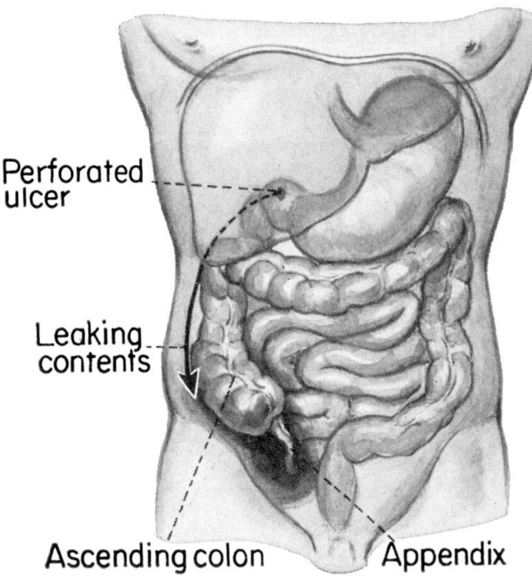

FIG. 155. Acute appendicitis or perforated peptic ulcer? These 2 conditions may be confused, because leaking contents from the ulcer may pool around a normal appendix, producing a "serosal appendicitis."

under the left hemidiaphragm is free intraperitoneal air, the thickness of the diaphragm is less than a quarter of an inch; whereas, if it is gastric air, the thickness includes both the diaphragm and the stomach wall and appears to be thicker.

Obliteration of liver dullness can be demonstrated by percussion if a large amount of intraperitoneal air is present.

FORME FRUSTE ULCER

This is a pinpoint perforation that is sealed rapidly. The rapid closure is brought about by plugging of the perforation or obliteration by the under surface of the liver or by the gallbladder. Since the perforation is small and the sealing rapid, the leakage is minimal. The peritoneum usually can cope with a small amount of soiling, which is chemical and relatively sterile; hence, the clinical manifestations are minimal or absent (Fig. 154). The patient may walk about, the pain is slight, tenderness is absent or deep, the bowel sounds are usually present, and the spontaneous pneumoperitoneum (air bubble)

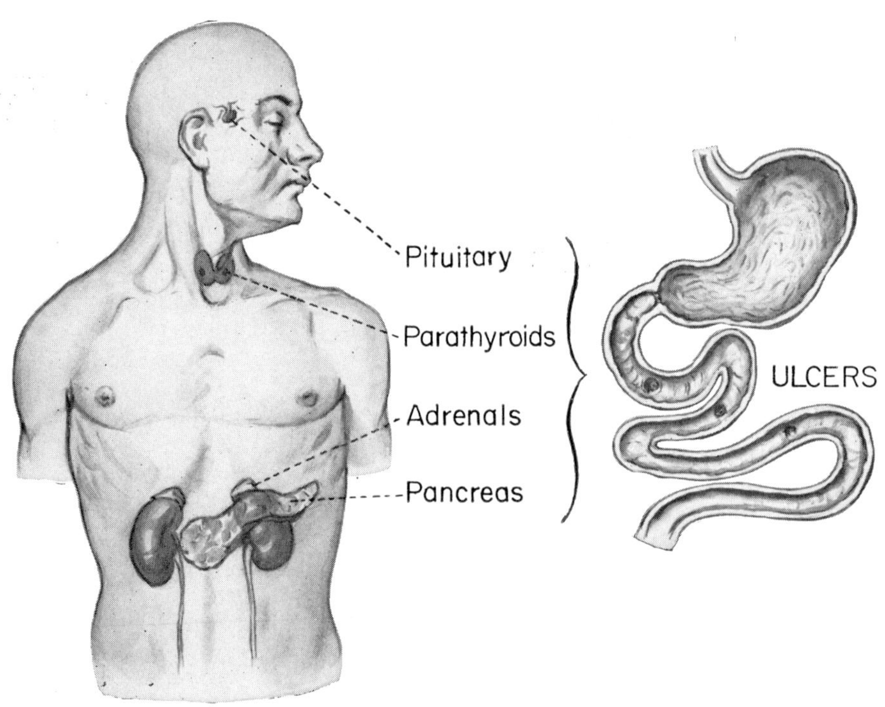

FIG. 156. Ulcerogenic lesions of some endocrine glands must be considered in atypical peptic ulcer response.

is lacking. These are the cases that are most likely to escape detection. Patients with this type of perforation reperforate with their next meal. With the 2nd perforation the classic picture usually becomes manifest. Perforated peptic ulcer may be confused with appendicitis (p. 143) when the upper abdominal pain shifts to the right lower quadrant. Such shifting in perforated ulcers is due to the gravitation of escaped duodenal or gastric contents along the "paracolic gutter" of the ascending colon. The contents pool around the appendiceal area and produce a "serosal appendicitis" (Fig. 155). These patients have right lower quadrant or McBurney point tenderness. Such errors should be infrequent if the physician recalls that the patient with a perforated peptic ulcer is much sicker, has tenderness along the entire "paracolic gutter," absence of bowel sounds, air in the peritoneal cavity, and usually an antecedent ulcer history.

Occasionally, a perforated peptic ulcer is seen in infants. The etiology is unknown.

Polyendocrine Aspects of Peptic Ulcer

The so-called Zollinger-Ellison syndrome was reported by these 2 surgeons in 1955. This added a new facet to the duodenal ulcer problem. They described intractable peptic ulcers seemingly associated with noninsulin-producing islet cell tumors of the pancreas. The syndrome is associated with severe hypersecretion (over 2,500 ml.) as determined by overnight gastric suction, ulcers in atypical locations, and an excessively high incidence of recurrence regardless of the type of therapy. Many such cases end fatally as a result of perforation and/or hemorrhage. Recent evidence suggests that this is only one manifestation of a widespread endocrine disorder. Such ulcerogenic adenomas or abnormalities have been reported in the pituitary, the parathyroids, the adrenals and even the duodenum (Fig. 156). Duodenal wall adenomas are histologically similar to the adenomas occurring in the pancreas. They have been referred to as duodenal "islet cell" adenomas.

The use of cortisone and related compounds can produce gastroduodenal ulcers or exacerbations of older ones. Massive gastrointestinal hemorrhage is the chief complication.

In patients demonstrating atypically located ulcers (esophagus, 2nd and 3rd portions of the duodenum, jejunum), severe intractability and recurrences, this syndrome must be considered. A high index of suspi-

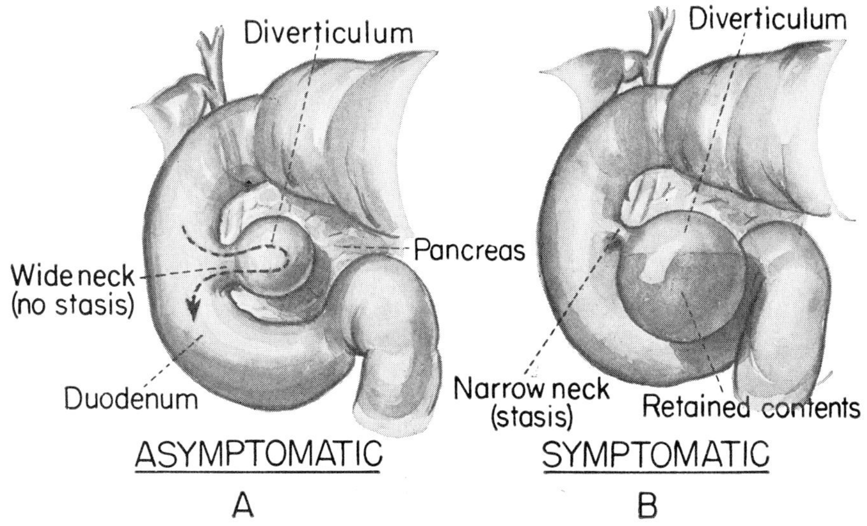

Fig. 157. Duodenal diverticulum. (A) If the neck of the diverticulum is wide, contents may enter and leave without producing stasis. (B) If the neck of the diverticulum is narrow, gastrointestinal contents become entrapped and produce stasis, which in turn results in inflammation and its sequelae.

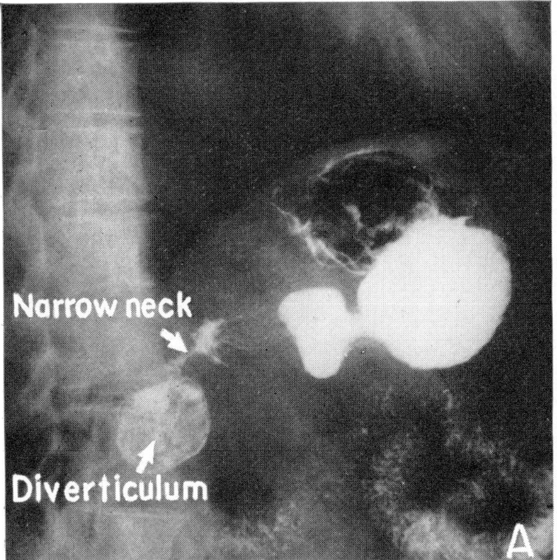

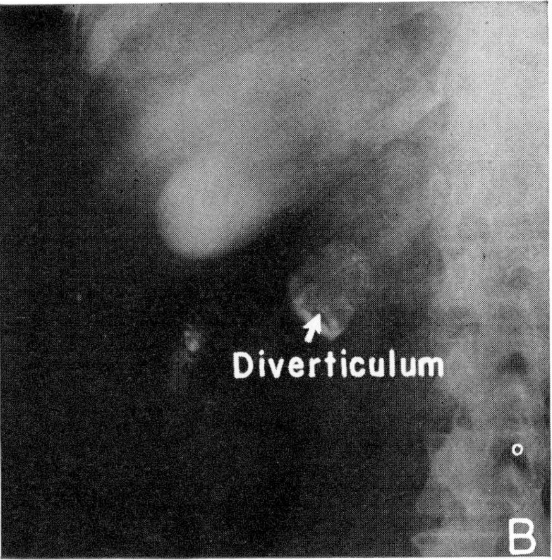

Fig. 158. Roentgenogram of a diverticulum of the descending part of the duodenum. (A) The narrow neck of the diverticulum should be noted. (B) Retention of barium in the diverticulum 24 hours after ingestion of the meal.

sion on the part of the clinician will be most rewarding. These ulcerogenic tumors have a tendency to become malignant.

Duodenal Diverticulum

These diverticula are present in from 2 to 5 per cent of all persons past 50 years of age. The exact cause is unknown, but there is general agreement that a point of weakness is present where blood vessels, nerves and ducts enter and leave the bowel. The frequent occurrence in the 2nd part of the duodenum, particularly about the ampulla, is believed to be due to a weakness of the wall caused by the passage of the common bile and pancreatic ducts at this site (Fig. 157). The diverticulum may vary in size from the size of a pea to that of a pear; it is characteristically ovoid in shape. The vast majority project from the concave aspect of the duodenum in the 2nd, the 3rd and the 4th portions.

No characteristic symptoms exist. The condition may be symptomless and found coincidentally in the course of a roentgenologic examination. Symptoms, if present, may mimic those of gallbladder or gastric diseases. The most common symptom is pain or discomfort of varying intensity in the region of the upper abdomen, usually the right upper quadrant or the epigastrium. It is usually related to the intake of food. A change in position may bring about drainage and relief. Also attributable to duodenal diverticulum is melena, hematemesis, diarrhea and nausea. It remains for careful roentgenographic study to demonstrate the lesion (Fig. 158). A 4- or 6-hour retention film is of value to determine the presence or the absence of *stasis*. The symptoms of the diverticulum are due to distention, pressure or mechanical interference. Inflammation occurs with stasis; this results in diverticulitis with its associated sequelae of erosion, hemorrhage, perforation and peritonitis.

Malignancy in a duodenal diverticulum has been reported.

Tumors

Benign tumors are uncommon, the most usual types being leiomyomas, lipomas and polyps. Primary carcinoma of the duodenum is rare. As the tumor enlarges, the symptoms produced are not unlike those of carcinoma of the pyloric end of the stomach (p. 123). Roentgenographic investigation permits detailed study of the lesion.

H. A. Oberhelman, Jr., *et al.* have reported 6 personal cases of ulcerogenic tumors of the duodenum. These solitary tumors were presumably of pancreatic islet cell origin and associated with intractable peptic ulcerations.

Ampulla of Vater

This area of the duodenum is important, because carcinoma occurs here with relative frequency. Obstructive jaundice is usually the first, if not the only, sign or symptom to appear. This requires differentiation from a stone in the common duct, a stricture of the common duct, and a carcinoma of the head of the pancreas (p. 236). Since the pancreatic duct also opens at the ampulla, the pancreatic digestive enzymes may be absent in the intestinal tract also. This results in pancreatic insufficiency, which can be diagnosed when the feces reveal microscopic undigested striated meat fibers. This indicates an absence of the proteolytic enzyme trypsin (Fig. 159). Continuous but slight bleeding may be present; hence, melena is a common manifestation. At times the hemorrhage may be massive. A careful roentgenographic study of the duodenum, particularly in its descending portion where the ampulla is located, may reward the clinician in making as early a diagnosis as possible.

Foreign Bodies

The old teaching that anything that passes by mouth will pass per rectum is usually correct. If the object is sharp, it may penetrate anywhere along the esophagogastrointestinal tract; there are 3 sites of predelection for such penetration. They are the pylorus, the duodenojejunal flexure and the ileocecal region. It is imperative, therefore, that the progress of foreign bodies be studied by repeated roentgenographic or fluoroscopic examinations. If an object remains stationary, usually for 24 hours, and if tenderness is present at the foreign body site, surgical removal becomes necessary.

JEJUNO-ILEUM

Diverticula

Diverticula of the jejuno-ileum, if asymptomatic, are discovered by the radiologist. They can produce symptoms ranging from

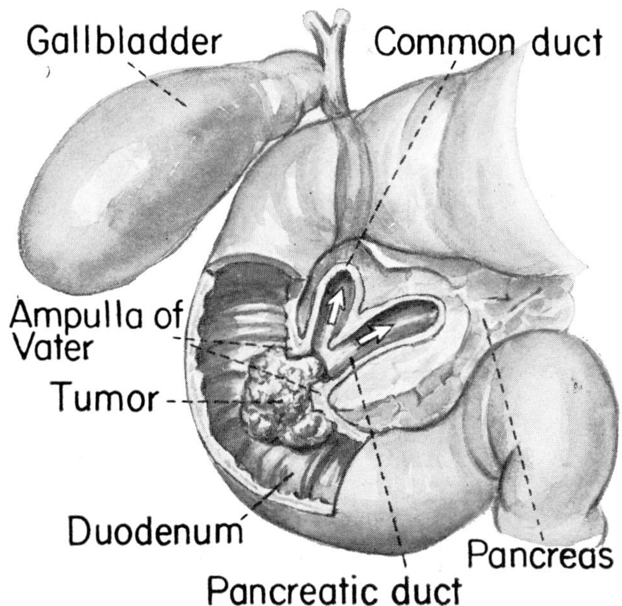

Fig. 159. Carcinoma of the ampulla of Vater. A relatively small tumor at this site can obstruct the common bile duct and the pancreatic duct. This results in obstructive jaundice and pancreatic insufficiency.

vague epigastric distress to severe intestinal bleeding. They are easily overlooked at the operating table, because they are hidden within the leaves of the mesentery. Therefor, they should be sought on the mesenteric side of the bowel (Fig. 160). In this way they differ from diverticula of the large bowel which are found along the antimesenteric border (p. 156).

Any patient suffering from epigastric distress or gastrointestinal bleeding, in whom the commoner esophagogastrointestinal diseases have been excluded, should be examined for such diverticula. Careful roentgenographic study following the progress of the barium meal at half-hour intervals can be most rewarding. Symptoms may be due to mechanical pressure or to inflammatory changes (diverticulitis) and its complications.

Meckel's diverticulum is considered separately because of its relative frequency and specificity. It is a remnant of the obliterated vitelline duct of embryonic life (Fig. 185). The proximal part of the duct that enters the primitive gut fails to become completely obliterated and forms this pouch.

The author has found it helpful to discuss this entity as the "disease of 2's" (Fig. 161). It is found approximately in *2 per cent* of all individuals; it favors males *2 to 1*; it is *2 feet* away from the ileocecal valve; it is usually *2 inches* long; it is confused with *2* surgical conditions, namely, appendicitis and peptic ulcer; it may contain one of *2* types of ectopic tissue, gastric or pancreatic, and is associated with *2* complications (hemorrhage and perforation). The condition may be symptomless or act as any other diverticulum in that a variety of symptoms may be produced by it. It predisposes to intussusception, torsion, or bands which lead to intestinal obstruction. When a Meckel's diverticulum is found in an inguinal hernial sac, it is known as a *Littre's hernia* (p. 254).

Regional Enteritis (Crohn's Disease)

This is a mysterious and remarkable disease. It was described as a clinical entity by Crohn, Ginzburg and Oppenheimer in 1932. Although many theories exist as to its causes, nothing definite has been established. Climate and geographic distribution seem to be factors; the disease is uncommon in the region of the Gulf of Mexico and the Caribbean Sea. The average age group affected is that between 25 and 35 years, although it has been encountered in practically every decade.

The disease is characterized by scarring inflammatory changes and destruction which

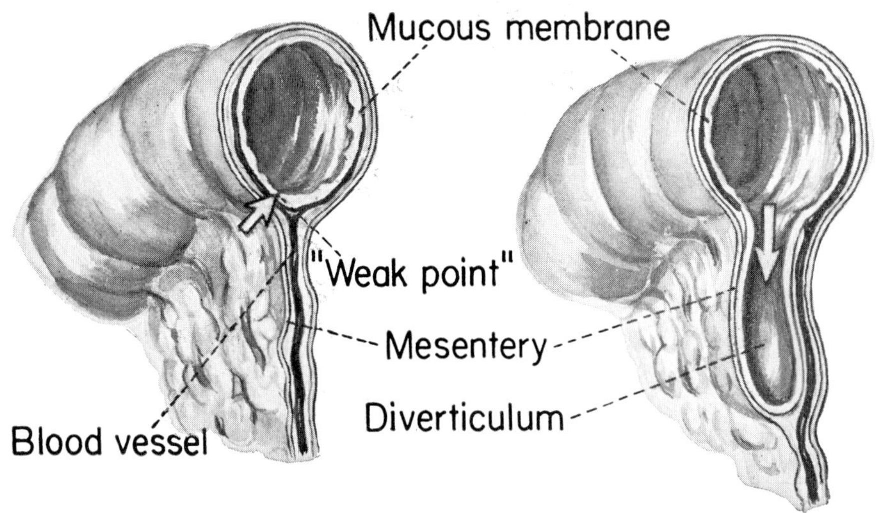

Fig. 160. Jejuno-ileal diverticula. These are easily overlooked at the operating table, because they are located and hidden within the leaves of the mesentery.

involves the wall of the small intestine, its mesentery and regional lymph nodes. As originally described, it was thought that it involved only a few inches of terminal ileum —hence the term "terminal ileitis." It became apparent, however, that the disease could affect any segment of the bowel. Multiple foci throughout the jejuno-ileum are occasionally present with apparently normal bowel intervening; the latter sections have been called "skip areas."

The clinical picture is varied, the prominent features being diarrhea, fever and loss of weight; diffuse lower abdominal distress and progressive anemia frequently are present. Because of the lack of conformity to any specific clinical pattern it is best to consider the condition in 4 stages (Fig. 162).

Stage 1 is the **inflammatory** stage. This is frequently mistaken for acute appendicitis, any many times the true condition is not revealed until laparotomy has been performed. The complaint is one of generalized abdominal distress associated with pain and tenderness which may be localized in the right lower quadrant. Low-grade fever and leukocytosis are also present. The clinician should suspect something unusual when the history reveals an insidious onset. A mass is usually palpable in the right lower quadrant; frequently this is detected rectally. If the patient is operated upon during the inflammatory phase, particularly if the terminal ileum is involved, the condition should be diagnosed immediately because of the edematous and hyperemic appearance of the involved

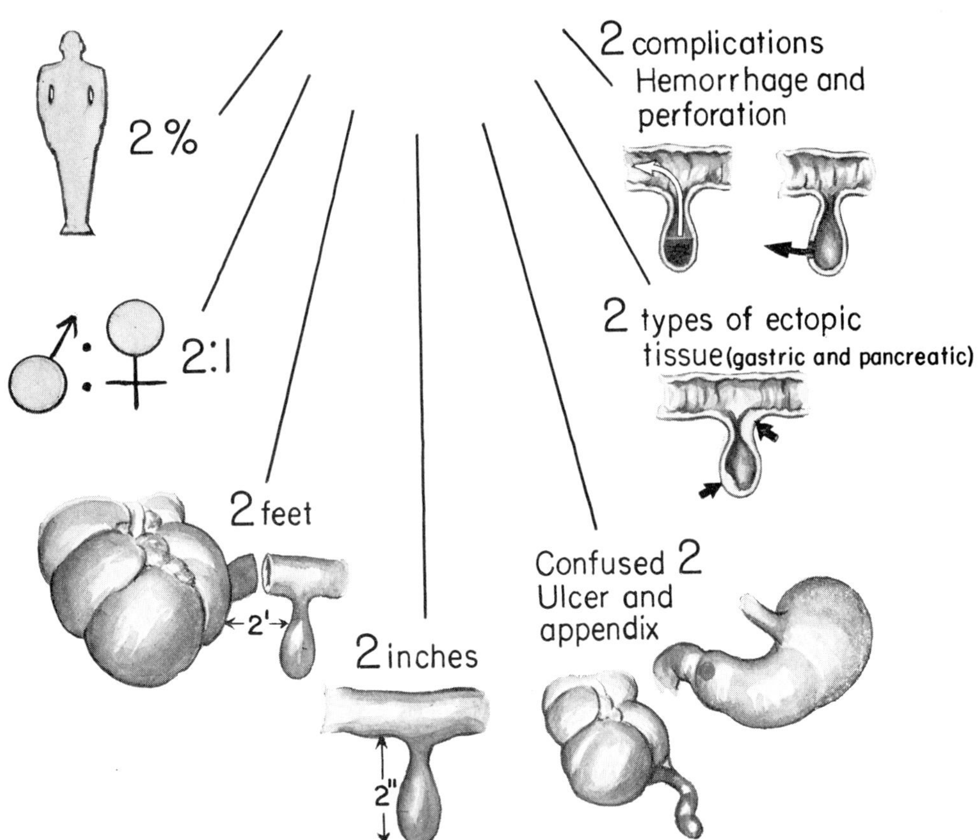

FIG. 161. Meckel's diverticulum. This is the disease of "2's."

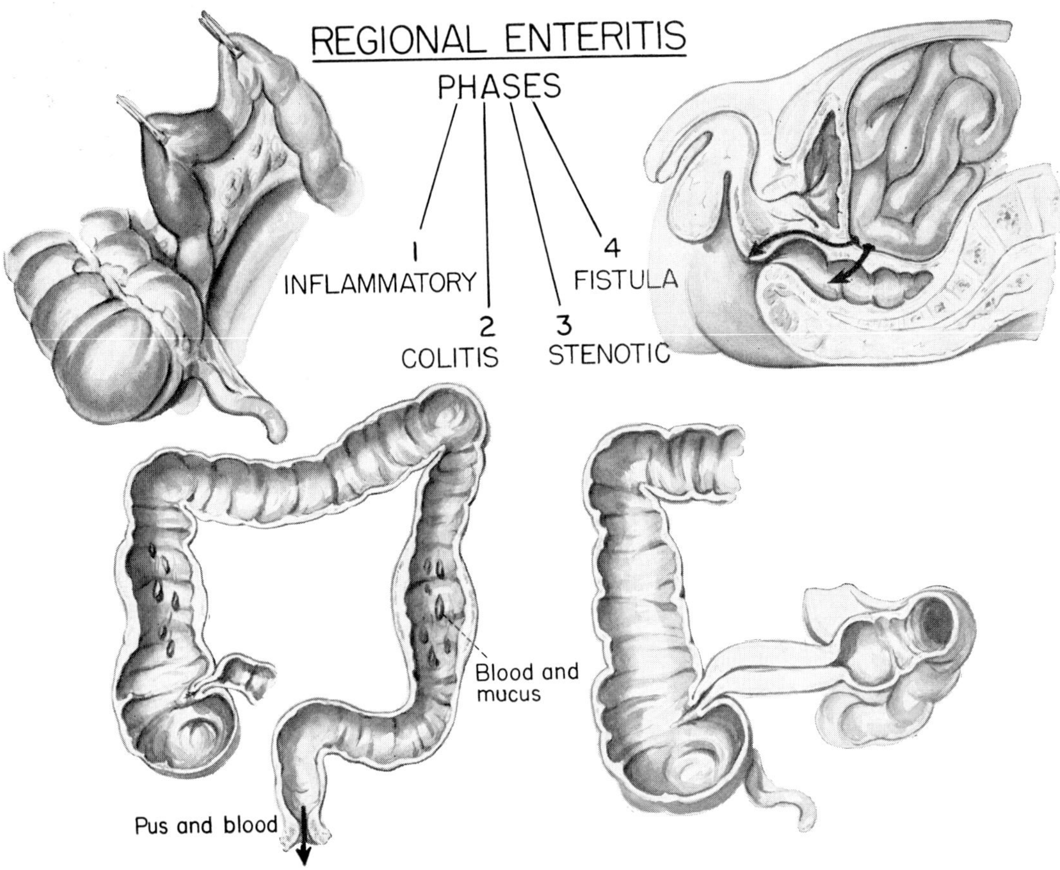

FIG. 162. The 4 phases (stages) of regional enteritis. These stages gradually merge with each other and may overlap.

bowel. The adjacent mesentery is thickened and edematous, and the regional lymph nodes are enlarged and friable. Occasionally, an abscess may be present in the mesentery. When regional enteritis is discovered, removal of the appendix is contraindicated. If appendectomy is performed in the presence of terminal ileitis, a so-called "fecal fistula" frequently results which can continue to drain until the true nature of the disease is discovered and, if possible, eradicated.

Stage 2 is the **colitis** stage. This stage probably results from the spread of the disease across the ileocecal valve to the cecum and the colon. These patients present a chronic history of a persistent diarrhea which contains mucus and blood. A low-grade fever, loss of weight and strength are noted, and the patient presents an anemic appearance. In this stage the abdominal cramping distress is not severe.

Stage 3 is the **stenotic** stage in which the signs and symptoms are those of small bowel *obstruction*. Cramps, nausea, vomiting and at times visible peristalsis are present. Constipation is the rule. A mass in the right lower quadrant is almost always palpable in this stage.

Stage 4 is the **fistula** stage. This late stage is characterized by fistulas which may extend from one segment of bowel to another. Fistulas also occur externally through the abdominal wall, particularly in an abdominal scar. The perineum is not an unusual location for such abnormal openings. Anal fistulas may be directly connected to diseased bowel in the pelvis or may result from local inflammation and irritation produced by the diarrhea. Such fistulas always should suggest regional enteritis to the clinician. The fistula phase has been confused with tuberculosis and actinomycosis as well as other chronic specific granulomas.

When the condition is suspected, fluoroscopic and roentgenographic examinations usually will reveal the classic changes. The terminal ileum is involved for a distance of several inches; this is characterized by stiffness of the bowel wall, narrowing of the lumen, and alteration of the normal mucosal pattern. Occasionally, frank ulcers can be demonstrated. The so-called "string sign" is present in the late stages of the disease.

The prognosis must be guarded. A period of several years of apparent good health may be followed by exacerbations. The disease is a discouraging one and extremely difficult to treat.

Ulcers

Both nonspecific and stomal ulcers can involve the small bowel.

Gastrojejunal ulcers have been referred to as stomal or marginal ulcers. This is a distressing postoperative complication which usually follows gastrojejunostomy. Less frequently it is encountered as a complication of gastric resection. It is directly related to the persistent ability of the remaining stomach to produce excessive amounts of gastric acid. The clinical manifestations are similar to those described under gastric and duodenal ulcers (p. 127) but are more severe. The pain usually is located to the left of the midline of the abdomen and is associated with tenderness at this point. Such ulcers have the same complications as peptic ulcers elsewhere, namely, hemorrhage, obstruction and perforation. Since the anastomosis is close to the transverse colon, perforation of a stomal ulcer may occur into the transverse colon and result in a gastrojejunocolic fistula. Definitive diagnosis is made roentgenologically. The diagnosis is important, since most gratifying results are obtained with vagotomy.

Nonspecific ulcers of the jejuno-ileum constitute one of the rare and enigmatic diseases of the abdomen. Little is known of their etiology, and the clinical picture is vague and confusing. The complications are the same as those of ulcers described elsewhere. Here, too, tumors of the endocrines (pituitary, parathyroids, pancreas and adrenals) must be considered as possible etiologic factors (p. 236).

Tumors

Both benign and malignant tumors of the jejuno-ileum occur in approximately the same frequency.

Benign. The benign tumors are usually lipomas, leiomyomas, fibromas, and polyps; they are often the cause of an intussusception.

The symptoms vary greatly. When they become large, they present the picture of small bowel obstruction. With perfection in roentgenologic technics it is likely that these lesions will be identified more frequently before the development of obstruction.

Malignant. The malignant tumors of the jejuno-ileum are either carcinoma or sarcoma. Most *carcinomas* are found in the jejunum but appear at an earlier age than colonic carcinomas. Symptoms, if present, are associated with varying degrees of obstruction. They may spearhead an intussusception. Although the jejuno-ileum can be involved in generalized polyposis, it is rare for carcinoma to develop in the small intestines. This is unlike the behavior of multiple polyposis in the large bowel. The clinical picture and course are somewhat similar to those described under occlusion of the superior mesenteric artery (p. 142).

Carcinoids are argentaffinomas which are found throughout the intestinal tract; they appear commonly in the appendix (p. 150). They are called argentaffinomas because of the affinity of these neoplastic cells to pick up silver salts. Appendiceal carcinoids rarely if ever metastasize, but the carcinoids involving the bowel appear to act totally different, both biologically and clinically. Extra-appendiceal carcinoids behave as do carcinomas elsewhere, metastasizing to regional lymph nodes and frequently to the liver, the lungs and the bones. Carcinoids produce the so-called *serotonin syndrome*. This has been referred to as "serotonin toxicity" and is characterized by a lobster-red flushing of the face, occasionally dusky cyanosis, severe diarrhea, ascites, malnutrition and lesions of the right heart. Since this syndrome signifies the presence of large tumors which elaborate excessive amounts of serotonin, the prognosis is bad. Increased levels of 5-hydroxyindoleacetic acid (5-HIAA) are excreted in the urine.

Sarcoma of the small intestine is a rare disease and occurs more frequently in males. Unlike carcinoma, the lesions are often multiple. The symptoms are those associated with obstruction, ulceration or intussusception.

Vascular Accidents

Intestinal infarction due to vascular occlusion may be arterial or venous. Involvements of the superior mesenteric vessels are particularly serious. Emboli in the superior mesenteric artery usually represent fragments of vegetations from cardiac valves on the left side of the heart. Superior mesenteric vein thrombosis usually is associated with inflammation within the area drained by this vessel. Thrombi may be propagated in a retrograde manner from the portal vein.

Embolic occlusion of the superior mesenteric artery usually is seen in elderly people with advanced arteriosclerosis. Males are affected more commonly than females. The clinical picture is characterized by dramatic suddenness with severe abdominal pain and shock. Frequently it is diagnosed as intestinal obstruction. The "obstruction phase" predominates because of the rapidity in development of abdominal distention, obstipation and prostration. An extensive generalized peritonitis is soon evident. The bowel supplied by this vessel becomes gangrenous; unless it is resected, multiple perforations develop, and the patient succumbs rapidly. If the occlusion involves the main trunk of the superior mesenteric artery, the entire jejunoileum and the right half of the colon are involved. If lesser branches are affected, smaller areas of infarction result; the latter respond well to early resection and anastomosis. More recently, restoration of blood flow has been attempted by means of embolectomy and thrombectomy. The prerequisite of successful embolectomy is early diagnosis. Mesenteric angiography may provide a helpful adjunct in such cases.

Thrombosis of the Superior Mesenteric Vein. These venous thrombi usually are associated with an inflammatory process, particularly acute appendicitis, regional enteritis, ulcerative colitis and diverticulitis. Also, bowel distention may produce thrombosis.

Thrombophlebitis can originate in the small veins about an acutely inflamed appendix even after the removal of the infected appendix. The process continues proximally and involves larger tributaries of the portal system. Should this propagation continue, the thrombosis reaches the portal vein (pylephlebitis) via the superior mesenteric vein. The amount of damage to the bowel wall varies with the rapidity with which the process spreads. If there is slow propagation, or if there has been a pre-existing portal obstruction, sufficient collateral circulation may have developed to protect the bowel from gangrene. Distention is marked and is mistaken for a postperitoneal bowel obstruction. If the patient passes dark bloody fluid per rectum, the clinician should consider superior mesenteric vein thrombosis or thromophlebitis in the differential diagnosis.

The inferior mesenteric artery is rarely the site of an embolus. However, if this should occur, it is rarely fatal, because the anastomosis of this vessel with the superior mesenteric and hemorrhoidal vessels form adequate collaterals to the involved segment of bowel.

It has been the author's experience to suspect mesenteric thrombosis or embolus in any case of *small bowel* intestinal obstruction in which no scar from previous abdominal surgery is present, particularly if the patient is past 50.

Cysts

So-called gas cysts of the intestines occur in clusters and resemble "soapsuds." On puncture they sometimes produce an audible popping sound.

Enteric cysts or duplication cysts have been found throughout the length of the bowel. They are developmental anomalies and are uncommon. They appear along the antimesenteric border of the bowel. If such a cyst increases in size, it may retain its original submucosal position and replace the lumen of the bowel by inward displacement of the mucosa. These patients present a clinical picture of intestinal obstruction.

Lymphatic cysts are also of congenital origin; they are rare.

Acute Mesenteric Lymphadenitis

The etiology of this condition is obscure. It occurs chiefly in children and in those who have had a recent upper respiratory infection. It is difficult, and at times impossible, to differentiate from acute appendicitis. The clinical picture presents abdominal pain, nausea, vomiting and tenderness in the right lower quadrant, particularly in the region of McBurney's point. The glands involved are particularly in the mesentery of the terminal ileum. If one can be certain of the diagnosis, the treatment should be conservative and not surgical. Chronic mesenteric lymphadenitis usually is associated with a specific granulomatous disease.

Congenital Defects

These defects result from abnormalities in the rotation of the bowel. If intestinal obstruction results, symptoms become evident, and early intervention is necessary. The patient is usually a child in whom vomiting is the cardinal symptom. Since most of these conditions occur distal to the ampulla of Vater, bile is present in the vomitus. Intestinal obstruction in children should suggest such a congenital condition. (See Intestinal Obstruction, p. 176.)

APPENDIX

Appendicitis

Acute appendicitis was first described in 1886 by Reginald Fitz. The literature, which contains thousands of reports, is replete with every aspect of this disease.

Incidence. Typically, the disease appears in the 2nd and the 3rd decades but may occur at any age. If present in children or the aged, the clinical picture is altered and is more difficult to interpret. After the age of 40 acute appendicitis becomes less frequent.

Etiology. Although the exact cause is unknown, *stasis* plays an important role in the etiology. Such stasis may be due to a fecalith, a kink, a congenital band, or edema. Bacteria, which are omnipresent, increase in number with stasis, and inflammation results. Within the first 24 hours following obstruction, the appendiceal wall becomes thick and edematous, and the lumen may be filled with

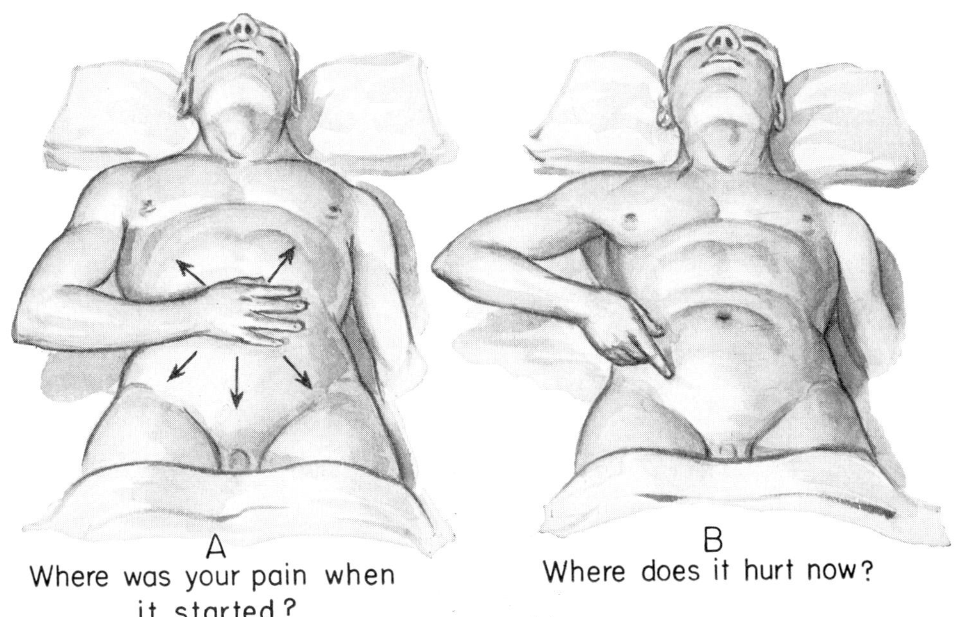

Fig. 163. The 2-question test. (A) The patient demonstrates a pattern of diffuse abdominal distress in answer to the 1st question. (B) In answer to the 2nd question he pinpoints his tenderness to McBurney's point.

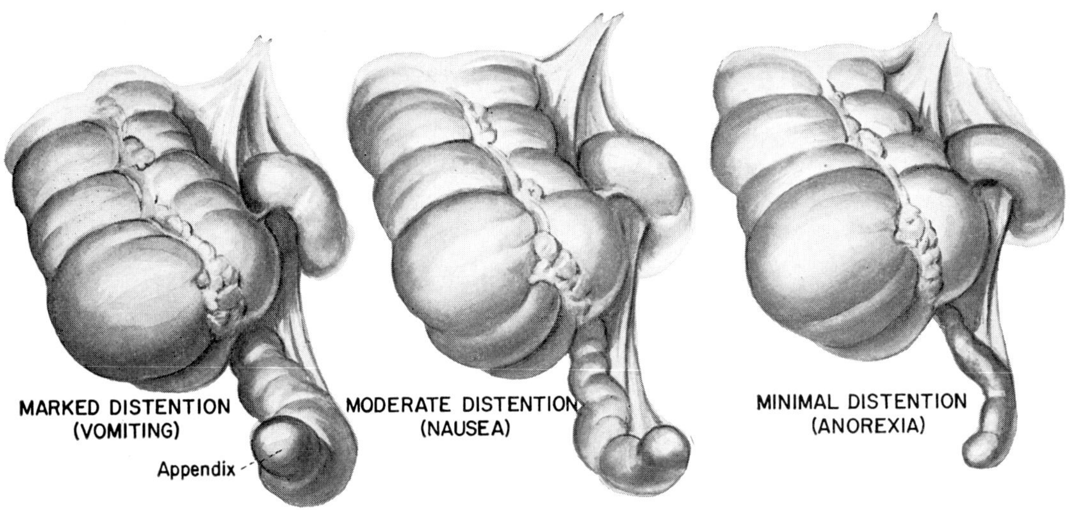

FIG. 164. Anorexia, nausea and vomiting are 3 degrees of one symptom; they are dependent on the amount of distention in the appendix.

pus. Should the appendiceal outlet suddenly open and the contents be discharged into the bowel, the acute phase of the attack subsides spontaneously; if, however, the lumen remains obstructed, the disease progresses. After 24 hours, in the typical case, the serosa becomes covered with exudate, and cloudy fluid appears in the peritoneal cavity.

SYMPTOMS. The symptoms in the typical case follow a definite pattern. *Any diffuse epigastric distress that localizes to the right lower quadrant within 24 hours is acute appendicitis until proved to be otherwise.* However, this is not the terminology that a patient uses. He complains of a "bellyache," "gas pains" or a "spoiled stomach." Being certain that it is "something I ate," he unfortunately takes the advice of a well-meaning friend or relative and attempts to relieve his "bellyache" with a cathartic. This unfortunate act is largely responsible for the still high mortality in this condition. The cause of mortality in acute appendicitis is closely associated with the three "P's," namely, *P*urgation, *P*rocrastination and *P*oor surgical judgment. In only 10 per cent of the cases is the pain colicky, and in a much smaller percentage is the pain severe enough to require sedation. If the patient requires sedation for pain, the condition is rarely appendicitis. Pain that begins in the lower abdomen and remains there is more suggestive of pelvic disease than appendicitis.

DIAGNOSIS. The *2-question test* permits one to diagnose acute appendicitis rapidly in over 80 per cent of cases (Fig. 163). It is conducted in the following way: *Question No. 1:* "Where was your pain when it started?" In answer to this the patient points to his entire abdomen or periumbilical region. *Question No. 2:* "Where is your pain now?" In answer to this the patient points to his right lower quadrant. If the 2-question test is positive, the condition must be considered one of appendicitis until proved to be otherwise.

A frequent complaint is the sensation of a desire to defecate but the inability to do so. The patient feels that if he could have a bowel movement, he would feel much relieved.

Nausea and vomiting are exceptions rather than the rule. It is unfortunate that the importance of *anorexia* has not been stressed. Anorexia, nausea and vomiting should be considered as 3 degrees of one symptom (Fig. 164). If a patient has a markedly distended appendix, vomiting may be present; if there is moderate distention, nausea usually is present, and since all patients with acute appendicitis have microscopic distention of the appendix, then, theoretically at least, all patients with appendicitis have anorexia. This is so typical and constant that when a patient states that he is hungry, acute appendicitis is rarely the cause of his trouble.

There is usually a change in the daily stool habit; constipation is the rule. Diarrhea is most unusual in acute appendicitis in adults; however, it is frequently present in children. Chills (not a chilly sensation) are rarely found in appendicitis. If a true chill is present, this suggests an empyema of the appendix or an appendiceal abscess.

PHYSICAL FINDINGS. An elevated *temperature* is rare in acute appendicitis. Fever, when present, is due to peritoneal soiling. The *pulse* is of little diagnostic value in that it is usually normal or maintains a given ratio with the temperature. For every degree rise in temperature there is a 10-beat increase in pulse.

Tenderness is present *at McBurney's point* (Fig. 165). This is located by drawing an imaginary line between the right anterior superior iliac spine and the umbilicus; this line is trisected; McBurney's point is located 1 cm. below the outer trisection point. Although some (neuroanatomists) insist that this point remains constant regardless of the location of the appendix, the author is convinced that the tenderness is located wherever the involved appendix is located. An almost infallible diagnostic rule is the following: pain, a symptom, may be referred anywhere along its nervous path; but tenderness, a physical finding, remains at the site of the lesion. It is advantageous to permit the patient to identify the spot that is most tender.

Cough tenderness may be helpful in eliciting a point of maximum tenderness. The patient is asked to cough, and a sharp twinge of localized pain will occur in the involved area. Following coughing, the patient should be asked to pinpoint with 1 finger the exact area of greatest pain. The position of the vermiform appendix varies considerably. When the appendix remains in the right lower quadrant, difficulties in diagnosing are minimized. When appendicitis is associated with a nondescent of the cecum, appendiceal

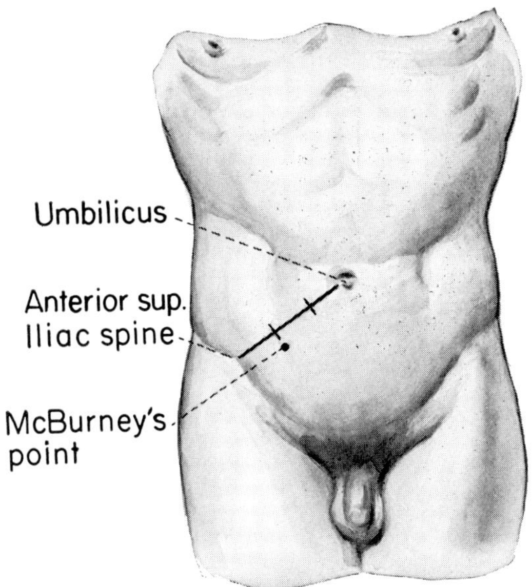

FIG. 165. McBurney's point. The point of tenderness of an acute appendix is not constant, since it is dependent upon the location of the inflamed organ.

tenderness may be in the right upper quadrant; if associated with malrotation of the cecum, the tenderness is in the left upper quadrant.

It is not the desire of the author to confuse when he states that acute appendicitis does *not* produce right rectus rigidity. This sign has been mistaken for muscular defense. If one exerts pressure over an inflamed appendiceal region, both recti must contract simultaneously. This is *muscular defense* (Fig. 166). It is impossible for most people to contract one rectus muscle voluntarily without contracting the other. Therefore, to elicit true *right rectus rigidity*, both hands must be placed on the abdomen at the same time. If upon so placing both hands the physician demonstrates that one rectus is relaxed whereas the other remains rigid, this is true unilateral rectus rigidity. The demonstration of such a phenomenon indicates the presence of a mass (Fig. 167).

DIAGNOSTIC AIDS. Too many signs have been described as aids in the diagnosis of acute appendicitis. To enumerate these would be merely a display of "cerebral muscle."

However, a few important and practical signs will be discussed.

Rovsing's sign is positive if the patient experiences pain in the right lower abdominal quadrant when pressure is made over the left lower quadrant. Presumably this is the result of a displacement of colonic gas to an inflamed appendiceal or cecal region.

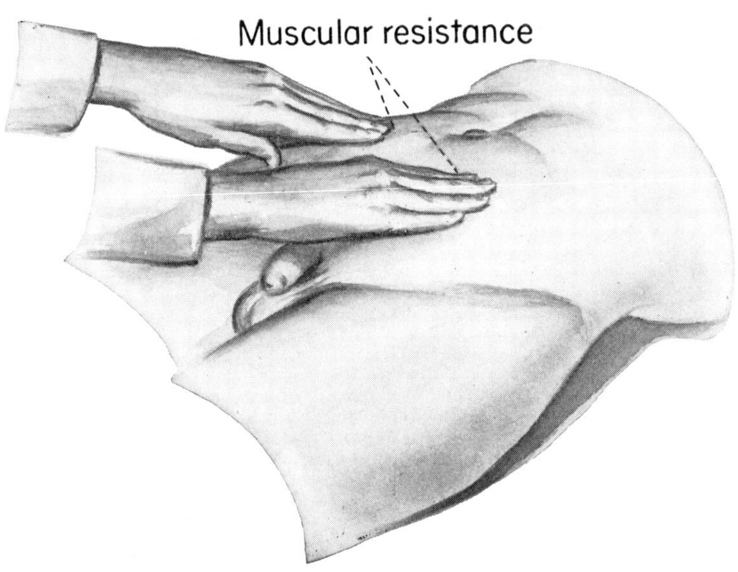

FIG. 166. Muscular defense. This must not be confused with right rectus rigidity. The former is demonstrated by placing *both* hands on the abdomen simultaneously and feeling the resistance of both recti.

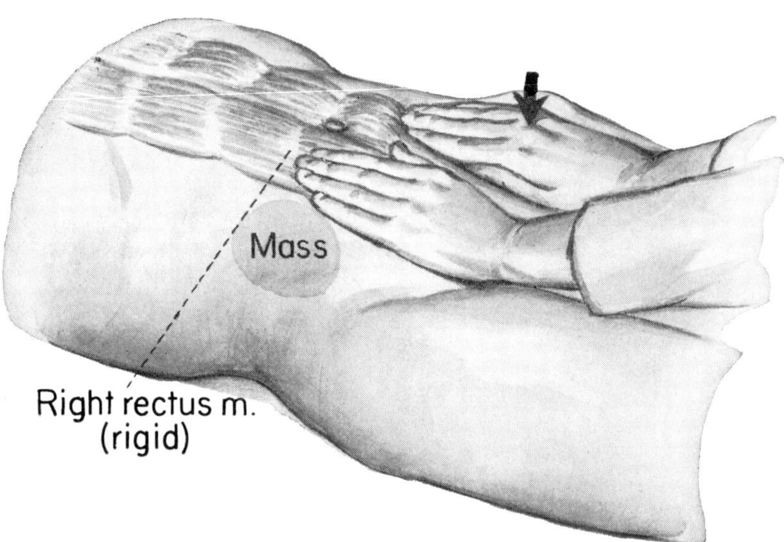

FIG. 167. Right rectus rigidity. With both hands placed on the recti simultaneously, the examiner detects that the left rectus is relaxed, but the right rectus is tense. This is produced by an underlying mass (inflammatory or neoplastic.)

The *psoas* and the *obturator signs*, although usually described with acute appendicitis, do not diagnose this condition but rather *locate* an inflamed appendix. The *psoas sign* is elicited by placing the patient on his left side and hyperextending the right leg. This stretches the psoas muscle and elicits pain if an associated fasciitis is present with a *posteriorly placed* inflamed appendix (Fig. 168). The *obturator sign* is elicited by internal rotation of the flexed right thigh. This stretches the obturator internus muscle and fascia (Fig. 169). If this maneuver elicits pain, it suggests an obturator internus fasciitis and an inflamed pelvic appendix.

Peritoneal rebound implies the presence of a peritonitis, regardless of the cause (Fig. 170). The physician should explain to the patient what he is about to do, so that the sudden release of abdominal pressure does not frighten the patient and produce a false response.

A *rectal examination* must be included if the patient is to be examined thoroughly. At times a palpable mass or tender area will be felt on the right side (Fig. 171). In children and in thin individuals with generalized visceroptosis, inflamed appendices are palpated easily. The *bimanual examination* should be included to rule out pelvic disease; however, more important than the latter is the *bidigital examination*. This is conducted by placing one finger in the vagina and another finger in the anal orifice with the perineum between (Fig. 172). This differentiates feces from cervix, adnexal and uterine enlargement, or intraperitoneal pelvic masses.

Laboratory Tests. These procedures should be considered last and least important; they supply corroborative evidence. The *leukocyte count* usually is elevated, being over 12,000 in more than half of the cases; however, it is well known that acute gangrenous appendicitis can occur with a normal white blood cell count. The differential blood count may be more helpful than the total white count. *Urinalysis* is done routinely. However, an acute appendix located close to the bladder, the right ureter, or the lower pole of the right kidney may produce an inflammatory response around the bladder, the ureter or the kidney that results in a hematuria. The *flat roentgenogram* should be used only when the diagnosis is doubtful. Rarely is a spontaneous pneumoperitoneum produced by a perforated appendix (p. 132). If this is found, then one must assume that the appendix was of tremendous size and greatly distended.

The late (neglected) cases of acute appendicitis manifest the following complications: local or generalized peritonitis, subdiaphragmatic abscess, intestinal obstruction,

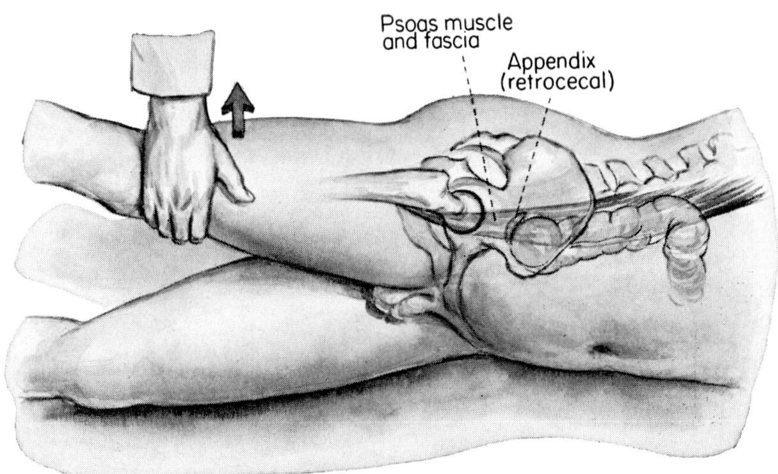

Fig. 168. The psoas sign. This does not diagnose but rather locates an inflamed retrocecal appendix.

jaundice and pylephlebitis. (These conditions are discussed under their specific headings.)

Differential Diagnosis. The differential diagnosis of acute appendicitis is in reality the differential diagnosis of the "acute abdomen." To list and discuss 80 or 100 conditions which by the stretch of the imagination might simulate an acute appendicitis is most impractical. Seven conditions constitute 90 per cent of the diagnostic errors. These

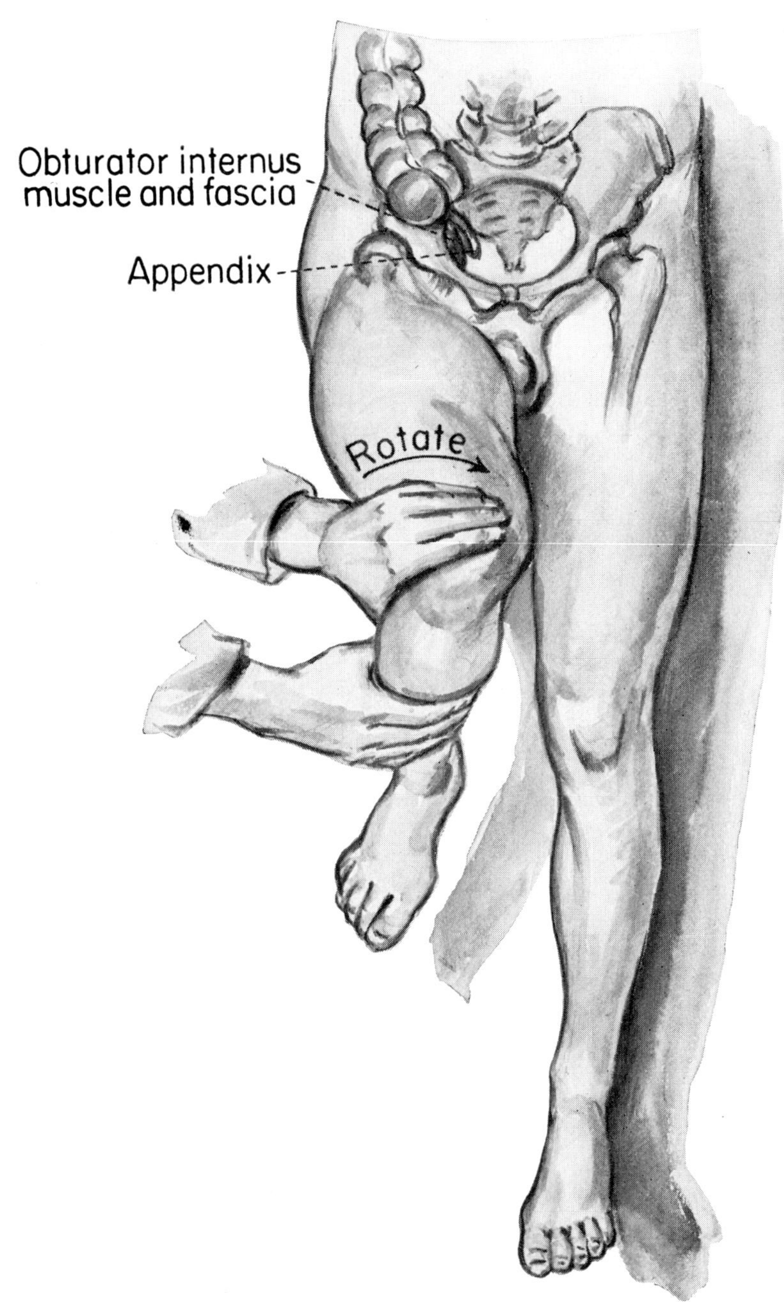

Fig. 169. The obturator sign. This does not diagnose but rather locates an inflamed pelvic appendix.

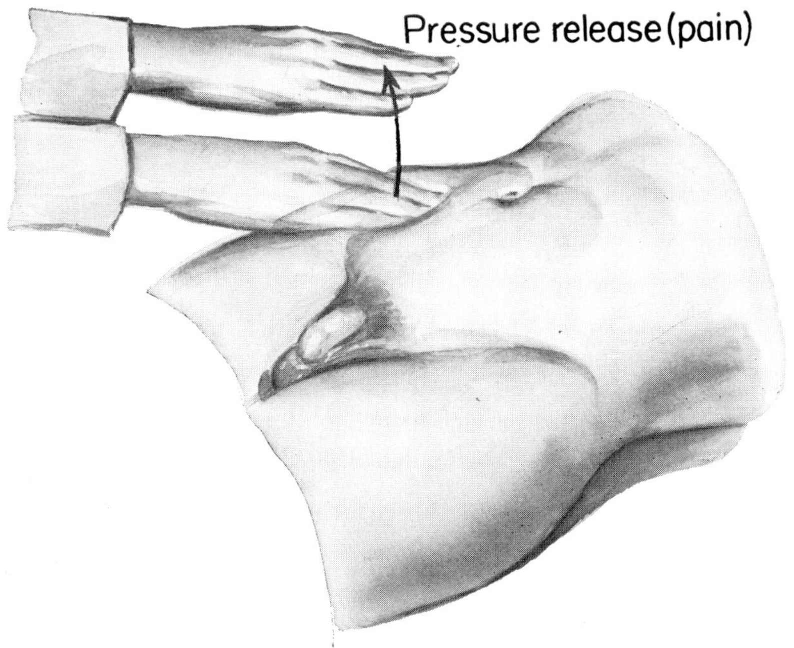

FIG. 170. Peritoneal rebound. When present, this sign suggests peritonitis regardless of the cause. It may be executed in any abdominal quadrant and is demonstrated best by making firm, steady, yet gentle pressure with one hand and then suddenly releasing. The complaint of pain with release of pressure suggests peritonitis.

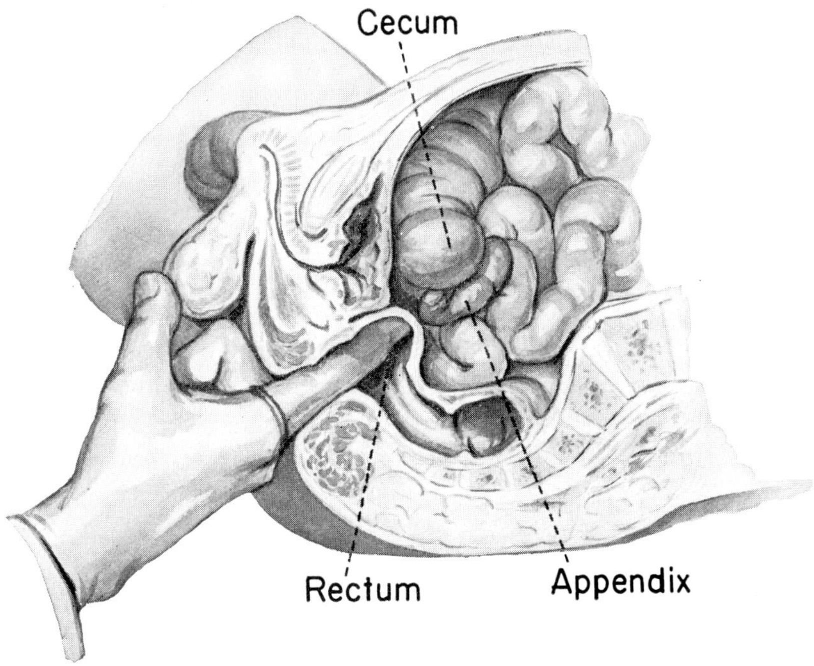

FIG. 171. The importance of the rectal examination cannot be overstressed. It may be the only positive finding in acute appendicitis, particularly in children and in pelvic appendicitis.

are acute cholecystitis, renal and/or ureteral colic, perforated peptic ulcer, acute hemorrhagic pancreatitis, pelvic inflammatory disease, pneumonia and coronary disease. These conditions are discussed under their own headings.

An *appendiceal abscess* should be suspected if the case is over 2 or 3 days in duration and presents a septic syndrome. By septic syndrome is meant an "iceberg" fever, chills, profuse sweats and a leukocytosis over 18,000 to 20,000.

Subacute appendicitis is the designation applied to an appendix which was acutely inflamed some weeks or months prior and is now quiescent or subsiding.

Chronic appendicitis is still a debatable condition. It must be admitted, however, that the appendix, like any other organ, can be chronically inflamed as the result of previous acute attacks. In the absence of chronic inflammatory changes, which should be demonstrable microscopically, what is meant by chronic appendicitis? The appendix may become obstructed, as in the case of any other organ that has a lumen. Such obstruction results in *appendiceal colic* but inflammatory changes may be lacking, particularly if the obstruction is overcome spontaneously. Although such appendices might not reveal inflammatory signs, early relief is obtained after appendectomy.

Miscellaneous Conditions

Tumors rarely affect the appendix. The carcinoid tumors which involve it consist of glandular and embryonal elements and have been referred to as *argentaffinomas*. Although histologically these are the same as the argentaffinomas found in the small and the large intestines (p. 141), appendiceal involvement rarely if ever metastasizes and therefore does not produce the so-called "serotonin syndrome" (red face, dusky cyanosis, diarrhea, and right-heart manifestations). Enzyme action on serotonin produces 5-hydroxyindoleacetic acid. When this is detected in the urine, it implies metastases and a poor prognosis.

True carcinoma of the appendix is rare; these, too, are usually found accidentally. The so-called *mucocele* of the appendix is present not infrequently; it results from an overabundance of obstructed mucuslike material that has become entrapped in the appendiceal lumen. Usually it is diagnosed as

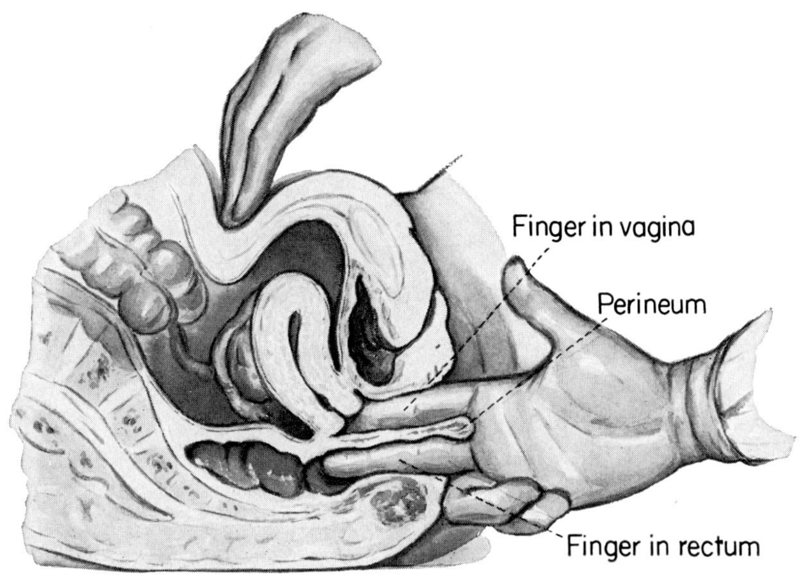

Fig. 172. The bidigital examination. With 1 finger in the vagina and 1 finger in the rectum, one can differentiate feces, adnexal and uterine masses from other intraperitoneal pelvic enlargements.

"chronic appendicitis." The appendix may be involved in tuberculosis, actinomycosis and other granulomatous conditions.

COLON

Carcinoma of Right Half of Colon

The clinical picture of carcinoma of the right half of the colon and the cecum is entirely different than that of the left half. There are 2 reasons for this: (1) the lumen of the large bowel diminishes from cecum to sigmoid; (2) the contents of the right half of the colon are liquid, and those of the left half are solid (Fig. 173). Since the right side of the colon has a large lumen and liquid contents, the obstructive phase is almost completely lacking.

It usually occurs in the 4th, the 5th or the 6th decade. Frequently, the earliest symptom is a mild, intermittent nondescript discomfort in the right lower quadrant. Unfortunately, this rarely is severe enough to warrant an examination. Less specific complaints are nausea, anorexia, epigastric distress and possibly low-grade fever. Bowel habits may be altered (constipation and diarrhea), although this change never is as marked as that observed with tumors on the left side of the colon. Loss of strength and weight are late signs. Unfortunately, the condition progresses insidiously until the patient becomes aware of increasing weakness, pallor or a palpable mass. Right-sided carcinomas, particularly those affecting the cecum, ulcerate and assume a polypoid form. They bleed readily. Some of these anemias are so severe that the patient resembles a case of pernicious

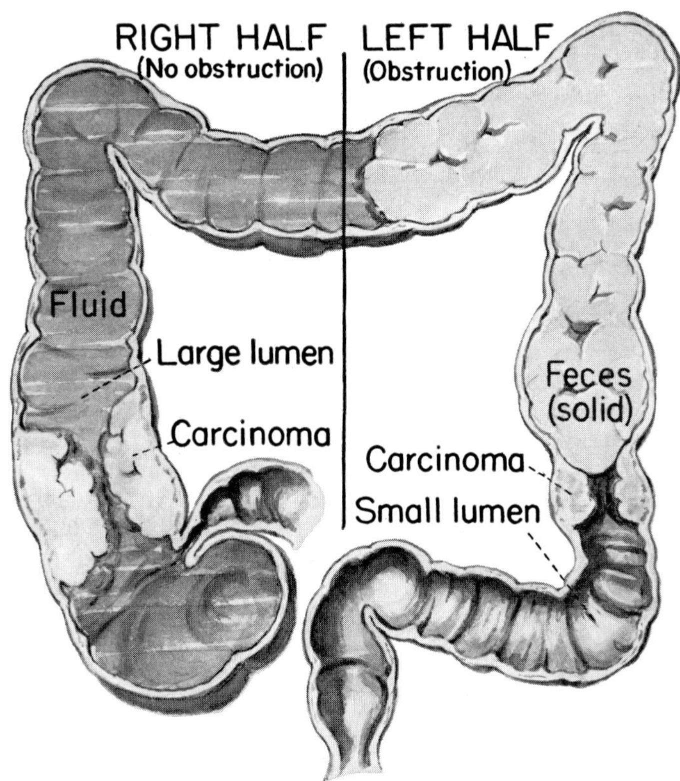

Fig. 173. Carcinoma of the *right* side of the colon does not produce obstruction, because the intestinal contents are liquid, and the lumen is large. Carcinoma of the *left* side of the colon frequently is associated with obstruction, because the intestinal contents are solid, and the lumen is small.

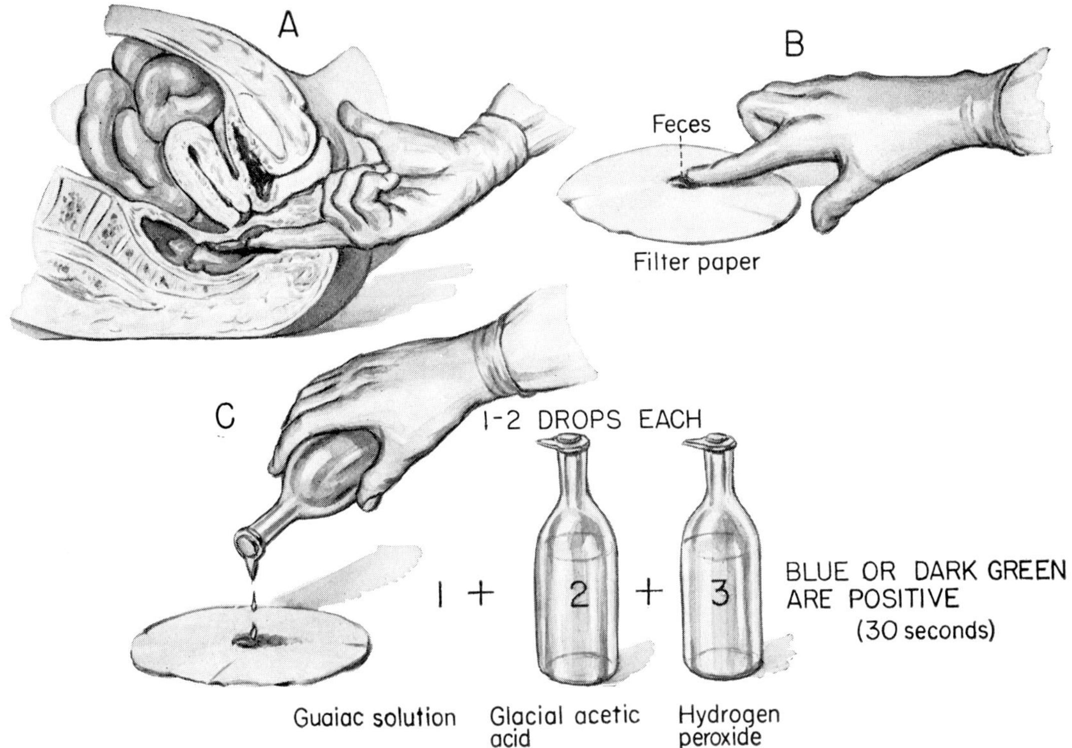

FIG. 174. The guaiac test for occult blood in the feces (see text).

anemia. Although blood may not be visible on gross examination of the stool, it is invariably detectable with chemical analysis.

An office technic which is simple for the detection of occult blood in the feces in unprepared patients is worth while (Fig. 174). The benzidine and the orthotoluidine tests are too sensitive for routine use in patients who have not been prepared with a meat-free diet. The guaiac test appears to be the best for this purpose. It can be carried out in the following way: the 3 reagents necessary are guaiac solution, glacial acetic acid and hydrogen peroxide. These can be kept easily in small standard drop bottles. A saturated solution of guaiac crystals in 95 per cent alcohol is satisfactory. One or 2 drops of each solution are placed in sequence, and the test is read within 30 seconds. Other color changes or delayed color changes are to be regarded as negative. No test is foolproof, however; positive reactions with this simple procedure warrants a thorough study of the case.

Physical examination reveals a palpable mass in approximately 25 per cent of these patients; the mass is firm and somewhat nodular. Some vague local tenderness is usually present in the region of the tumor.

It is fortunate that carcinoma of the right colon, particularly the cecum, has a marked tendency toward localization. Spread occurs late in the course of the disease, either to regional lymph nodes, via the portal vein to the liver, or direct extension by contiguity to surrounding structures.

Fluoroscopic and roentgenographic examinations with retrograde instillation of barium into the colon and by contrast air studies usually confirm the diagnosis.

Five-year survivals (note the word "cure" has not been used) as high as 75 per cent have been reported following radical surgical therapy.

It is important to emphasize the relationship of the appendix to right-sided carcinoma. Since the earliest symptoms of carcinoma of the cecum are associated with the right lower quadrant, the physician might suspect appendicitis. If the patient is subjected to appendectomy, the appendix usually is found to be normal, although various types of appendiceal changes have been reported which occur secondary to the cecal lesion. Particularly confusing is the presence of a gangrenous appendicitis which can result from carcinoma obstructing the appendiceal lumen. Then an appendectomy may be performed, and the carcinoma overlooked. Localized peritonitis and periappendiceal abscesses have been drained, and the primary carcinoma has been overlooked.

Although bowel obstruction is most unusual in right-sided carcinoma, it may occur in the late case when the tumor has assumed tremendous size, or if the ileocecal valve has been invaded.

Carcinoma of Left Half of Colon

Carcinoma of the left side of the colon is considered separately, because the outstanding findings are those of obstruction. This is in contradistinction to the nonobstructive carcinoma of the right side of the colon. The reasons for the obstructive manifestations in the left colonic segment are due to the smaller size of the lumen and the solidity of the contents (Fig. 173).

Little is known of the etiology; however, some benign lesions are known to be complicated by carcinoma. Benign polyps may undergo malignant degeneration. The incidence of malignancy in multiple polyposis of the colon is so high that radical resection must receive serious consideration. Chronic nonspecific ulcerative colitis also is associated wtih carcinomatous degeneration.

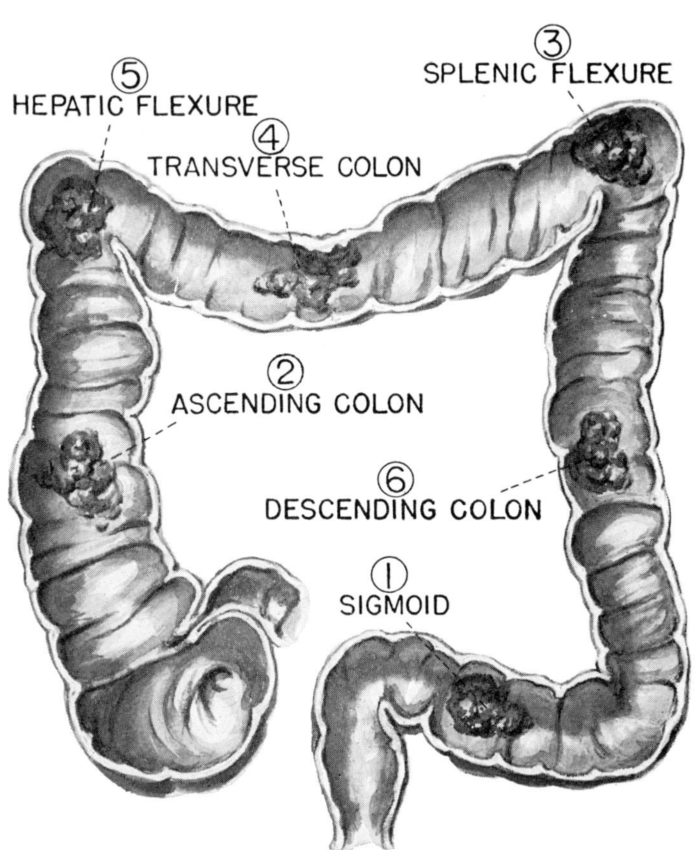

Fig. 175. Frequency of locations in carcinoma of the colon. The rectosigmoid junction is by far the most common site.

Approximately half of all colon carcinomas occur in the sigmoid region. In frequency this is followed by the ascending colon, the splenic flexure, the transverse colon, hepatic flexure and the descending colon (Fig. 175).

Carcinomas of the left colonic segment are usually of the infiltrative type and produce a so-called "napkin ring" type of deformity. The most common and possibly the earliest complaint is a *"change in stool habit."* Most people have a stool habit, whether the bowel movement is once a day or once a week. Whenever this pattern changes, carcinoma of the colon must be ruled out. Constipation is the rule, but this may alternate with diarrhea. Narrowing of the lumen produces "ribbon-like" stools; however, this is a late and over-emphasized sign of carcinoma. Cramping or colicky distress is usually present. The onset is insidious and mild, and unfortunately much valuable time is lost in discovering the tumor. Often on the surface of the stools are streaks or flecks of bright-red blood. It is unfortunate that the patient may associate such bleeding with "piles"; also, the physician may confirm the presence of piles. A good rule to follow is that the presence of blood in the stool, particularly if hemorrhoids are present, should be considered carcinoma until proved to be otherwise. Frequently, carcinomas at the so-called rectosigmoid junction can be palpated rectally. At times the tumor is palpable abdominally.

The colon proximal to the obstruction becomes dilated, edematous and friable. The patient presents the picture of a nonstrangulated large bowel intestinal obstruction (p. 176). If the obstruction is unrelieved, stercoral ulceration develops which leads to bowel perforation and peritonitis. The tumor itself may perforate the colonic wall. Surrounding structures are involved by contiguity, particularly the abdominal wall and the small intestine. If ulceration and secondary infection supervene, a septic course appears with fever, chills, sweats and an elevated leukocyte count. Although carcinoma of the left half of the colon produces obstruction, these patients may have secondary anemia also. The tumor may spread via the regional lymph nodes or the blood stream.

The diagnosis can be established with a fair degree of accuracy by means of the roentgenographic examination after the retrograde instillation of barium. It is unwise whenever suspecting a colon or an obstructing lesion to give the patient barium by mouth, since this may obturate the lumen. Double contrast air technics are particularly valuable in evaluating lesions of the hepatic and the splenic flexures. Proctoscopic examinations are helpful in diagnosing carcinoma of the rectosigmoid junction and the lower sigmoid colon (p. 171).

The discovery of one carcinoma does not rule out the existence of another. Five per cent of all colon carcinomas are multiple.

Resection is possible in over 80 per cent of patients with colon carcinoma, and approximately 50 per cent of such patients are alive 5 years later; this picture is a happier one than carcinoma of the stomach. Since this is one of the more favorable visceral cancers, early diagnosis is imperative, thorough study is vital, and energetic therapy is mandatory.

Prognosis in carcinoma anywhere must be extremely guarded. To discuss "5-year cures" seems to be erroneous when one realizes that 20-year survivals with metastases are recorded.

Benign Tumors of the Colon

The 3 most common benign growths are the adenomatous polyp, the papilloma and the lipoma. Uncommon benign tumors are fibromas, hemangiomas, leiomyomas, neurofibromas and melanomas.

The adenomatous polyp may be seen at any age and in any portion of the colon; it is situated most commonly in the sigmoid and the rectum. Every adenoma must be considered as a malignant growth until proved to be otherwise. In children they have a tendency to occur singly and produce prolonged intermittent bleeding. In adults they are usually multiple. They may be the basis for acute or chronic obstructions and they form an ideal spearhead for an intussusception (p. 182). Endoscopic, as well as roentgenographic examinations are helpful in determining the diagnosis and the progress of these tumors, particularly when they are pedunculated and removed locally.

Lipomas can occur anywhere in the gastrointestinal tract but are found most commonly on the right side of the colon (cecum, ascending and transverse colons). There is no clinical syndrome that is pathognomonic of such tumors. Symptoms referrable to intestinal obstruction or intussusception may be present. Obstructions may be acute, subacute or chronic. When chronic, the symptoms are present for months or years and consist of vague abdominal distress; there are frequent remissions and exacerbations. Ulceration of the mucosa produces occult or visible hemorrhage. A positive diagnosis is rarely made preoperatively. It is usually thought to be a malignant neoplasm.

Papilloma of the colon is found almost exclusively in adults. It is located most frequently in the rectum. Since it bleeds readily, its presence becomes manifest with rectal bleeding. These lesions can produce a hemorrhage that is alarmingly profuse. Large papillomas often are malignant.

Carcinoid Tumors

The exact nature of these tumors is still unknown. They have been referred to as argentaffin tumors, because they often contain silver-reducing granules. Although frequently encountered in the appendix and the lower ileum, they have been observed in the colon also, as well as in other parts of the gastrointestinal tract.

The average age of patients with carcinoids of the intestines is in the 4th and 5th decades; however, appendiceal carcinoids are encountered usually in the 2nd decade. The most common symptom in carcinoids of the intestines are those of intestinal obstruction.

These tumors should not be considered as

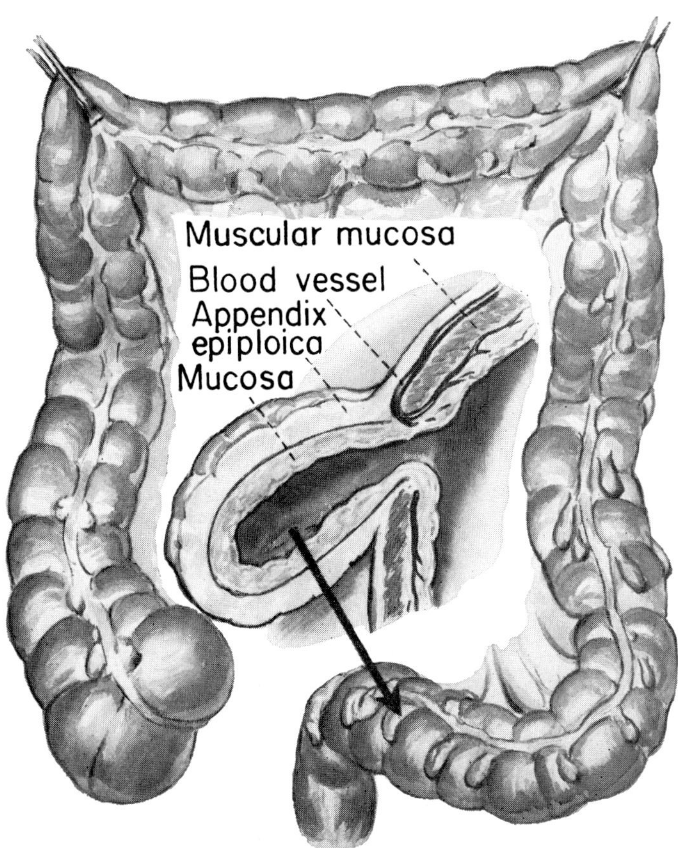

Fig. 176. Diverticula of the colon are difficult to find during surgery, because they are located in and hidden by the appendices epiploicae.

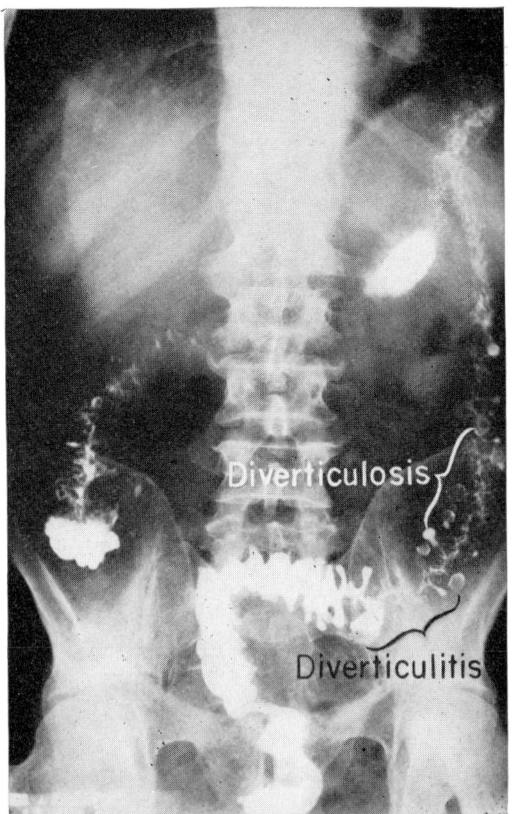

Fig. 177. Roentgenogram of diverticulosis and diverticulitis of the colon. The noninflamed diverticula are round and smooth, but those that become infected and inflamed become narrow, rigid and "serrated."

benign. It is the consensus that from the very start they are malignant, but that they grow slowly and metastasize late. Microscopically, the tumor can be suspected when the cut surface appears *yellowish* and homogenous.

Serotonin is secreted by the tumor, and trytophan is its precursor. Diagnosis can be made, particularly of large and small bowel lesions, by examination of the urine for 5-hydroxyindoleacetic acid, which is produced by enzyme action on serotonin. When this is found, it usually signifies very large tumors and/or metastases and a poor prognosis (see p. 150).

Diverticulosis and Diverticulitis

Diverticula or tiny pouches of the colon are found frequently in people past 40. They appear most frequently in the sigmoid. Men are afflicted twice as commonly as women, and obesity is a contributing factor. Colonic diverticula differ from those in the small intestine in that the former arise from various parts of the circumference of the bowel, not being confined to the line of mesenteric attachment, as are those of the small bowel. Their origin is unknown; however, they occur through weak areas in the muscle coat at the site of the entrance of blood vessels. The longitudinal muscle bundles afford some protection; hence, these diverticula tend to occur in 3 longitudinal rows which coincide with the intervals between the taenia coli. The diverticulum is a herniation of mucosa and thinned muscularis mucosae which in no way differs from the bowel structure. They are difficult to see when the exterior of the bowel is examined, because they arise in the region of the appendices epiploicae and are hidden by these fatty caps (Fig. 176).

By the term *diverticulosis* is meant the presence of diverticula; by the term *diverticulitis* is meant inflammation of the diverticulum. The incidence of diverticulitis in cases of diverticulosis is not known definitely. However, physiopathology is more important than the statistical relationship. So long as the neck of the diverticulum is wide and permits entrance and exit of colonic contents, inflammation rarely occurs. If the neck becomes constricted, it produces obstruction, stasis and inflammation (Fig. 158).

Most individuals who have diverticula are unaware of their presence. It is the complications of these pouches that produce symptoms; these vary greatly in their severity from mild indigestion to severe abdominal distress. The complications of diverticulitis are associated with obstruction, inflammation and ulceration.

A markedly inflamed diverticulum causes pain and tenderness; these subside spontaneously if the diverticulum evacuates itself. If the inflammatory process persists, tenderness is demonstrable in the left lower quadrant (sigmoid); this has been called "left-sided appendicitis." A pericolic abscess may result; it is sharply localized and can become quite large. Perforation results in peritonitis. The most common cause of vesicosigmoidal fistula is diverticulitis of the sigmoid colon. Should this occur, the patient is aware of gas

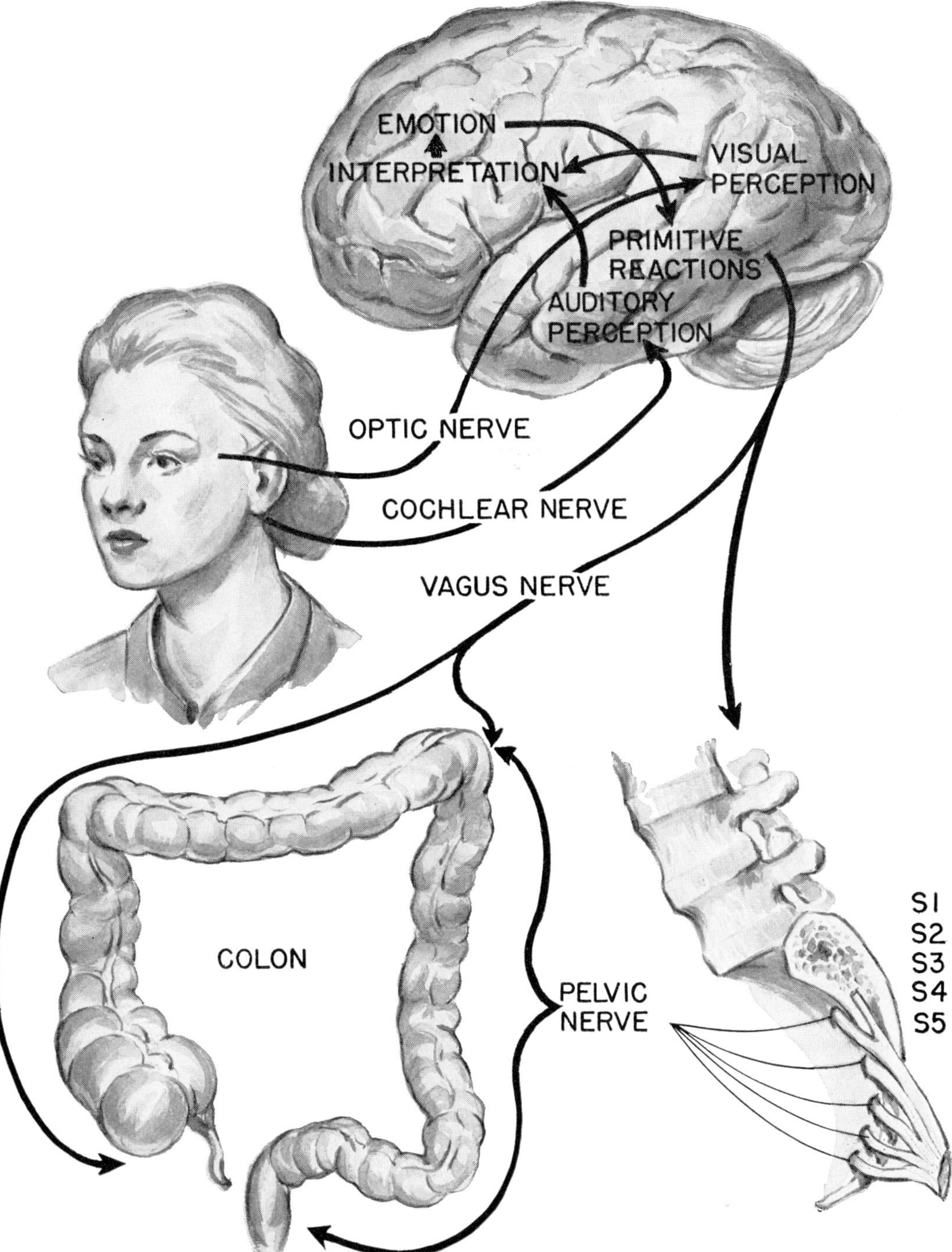

FIG. 178. Nonspecific ulcerative colitis. The emotional phase of this condition plays an important part. Since both halves of the colon are involved, there apparently is some communication between the vagal component (worry nerve) and the sacral nerves.

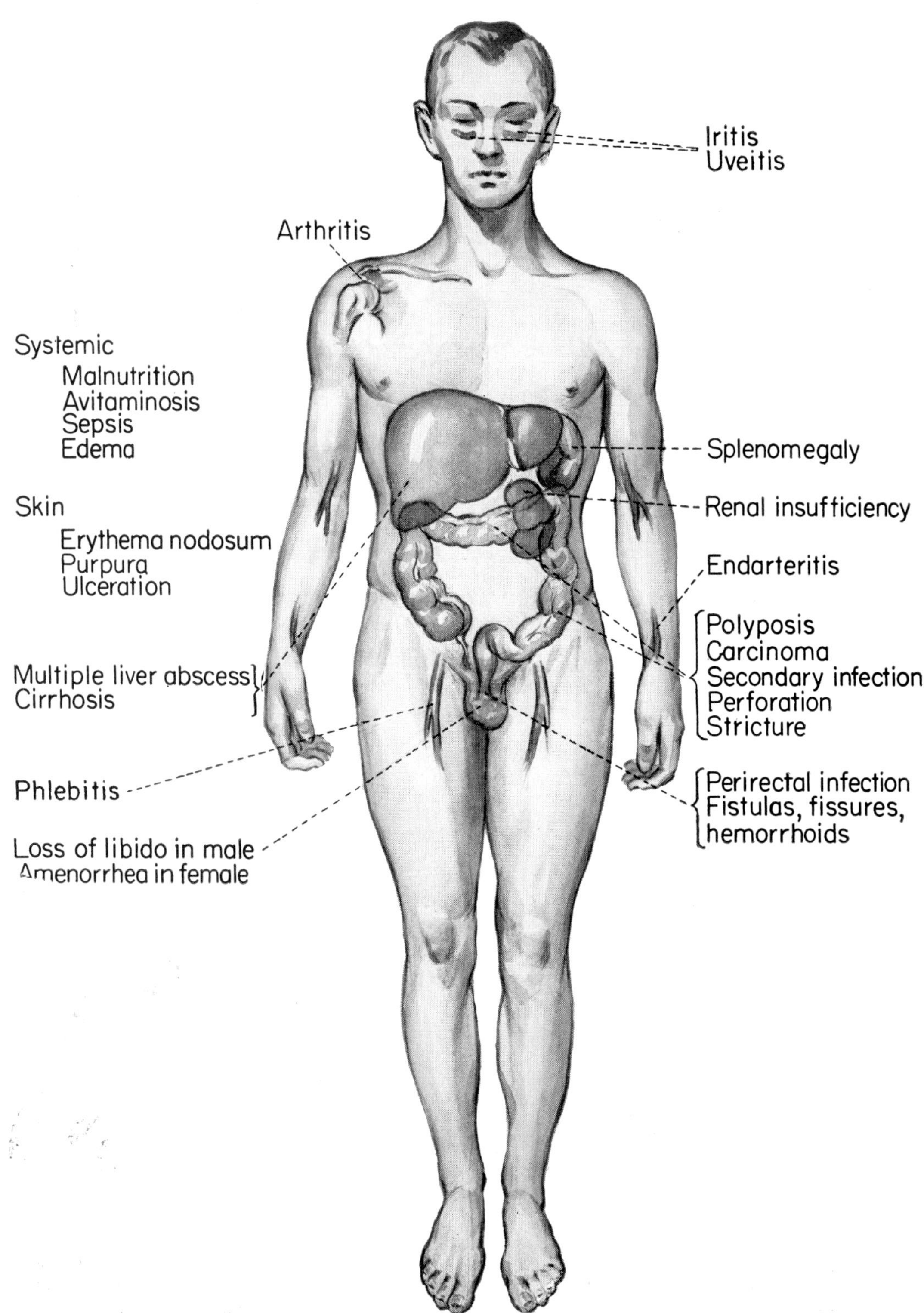

FIG. 179. Complications of chronic nonspecific ulcerative colitis.

being passed when he urinates. Scar tissue may deform the involved segment of colon and produce obstructive manifestations. This may be difficult to differentiate from carcinoma; however, the involved segment is usually longer than that found with a malignant neoplasm. *Hemorrhage* is worthy of special mention in cases of diverticulitis. Although the bleeding it usually mild or occult, it may be massive and critical.

The presence of diverticula is ascertained best by roentgenographic examination. The residual barium in these diverticula usually is expelled within 24 hours. If this fails to take place, stasis is suspected (Fig. 177). Diverticula may escape detection, even with a careful roentgenographic technic, when they are filled with feces or inspissated mucus and prevent the entrance of the barium.

Chronic Nonspecific Ulcerative Colitis

This name applies to a group of chronic ulcerating inflammations of the colon for which no definite etiology has been established.

Etiology. Various bacteria have been condemned, the allergic theory has its proponents, and there are those who consider nutritional deficiencies as the cause rather than the effect of the disease. The neurogenic theory is currently popular, since these patients often display emotional instability. The frequent location of the ulcers along the course of the taeniae coli suggests that spasm along longitudinal muscle bundles may be a factor in the development of these ulcers. There is evidence which indicates that deleterious changes may occur in the colon by way of impulses reaching it via the vagus or the pelvic nerves (Fig. 178). The author has advocated vagotomy in the treatment of this disease. Although this therapy is to be attempted with much trepidation and thought, it nevertheless warrants investigation. The condition usually begins in early adult life and affects both sexes with equal frequency. Its course is interrupted by remissions; unfortunately, exacerbations recur, and the disease continues in a progressive downhill course.

The symptoms consist of "colicky" abdominal pain and diarrhea. The stools are semisolid or liquid and contain excessive amounts of mucus, pus and blood. Rectal pain results from the frequent passage of copious liquid stools. As the disease progresses, impaired digestive functions produce malnutrition and dehydration.

Physical examination reveals intermittent fever, anemia and tenderness, particularly in the region of the sigmoid and the upper rectum. Localized abscesses are prone to form, and these may perforate externally or into adjacent organs. Fistulous communications between the colon and the small intestine, the vagina, the uterus and the urinary bladder are not infrequent. The external fistulas are encountered most frequently in the perianal region.

Fluoroscopic, roentgenographic and endoscopic examinations are most helpful. Proctoscopic examination reveals a mucosa that is hyperemic, ulcerated, and bleeds readily. Roentgenographic findings with barium instillation reveal a colon that is less distendable than normal and a narrowed lumen. These findings may be local or general. The haustral markings are usually absent or less prominent, motility is diminished, and the length of the organ is reduced. The margin of the colon has an irregular or "moth eaten" appearance due to the presence of edema and ulcers. Later in the course of the disease the cicatricial narrowing of the lumen makes differentiation from carcinoma extremely difficult. Particularly is this so since malignant degeneration is in itself a complication of ulcerative colitis. The process may extend across the ileocecal barrier and into the terminal ileum (p. 138). Pseudopolyps, a result of edema, may become so numerous as to fill the lumen of the bowel. If marked, this produces a cobblestone appearance.

The complications are legion. The study of Figure 179 will reveal many of the numerous complications associated with this condition.

The differential diagnosis must include bacillary and amebic dysentery, intestinal tuberculosis, benign and malignant tumors, congenital polyposis and venereal lymphogranuloma. True polypi microscopically reveal the characteristic adenomatous changes, whereas pseudopolyps are inflammatory. Venereal lymphogranuloma is associated with a positive Frei test and an elevated serum

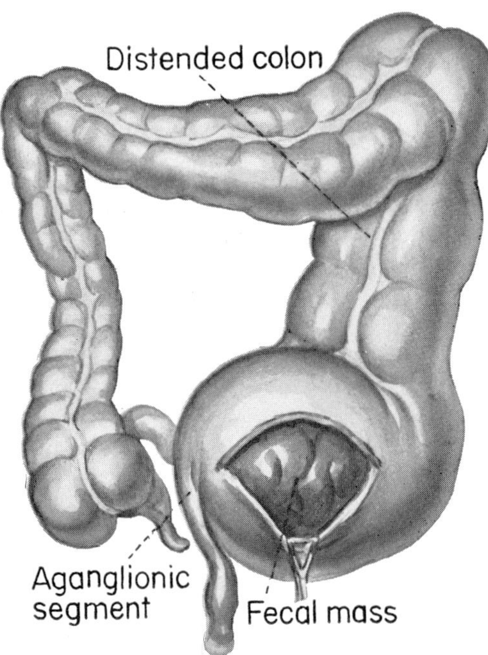

FIG. 180. Megacolon is supposed to be due to an aganglionic segment which usually appears in the rectosigmoid region. This results in massive dilatation proximal to this point of functional obstruction with the formation of large collections of inspissated feces.

globulin. Bacteriologic study of exudate from infected inguinal glands and biopsy of the involved rectal mucosa are also contributory.

The prognosis of ulcerative colitis always must be guarded.

Polyposis of the Colon

Polyps can be found in any portion of the bowel; however, there is a predilection for the rectum. They are encountered frequently in the alimentary tracts of children. There appears to be a familial tendency, particularly when the polypi are numerous.

The most common complaints are bleeding and/or diarrhea.

Thorough endoscopic and roentgenographic examinations aid in their detection, location and number. Removal of either a solitary polyp of a large segment of colon in the case of multiple polyposis is mandatory because of the tendency to malignant changes.

Congenital familial multiple polyposis (Peutz-Jeghers syndrome), also known as melanosis coli (p. 14), is an uncommon yet important disease. It is characterized by a familial predisposition in which the bowel mucosa, particularly of the large intestines, is totally covered by numerous small pedunculated polyps. The occurrence of melanin deposits about the lips and the oral cavity commonly is associated with this condition (p. 14). In some instances the polyps extend through the entire intestinal tract and even involve the stomach. Such polyps apparently develop after birth; cases have been described in children as young as 2 years of age. Frequently, the disease is discovered by chance, but attention may be called to it because of bowel symptoms, such as bleeding or disturbances of bowel function. Since polyps of the large bowel are known for their tendency toward malignant degeneration, this disease is believed to be almost 100 per cent premalignant. It is unfortunately true that many of these cases remain undiagnosed until the malignancies develop. It is not unusual for several primary lesions to be found in a given specimen.

Megacolon

This has been referred to as aganglionosis and Hirschsprung's disease. It is encountered most frequently in infants and children. The type that occurs within the first 2 decades of life presumably is due to a congenital defect in the bowel wall; it is described also as *idiopathic congenital megacolon.* Swenson demonstrated that a segment of large bowel just distal to the dilated colon revealed an absence of the myenteric plexus of Meissner and Auerbach. In the most common pattern only a short segment at the rectosigmoid junction is aganglionic. Since peristaltic waves cannot traverse such a segment, the bowel proximal distends (functional obstruction). Occasionally, the enire rectum is aganglionic, and rare cases of total aganglionic colons have been described. *Acquired* megacolon presents a different problem in that the ganglia are present in most of these adult patients. Numerous theories regarding the etiology of this type of megacolon include achalasia, malrotation, nutritional and avitaminotic disturbances in bowel motility.

Symptoms. These result from progressive dilatation of the colon. The left side of the large bowel is affected first, but the entire colon may become involved as far as the ileocecal valve. In the type that begins in infancy marked disturbances in bowel function appear early. Obstipation may progress to the point of total obstruction. Abdominal distention is marked, and vomiting may occur. Rectal examination, particularly in infants and children, is essential and informative. If a considerable quantity of green sticky meconium is present on the examiner's finger, the gastrointesinal tract is almost certain to be patent. The expulsion of large amounts of gas and liquid stool in any infant with a distended abdomen is suggestive of Hirschsprung's disease (Fig. 180). If the condition is not corrected, extreme nutritional deficiencies with marked loss of weight and cachexia result. Fluoroscopic and roentgenographic studies reveal colonic dilatations that may assume tremendous proportions (Fig. 181). The entire colon or any segments of the colon may be dilated. Persistent fecal impaction with obstruction and perforation occurs in the neglected cases. Volvulus and strangulation of the bowel have been reported.

The diagnosis is confirmed by *biopsy* of the bowel wall in the region of the rectosigmoid and upper rectal segment, which reveals an absence of the myenteric plexuses.

Other organs also may be involved. Mega-esophagus, mega-ureter and megaduodenum have been known to occur concomitantly.

Foreign Bodies

Foreign bodies may become lodged in the colon after their ingestion or after their placement per rectum. Symptoms of obstruction may develop; if the object is sharp, perforation can occur; this may lead to peritonitis and/or abscess formation. Frequently, such abscesses are misdiagnosed; the preoperative diagnosis is usually appendiceal abscess or an abscess due to diverticulitis. The true nature of the condition may be discovered

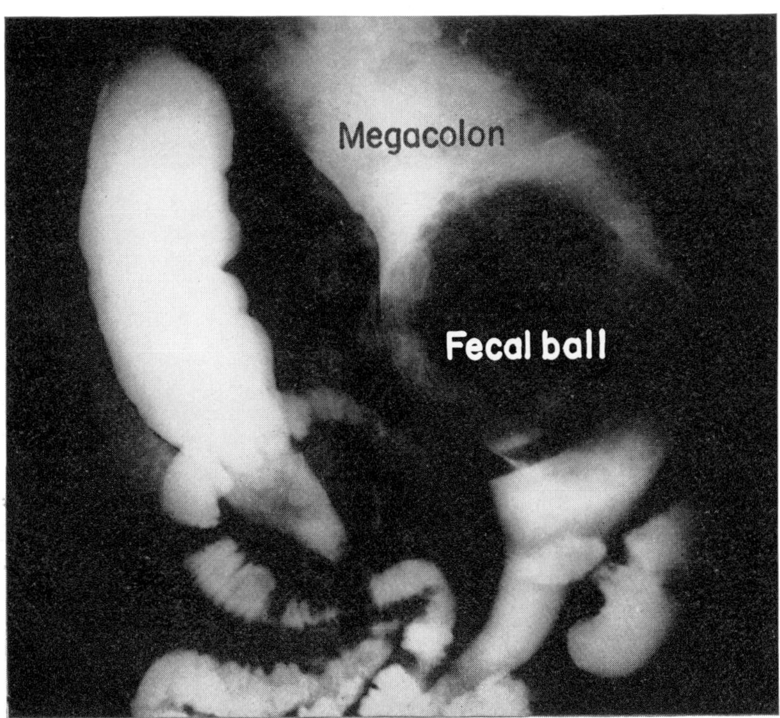

Fig. 181. Roentgenogram of congenital megacolon (Hirschsprung's disease).

only at the time of exploration when the foreign body is found. Fortunately, many of these objects are radiopaque. Figure 182 illustrates a screwdriver that was inserted into the rectum by the patient for the supposed purpose of reducing his prolapsed piles. It had traveled in a retrograde direction to the splenic flexure and was removed by incising the descending colon.

Specific Granulomas

Tuberculosis and actinomycosis must be mentioned; the latter seems to be appearing with increased frequency. These will produce symptoms similar to any ulcerating bowel condition. Actinomycosis usually is associated with the ultimate development of a mass and multiple fistulous openings. Tuberculous ulceration of the cecum comprises one half of all intestinal tuberculosis. Most of these patients have an active pulmonary lesion. In any draining sinus the specific granulomas must be considered.

Amebiasis

Several aspects of amebic dysentery are of surgical importance. The disease appears in endemic forms, but epidemic outbreaks do occur. These usually are due to a contaminated water supply or fly transmission. The trophozoites are of no great importance in the epidemiology of the disease, since they rarely survive exposure to hydrochloric acid, digestive enzymes, or life outside of the body. However, the encysted forms are resistant and responsible for transmission, which takes place in 1 of 4 ways: the house fly, polluted water, vegetables, and direct contact with human carriers (Fig. 183). This condition should be kept in mind in any resistant case of gastrointestinal disease regardless of geographic distribution.

Ingested cysts of *Endamoeba histolytica*, upon reaching the intestinal tract of the new host, excyst. The resulting trophozoites penetrate the host's tissues. Lesions are found most commonly in the cecum, the ascending colon, the sigmoid and the rectum. Since this stage is associated with abdominal pains and cramps and possibly tenderness in the right lower quadrant because of cecal involvement, these cases may be mistaken for acute appendicitis. Invasion of the submucosa may be followed by entry of the amoeba into radi-

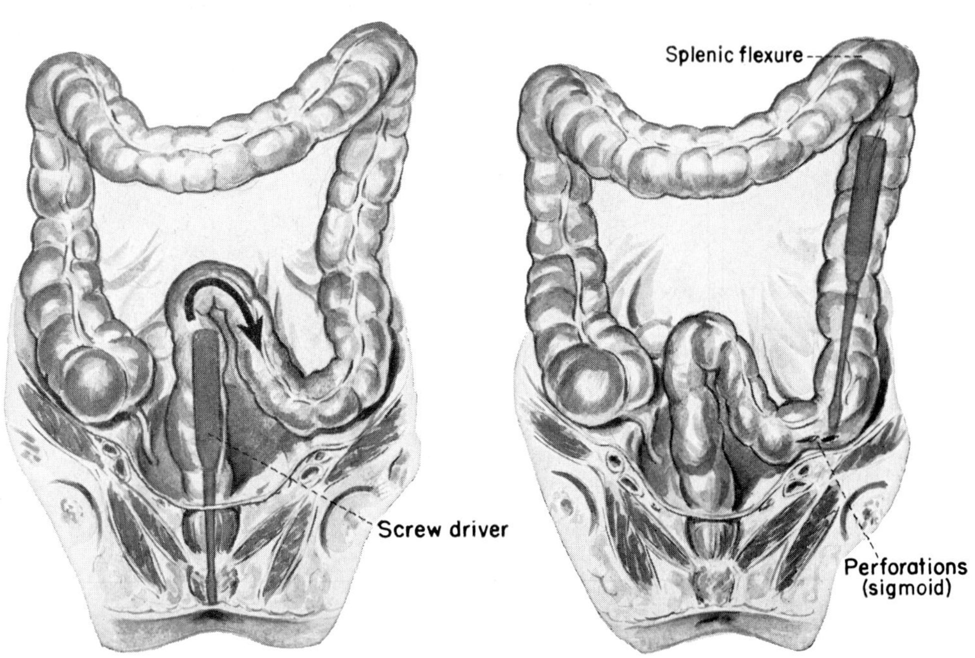

Fig. 182. Self-introduced screwdriver which caused perforations of the colon.

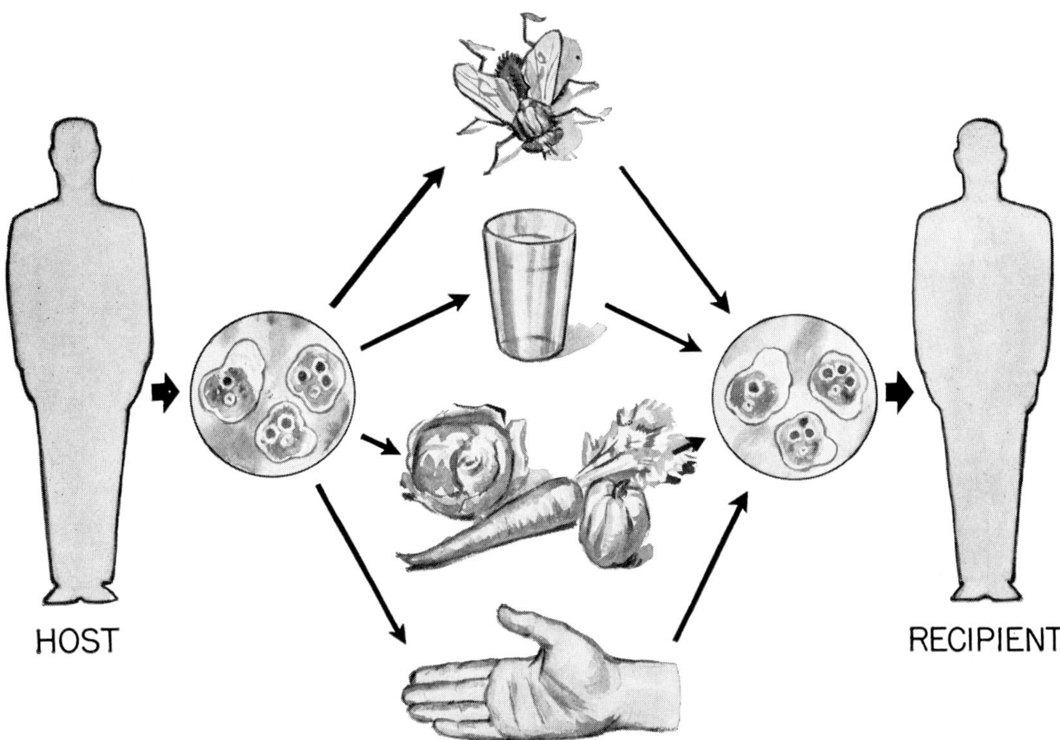

FIG. 183. Amebiasis. The encysted forms are the resistant ones. They are transmitted to the new recipient by the house fly through drinking water, fresh vegetables or direct contact. Several aspects of amebic dysentery are of surgical importance.

cals of the portal vein and metastases to the liver. Amebic hepatitis or abscess of the liver is by far the most frequent and important complication. Such abscesses may be single or multiple, acute or chronic. Right-lobe liver abscesses can extend upward, penetrate the diaphragm and rupture into the lung. They also have reached the brain, skin, bladder, uterus and vagina (Fig. 184). These may be associated with amebic sinuses.

Pseudomembranous Enterocolitis

This is an uncommon but extremely serious disease. Staphylococci usually are demonstrated growing abundantly and relatively alone in the feces (staphylococcal enteritis). It frequently follows antibiotic treatment with broad-spectrum drugs, particularly if the drugs have been used orally and prophylactically. These drugs eliminate coliform organisms. The resistant staphylococcus presumably prospers because of the absence of competing bacteria which normally are present in the intestinal tract; in other words, the bacterial balance of power is disturbed. The disease was known before antibiotics were used and still occurs in patients who have not received such medication.

Symptoms. These consist of severe cramping abdominal pain, nausea, vomiting, distention, continuous watery diarrhea and early prostration. The stools are voluminous. Usually, fever is present, and there is a rapid drop in blood pressure secondary to excessive loss of fluids. Stool cultures reveal an almost pure culture of a resistant coagulase-positive *Staphylococcus aureus*. It is dangerous and unnecessary to await the results of cultures, as the diagnosis can be established on direct smear and gram stain of the liquid stool. The process may involve the entire colon and parts of the ileum. The diarrhea and watery stool frequently contain "rice bodies" which represent desquamated membranous mucosa.

It is imperative that an early diagnosis be

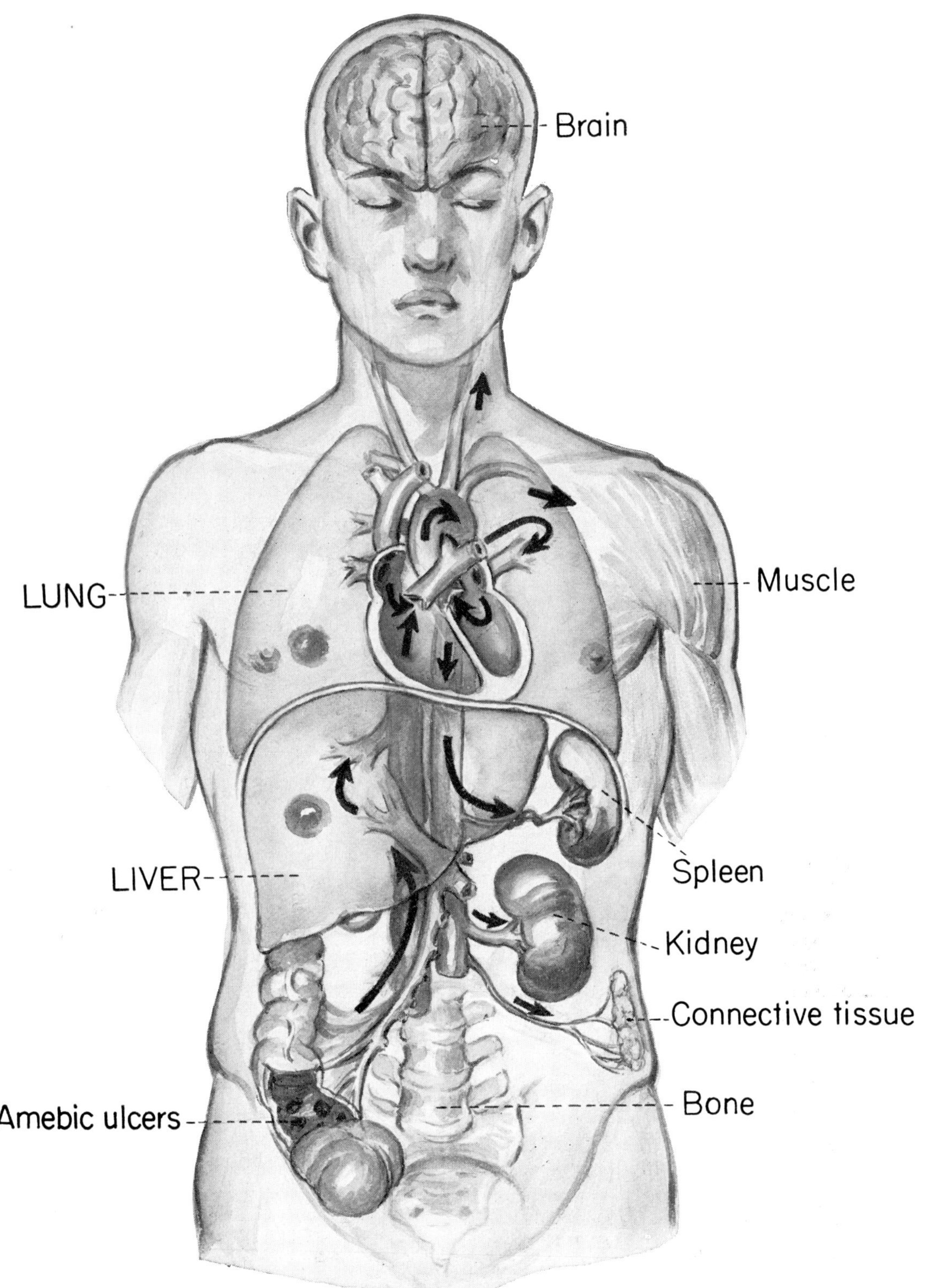

FIG. 184. Amebic ulcer and some of the possible paths of extension and development of amebic abscesses.

made, since the mortality is high if the condition is untreated. Recently, dramatic recovery has been observed with the introduction of suspensions of stool from normal persons. Such suspensions have been introduced by a rectal catheter or by inlying nasogastric tubes.

UMBILICUS

The vitelline duct, the urachus and the umbilical vessels traverse the umbilicus. Only the first 2 are clinically important.

Vitelline Duct

The vitelline (omphalomesenteric) duct is a short-lived structure but is important in the normal development of the embryo. It acts as the communication between the embryo and the yolk sac and is obliterated by the 7th week of fetal life. All or any part of

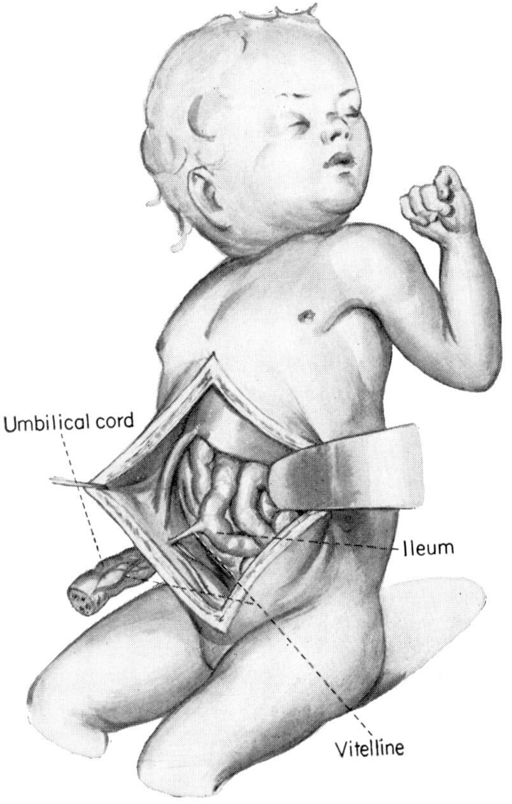

Fig. 185. The vitelline duct normally becomes obliterated by the 7th week of fetal life, but all or any part of it may persist.

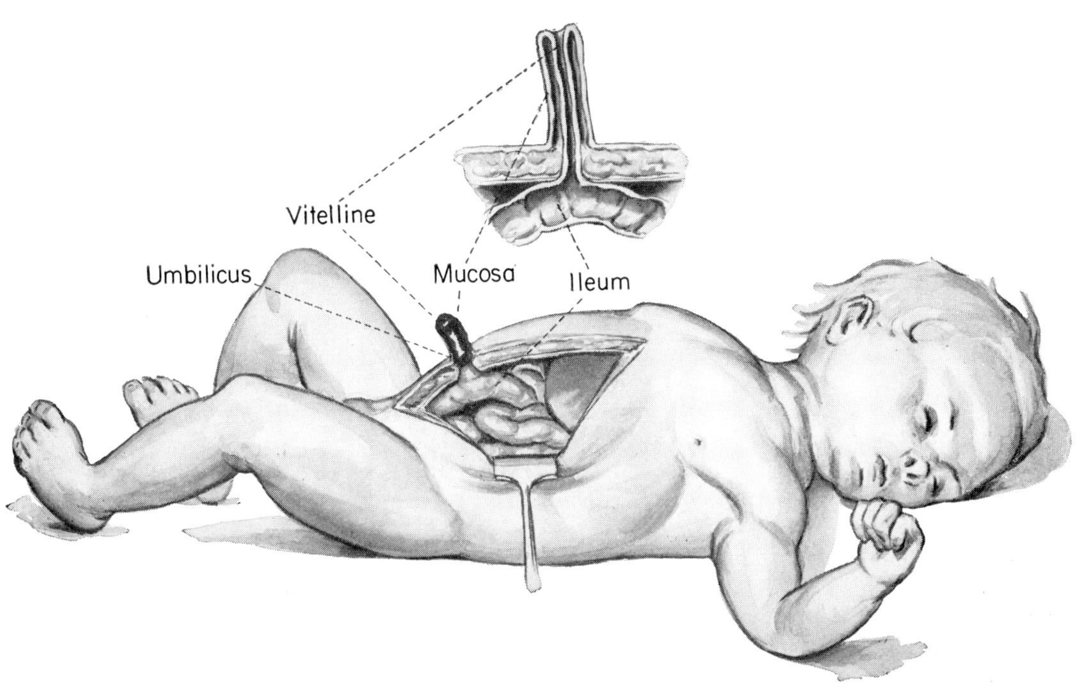

Fig. 186. Persistence of the entire vitelline duct.

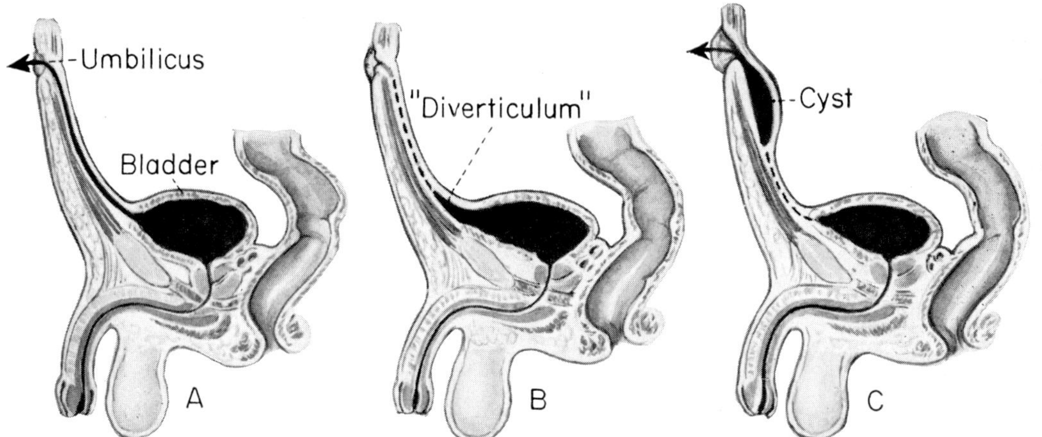

FIG. 187. Disorders of the bladder and the umbilicus of urachal origin. (A) Congenital patent urachus (complete). (B) Vesicourachal "diverticulum," which opens internally. (C) Cyst and sinus which open at the umbilicus.

this duct may persist (Fig. 185). When the proximal portion persists, the resulting outpouching which arises from the ileum is known as a *Meckel's diverticulum* (p. 138). When the distal portion persists, a *superficial umbilical adenoma or polyp* forms; this may be related to an incomplete sinus. If the central portion persists, a *vitelline cyst* forms beneath the umbilicus or in the leaves of the mesentery of the ileum. When the entire duct persists, a patent tube results which forms a *fistula* between the bowel and the umbilicus (Fig. 186). If the lumen is small, a watery mucoid discharge appears at the umbilicus, but if the lumen is large, a fecal fistula results.

The direct and the differential diagnosis of persisting draining umbilical lesions is important. In uncomplicated cases radiopaque material may be injected into the tract to determine its origin. Probing is dangerous, since it does not give adequate information and may easily perforate the intestinal wall.

Omphalitis

Omphalitis is due to uncleanliness. It produces a red weeping lesion at the umbilicus which must be differentiated from persistent granulating tissue, concretions, endometriosis, and primary or secondary tumors.

Congenital Umbilical Hernia (Omphalocele)

Congenital umbilical hernia differs from a prolapsed patent duct in that there is a transparent covering over the nonprolapsed herniated bowel. A patent urachus is identified readily by the fact that urine leaks from the umbilicus; a cystogram corroborates the diagnosis. Occasionally, a loop of intestine herniates into the umbilical cord and is included inadvertently as the cord is tied. This produces an *umbilical fecal fistula.* Abdominal exploration is the only way that this condition can be identified with certainty and corrected.

Urachus

Embryologically, the urachus is part of the bladder. In adult life it appears as an obliterated cord between the umbilicus and the dome of the bladder. Hinman suggests the following classification of urachal embryologic defects: (1) congenital patent urachus; (2) vesicourachal "diverticulum"; (3) umbilical cyst and sinus; (4) alternating urachal sinus (Fig. 187).

The congenital patent urachus is completely open and presents a communication between the dome of the bladder and the umbilicus. In some cases drainage occurs only with abdominal pressure, and in other cases urine flows from the umbilicus with each act of micturition. When pressure over the bladder produces umbilical urinary flow, the diagnosis is certain. Lateral cystograms reveal the defect. Urachal lesions must be distinguished from omphalitis and patent omphalomesenteric duct. Vesicourachal "diverticulm" presents only an internal opening into the bladder. Urachal cysts usually open externally. This is generally in combination with a sinus. Infected umbilical cysts tend to remain subumbilical. Urachal cysts produce manifestations of a localized intra-abdominal mass which is present in the midline.

Neoplasms

Umbilical neoplasms, particularly primary squamous cell carcinoma as well as metastatic carcinoma, have been reported. Any firm node in the region of the umbilicus should be removed for microscopic study, since these may be metastatic carcinomas from the gastrointestinal tract or the ovary.

RECTUM AND ANUS

The incidence of anorectal diseases is high. Every patient complaining of rectal symptoms, particularly bleeding, constipation, pain and tenesmus, must be examined

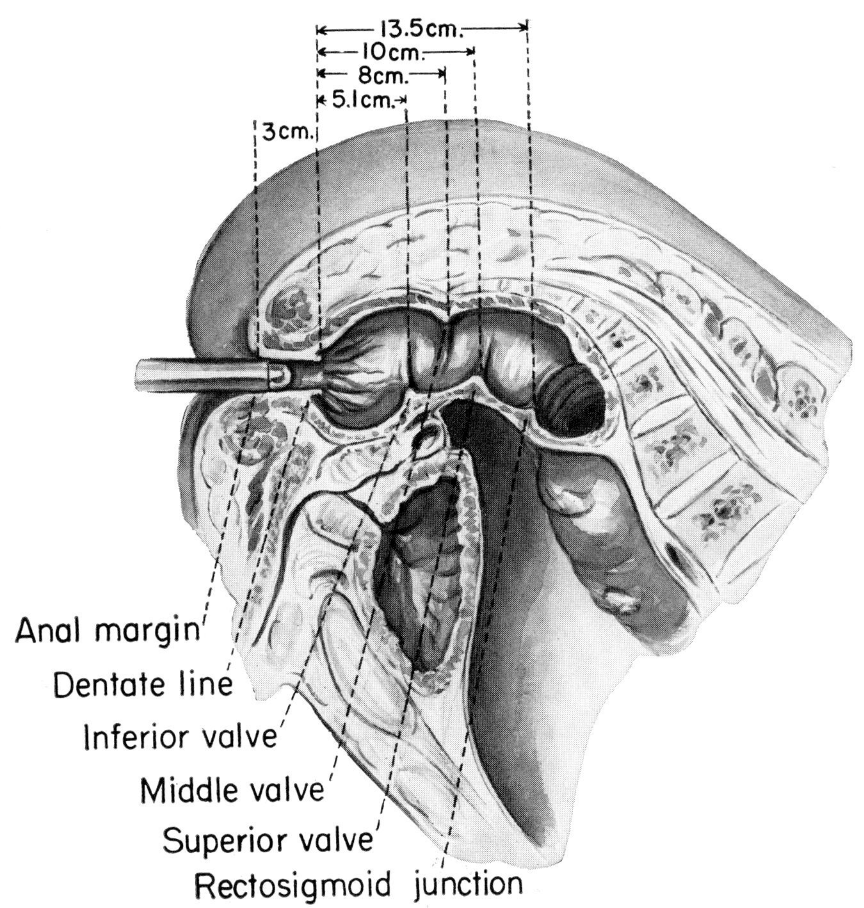

Fig. 188. The anatomy of the anorectal region. The important anatomic landmarks and their locations are shown.

carefully. The importance of rectal examinations has been stressed repeatedly. This is accomplished best with the patient on his left side or in the knee-chest position. Direct inspection with appropriate armamentarium and light is an indispensable part of the examination; both the anoscope and the proctoscope are necessary. If blood, pus and/or mucus are seen in the ampulla of the rectum with no visible lesion to account for the findings, a careful roentgenologic study is required. The examining physician should acquaint himself with the anatomy of this region so that he may be able to interpret the lesion and the location properly (Fig. 188).

Hemorrhoids (Piles)

These are varicosities of the hemorrhoidal veins. A simple classification into internal and external varieties is adequate. An *internal hemorrhoid* is covered with mucous membrane and therefore is proximal to the dentate line. An *external hemorrhoid* is covered with skin and is distal to the dentate line. Internal hemorrhoids usually appear as 3 primary piles. These are the accompanying veins of the terminal branches of the superior hemorrhoidal artery.

The etiology is obscure; however, they often occur after childbirth, or they represent chronic venous hypertension which is associated with such extrinsic factors as prostatic hypertrophy, uterine enlargement or pelvic tumors. Always to be considered is the possibility of venous obstruction due to rectal carcinoma. Undoubtedly, there is a congenital deficiency which predisposes to the formation of hemorrhoids. Hemorrhoids may be nature's portacaval shunts and attempt to bring about a collateral circulation (cirrhosis of the liver). Whenever an individual is examined who has piles and no hair on his chest (cirrhotic habitus), one should be suspicious of cirrhosis of the liver. Such

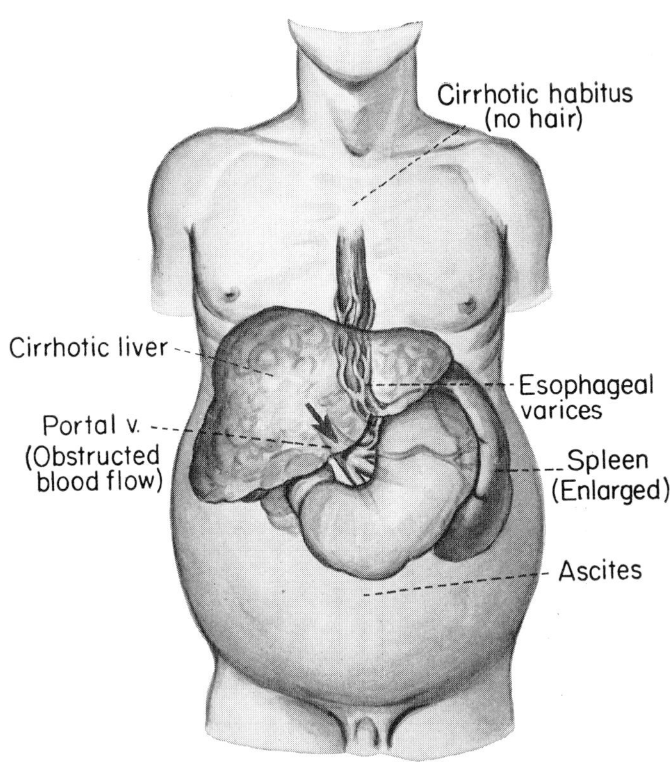

Fig. 189. The cirrhotic habitus. Note the absence of hair of the chest.

hemorrhoids, if possible, should not be disturbed (Fig. 189).

Hemorrhoids *do not* cause pain. Internal hemorrhoids protrude, bleed or produce itching. If pain is present, it is due to infection, ulceration, thrombosis or prolapse with strangulation. External hemorrhoids rarely produce symptoms unless they become acutely inflamed or thrombosed. A thrombotic pile produces sudden localized pain, usually after defecating. This may be severe enough to be completely disabling and may require sedation. The diagnosis is obvious on inspection. Internal hemorrhoids may not be felt on digital examination, since the finger compresses the vein. Demonstrable evidence should be sought with the anoscope.

Since internal hemorrhoids are above the dentate line, they are not related to sensory nerve fibers and therefore cause no pain. External hemorrhoids occur below the dentate line in an area supplied by sensory pain fibers; if they become thrombosed, they produce severe pain. The blood that is associated with hemorrhoids is bright red; this is seen on the toilet tissue or in the commode. The bleeding may disappear and not reappear for varying periods of time. A hard or voluminous stool, usually following a period of constipation causes the blood to reappear. Anemia may be absent or severe. Because of the paucity of symptoms these cases are often neglected.

Cryptitis, fissure-in-ano, ischiorectal abscess and fistula-in-ano are considered together, since they are frequently related. Some are of the opinion that a fistula-in-ano is the 4th or last stage of a cryptitis.

Cryptitis

Tiny little crypts of Morgagni encircle the rectum just inside of the anal canal at the dentate line. These are identified easily on anoscopic examination. The etiology of cryptitis is still moot; however, some are of the opinion that it results from broken-off bits of constipated stool which become entrapped in the crypt. Others blame plugged anal glands which are associated with these crypts. In either event stasis plays an important role. Cryptitis produces anal spasm, painful defecation, pruritus ani and tenesmus. Anoscopic examination reveals an inflamed circular area representing the base of the crypt and frequently an elongated inflamed papilla directly in continuity with it.

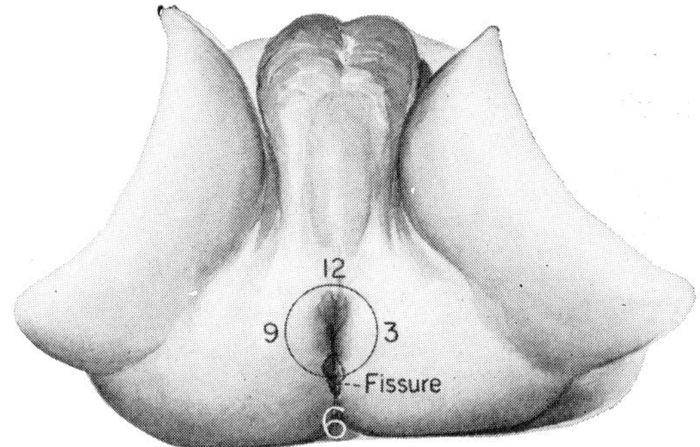

Fig. 190. An anal fissure is located in the 6 o'clock position.

Fissure-in-Ano

This represents the most frequent cause of painful rectal bleeding. It is a break in the anal skin which frequently fails to heal. An associated infected crypt always should be sought for. The pain produces sphincteric spasm which leads to further constipation, and a vicious circle results. Almost all anal fissures occur at the posterior commissure; this would correspond to the 6 o'clock location when the patient is in the lithotomy position (Fig. 190). The pain is quite characteristic in that it is sharp and tearing and is initiated by a bowel movement. Bleeding appears as a spot of fresh blood seen on the toilet tissue or on the stool.

Anal ulcer is the result of repeated attacks of anal fissure. The pain now becomes more intense and continuous. Examination reveals, instead of the linear abrasion characteristic of the fissure, an oval undermined loss of continuity of the lining of the anus. External to this the characteristic "sentinel tag" is noted. This results from an edema of the marginal skin due to blockage of the lymphatics and has been referred to erroneously as a sentinel "pile." It is not a hemorrhoid. Infected adjacent anal crypts may undermine the ulcer. Such infected crypts are important, both diagnostically and therapeutically (Fig. 191).

Ischiorectal Abscess

This common and painful infection usually results from an infected crypt. Such abscesses may be divided into those that occur above or below the levator ani muscles.

The so-called **deep or supralevator infections** are fortunately the uncommon variety. They occur in a space bounded by the levator muscles below, the wall of the rectum medially, and the peritoneum above. Since this space is situated away from the sensory nerve supply, localizing symptoms appear notoriously late. Peritoneal irritation may be produced, and such cases have even been mistaken for acute appendicitis.

The **superficial or infralevator type of abscess** is the one encountered most commonly. The clinical manifestations consist of severe local pain and tenderness which produce rapid and complete disability. The patient prefers to lie on his side or abdomen. Fever and leukocytosis usually are elevated. Physical examination reveals an area of redness and induration in the involved buttock. Rectal examination is frequently impossible because of the severe spasm and pain. If an ischiorectal abscess breaks into the rectum or through the outside skin on the gluteal surface, immediate relief is obtained, and the acute symptoms disappear spontaneously. When an ischiorectal abscess communicates with the exterior through the gluteal skin a fistula-in-ano results.

Fistula-in-Ano

It is helpful to consider this condition through 4 stages in its development (Fig. 191):

Stage 1. Cryptitis
Stage 2. Burrowing
Stage 3. Ischiorectal abscess
Stage 4. Fistula-in-ano

A fistula-in-ano frequently starts as an infected crypt. For total eradication of such fistulas the entire tract and the involved crypt must be removed. An infected crypt burrows either above or below the levator ani. An ischiorectal abscess then develops.

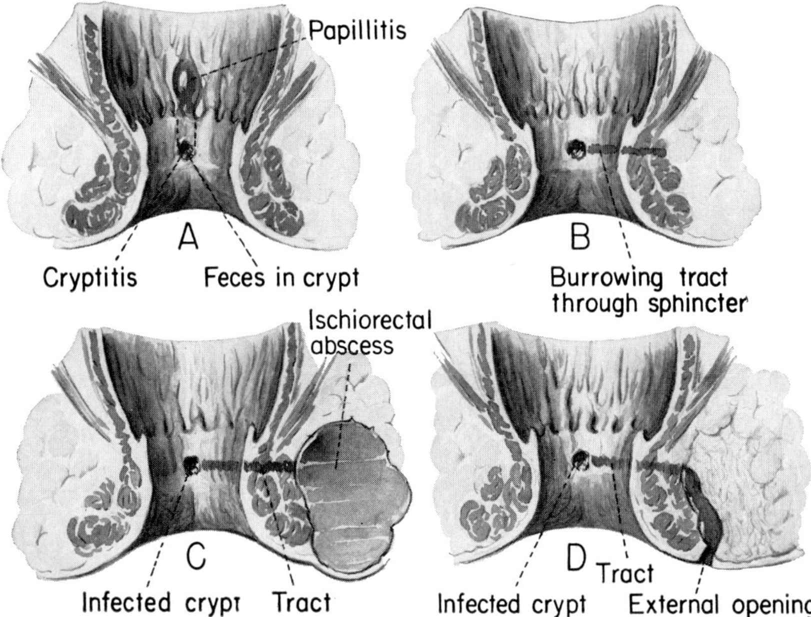

Fig. 191. The 4 stages in the development of a fistula-in-ano. (A) The cryptitis-papillitis stage usually is associated with constipation. (B) Burrowing of the infection may pass above, below or through the sphincter muscle. (C) Infection in the fatty ischiorectal space leads to the development of an ischiorectal abscess. (D) The ischiorectal abscess after rupturing gives rise to the fully developed fistula-in-ano.

This finally communicates with the external or gluteal surface either spontaneously or surgically, and the fully developed fistula-in-ano is formed. Occasionally, the infection spreads throughout the tissues of the perineum and produces numerous openings (waterpot type). Rectal strictures may develop. The symptoms, besides those of recurrent abscesses, consist of a continuous annoying discharge; pain and systemic evidence of infection occur. Bowel movements are painful. The lesion varies in extent and location. The communication with the rectum may be microscopic and difficult to determine because of healing of the infected crypt. If the fistula is distal to the sphincter ani, it is subcutaneous; however, these tracts may course through or above the sphincter muscles. Formerly, such fistulas were thought to be associated with tuberculosis, but such cases are rare.

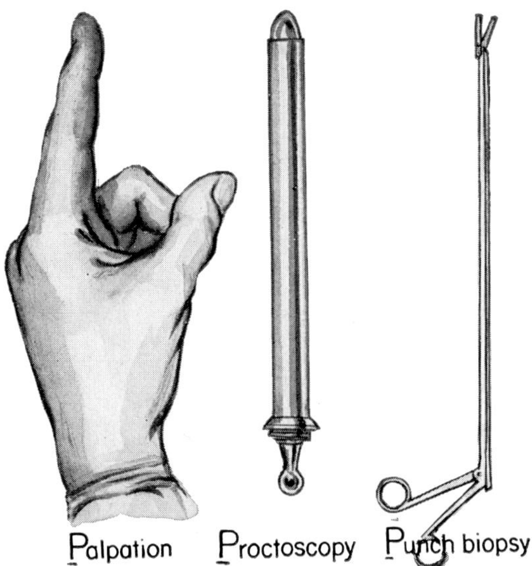

FIG. 192. Every patient with an anorectal or bowel complaint is entitled to the simple and accurate 3 "P" examination (palpation, proctoscopy and punch biopsy).

BENIGN STRICTURE OF THE RECTUM

This acquired condition may follow trauma, radiation therapy, particularly of the cervix uteri, or may result from specific diseases, especially lymphogranuloma venereum. The symptoms of an associated abscess may overshadow the underlying cause.

Clinical manifestations are characterized by the passage of pus, mucus and blood in the stool; later symptoms are obstructive ones. Those cases associated with the venereal disease known as lymphogranuloma venereum usually have a primary lesion located on the vulva, the pubis, within the vagina or the rectum. Nodes about the lower rectum become the site of secondary involvement. Perirectal abscess formation and mucosal ulceration occur which give rise to strictures. This latter condition is due to a specific virus from which a worthwhile antigen may be prepared. The Frei test is a valuable diagnostic aid which should be utilized in all suspected cases of benign stricture of the rectum.

RECTAL PROLAPSE

The etiology is unknown; however, 2 possible factors have been mentioned, namely, a loose fixation of the rectum and a deep cul-de-sac. If the anterior rectal wall prolapses, it may bring with it a downward projection of the peritoneum containing loops of small intestine. The condition usually is seen in infants or in the aged; it is more common in women. Venous obstruction which results from contraction of the anal sphincter produces marked congestion. This makes reduction difficult or impossible, and necrosis may develop.

CARCINOMA OF THE RECTUM

This condition is as frequent as the combined cancers of the rest of the colon. It appears between the rectosigmoid junction and the anus (anal carcinoma is of the squamous type). The growth may be silent, but in the majority of cases *bleeding* is the first sign. The blood varies in color, depending on the length of time it remains in the rectum. It is usually bright red.

Change in bowel habit may precede bleeding and is a symptom that warrants immediate investigation. A sense of incomplete evacuation, looseness of the stool or a frequent desire to defecate must be considered as carcinoma until proved to be otherwise. This is particularly true of the patient with hemorrhoids, since both the patient and the

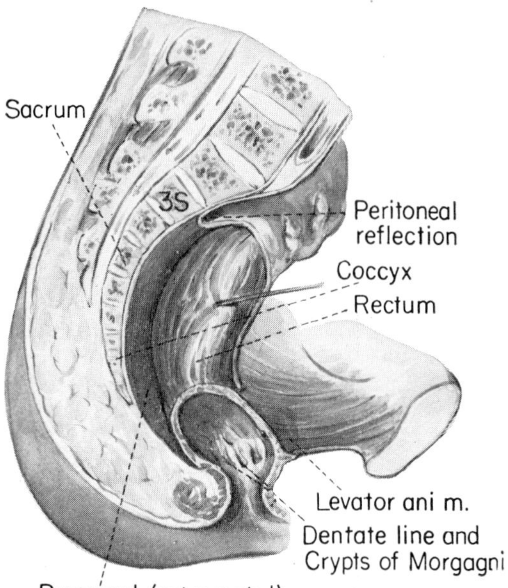

FIG. 193. The presacral (retrorectal) space.

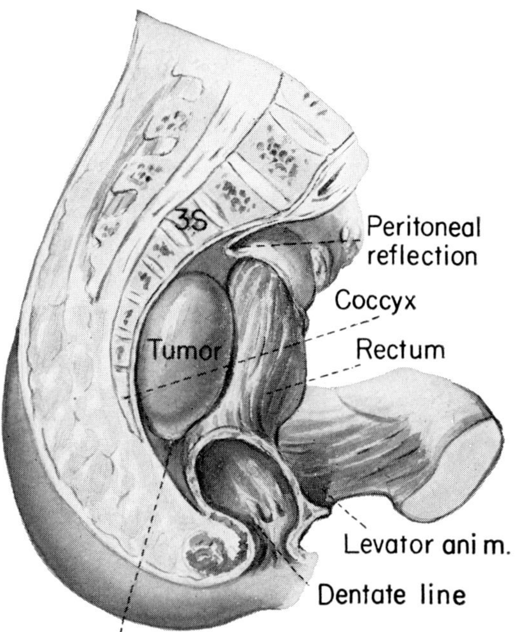

FIG. 194. A mass involving the presacral space and causing pressure and bulging of the posterior rectal wall.

physician may be guilty of attributing these signs and symptoms to the piles.

Obstructive symptoms are the first manifestation if the tumor encroaches upon the bowel lumen. Cramping pain in the left lower quadrant and distention occur (see Intestinal Obstruction, p. 176). Total obstruction is rare in carcinoma of the rectum proper; however, it does occur when the tumor is located at the rectosigmoid junction. Loss of weight, anemia, and pain in the region of the sacrum are manifestations of late carcinoma.

Diagnosis. *Every patient is entitled to digital and proctoscopic examinations* (Fig. 192). Though roentgenologic studies are of great value in diseases above the rectosigmoid, little reliance should be placed on these technics in a patient with rectal carcinoma.

Since these lesions are well within reach of the examining finger, it is incumbent on the physician to assume full responsibility for the identification of the tumor and institution of early therapy.

Carcinoma of the Anus

This carcinoma is of the squamous cell type. It is rare, occurring only 1/20th as common as carcinoma of the rectum.

It differs from carcinoma of the rectum in many respects. Because of its location, near the anal sphincter, and in an area richly supplied with pain fibers, pain and anal spasm are early and significant symptoms. These lesions are prone to early infiltration of the perirectal connective tissue and the vaginal wall. They metastasize to the inguinal lymph nodes in contradistinction to carcinoma of the rectum, which spreads to the deeper pelvic nodes. Bleeding is usually present. The prognosis is poor.

Retrorectal Tumors

These are extrarectal tumors that occur in the presacral (retrorectal) space. They are important, because they are more common than was previously thought. Many of these masses are asymptomatic; however, they may be associated with draining sinuses or fistulas.

The presacral (retrorectal) space has the following boundaries (Fig. 193): anteriorly, the rectum; posteriorly, the sacrum and the coccyx; cephalad, the peritoneal reflection, which is usually at the 2nd or the 3rd sacral segment; caudad, the levators ani; laterally, the peritoneal reflection and the lateral rectal stalks. This space contains branches of the sacral and the sympathetic nerves, the middle sacral, ileolumbar and middle hemorrhoidal vessels and lymphatics.

The number of conditions that involve this space are 5: (1) inflammatory, (2) congenital, (3) neurogenic, (4) osseous and (5) miscellaneous.

The inflammatory mass is by far the most common. Infected dermoids and teratomas are not included in this group. These masses can result from an infected crypt of Morgagni which spreads upward into the space (Fig. 194). Such an abscess may rupture higher up in the rectum or may drain through its primary source. Chemical tumors (oleomas) result from the injection treatment of hemorrhoids or prolapse. The mineral oil base in these solutions is the offender.

Symptoms vary from low back pain to a feeling of fullness and pressure in the rectum; in some instances a purulent discharge from the anal canal is noted. Proctoscopic examination reveals a bulging into the rectum; this is covered by a normal mucosa. In some instances a draining sinus in the posterior wall of the anal canal may cause confusion. A definite diagnosis is arrived at on examination with the patient under anesthesia and exploration or biopsy of the mass. The prognosis for patients with inflammatory tumors is excellent, since adequate drainage results in cure.

Congenital tumors constitute the greatest number of retrorectal neoplasms. These consist of chordomas, teratomas, dermoid cysts and meningoceles. *Chordomas* are fetal remnants of the notochord. Dysfunction of the bladder is a constant complaint. Pain is present in the rectal, the gluteal, the low back or the perineal areas; this may extend along the sciatic nerve. Roentgenographic study reveals destruction of the sacrum and the lower sacral segments if the lesion is large. *Teratomas* have been referred to as Middeldorpf tumors. These represent more than one germ layer and are complex in structure, containing such materials as bone, cartilage, muscle, teeth, nerve, fat and intestinal mucosa. This type of tumor is seen most often in infants and newborns. On occasion a proctoscopic examination may reveal a protruding tooth or bone. The prognosis is poor, since complete removal is seldom accomplished because of size, secondary infection and extension into adjacent structures.

Dermoid cysts frequently constitute the etiologic basis for so-called recurrent fistulas. These cysts rarely produce symptoms until they have become infected. The differential diagnosis is concerned principally with anorectal fistulas. Roentgenographic studies of the bony region may show the result of pressure erosion on the anterior aspect of the sacrum. Prognosis as to life is good, but the condition is resistant to therapy, and repeated surgical interventions may result in rectal incontinence.

Neurogenic Tumors

These tumors have their genesis in nerve tissue and are either neurofibromas or neurilemmomas. The radiologist may demonstrate erosion of the sacral canal or the sacral foramina. Although frequently asymptomatic, they may cause pain along nerve roots which is accompanied by dysfunction of the rectum and the bladder. The prognosis is good if the tumor is removed completely. Ependymomas arise from the cauda aquina. Pain is marked and referable to nerve root irritation, producing rectal and vesicle dysfunction. The prognosis of these tumors is not good. The prognosis of neurilemmoma, however, is better.

Osseous Tumors

These include osteogenic sarcoma, cartilaginous tumors and giant cell tumors.

Miscellaneous Tumors

Any tumor may arise in this space consistent with the tissues contained herein. Hence, lipomas, hemangio-endothelioma, fibrosarcoma and metastatic tumors, as well as others, have been reported.

Congenital Malformations of the Rectum and the Anus

These malformations comprise an important group of anomalies in infancy. They involve the rectum, the anus, the urogenital organs or any combinations of these.

Classification. The most practical classification is the one suggested by Ladd and

Gorss. They have described 4 types (Fig. 195):

TYPE I: Presents a stenosis at or directly above the anus.

TYPE II: Represents an imperforate anus, the obstruction being membranous in character.

TYPE III: This is the most common type and is represented by an imperforate anus, the rectal pouch ending blindly some distance above the anus.

TYPE IV: Reveals a normal anus and anal pouch, but the rectal pouch ends blindly in the hollow of the sacrum.

Many infants with these anomalies also have communications between the rectum, the genito-urinary organs, or the perineum. These may be rectovesical, recto-urethral, rectovaginal or rectoperineal.

Clinical Diagnosis

TYPE I: These patients present symptoms soon after birth or later, depending on the degree of stenosis. Defecation is difficult, and ribbonlike stools may be noted. The abdomen becomes distended, fecal impaction is present, and megacolon results. The diagnosis is evident upon inspection and digital examination.

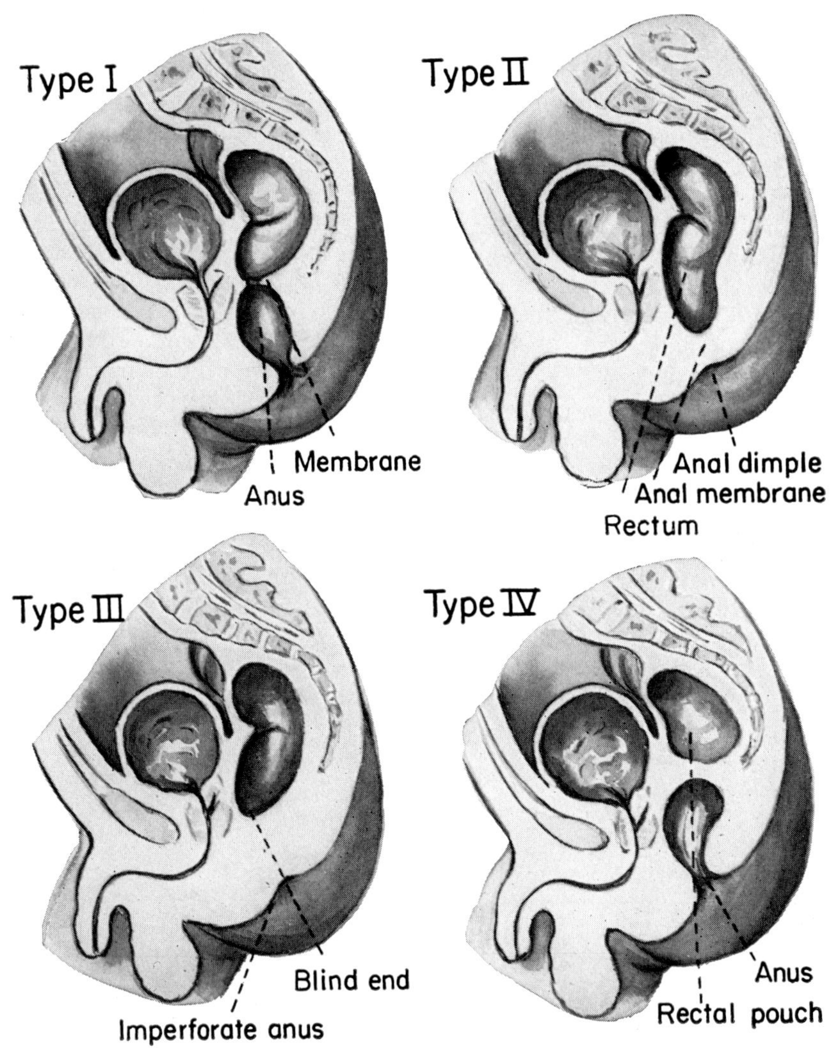

FIG. 195. Congenital malformations of the anorectal region.

TYPE II: This type is apparent soon after birth. A thin bulging membrane is seen which looks dark because of the meconium lying directly behind it. Since no meconium is passed, signs of intestinal obstruction develop within 48 hours *unless* there is an associated fistula which permits the bowel to empty elsewhere. This thin membranous obstruction is rare and must be differentiated from the common Type III, particularly since the therapy differs.

TYPE III: This is the most common type, accounting for 70 to 80 per cent of the cases. It is represented by a depression at the anal dimple. Puckering can be seen at this point when the anal sphincters contract. When the infant cries or strains the area bulges forward, particularly if the rectal pouch is low. External fistulas should be sought for. The passage of flatus or meconium through the urethra is pathognomonic of a recto-urinary fistula. These fistulas are not clinically evident if they become plugged with inspissated meconium. Signs and symptoms of intestinal obstruction develop in cases that are unassociated with fistulas or in which the fistula is plugged or too small for adequate drainage of bowel contents.

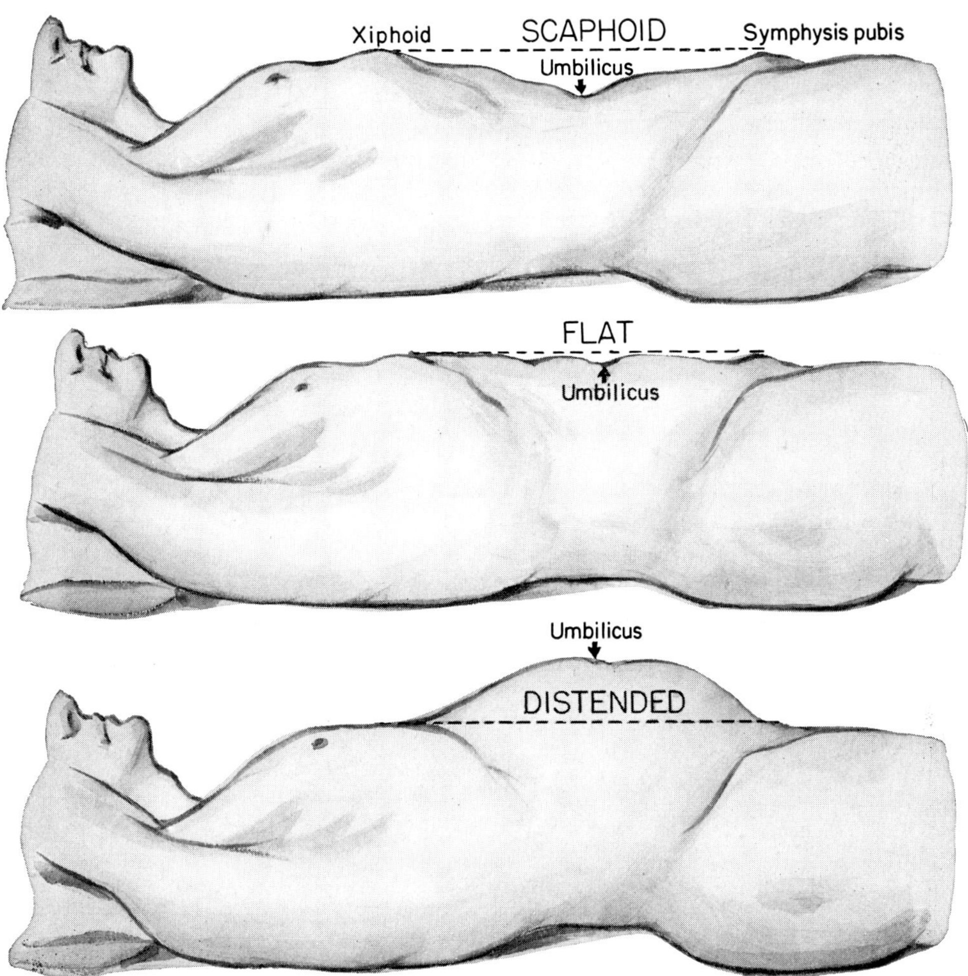

FIG. 196. The differentiation between a scaphoid, a flat and a distended abdomen is made readily if one compares the relationship between the umbilicus and the xiphopubic line (see text).

TYPE IV: In this type the anus appears to be normal, and the diagnosis can be overlooked for some days. However, no meconium is passed per anus, and signs of intestinal obstruction appear. The diagnosis is made when digital examination reveals the blind end of the anal pouch.

Roentgen diagnosis is helpful if the baby is placed in the upside-down position as recommended by Wangensteen and Rice. In this inverted position the colonic gas rises to the rectal pouch, and if a lead marker is placed at the anal dimple, one usually can estimate the distance between the end of the pouch and the anal skin. Lateral views may be particularly helpful. This method is useless if an associated fistula is present which permits deflation; it is also of little help in Type I. One may be misled if meconium at the distal end of the pouch prevents flatus from outlining the most distal portion. If a colostomy has been performed, roentgenograms are particularly useful by introducing contrast media into the distal colostomy loop. Associated fistulas also have been demonstrated by this method.

INTESTINAL OBSTRUCTION

Intestinal obstruction may result from a mechanical block of the bowel (dynamic), or from a neuromuscular inhibition of intestinal motility (adynamic). Formerly, the term "ileus" was used synonymously with intestinal obstruction; however, it is now reserved for those types in which no local organic lesion exists. So-called *adynamic ileus* may affect both the small and the large bowel; it occurs after laporotomy, peritonitis, renal and ureteral lesions, fractured spine, pneumonia, and as a terminal state.

ETIOLOGY

Mechanical obstruction or that type which is associated with a definite lesion at a given point is frequently caused by hernias and postoperative adhesions. *Age* is an important diagnostic factor. In infants intussusception and congenital anomalies are the chief causes of obstruction; in young adults the most frequent cause is postoperative adhesions; in later life neoplasms constitute the usual cause.

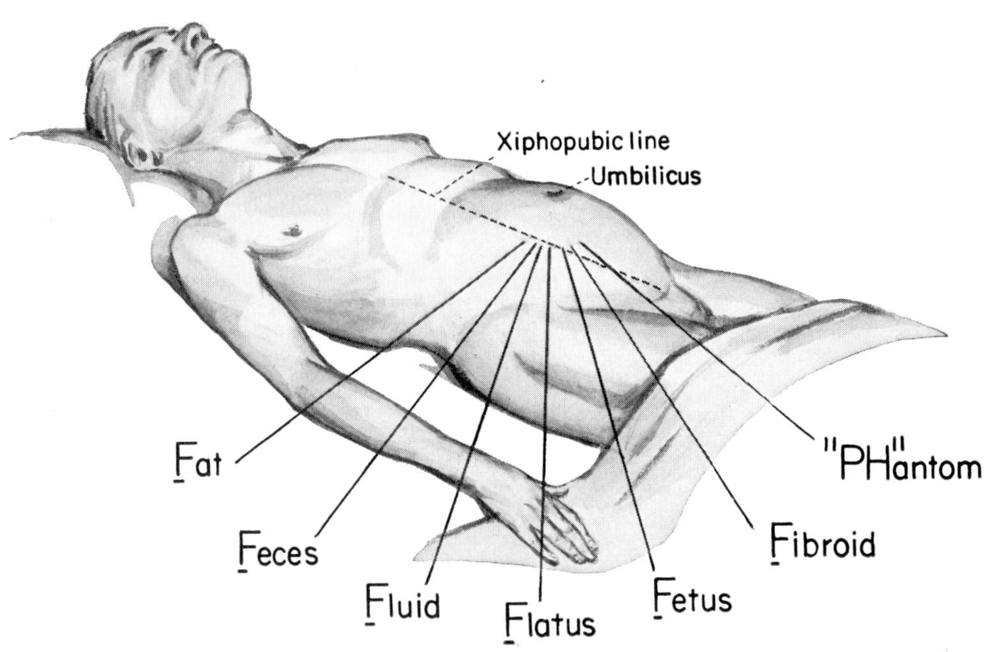

FIG. 197. The 7 "F's" in the differential diagnosis of abdominal distention.

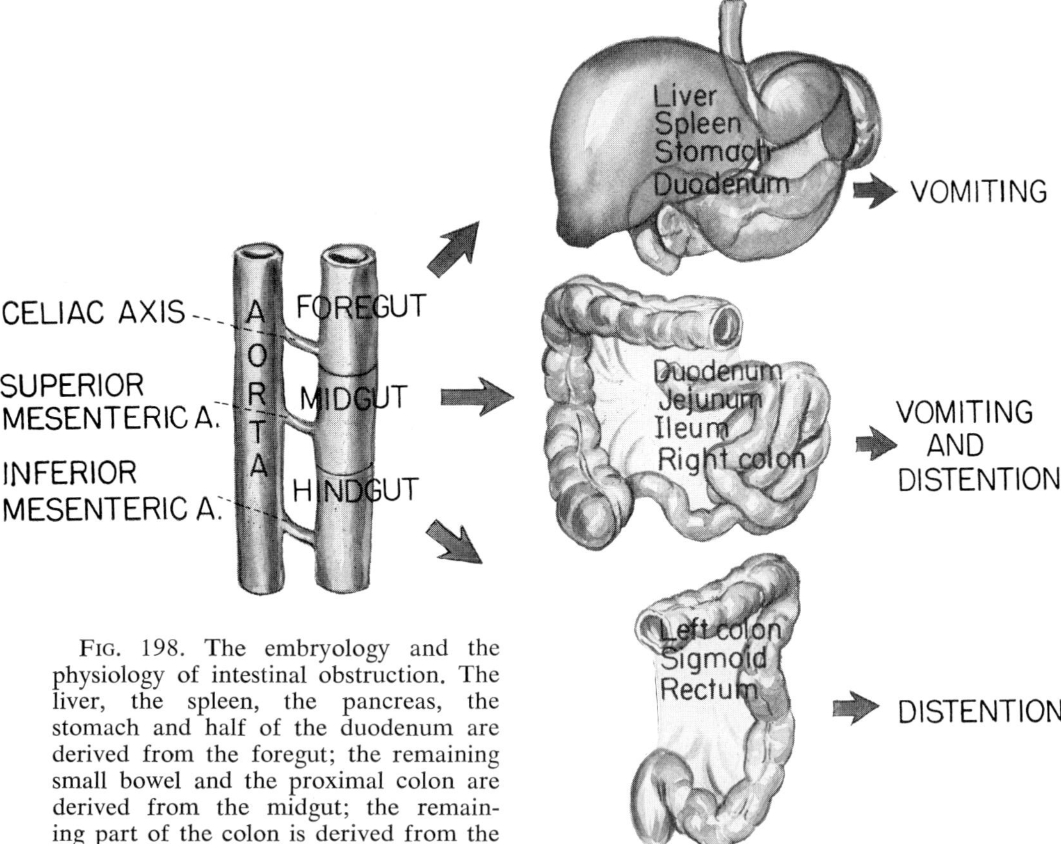

FIG. 198. The embryology and the physiology of intestinal obstruction. The liver, the spleen, the pancreas, the stomach and half of the duodenum are derived from the foregut; the remaining small bowel and the proximal colon are derived from the midgut; the remaining part of the colon is derived from the hindgut. If an obstruction involves that part of the gastrointestinal tract that is derived from the foregut, then vomiting is the outstanding symptom; if midgut bowel is involved, then both vomiting and distention are present; if that part of the colon that is derived from the hindgut is involved, then distention is the outstanding finding.

DIAGNOSIS

Intestinal obstruction is *not* a disease. It is a symptom complex. A proper diagnosis can be made after obtaining an answer to the following 4 questions:

1. Is this an intestinal obstruction?
2. Is this a large bowel or a small bowel obstruction?
3. Is this a strangulated or nonstrangulated obstruction?
4. Is this a complete or incomplete obstruction?

Question No. 1: "Is this an intestinal obstruction?" Nearly all of these patients at some time in the course of the condition experience pain, vomiting, distention and/or obstipation. However, these findings may be present only in part or may be lacking.

Pain synchronized with sound is the most pathognomonic finding in intestinal obstruction. When pain and audible peristalsis (stethoscope) occur simultaneously, intestinal colic is present. No other colic will produce this.

Distention of the abdomen is usually present unless the obstruction is very high, or if the bowel can be emptied distal to a large bowel lesion. "What is distention?" Since no anatomically adequate definition has been found, the author prefers to utilize the anatomy of the anterior abdominal wall as an index to distention (Fig. 196). If an imaginary line is drawn between the xiphoid and the symphysis pubis, it will be noted that the umbilicus normally lies beneath (dorsad) this xiphopubic line. This is a *scaphoid* abdomen. If the umbilicus is on the xiphopubic line, the abdomen is described as being *flat*. If the umbilicus is above the xiphopubic line, the abdomen is *distended*. If we utilize this method, we have a specific diagnostic aid that is most accurate in discovering early distention and its progress. If the umbilicus is on or above the xiphopubic line—in other words, if an abdomen is flat or distended—the differential diagnosis includes the 7 "F's," namely, Fat, Feces, Fluid, Flatus, Fetus, Fibroids and "Phantom" tumors (Fig. 197).

Obstipation or the absence of bowel movements may be present or absent in intestinal obstruction. If the obstruction is incomplete, both flatus and feces will pass per rectum. Early in the course of a complete obstruction the intestinal contents may be expelled distal to the lesion, either spontaneously or with an enema, thus giving the patient relief, and the doctor a degree of false security. In some incomplete strangulated obstructions, such as that which occurs in Richter's hernia, only part of the circumference of the bowel is strangulated; in such cases diarrhea, a result of hyperperistalsis, may be present.

Vomiting, if interpreted properly, is a helpful diagnostic aid. Dogma may be dangerous; however, when reasonably applied it serves the purpose of emphasis. Patients with

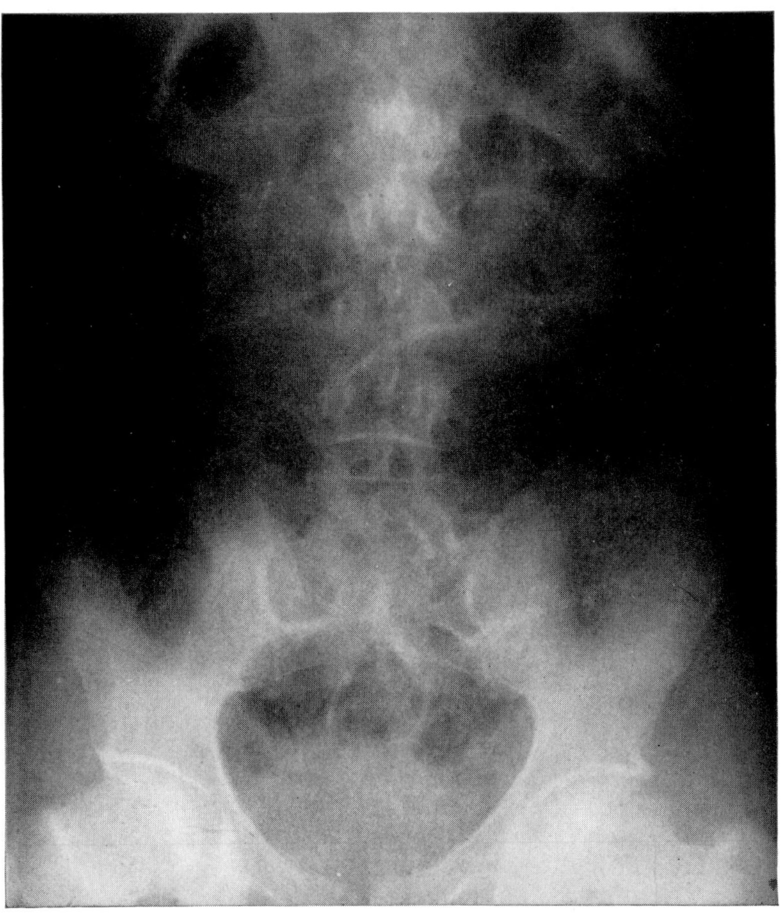

FIG. 199. Flat roentgenogram demonstrating the absence of gas in the true pelvis. This is suggestive of a complete intestinal obstruction.

large bowel obstructions do *not* vomit, but patients with small bowel obstructions *do* vomit. There are exceptions to every rule; any organ that twists on its base might produce vomiting. Therefore, large bowel obstructions due to volvulus (sigmoid and transverse colon) may be associated with vomiting. The higher (cephalad) the lesion, the earlier the vomiting. This will be discussed in detail under Question No. 2.

Abdominal auscultation not only is important in discovering synchronization of pain and sound but also aids in the identification of abnormal bowel sounds that are diagnostic of obstruction. Normally, intestinal sounds are heard as clicks or gurgles, but in intestinal obstruction distinct metallic tinkles can be heard which are called *obstructive borborygmi.* These are pathognomonic of intestinal obstruction. If intestinal sounds are totally absent, one must suspect bowel paralysis from toxemia or peritonitis.

Question No. 2: "Is this a large bowel or a small bowel obstruction?" In the vast majority of cases, if vomiting is an early and outstanding symptom, the patient has a small bowel obstruction. Vomiting is a late and unimportant complaint in patients who have a large bowel obstruction; however, distention is present early (Fig. 198). The vomitus first consists of gastric contents, then bile, then the contents of the upper intestine and finally contents of the terminal ileum. The last has a distinct fecaloid odor and appearance. The word "fecal vomiting" should not be used, since this is not true feces that the patient vomits. When true fecal vomiting occurs, it is pathognomonic of a gastrocolic fistula. Vomiting is not present in colonic obstruction, because most people have a

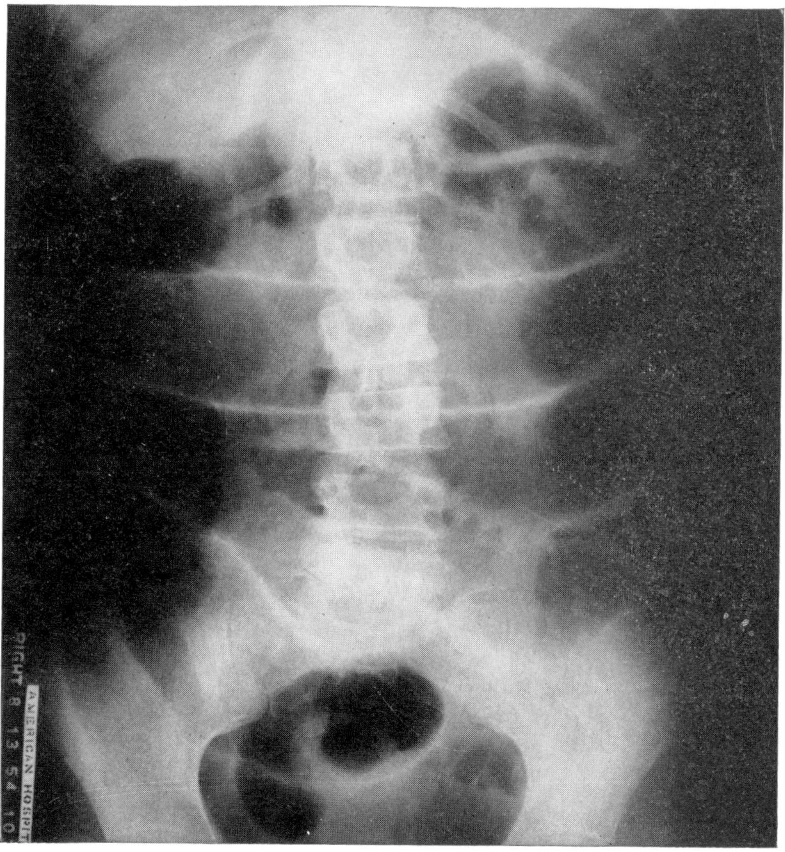

FIG. 200. Flat roentgenogram demonstrating a "stepladder" pattern in a case of small bowel obstruction.

competent ileocecal valve. The *flat roentgenogram* is a most useful adjunct in differentiating large bowel from small bowel obstructions. The film should include the diaphragm and the pelvis. It should be taken as soon as intestinal obstruction is suspected and before nasogastric siphonage or enemas are started. Gas in the ampulla of the rectum (sacral area) is absent when a complete mechanical obstruction exists (Fig. 199). This is particularly true if this is present after an enema is given. Normally, gas is not present in the small bowel except in infants, aged patients and air-swallowers. When gas is present in the small bowel, it usually assumes a "stepladder" pattern (Fig. 200). Small bowel is identified further by the fact that the transverse striations (valvulae conniventes) extend completely around the intestines. In large bowel obstruction, the roentgenogram reveals a horseshoe or inverted "U" arrangement if the obstruction is on the left side (Fig. 201). This is due to distention of the descending, the transverse and the ascending colons. The large bowel can be identified further on the roentgenogram in that it occupies the lateral aspects of the abdomen, it runs in a vertical direction (with the exception of the transverse colon), and the incomplete transverse striations and haustra are demonstrable. When isolated segments of bowel are noted on the roentgenogram, particularly small bowel, one should suspect acute pancreatitis (p. 227). If an acute inflammatory process

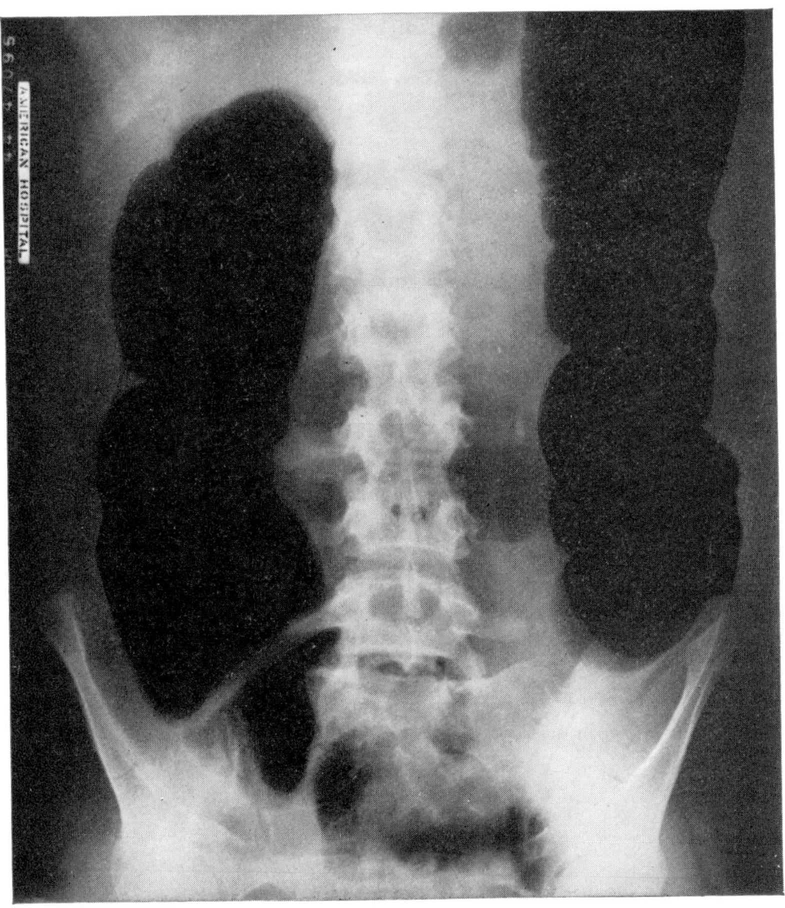

FIG. 201. Flat roentgenogram demonstrating the inverted "U" or horseshoe pattern in a large bowel obstruction caused by a carcinoma of the rectosigmoid.

can be ruled out, and if peritonitis is not present, a barium enema may be given to obtain specific isolation of a large bowel lesion. The usage of barium by mouth is dangerous.

The *history* is helpful in differentiating large bowel from small bowel obstructions. A slow progressive chronic increasing constipation suggests a large bowel obstruction, whereas an acute violent attack of pain with obstruction signifies a small bowel obstruction. The presence of a scar on the anterior abdominal wall from previous abdominal surgery is strong evidence in favor of a small bowel lesion. The author has not seen a large bowel obstruction caused by postoperative adhesions; although these have been reported, they are extremely rare.

Question No. 3: "Is this a strangulated or nonstrangulated obstruction?" Strangulation rarely occurs in large bowel obstructions, with the exception of volvulus. When strangulation is present, *tenderness* can be elicited at the site of the lesion. This must not be confused with pain. Strangulation, if untreated, results in shock. When a segment of bowel becomes strangulated, both intra-intestinal and intraperitoneal hemorrhage occur. A strangulated loop of bowel may be detected by the roentgenogram, because it appears as an isolated loop and assumes a vertical position. Since blood is present in its lumen, the characteristic valvulae conniventes are absent (Fig. 202).

Question No. 4: "Is this a complete or incomplete intestinal obstruction?" In a com-

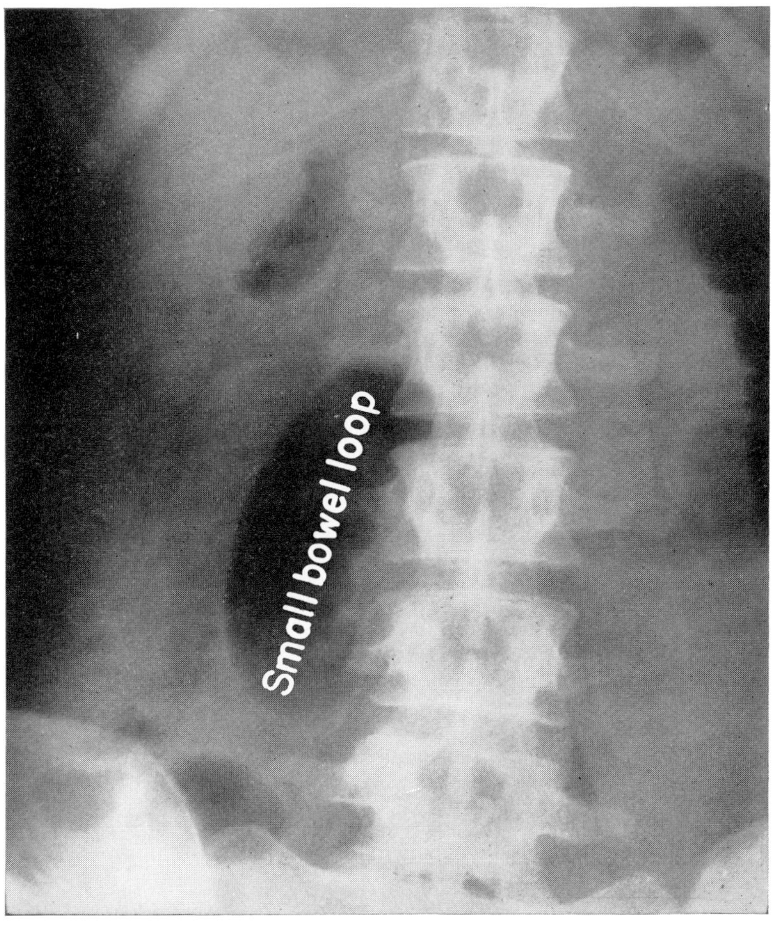

FIG. 202. Flat roentgenogram demonstrating a strangulated loop of small bowel.

plete obstruction neither flatus or feces passes per rectum. The exceptions to this have been stated. The so-called "scout" roentgenogram of the abdomen is particularly helpful in that no gas is noted in the true pelvis (Fig. 199). These patients look very sick and deteriorate rapidly if treatment is delayed.

Laboratory findings are of little help in the diagnosis of bowel obstruction. Urinalysis may aid in revealing sugar, albumin or a ketonuria. The blood reveals changes indicative of dehydration if this is present. A rise in the red and the white blood cell counts, the hematocrit and the hemoglobin also reveal dehydration. There is a marked loss of chlorides. Alkalosis is determined by an increased CO_2 combining power.

Specific Causes of Obstruction

Intussusception. This is a telescoping of one portion of the bowel into another. When an intussusceptum has been drawn into its intussuscipiens, the process will be a progressive one until relief is obtained or death supervenes.

Incidence. Intussusception is one of the most frequent surgical emergencies in infancy. In adults it usually results from some abnormality, such as a tumor, but in childhood and infancy such factors are usually lacking.

Classification. It is helpful to divide intussusceptions into simple and mixed varieties (Fig. 203). The simple include enteric, ileocolic, ileocecal and colic. The mixed in-

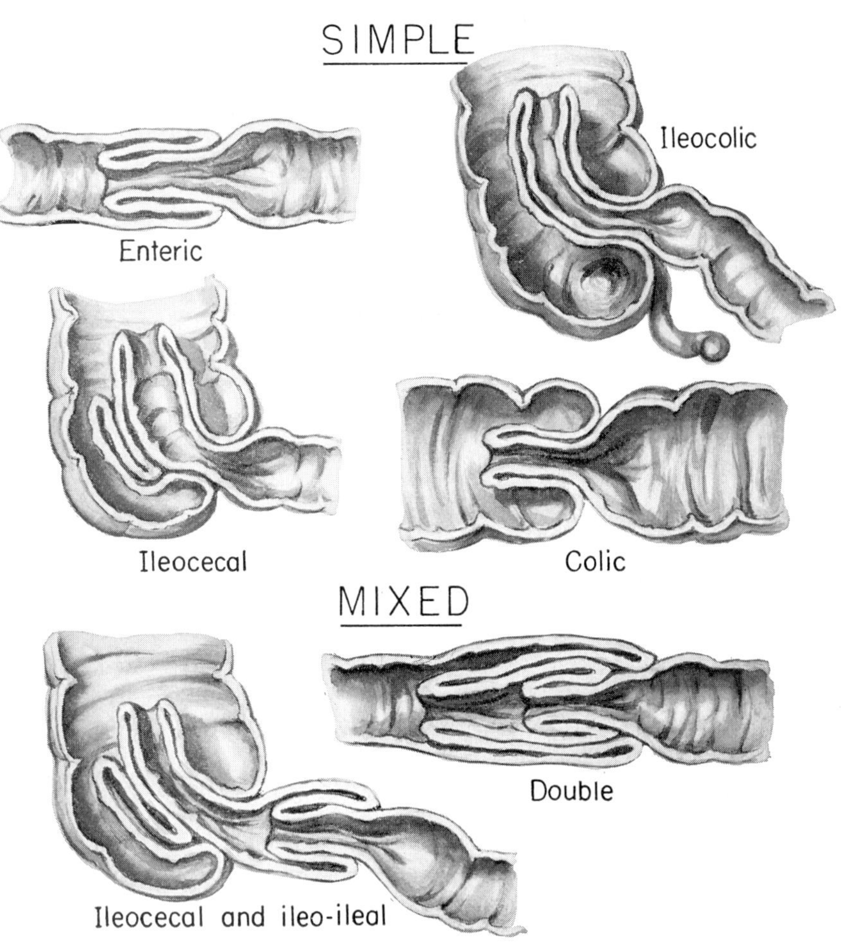

Fig. 203. Classification of intussusception.

clude ileocecal and ileo-ileal and double. In the ileocolic type the ileum prolapses through the ileocecal valve, which remains at a relatively fixed point. In the ileocecal variety, however, the ileocecal valve and/or the adjacent cecum is the spearhead and invaginates the ascending colon, drawing the ileum behind it (Fig. 204).

Intussusception has been classified also as acute, subacute and chronic. These variations are due to the relative looseness or tightness with which the intussusceptum is held by the intussuscipiens. The tighter it is held the greater is the constricting effect upon the mesentery, and the more rapid is the development of strangulation and necrosis.

Symptoms. The symptoms vary somewhat in children and adult. In adults the symptoms are those of partial or complete bowel obstruction and are associated with abdominal cramps, nausea and vomiting. Bowel movements may be normal, and at times a diarrhea is present. There is little or no evidence of tenderness or peritoneal irritation, since the involved or necrotic intussusceptum is encased within the essentially normal intussuscipiens, thus protecting the general peritoneal cavity. A mass is usually palpable. Rectal examination frequently reveals so-called *"currant jelly feces"* on the gloved finger; this is due to an admixture of blood and mucus. When the intusssusception is enteric, there is usually roentgenologic evidence of a small bowel intestinal obstruction (p. 179). These findings may or may not be present when the condition involves the colon. Barium enema in these cases reveals an obstructing lesion at the apex of which the so-called "coiled spring" pattern may be seen. This results from the barium streaking between the layers of the intussusceptum and the intussuscipiens.

When children are affected, the parent notices that the child becomes pale, doubles up and draws his legs up because of severe pain. After the paroxysm ceases, the child

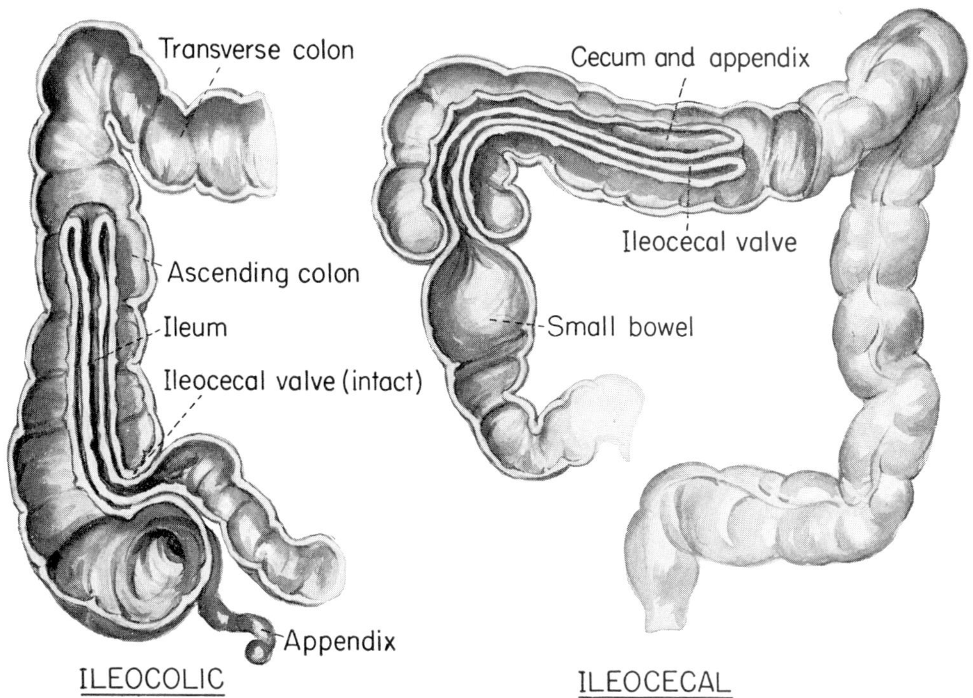

Fig. 204. In the ileocolic type of intussusception the ileocecal valve remains in its normal fixed position. In the ileocecal type, the ileocecal valve acts as the moving spearhead.

resumes a playful attitude and appears to be quite normal, but later he has a recurrence of the painful episode. As the obstruction progresses, pallor, sweating, dehydration and shock appear. In rare cases the intussusceptum may protrude from the anus. This is differentiated from rectal prolapse by passing a finger into the rectum and then between the intussusceptum and the surrounding anal sphincter. In a prolapse of the rectum such a maneuver is impossible because no such space exists.

There are cases of congenital polyposis of the gastrointestinal tract primarily involving the small intestines which are associated with dark pigmented melanin spots of the buccal mucosa, the hard palate and the lips. These spots look like freckles but are darker; they may be found also on the fingers and the toes. The two associated lesions comprise a syndrome which is familial in nature, inherited as a mendelian dominant. These cases are predisposed to intussusception. This entity has been discussed under the heading of Peutz-Jeghers syndrome (p. 160). Meckel's diverticulum is another cause of intussusception. Hypertrophied Peyer's patches, polyps and malrotations also are possible etiologic factors.

VOLVULUS

Volvulus consists of a twist (torsion) of a loop of intestine around its mesentery. It occurs more frequently in the colon than in the small intestine.

Volvulus of the Sigmoid

This twist is most likely to occur in patients who have a long sigmoid loop and a narrow mesenteric attachment (Fig. 205). Because of this, the bowel rotates around the fixed point. Cases become subacute and recurrent if the loop rotates and then returns to its normal position. The direction of rotation varies.

Signs and symptoms of intestinal obstruction are present; the distention may be enormous. Vomiting is an early symptom; this differs from other types of *large* bowel obstruction. Tenderness in the left lower quadrant appears when the blood supply is interfered with, and gangrene develops. The

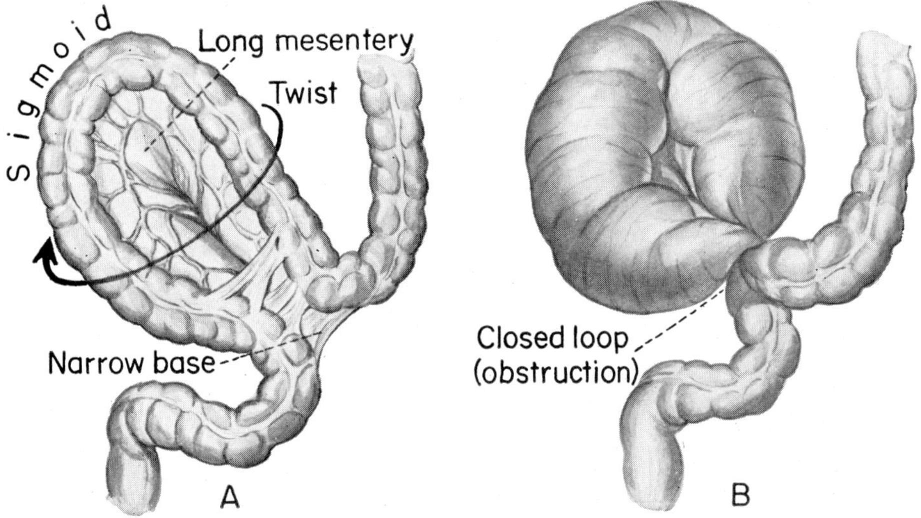

Fig. 205. Volvulus of the sigmoid. The 2 anatomic factors which predispose to this condition are a long elongated sigmoid loop and a narrow mesenteric attachment. Some fibrosis may occur at the base of the mesosigmoid, accentuating its narrowness. When the twist is complete, a closed loop type of obstruction results.

roentgenogram usually presents a tremendously distended loop of large bowel rising out of the pelvis. Absence of fluid levels and the loss of haustral markings are most suggestive. The "ace of spades" sign becomes apparent as barium enters the region of the twist.

Volvulus of the Cecum

This designation is misleading, because in almost all of these cases some part of the terminal ileum and the ascending colon also are involved. In most cases the rotation is in a clockwise direction. The clinical picture is that of bowel obstruction; however, in the current type the symptoms may be confused with acute appendicitis. The anatomic prerequisite for such volvulus is abnormal mobility of the cecum and the ascending colon. A roentgenogram that reveals a dilated cecum, abnormally placed, should make one suspicious of this condition. Tenderness over the massively dilated cecum is usually present.

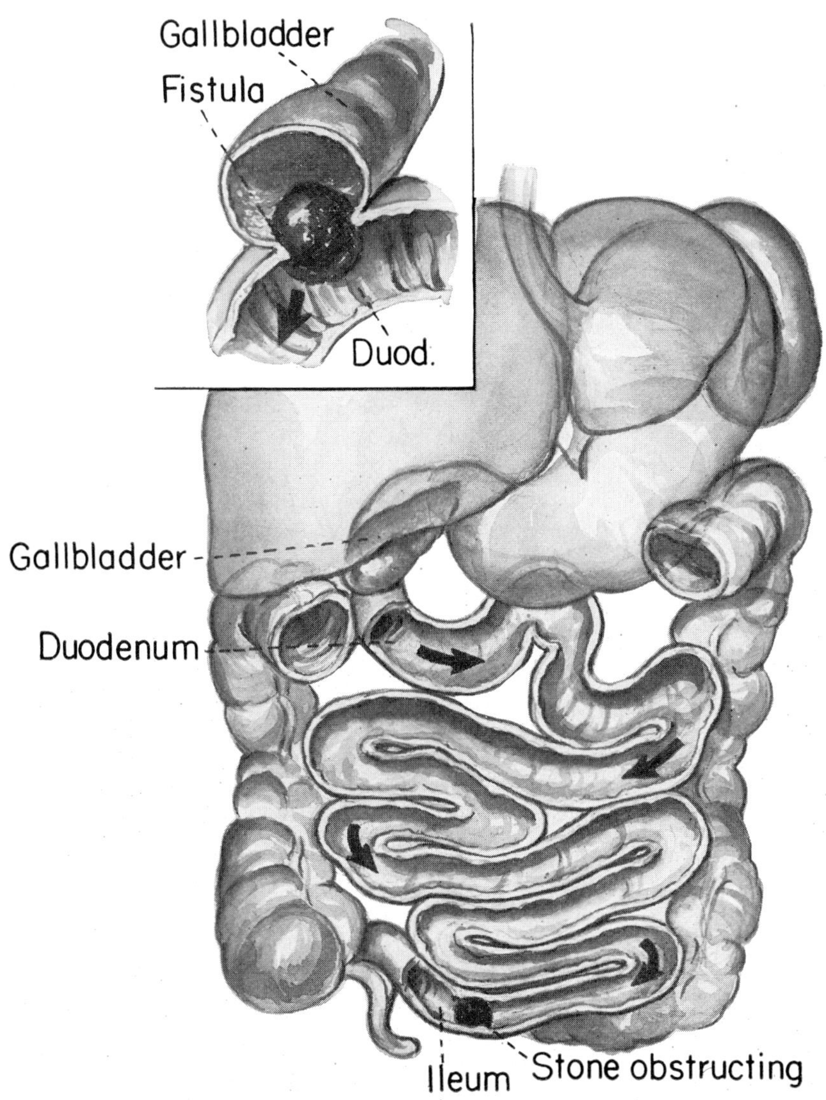

Fig. 206. The physiopathology of gallstone ileus.

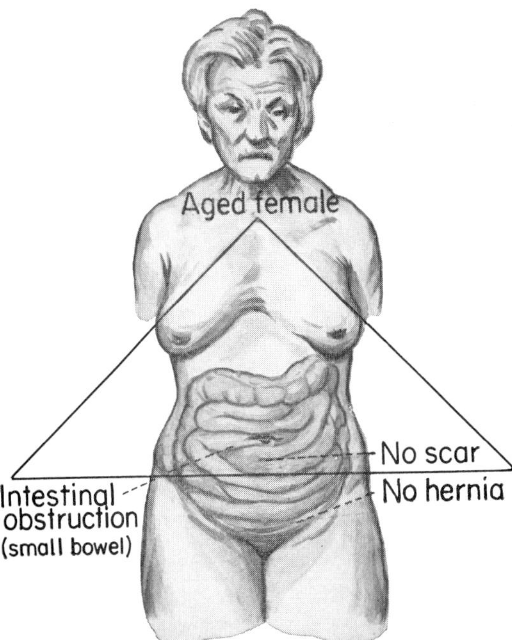

FIG. 207. Gallstone ileus can be diagnosed if this triad is apparent.

GALLSTONE ILEUS

The occurrence of this condition is relatively rare. It is a type of small bowel obstruction that occurs in the later years of life (6th decade and later). The calculus usually gains entrance to the small bowel following the development of a cholecystoduodenal fistula. Such a fistula is the result of repeated attacks of cholecystitis, plus pressure necrosis from a gallstone (Fig. 206). Almost all stones become impacted in the distal ileum, because the lumen is smallest here. As the stone travels distally in the bowel, it may become engaged temporarily and then disengaged; then the obstructive signs and symptoms would alternate also. A correct diagnosis of gallstone ileus can be made in most instances preoperatively. This is possible if the following desiderata are met (Fig. 207):

1. The patient is past the 6th decade (usually a female).
2. Signs of *small bowel* obstruction are present.
3. No scar on the abdomen from previous surgery and no visible external strangulated hernias.

If one is fortunate enough to have a flat roentgenogram that reveals air or contrast media in the biliary tract, the diagnosis of cholecystoduodenal fistula is definite (Fig. 208).

MESENTERIC VASCULAR OCCLUSION

Occlusion of the mesenteric vessels may involve either the artery or the vein; often a

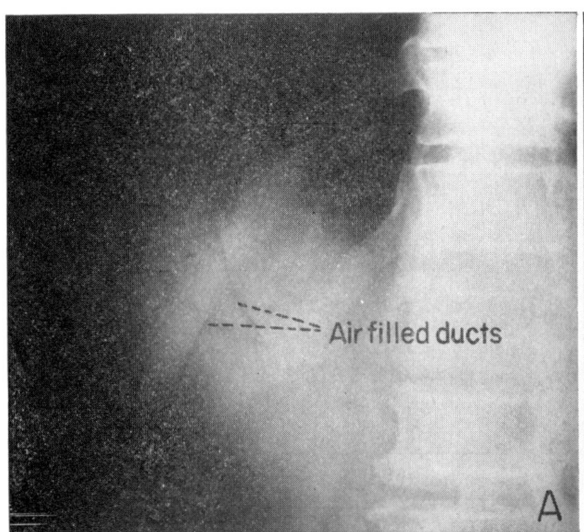

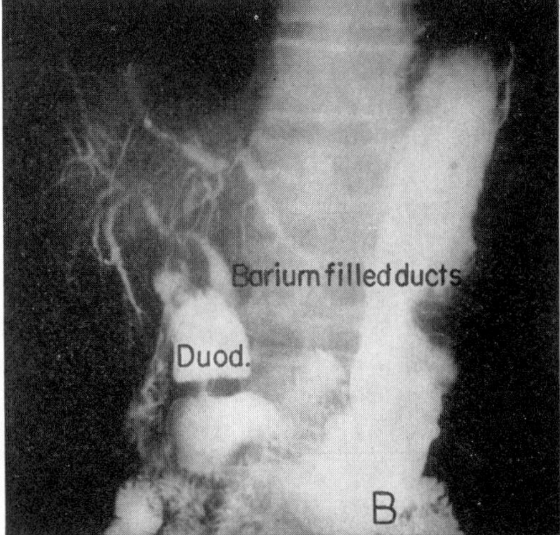

FIG. 208. Roentgenogram of a spontaneous cholecystoduodenal fistula.

combination exists. The picture of intestinal obstruction usually develops.

Mesenteric venous occlusion accounts for over three fourths of the cases of mesenteric occlusion. There is usually a history of some infection (appendicitis, diverticulitis, peritonitis or thrombophlebitis). There may be a prodromal period in which intermittent colicky abdominal pain has been present. When the bowel becomes devitalized, the pain becomes intense and continuous. Such occlusion may involve the accompanying artery. Melena is usually present. Of importance is exquisite abdominal tenderness over the involved segment; however, rigidity may be absent. Shock or impending shock is common. Blood noted with the rectal examination may give the first clue. The flat roentgenogram reveals an indefinite small bowel gas pattern or isolated loops in which the valvulae conniventes are obliterated.

Mesenteric arterial occlusion is present in either elderly patients with cardiovascular disease or in young patients with valvular heart conditions. The onset is sudden and dramatic with severe abdominal pain. The degree of shock is dependent on the severity and the extent of the occlusion. Bowel sounds disappear rapidly, and the abdomen becomes distended. Signs and symptoms of intestinal obstruction develop. In the absence of a scar on the abdomen or a visible strangulated hernia, mesenteric thrombosis must be considered seriously; it must be differentiated from gallstone ileus (p. 186).

Endometriosis involves the small and/or the large intestine. It can produce intestinal obstruction, and since it is a benign condition that exhibits marked infiltrative tendencies, it is readily mistaken for a malignant lesion. *Acquired dysmenorrhea* and/or *acquired dyspareunia* are particularly suggestive of endometriosis. Menstrual irregularities also might be present. If the sigmoid is involved, it may be narrowed, but the mucosa appears to be normal. The possibility of this condition must be kept in mind in every case of intestinal obstruction in women between the ages of 30 to 50. Since the prognosis is good, and the surgical mortality is low, such patients should be explored in the hopes of finding this benign condition.

Irradiation may be the cause of a stenosing and obstruction lesion of the bowel. Frequently the sigmoid and the terminal ileum are involved. When a history of irradiation is obtained, and when signs and symptoms of bowel obstruction are manifest, one should keep this possibility in mind.

Regional enteritis has been discussed elsewhere (p. 138). It must be considered in cases of bowel obstruction, particularly those involving the small intestines.

Internal hernias can produce bowel ob-

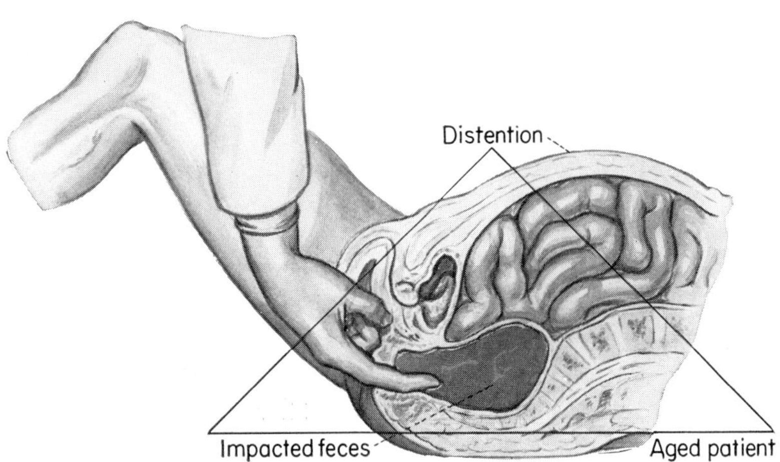

FIG. 209. Fecal impaction should be suspected in the aged patient with large bowel obstructions.

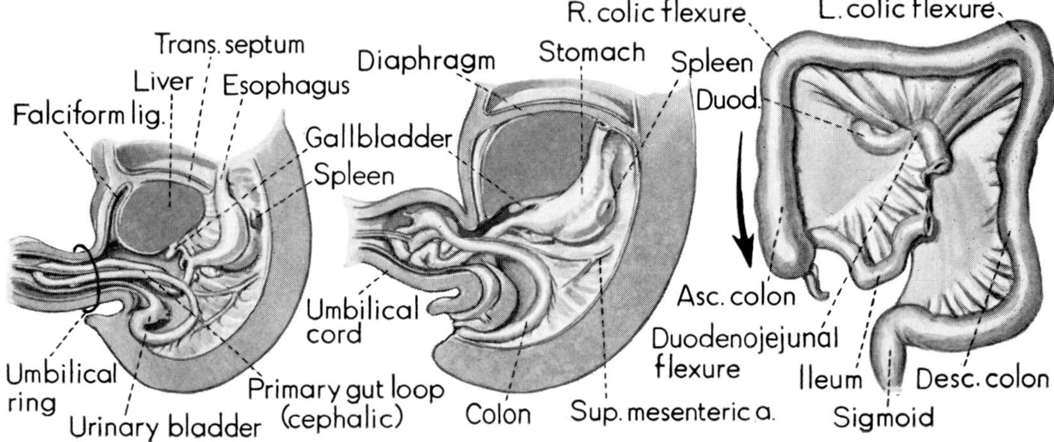

FIG. 210. Embryology of intestinal rotation. It is convenient to divide this into 3 arbitrary stages. (A) The 1st stage deals with a physiologic umbilical hernia in which the midgut is herniated into the extra-embryonic celom. (B) The 2nd stage is the stage of rotation, in which the midgut rotates and returns to the celomic cavity. (C) The 3rd stage results in the fixation of the bowel to the posterior parietal wall and the descent of the cecum.

structions; however, the incidence of these is less than 1 per cent. The mortality is high, because a large percentage of these cases are associated with early strangulation, and the diagnosis is delayed.

Fecal impaction can cause a large bowel obstruction, particularly in older patients (Fig. 209). It is most embarrassing when this common condition is overlooked, particularly if the patient is operated upon unnecessarily. Such obstructions are rarely acute, and the diagnosis is made readily by rectal examination. The flat roentgenogram shows a mottling (fecal masses) of the large bowel.

The **superior mesenteric artery syndrome** is an unusual form of high intestinal obstruction. It represents a compression of the

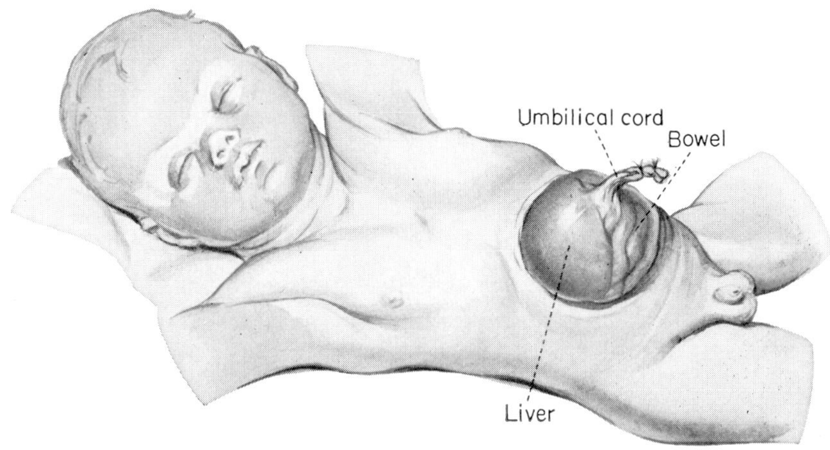

FIG. 211. The anomaly that results from a derangement of Stage 1 is omphalocele, in which the midgut and other viscera remain in the physiologic umbilical hernia.

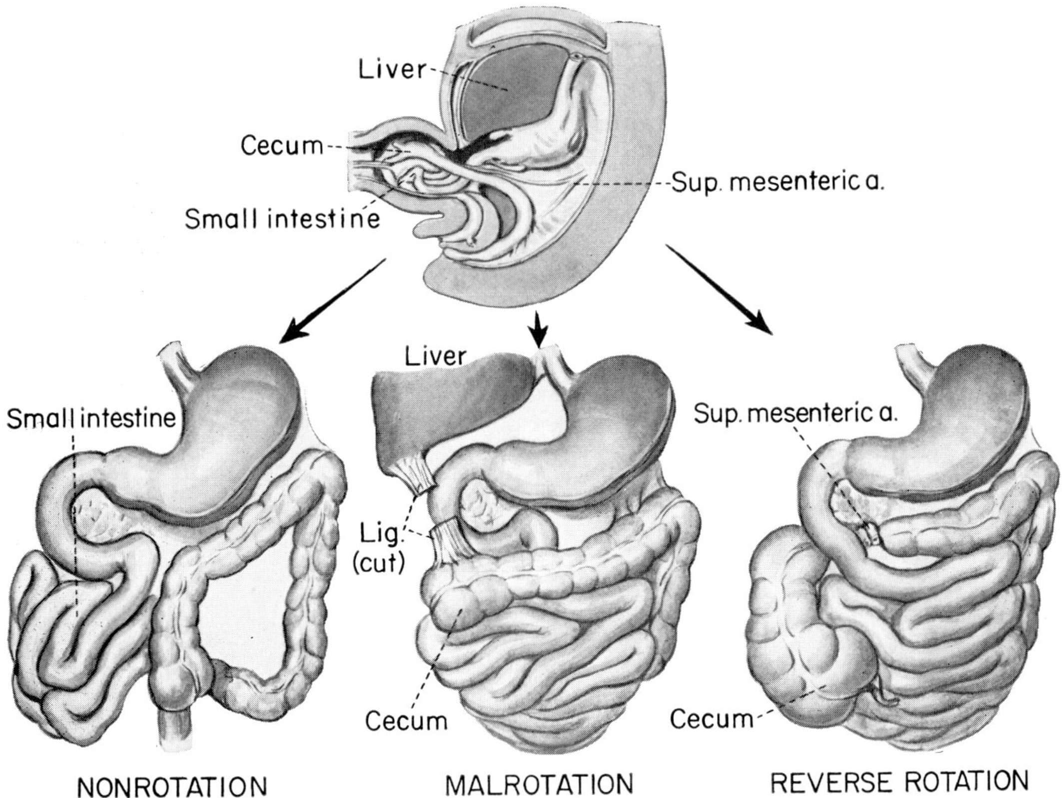

FIG. 212. Second-stage intestinal rotation varieties may conveniently be divided into 3 types. (A) Nonrotation, in which the midgut does not rotate after reduction into the celomic cavity. (B) Incomplete rotation (malrotation), in which the midgut rotates in a normal direction but is arrested along its normal course. The all-important congenital band or attachment plays an important part in this type. (C) Reversed rotation, in which the midgut rotates in a clockwise direction around the superior mesenteric artery.

fixed 3rd portion of the duodenum by the superior mesenteric neurovascular bundle anteriorly and the aorta and the vertebral column posteriorly. The upright posture of man predisposes to this anatomic "nutcracker." Postprandial distention, pain, nausea and vomiting are suggestive symptoms. Food ingested 24 hours previously may appear in the vomitus. Because of this consequence patients eat less and develop malnutrition and avitaminosis. The acute form of the condition starts as a high intestinal obstruction with marked gastric dilatation and bile-stained vomitus. The roentgenogram reveals a marked dilatation of the duodenum through its 2nd portion with a sharp demarcation at the midline.

Anomalies of Intestinal Rotation. Congenital anomalies of intestinal rotation are encountered more frequently in infants and children. If unrecognized, surgical errors, such as an inadvertent gastroileostomy, may occur, or the appendix may be extremely difficult to locate.

EMBRYOLOGY OF INTESTINAL ROTATION. Consideration of this subject in 3 convenient though arbitrary stages (Fig. 210) will aid in understanding these anomalies. *Stage 1* is the physiologic (umbilical) herniation phase. It occurs between the 5th and the 10th weeks of embryonic life and involves primarily the midgut. *Stage 2* takes place at the 10th and the 11th weeks when the midgut returns to the celomic cavity. During this stage rotation (twisting) occurs in counterclockwise direction, the central axis of the twist being the superior mesenteric artery. The cranial limb rotates in a counterclockwise fashion, first inferior and then to the left of the superior mesenteric artery, making an arc of 180°. The caudal limb at the same time rotates counterclockwise left 90° superior and then a further 90° to the right of the superior mesenteric artery. The duodenum thus comes to lie behind the transverse colon. *Stage 3* is the stage of fixation and descent, during which the cecum, the ascending and the descending colons become fixed to the posterior abdominal wall. There is also fixation of the base of the small bowel mesentery from the ligament of Treitz to the ileocecal junction. With this oversimplified and yet practical understanding of intestinal rotation we may review the anomalies that occur during the various stages.

STAGE 1. The anomaly that occurs in the 1st stage is an *omphalocele* (Fig. 211). Here the midgut fails to return to the celomic cavity from its umbilical location. Since the midgut remains in the umbilical sac, it may be accompanied by the liver, the stomach, the spleen, and the pancreas. This is a disease of the neonatal period that requires immediate surgical attention.

STAGE 2. Three types of anomalies may occur from faulty rotation during the 2nd stage: *nonrotation, malrotation* and *reversed rotation* (Fig. 212).

When the midgut fails to rotate, *nonrotation* results (Fig. 212, *left*). In this type of anomaly the duodenum descends downward in a straight line to the right of the superior mesenteric artery and in direct continuity with the small bowel, all of which is located in the right half of the abdominal cavity. The colon is located mainly in the left half; frequently, the ligament of Treitz is absent. The terminal ileum enters the cecum by crossing the midline from the right side, which is contrary to its normal direction (normally the ileum enters from the left side). Nonrotation is one of the very rare anomalies.

The most common of these 3 anomalies is *malrotation* (Fig. 212, *center*). Many authorities have objected to the term "malrotation," because in this anomaly there is an incomplete rotation in which the midgut does not complete the 180° rotation counterclockwise. Rotation may be arrested at any point, so that the cecum stops at the splenic level, in front of the superior mesenteric vessels, or assumes its most common position, subhepatic. Some authorities believe that the difficulties result from an abnormal membrane that stretches across the duodenum. Such membranes or unusual attachments are practically always associated with malrotated cecums. These congenital bands are thin bloodless fibrous structures that can obstruct the duodenum. If such a band is cut transversely, the cecum and/or the transverse colon to which it was attached is loosened, and the organs continue their normal rotation and descent.

Reversed rotation is a rare anomaly (Fig. 212, *right*). Here the midgut instead of going through a counterclockwise movement rotates in a clockwise direction through an arc of 90°. The cecum and the transverse colon pass through the root of the mesentery behind the superior mesenteric artery and the duodenum. Frequently the opening in the mesentery is small, and the risk of obstruction is great.

STAGE 3. Anomalies in the 3rd stage deal with the lack of posterior attachment of the bowel and with nondescent. If the duodenum fails to adhere to the posterior abdominal wall, it becomes freely movable. A mobile cecum, although normally located, lacks its posterior attachment. If the jejunum and the ileum fail to attach, they hang freely on a long, narrow pedicle of mesentery.

The diagnosis of anomalies associated with intestinal rotation depends on the presence of symptoms. A history of chronic recurrent abdominal discomfort dating to childhood should arouse the surgeon's suspicion. Sudden severe abdominal pain results from volvulus of the bowel. The roentgenographic examination enables one to diagnose these conditions preoperatively. Intestinal obstruction is by far the most common complication; it is caused by volvulus or obstructing congenital bands.

7

Liver, Gallbladder and Bile Ducts

Numerous functions and chemical processes take place within the liver despite the fact that it has only one specific cell—the polygonal cell (Fig. 213). The functional derangement and the degree of disturbance depend on the nature and the severity of the disease, as well as the stage in which it is studied. To add to the difficulty of such a study is the fact that hepatic functions vary in different phases of a disease and in different patients. For these reasons no single test can be relied upon.

LIVER FUNCTION TESTS

Hepatic tests should be used in groups. Repetition of these tests is necessary, since they vary from day to day with no apparent change in the clinical condition. It must be emphasized that the hepatic tests are not specific for any particular type of hepatic disease but are utilized as an adjunct to determine the presence of hepatic pathology.

The table of tests on page 192, although not all inclusive, is recommended. The liver

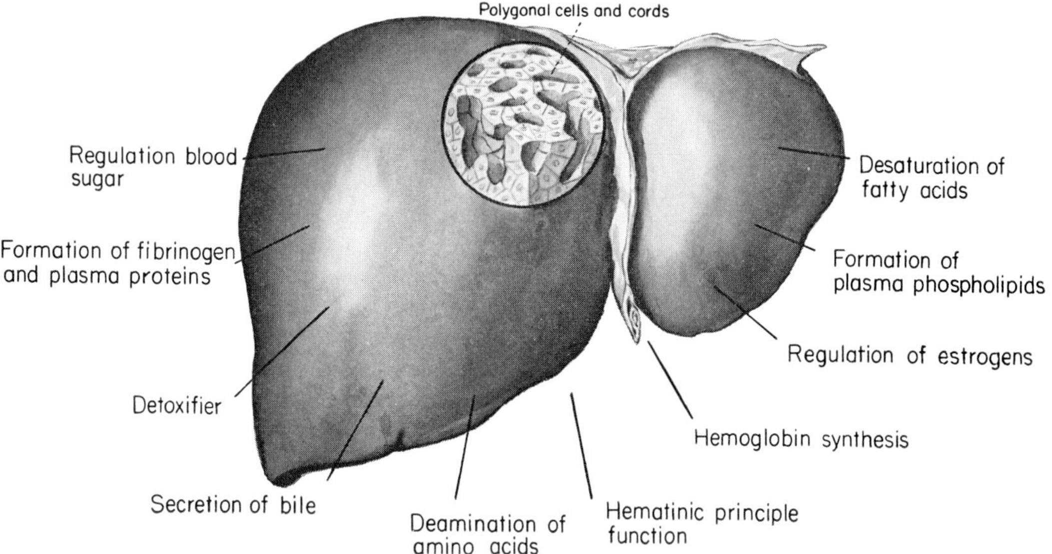

FIG. 213. The liver performs many important functions. Some of these are depicted here.

TABLE 5. HEPATIC FUNCTION TESTS

TEST	NORMAL VALUE
Transaminase (SGPT)	10-40 per ml.
Bromsulphalein (BSP)	0-5% retention at end of 40 minutes
Cephalin flocculation	0-1+ (at 48 hours)
Thymol turbidity	0-4.0 units
Bilirubin, direct (immediate)	0.1-0.2 mg. per 100 ml.
Bilirubin, indirect (total)	0.2-1.0 mg. per 100 ml.
Icterus index	1-6 units
Cholesterol, total	140-250 mg. per 100 ml.
Alkaline phosphatase	1.5-5.0 Bodansky units 0.8-2.3 Sigma units per ml.
Serum protein	
Total	6.5-8.0 Gm. per 100 ml.
Albumin	4.0-5.5 per 100 ml.
Globulin	1.5-3.0 per 100 ml.
A/G ratio	1.6-2.0
Fibrinogen	200-600 mg. per 100 ml.
Urine urobilinogen	1.0 Ehrlich units (2 to 4 P.M. specimen)

has a tremendous reserve capacity, so that only 15 per cent of its parenchyma is necessary to sustain life. Since most functions of the liver occur in the polygonal cells, and since they may perform some functions well and be defective in others, a number of tests may be necessary to determine a so-called "liver profile." No single test can be considered to be pathognomonic. These laboratory data do not replace the history and the physical examination.

Palpation. The liver normally is not palpable in the adult but may be felt readily when the organ is enlarged or displaced. Palpation is best from below upward, starting in the right lower quadrant and progressing upward toward the right costal arch. A *Riedel's lobe* is a tonguelike projection which juts forward and appears in the right upper quadrant (Fig. 214). It may simulate an enlarged gallbladder or a tumor of the liver. Also, *tendinous inscription* in a well-developed right rectus muscle has been mistaken for a pathologic liver or gallbladder. These conditions usually can be differentiated if the patient is examined in the supine position, with the knees elevated, the arms at the side, and breathing through the open mouth.

Biopsy. Particularly to be condemned as a diagnostic aid is the so-called "blind" liver biopsy. With so massive an organ as the liver, one wonders how often correct information can be obtained by taking a minute specimen. The method is not without danger. It is true that many favorable reports have appeared in the literature regarding the advantages of this method; however, whenever possible, exploratory laparotomy is the method of choice. If a biopsy is taken during the course of the laparotomy, one can at least see what is being biopsied, evaluate the macroscopic appearance of the involved organ and determine operability. This is impossible with the "blind" method. The liver biopsy which is taken in the presence of obstructive jaundice is particularly dangerous because of possible biliary leakage and peritonitis.

HEPATITIS

"Hepatitis" can be defined in a broad sense as damage to the liver cells which results from such etiologic agents as viral, chemical, physical, bacterial or protozoal agents. Some authors also include the reactive and the reparative phenomena. Those forms of hepatitis due to a transmissable, filterable agent are undoubtedly the most prevalent ones. These are the infectious types.

The two types that are of surgical interest are infectious hepatitis and homologous serum hepatitis. Whether these are one and the same condition produced by a specific virus or entirely different entities which present a similar clinical picture is unknown (Fig. 215).

The infectious hepatitis virus gains entrance to the body through the oral cavity with ingested contaminated foods. Contamination is usually brought about by contact with contaminated feces or urine. Also droplet infection may be an etiologic factor. The incubation period is usually less than 1 month; it unquestionably occurs in epidemics. A skin test has been devised which gives a uniformly positive response in patients who have had this disease.

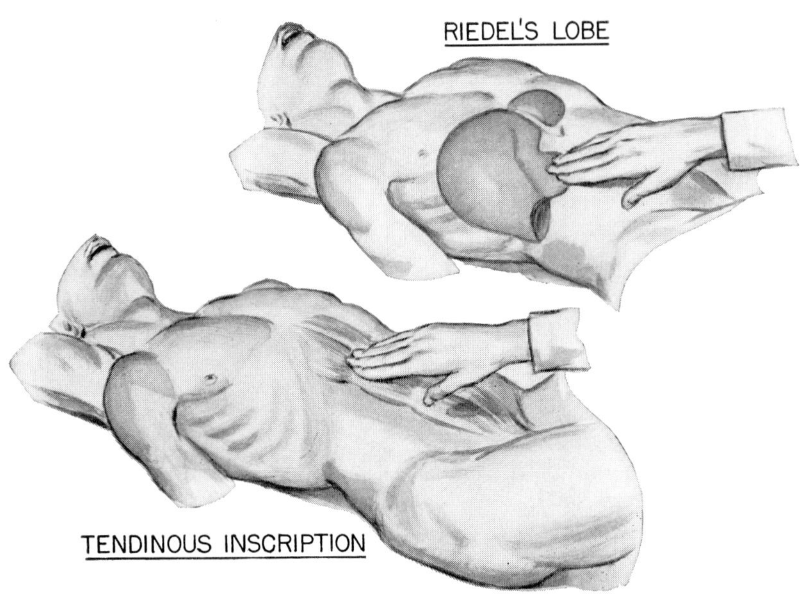

FIG. 214. A Riedel's lobe or a tendinous inscription may be mistaken for a diseased liver or gallbladder.

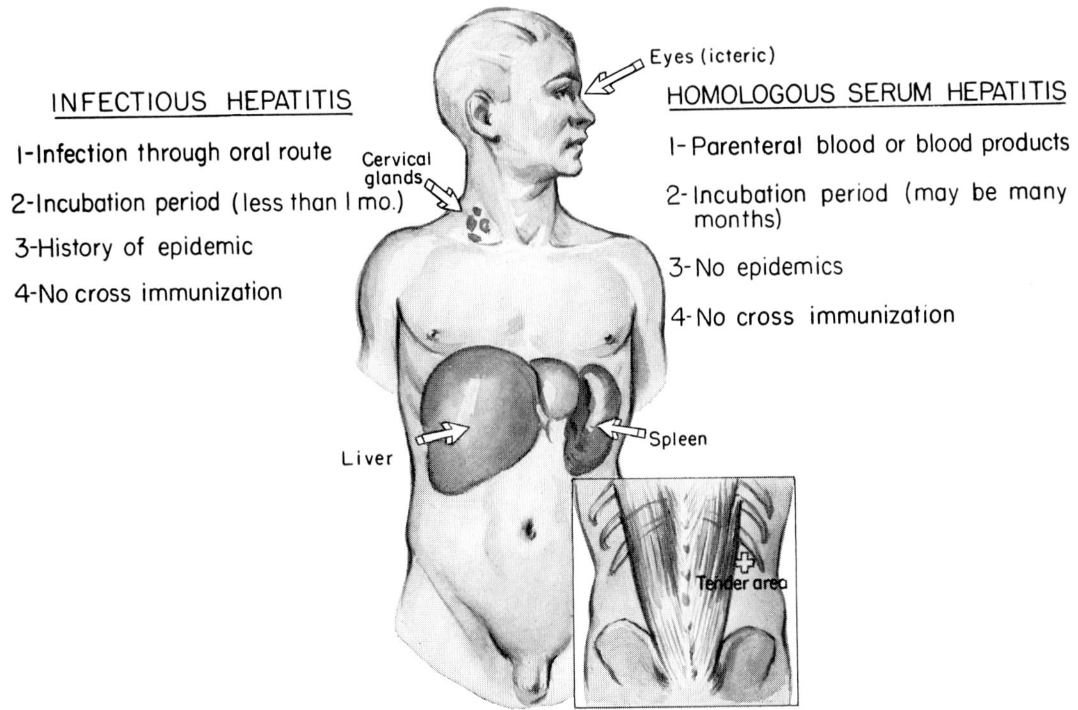

FIG. 215. Infectious hepatitis or homologous serum hepatitis? Some of the diagnostic and differential diagnostic features are tabulated in the illustration.

Homologous serum hepatitis has a longer incubation period, the symptoms appearing in 100 days or over. This hepatitis is transmitted parenterally following the use of serum or blood products administered subcutaneously, intramuscularly, intravenously or pharyngeally (sprays). This disease does not occur in epidemics. There is no cross immunity with infectious hepatitis.

Clinical Picture. Clinically, these 2 conditions present the same signs and symptoms. In the prodromal stage there are malaise, aching sensations, particularly in the extremities, anorexia, vomiting and constipation or diarrhea. Although visible *jaundice* is not present in all cases, symptoms usually subside if and when the icterus reaches its height. Pain is usually present in the right hypochondrium; this is increased by jarring or coughing. Fever and chills may be present. Enlargement of cervical lymph nodes may be noted, particularly on the right side. The liver is usually enlarged and tender to both palpation and percussion. The spleen is occasionally palpable but reveals the enlargement when percussed. If the condition becomes serious, bleeding from the body orifices occurs, nervous system symptoms appear, and serious cardiovascular damage becomes evident. Ascites frequently makes its appearance in those cases associated with fatal hepatitis.

Differential Diagnosis. The anicteric form of hepatitis frequently masquerades as influenza; it must be differentiated from other febrile conditions.

The liver function tests may indicate parenchymatous liver damage. The white blood count may be elevated and at times reveals a slight lymphocytosis.

The differential diagnosis of this condition involves the differential diagnosis of jaundice (p. 212). This is a medical rather than a surgical jaundice but must not be confused with gallbladder disease or lesions involving the head of the pancreas and the common bile duct.

The prognosis is comparatively good, since 95 per cent of cases of viral hepatitis recover fully. The mortality is approximately 0.5 per cent. From 4.5 per cent to 5 per cent of these patients acquire chronic sequelae such as

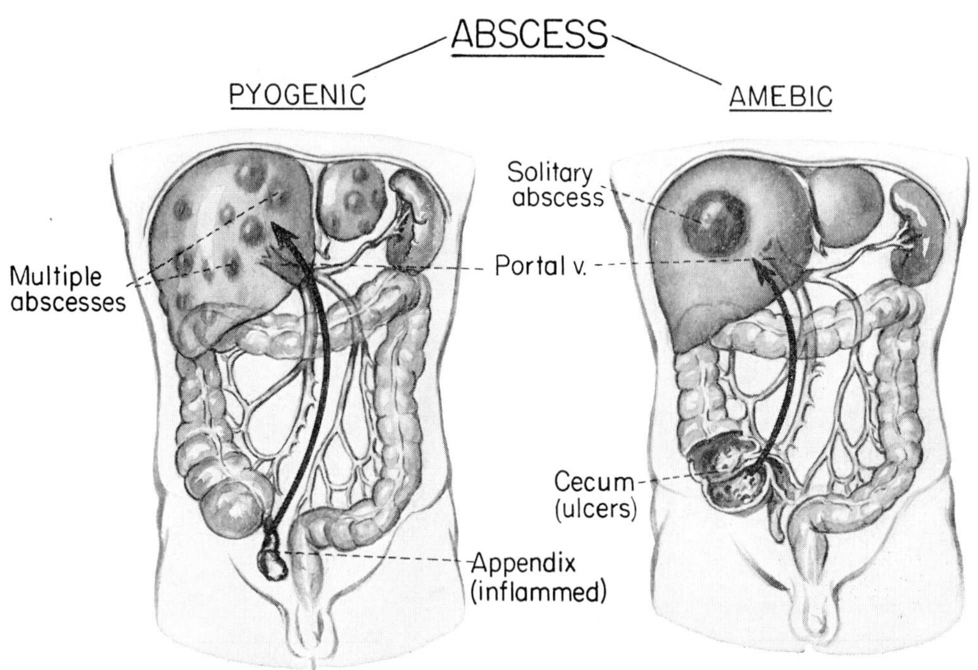

FIG. 216. Liver abscesses may be pyogenic (appendicitis, etc.) or amebic (*Endamoeba histolytica*). The infection usually travels to the liver via the portal vein.

chronic recurring hepatitis and portal cirrhosis (p. 196).

LIVER ABSCESS

For practical purposes liver abscesses may be divided into 2 types: pyogenic and amebic (Fig. 216).

Pyogenic Abscess

The pyogenic abscess is usually multiple and accompanies suppurative processes in the abdomen, such as appendicitis and ulcerative colitis, which produce pylephlebitis (thrombophlebitis of the portal vein). The offending organisms are usually hemolytic streptococci and the colon bacilli; however, other organisms may play a part. The portal vein is usually the path of entry to the liver, but the hepatic artery, infected bile ducts (cholangitis), or direct extension from adjacent organs also may be associated with the pathogenesis.

The symptoms include weakness, malaise, fever and chills, and mild pain in the right upper quadrant. The pain may be referred

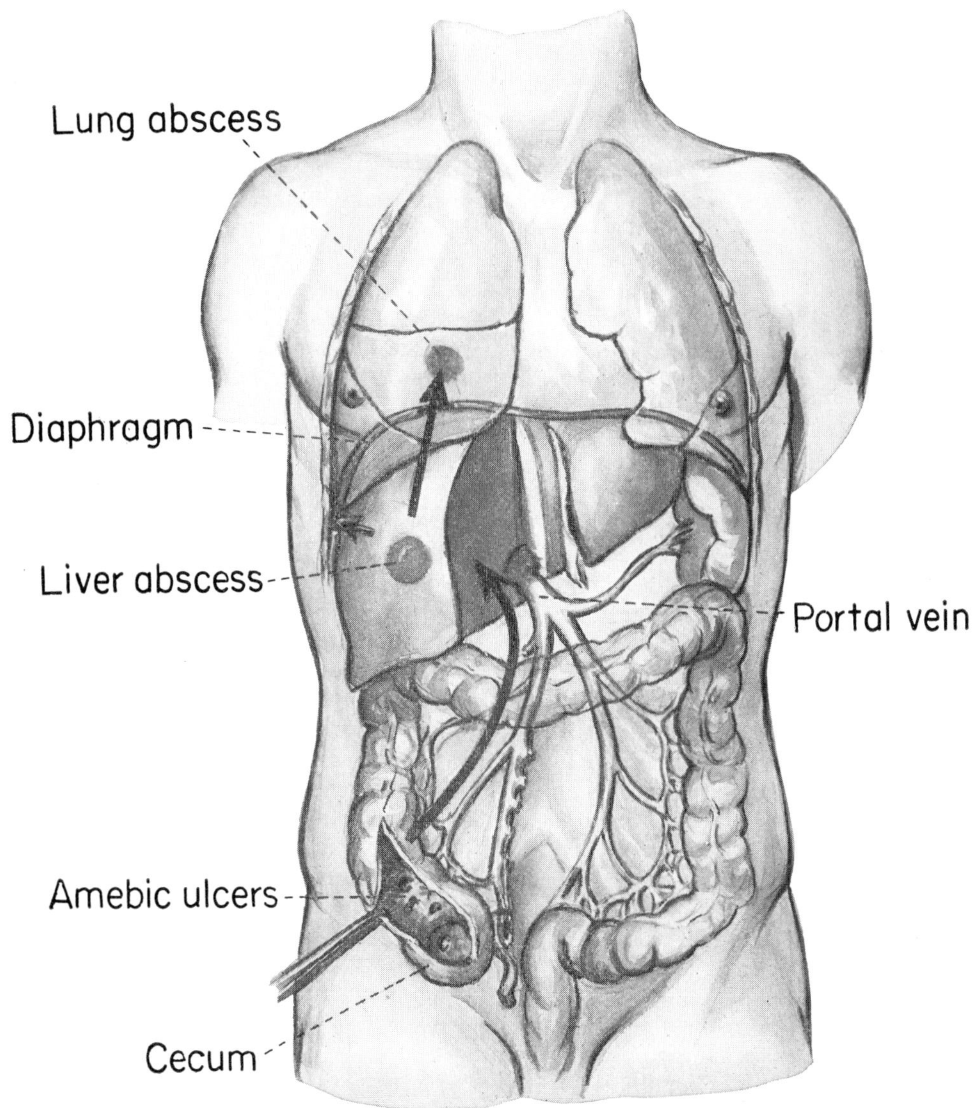

Fig. 217. The amebic liver abscess and its possible extension to the thoracic cavity.

to the right shoulder or the right side of the neck. With the advent of pylephlebitis, the signs of sepsis (chills, fever and sweats) dominate the clinical picture. If this extends into the right thoracic cavity, chest pain and cough develop.

Physical examination reveals liver enlargement and tenderness. Jaundice is the exception. Occult or hidden jaundice can be detected by a study of the serum bilirubin and the icterus index. A marked leukocytosis and secondary anemia are usually present. The fluoroscopic examination aids in detecting an elevated or fixed right hemidiaphragm. This must be differentiated from a subphrenic abscess (p. 202). In *liver abscess* the roentgenogram (AP view) reveals obliteration of the cardiophrenic angle. In *subphrenic abscess* the AP view reveals obliteration of the costophrenic angle, and the lateral view reveals an obliteration of the posterior costophrenic angle.

Liver function tests are helpful. The serum bilirubin and the alkaline phosphatase may be elevated.

The prognosis is guarded. Prior to the advent of chemotherapy and antibiotic drugs the mortality was stated to be as high as 50 to 95 per cent. However, due to modern therapy a more favorable outlook can be anticipated.

Amebic Abscess

The amebic liver abscess is usually solitary. It is encountered in both the temperate and the tropical climates. The causative organism is the *Endamoeba histolytica*; liver invasion is secondary to the intestinal disease. There is no primary amebic hepatitis or amebic abscess of the liver. It is likely that the causative agent reaches the right lobe of the liver via the cecum and the portal vein (Fig. 217). The time interval between the onset of the intestinal disease and hepatic complications has been estimated as less than 6 months in rare instances and occasionally as long as 57 years. Therefore, any patient who has had intestinal amebiasis is always in danger of hepatic complications.

Clinical Picture. Clinically, the difference between amebic hepatitis and amebic abscess is quantitative rather than qualitative. *Abdominal pain* is the most common symptom; this is usually present in the right upper abdominal quadrant but may be generalized. *Chest pain* is frequently present because of direct extension to the lungs or irritation of the diaphragmatic pleura. Increased respiration affects the intensity of the pain. Pleuropulmonary pain is more common with liver abscess than with hepatitis. The pain may radiate to the neck or the right scapula. *Physical findings* reveal liver tenderness and in most instances hepatomegaly. Exquisite pinpoint tenderness is present with abscess formation. Jaundice is infrequent.

Elevation of the right hemidiaphragm and limitation of its mobility may be seen fluoroscopically. The degree of the latter does not differentiate amebic hepatitis from amebic abscess. The stool should be examined for amebae. The complement-fixation test is still of doubtful clinical value. The pus, if aspirated or expectorated in the case of fistula formation, has the characteristic brick-red color. Liver abscesses, regardless of cause, may extend to the subphrenic spaces. Empyema thoracis, pneumonia, lung abscess, or pericarditis are fairly common complications. On occasion hepatic abscesses have ruptured into the thoracic duct or the inferior vena cava.

CIRRHOSIS OF THE LIVER

Cirrhosis is considered here for 3 reasons: it must be included in (1) the differential diagnosis of surgical diseases of the biliary tract, (2) the evaluation of liver function in determining the patient's ability to withstand surgical procedures, and (3) the recognition of portal hypertension.

Portal hypertension is particularly important, since some encouraging results are reported currently with surgical therapy. The hypertensive state in the portal system may be either intrahepatic or extrahepatic; these are differentiated with liver function tests (p. 192). Splenoportography may prove to be most helpful in the differential diagnosis of these conditions. The intrahepatic variety, which is more common, is discussed here.

Incidence

Portal cirrhosis is seen most commonly in men between the 5th and the 6th decades of life. The author has been impressed with the so-called cirrhotic habitus (Fig. 189). This is the male who has little or no hair on his chest; such males are predisposed to liver cirrhosis. Although no definite etiology has been established, toxic factors such as chronic alcoholism and an associated dietary deficiency are suspected. It is known, however, that this condition is seen also in the teetotaler.

Clinical Features

Esophageal varices usually produce hemorrhage, which can be mild, moderate or massive. If severe, the picture of shock is present. At times these varices are associated with enlarged gastric veins in the fundus of the stomach; they are demonstrable radiologically. If tremendously enlarged, they may produce dysphagia.

Hemorrhoids, in portal hypertension, are one of Nature's many ways of transferring blood from the portal to the caval system. Therefore, it is important to evaluate the condition of the liver in every case of hemorrhoids. Avoid hemorrhoidectomy in males who present a nonhirsute chest until the liver has been studied thoroughly. If hemorrhoidectomy is performed in cases of portal hypertension, important portacaval anastomoses are interrupted, and the patient may develop an ascites as a manifestation of portal decompensation.

The history may reveal alcoholism, malnutrition, previous jaundice, hepatitis, or chronic exposure to hepatotoxic agents. The size of the liver varies with the stage of the disease. In early cirrhosis the liver is enlarged and palpable, probably because of fatty infiltration; its enlargement upward can be demonstrated by percussion. As extensive fibrosis occurs, the liver shrinks; if palpable, it presents a hard, slightly nodular feel. In the late stage the characteristic atrophic "hobnailed" liver is present (Laennec's cirrhosis). Such a liver is not palpable unless ptotic. Liver function tests usually reveal severe damage.

The spleen is enlarged in all types of portal hypertension, but after an exsanguinating hemorrhage it decreases in size and may not be palpable. It becomes palpable, however, when the blood volume is restored. In portal hypertension with splenomegaly there may be an accompanying anemia, leukopenia and thrombocytopenia. This comprises the picture of so-called Banti's "disease." It is better to refer to this as Banti's syndrome. This phase of portal hypertension is discussed on

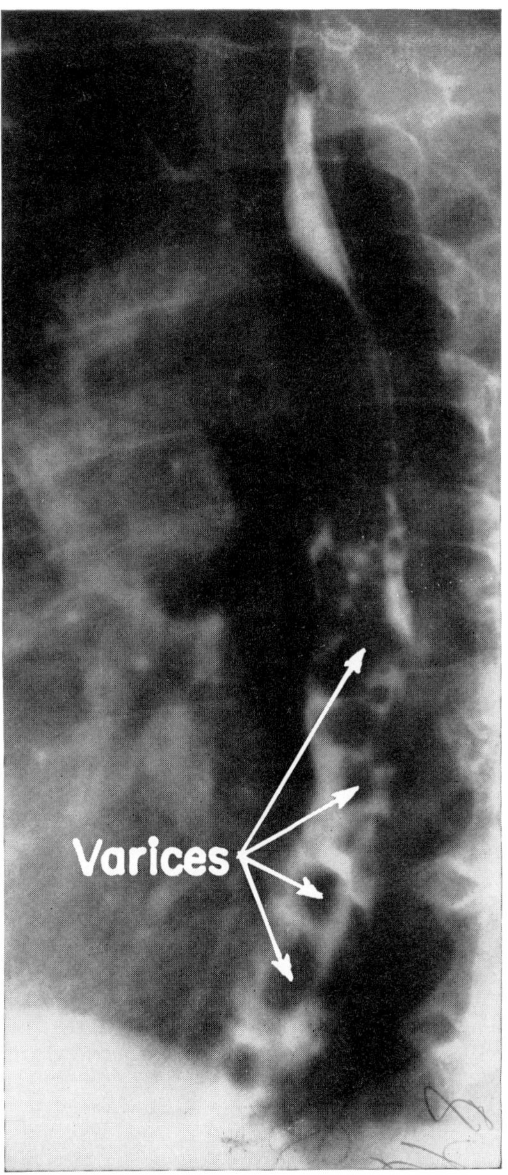

Fig. 218. Roentgenogram of esophageal varices. The patient has been given barium by mouth, and the characteristic "beaded" or "pearl-necklace" appearance is demonstrated.

page 249 under the heading of "Secondary Hypersplenism."

The skin may present telltale signs of hepatic disease. Jaundice usually appears late; it is rarely associated with pruritus. Engorged abdominal veins are visible, particularly around the umbilicus and over the lateral aspects of the abdomen. Such venous networks are readily demonstrable with infrared photography. *Spider naevi* frequently are present; they are usually noted about the head and the neck. *Palmar erythema* is also suggestive of hepatic disease.

Ascites is associated with lowered osmotic pressure and hypoalbuminemia. It constitutes one of the most distressing symptoms. The fluid is a transudate and is straw-colored. Carcinoma must be ruled out.

Bleeding esophageal varices can be present in a patient with minimal evidence of cirrhosis. The Bromsulphalein clearance test is probably the most sensitive in the early phase of cirrhosis, but it is of no value if jaundice is present. The gamma globulin test is also sensitive and may be of value when combined with other tests.

Diagnosis

Roentgenographic demonstration of esophageal varices should be attempted. It has been our custom to examine these patients roentgenologically soon after or even during mild bouts of hemorrhage. This, of course, must be done gently and expertly by one well trained in such cases. Almost all hypertensive esophageal varices are in the lower regions of the esophagus near the esophagogastric junction. When present, the typical so-called "beaded" appearance is demonstrable (Fig. 218). Varices in the upper third of the esophagus are usually congenital.

Endoscopy in the presence of hemorrhage has been advocated as a diagnostic aid; it is mentioned here to be condemned. This is far more traumatizing than a roentgenographic examination.

Portal venography or roentgenographic visualization after filling one of its branches with a radiopaque medium is recommended also. Time will prove its value.

The differential diagnosis is of vital practical importance, since the treatment differs tremendously in the various bleeding lesions of the esophagogastrointestinal tract. The *most common* site is the gastroduodenal segment; this constitutes the site of the vast majority of cases. Peptic ulcer is a common cause of *massive* hemorrhage, whereas a malignant neoplasm rarely causes this kind of hemorrhage. Other conditions which must be differentiated are hiatus hernia, severe hypertrophic gastritis, blood dyscrasia, and ulcerations from ectopic gastric and pancreatic tissues. If blood is coughed up and not vomited, it is frothy, bright red and alkaline to litmus paper. The surgical rarities and oddities have not been included in this differential diagnosis.

BENIGN TUMORS

Primary tumors of the liver, benign or malignant, are relatively rare. The benign tumors include hemangioma, adenoma, fibroma, teratoma and the so-called lipoma. Other tumors have been described; however, the 2 most frequent ones will be discussed, namely, benign hemangioma and adenoma.

Benign hemangioma is found more frequently in the liver than in any other internal organ. In most cases it is small, unproductive of symptoms, and frequently constitutes an incidental finding at surgery or necropsy. These hemangiomas communicate freely with the sinusoids of the liver; hence, they bleed briskly if incised. Frequently they are associated with hemangiomas of other organs, particularly the skin. If such a tumor is encountered during surgery, it may be mistaken for a metastatic lesion. Then such patients may be denied a curative or palliative resection. This is particularly true if the hemangioma is situated deep within the liver substance. Biopsy during surgery should be made whenever an unidentified hepatic nodule or tumor is discovered.

Benign adenomas of the liver are divided according to their cellular origin; hence, such terms as benign hepatoma, benign cholangioma and cholangiohepatoma are used. Tumors showing more than one cellular element are sometimes referred to as hamartomas.

The symptoms of benign tumors are usually mild or entirely absent. Dyspepsia, epigastric distress, distention and anorexia are common complaints. In over half of the cases the patient discovers the mass. Spontaneous rupture of such a lesion causes dramatic symptoms resembling an acute abdominal emergency. Auscultation over a benign hemangioma may reveal a bruit. Needle biopsy and peritoneoscopy are mentioned only to be condemned. The reason for this dogmatic stand is that the author considers these procedures a "peep show" laparotomy. Both of these adjuncts, particularly needle biopsy, predispose the patient to the danger of hemorrhage; furthermore, parasitic cysts are difficult to differentiate from tumor masses, and one surely would not wish to spread such cystic disease throughout the peritoneal cavity. Roentgenographic examination may reveal displacement of the stomach, the lower esophagus, or the colon, depending on the size and the location of the mass. Laboratory data are essentially noncontributory.

The author believes that the patient who presents an abdominal mass warrants a surgical exploration after a thorough study of the case. It is extremely difficult and in most instances impossible to differentiate a benign tumor, a malignant tumor, a metastatic tumor, a cyst, an abscess, or a specific granuloma (Fig. 219).

PRIMARY CARCINOMA OF THE LIVER

Incidence

Although infrequent in this country, this condition is often encountered among the natives of South Africa and the Orient. The predilection for certain geographic areas and racial groups is one of its most unusual features. The incidence in the American Negro is not nearly as high as that reported in African natives. The American Negro is a descendant of Africa, but it is the South African natives who show the highest incidence. Malignancies in general are less common in the colored race, but primary carcinoma of the liver seems to be the exception to this rule.

The condition occurs most commonly in the so-called "cancer age" between 50 and 60, but cases do appear in the extremes of life, having been reported in the 8th decade and in an infant on the 3rd day of life. Well over half of the adult cases are associated with a pre-existing cirrhosis. What these 2

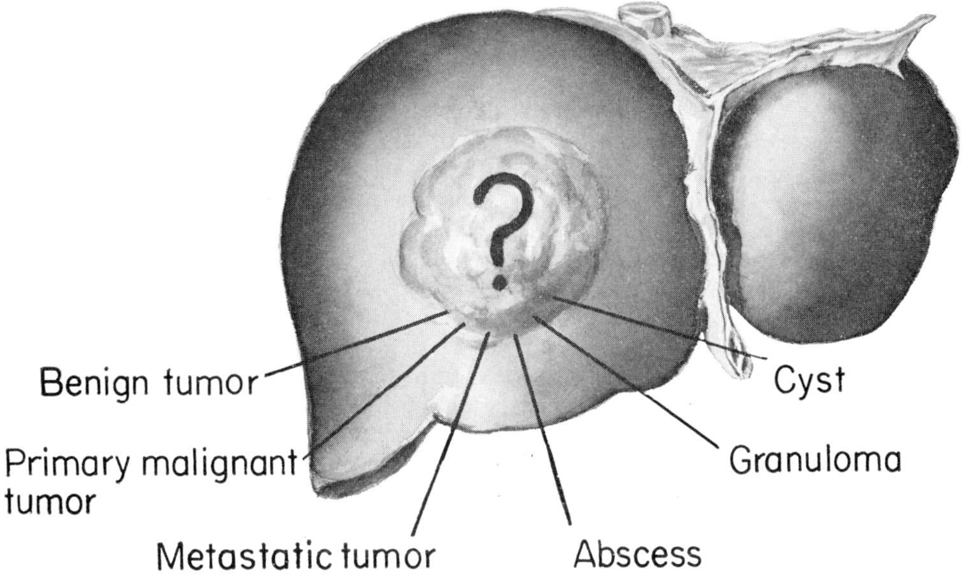

Fig. 219. Laparotomy is necessary to confirm a diagnosis of a liver mass in the majority of cases.

conditions have in common, if anything, is unknown. Methionine, one of the sulfur-containing amino acids, which is being used currently in the treatment of cirrhosis of the liver, seems to accelerate the development of these tumors in experimental animals. Therefore, some research workers suggest that such amino acids, which are necessary for normal growth, are necessary also for growth of these neoplasms.

Carcinomas of the liver may arise from the parenchymal epithelium or the epithelial lining of bile ducts; on this basis they have been designated as malignant hepatomas or cholangiomas. This distinction is of little clinical value and can be made only microscopically.

Clinical Features

Since the symptoms are not specific, they are not diagnostic. The condition may present itself in 1 of 5 ways:

1. The symptomatology suggests cirrhosis of the liver.
2. This group projects disorders involving the biliary tract.
3. The symptoms involve the gastrointestinal tract and at times are associated with internal hemorrhage.
4. This group is asymptomatic; the condition is discovered accidentally during the patient's lifetime.
5. This group includes those cases which are discovered at necropsy.

Pain is present in the majority of cases; it is rarely severe or cramplike, as when a hollow viscus is involved. It is usually situated in the right upper abdominal quadrant or epigastrium. The pain is due to enlargement of the organ which stretches Glisson's capsule. When the onset is severe and abrupt, with signs of peritonitis, perforation of a necrotizing tumor should be suspected.

Dyspepsia of varying degrees is present; nausea and vomiting are rare. *Hemorrhage* may manifest itself either as a bleeding esophageal varix, epistaxis or a bloody ascites. *Cachexia* and *asthenia* are present in over half of the cases. *Hepatic enlargement* depends on the location of the tumor. Malignancy should be suspected whenever a patient known to have cirrhosis suddenly presents a rapidly enlarging solitary liver nodule. If the mass is in the dome of the right lobe, that side of the diaphragm may be elevated. Such masses on the left side have been mistaken for an enlarged spleen. *Ascites,* if present, is due either to a pre-existing cirrhosis, thrombosis of the portal vein, or involvement of the visceral and parietal peritoneum. *Dependent edema* is due to hypoproteinemia or pressure on the inferior vena cava. *Jaundice* is a late sign. The *spleen* is palpable in about one fourth of the cases, but it is difficult to detect splenomegaly because of ascites, distention or hepatomegaly. The splenic enlargement is secondary to a pre-existing cirrhosis or to portal vein involvement by tumor tissue.

Diagnosis

Laboratory tests are of little value, since marked impairment of liver function can be demonstrated only when the tumor is a large one.

Roentgenographic examination is helpful in that it may demonstrate esophageal varices (Fig. 218), the size of the spleen and the liver, the presence of a mass in the region of the liver, and evidence of metastases. Displacement of the diaphragm, or gastric air bubble gives contributory evidence.

Surgical Exploration. Any or all of these cases that can withstand surgical intervention should have the value of exploration and possible alleviation of symptoms. The metastases of this tumor are remarkable in that they infrequently produce widespread or distant lesions. Although it has been shown that this primary tumor invades the hepatic and the portal veins relatively early, the infrequency of distant metastases is most surprising. This is particularly true of hepatoma. The most common sites of metastases when they occur are the lungs, the lymph nodes and the mediastinum. If the skeleton is involved, the vertebral column is the site of predilection.

SARCOMA

Sarcoma of the liver is rare. It appears to be associated with a pre-existing cirrhosis. Hepatic sarcoma usually pursues a rapidly fatal course; death occurs within a few months after the onset of this neoplasm. This

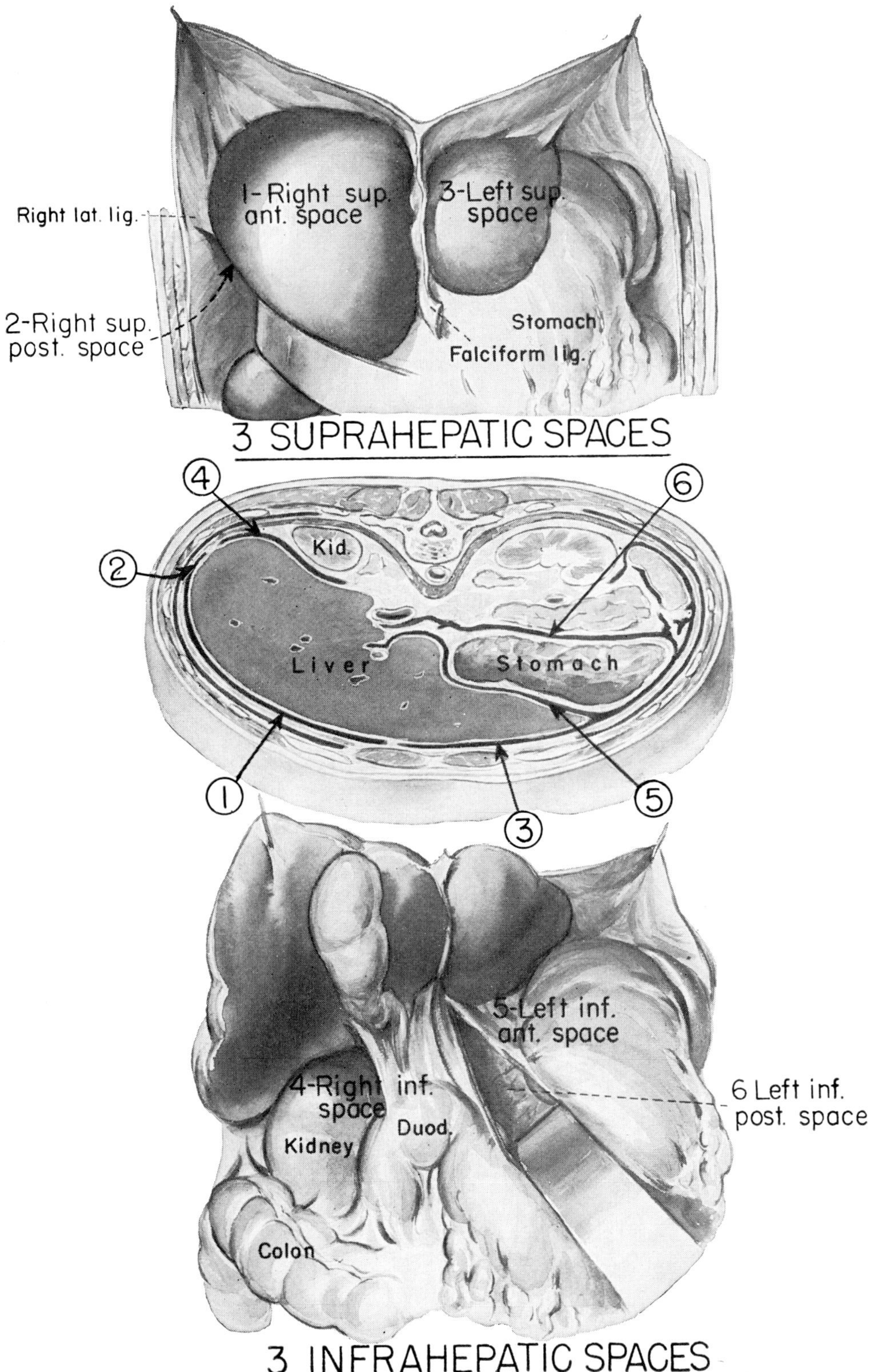

FIG. 220. The 6 subphrenic spaces. The signs and symptoms of subphrenic abscesses depend on which of these spaces are involved.

lesion is prone to disseminate widely throughout the liver and to metastasize via both the blood and the lymph channels. The clinical course is essentially similar to that of carcinoma.

METASTATIC TUMORS OF THE LIVER

Although the liver is a rare site for primary growths, it ranks second only to regional lymph nodes as a site for metastatic carcinoma. The abdominal organs, particularly the stomach and the colon, should be investigated carefully as a possible primary site for these metastases. The primary lesion can be symptomless and small, and the metastatic lesions attract attention first. The metastases gain access to the liver via the portal vein, arterial emboli, the lymph stream, or by direct extension. It has been stated that metastatic carcinoma of the liver carries an exceedingly poor prognosis, since 85 per cent of the patients die within a year of their discovery. One never should be too certain, since remarkable cases do exist. A case of metastatic carcinoma of the liver is recalled in which the patient is surviving 26 years after discovery of the condition.

Sarcomas of intra-abdominal organs are more rare than carcinomas, and when they do occur, they rarely metastasize to the liver.

SUBPHRENIC ABSCESS (SUBDIAPHRAGMATIC ABSCESS)

Divisions

The subphrenic area should be divided into 6 subphrenic spaces (Fig. 220). Three of these are suprahepatic, and 3 are infrahepatic. This is important clinically, because the signs and symptoms are altered according to the location. These spaces are:

1. Right superior-anterior space
2. Right superior-posterior space
3. Left superior space

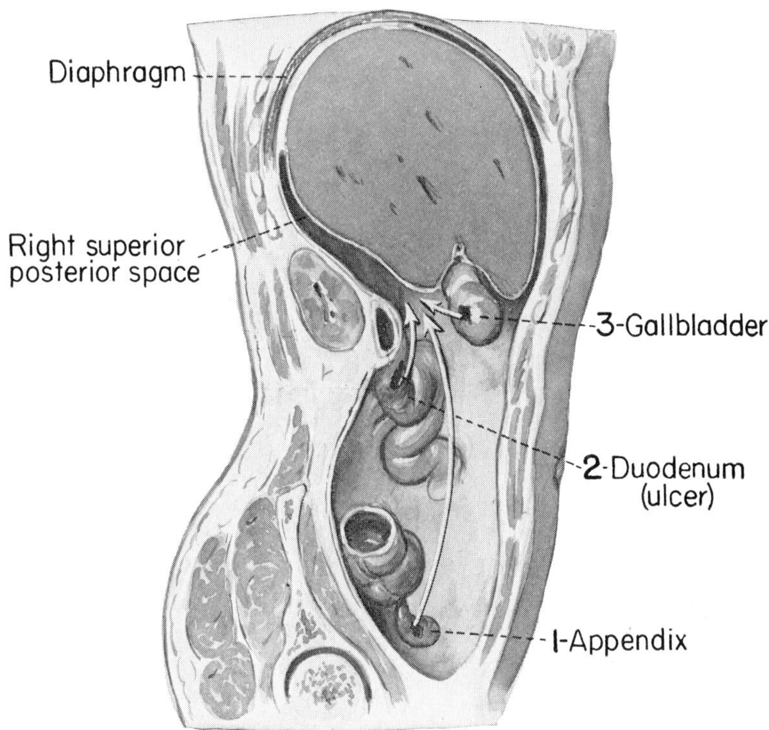

Fig. 221. The right superior-posterior subphrenic space is involved most frequently because the 3 most commonly affected abdominal organs (appendix, gallbladder and gastroduodenal segment) have access to it.

4. Right inferior space (Morison's pouch)
5. Left inferior-anterior space (perigastric space)
6. Left inferior-posterior space (retrogastric space)

Etiology

The majority of such abscesses are associated with perforated gastroduodenal ulcers, acute appendicitis or a diseased gallbladder. Because of this, the right superior-posterior space is the one that is involved most frequently (Fig. 221). Occasionally, these spaces may be infected from extension of an adjacent abscess (perinephric abscess); another mode of extension is from distant foci of infection.

Clinical Course and Diagnosis

The diagnosis is difficult at times because of a lack of localizing signs or symptoms. A *septic syndrome* is usually present; this consists of intermittent spiking fever, rigors, profuse sweating and leukocytosis (over 20,000). Such a syndrome signifies pus. *Pain* is often absent; if present, it appears as a dull, vague, deep ache in the right upper abdominal quadrant or the back. Shoulder pain is suggestive of diaphragmatic irritation. Physical signs are usually wanting but may

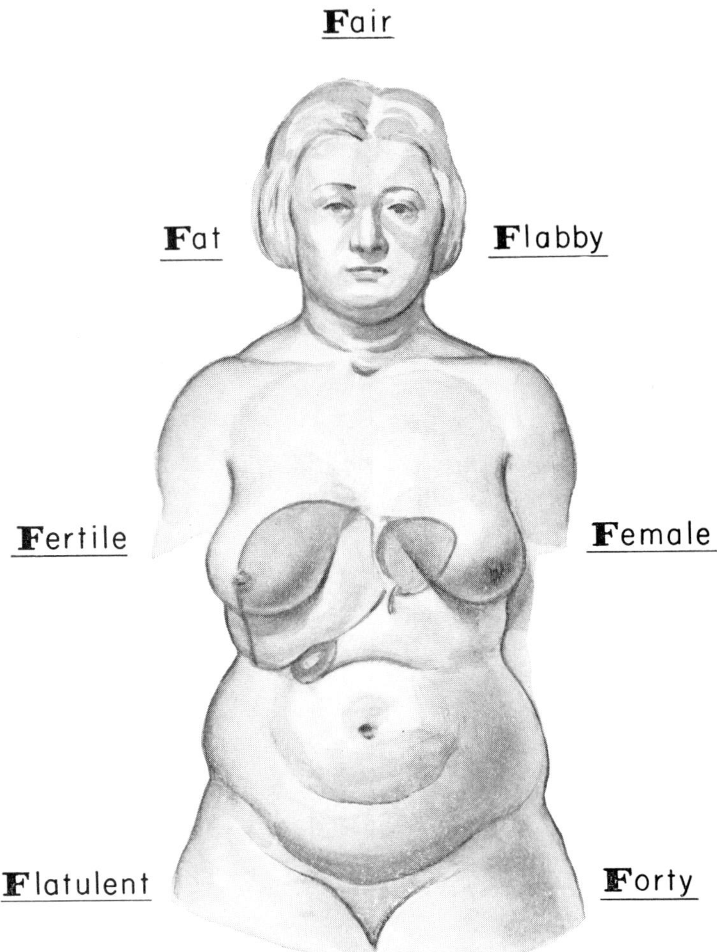

Fig. 222. The gallbladder patient usually corresponds to the 7-"F" type.

be associated with a slight amount of fluid in the pleural cavity. The author has not been able to elicit the so-called 3-layer percussion notes, even in large abscesses. If the abscess is in one of the anterior spaces, tenderness usually is found at the costal border; if posterior, there may be tenderness over the 12th rib on the involved side.

If untreated, resolution is rare; the abscess may rupture into the lungs, the pericardium, the stomach, the colon or through the parietes. Pleural or pulmonary suppuration is a common complication.

Diagnosis

Fluoroscopy is a most valuable diagnostic aid. If a subphrenic abscess is present, the hemidiaphragm on the involved side is either partially or totally immobile. If the abscess is large, the *roentgenogram* is helpful in that it reveals a high diaphragm; the abscess may be demonstrated if it contains gas and a fluid level. Postoperative pleural effusion suggests a possible subphrenic abscess. This is particularly true if a small amount of fluid is noted in the right costophrenic angle.

The use of aspiration or punctures as diagnostic aids is to be condemned because of the ease with which these abscesses are missed, and the danger of spreading the infection to the pleural and/or peritoneal cavities.

The differential diagnosis chiefly involves pleural empyema and liver abscess.

Prognosis

The prognosis is guarded, particularly if the diagnosis is made late, and the patient is in poor condition. The mortality can be lowered precipitously if early and adequate drainage is instituted.

GALLBLADDER AND BILE DUCTS

The gallbladder is an important organ which has numerous key functions to perform. Its removal is strictly contraindicated unless a definite indication is present. The clinical results following cholecystecomy are directly proportional to the amount of disease present in the organ.

Some of the more important *functions of the gallbladder* include:

1. Absorption: The gallbladder concentrates liver bile approximately 10 times.
2. Secretion: An important mucoid material is secreted by its mucous membrane.
3. Motor activity: Bile is delivered to the duodenum at the proper time and rate.
4. Change of pH of bile
5. Equalization of pressure within the entire biliary duct system
6. A reservoir for bile
7. Hormonal function (?)

Acute Cholecystitis

Incidence. The exact incidence of this condition is unknown because many such patients fail to consult a physician. The gallbladder type is the 7-"F" type: *F*air, *F*at, *F*ertile, *F*labby, *F*latulent, *F*emale of *F*orty (Fig. 222).

Etiology. Consensus points to an etiology that is primarily chemical; the role of bacteria is secondary. Stasis is the most important factor in the etiology of acute cholecystitis. Hypercholesterolemia and pregnancy seem to be associated with the formation of gallstones. Such stones obstruct the ducts and produce stasis and inflammation. It is true that there is a stoneless cholecystitis; but stasis can be produced by other factors such as spasm, swelling, kinks, anomalous vessels and bands.

When an excess of cholesterol is deposited on the mucosa of the gallbladder, the appearance is not unlike the seeds on a ripe strawberry. Because of this the term "strawberry gallbladder" has been applied. This is a cholesterolosis; it does not produce clinical signs or symptoms and does not require cholecystectomy.

The *organisms* encountered are usually those which normally inhabit the intestinal tract, namely, streptococci and colon bacilli.

Pathology. The appearance of the acutely inflamed organ is modified by the presence or the absence of pre-existing disease. Frank pus (empyema) is rarely encountered, even in an intensely inflamed gallbladder. Ulceration is usually related to calculi. Flimsy fibrinous or firm fibrous adhesions attach the gallbladder to the adjacent duodenum, colon and/or stomach. If the disease progresses, gangrene and perforation result with subsequent bile peritonitis.

Symptoms. Pain is the most prominent symptom. Its onset is usually sudden and often follows the ingestion of a heavy or

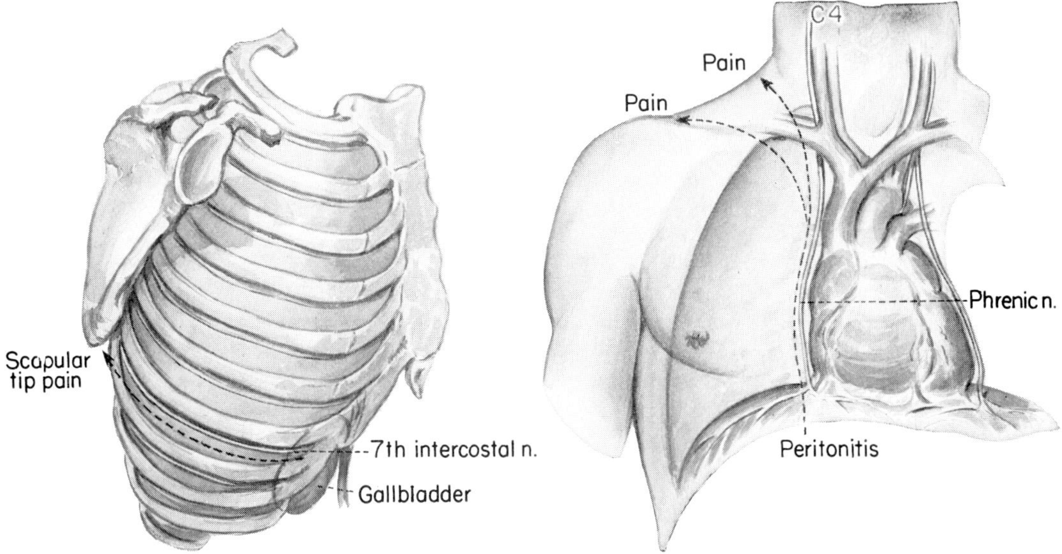

FIG. 223. Gallbladder pain or peritonitis? Gallbladder pain radiates to the tip of the right scapula. The pain of peritonitis radiates to the shoulder (phrenic nerve).

fatty meal. The pain may be one of 2 types: continuous if inflammatory, or colicky if associated with obstruction. It is important to differentiate these types of pain, because an inflammatory lesion may be treated conservatively, but an obstructed gallbladder demands immediate surgical relief. The pain is located most often in the right upper abdominal quadrant but may be in the epigastrium. It can be referred along its nervous path (splanchnic nerves); hence, gastrospasms may confuse the picture. If such a spasm is in the region of the gastric cardia, the condition may be confused with coronary disease. Gallbladder pain usually radiates to the tip of the right scapula or the interscapular area. This must not be confused with shoulder pain, which signifies irritation of the phrenic nerve and frequently is associated with peritonitis (Fig. 223).

Nausea and *vomiting* are extremely variable and of little or no diagnostic value. The presence of bile in the emesis merely denotes a patent pylorus.

The temperature may be somewhat elevated; however, many cases of acute cholecystitis are afebrile. It is important to emphasize that there is frequently little or no correlation between fever, pain and the severity of the disease.

Cardiac irregularities and gallbladder disease are thought to be associated. In acute cholecystitis, as in other inflammatory conditions, the pulse increases 10 beats for every degree rise in temperature.

Jaundice may accompany acute cholecystitis. If this is present, one must differentiate an associated hepatitis or obstruction of the common and/or hepatic ducts (see Jaundice, p. 212).

Tenderness, when present in the right upper quadrant, is a most important finding. If the gallbladder is distended and displaced downward, it may be palpable, particularly if the patient is thin. This habitus is infrequent in gallbladder patients. After 36 or 48 hours, an inflammatory mass (omentum wrapped around the gallbladder) may become palpable. If the gallbladder is large and distended, its fundus may reach to or below the umbilicus; if the liver is ptotic, the gallbladder also may assume a low position.

Diagnosis. Such low-lying inflamed gallbladders make differentiation from acute appendicitis difficult. Helpful in the latter differential diagnosis is the demonstration of triangular areas of hyperesthesia as related to the umbilicus (Fig. 224).

Some *laboratory tests* may be helpful adjuncts. The white blood cell count is usually

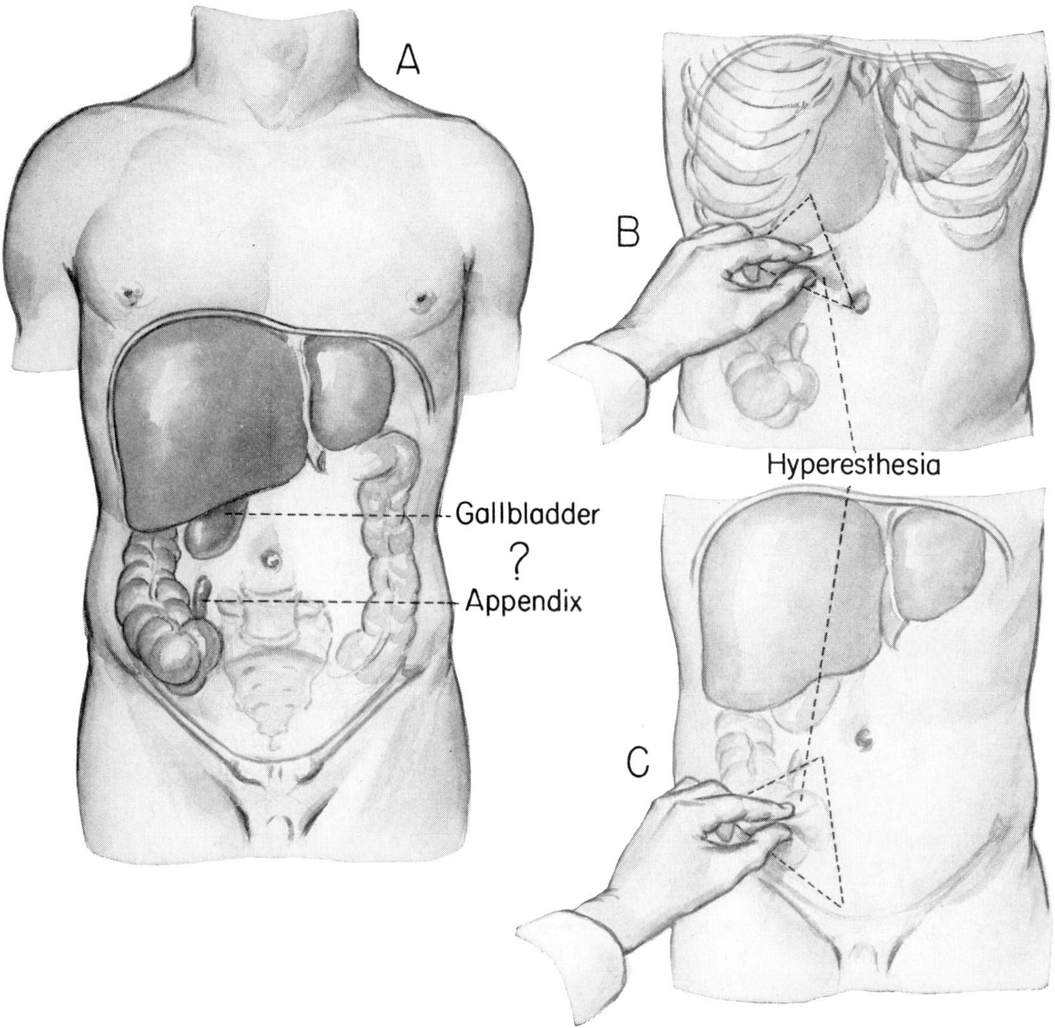

FIG. 224. Appendix or gallbladder? If an inflamed appendix is retrocecal and high, or if an inflamed gallbladder is situated low and on a level with the umbilicus, it may be difficult to differentiate the two. The detection of triangular zones of hyperesthesia as related to the umbilicus is of great help. If the gallbladder is at fault, the hyperesthetic triangular zone is directed upward from the umbilicus toward the right costal arch; if the appendix is inflamed, the zone is directed downward from the umbilicus toward the inguinal ligament.

elevated; if the leukocyte count is over 20,000, one may suspect a purulent cholecystitis or an empyema. The flat roentgenogram is particularly useful in detecting stones.

Differential Diagnosis. It is true that one may list numerous conditions that simulate acute cholecystitis. Such listings are merely a display of cerebral muscle. The following 6 conditions constitute 95 per cent of the diseases that are confused with acute cholecystitis:

1. Acute appendicitis (p. 143)
2. Perforated peptic ulcer (pp. 132-133)
3. Acute pancreatitis (p. 223)
4. Renal and ureteral colics (p. 266)
5. Acute salpingitis (pp. 273-274)
6. Coronary disease. This last diagnosis must be suspected, particularly in males, with

a history of hypertension or a previous story of organic heart disease. The typical picture offers no diagnostic difficulties, whereas atypical coronary conditions can be tragic if overlooked. If an absolute differentiation between biliary and cardiac pain cannot be made, the course of watchful expectancy is to be recommended.

Chronic Cholecystitis

Incidence. This condition is extremely common and at times difficult to diagnose. It may be associated with or without gallstones and is frequently a sequel to acute cholecystitis. The chronically inflamed gallbladder is thickened because of the deposition of scar tissue and at times calcium. Adhesions involve contiguous organs. If the cystic duct becomes obstructed, a hydrops develops (p. 218).

Symptoms. *Dyspepsia* is a common symptom. It includes a multitude of complaints such as epigastric distress, bloating, belching, heartburn, mild pain, distention, flatulence and anorexia. *Pain* is variable when present; it frequently occurs in intermittent attacks. It is usually localized to the right upper quadrant and may radiate to the tip of the right scapula or interscapular area. *Nausea* is frequent, and *vomiting* may occur during attacks. Certain foods are not tolerated well, particularly fried and fatty foods, raw apples,

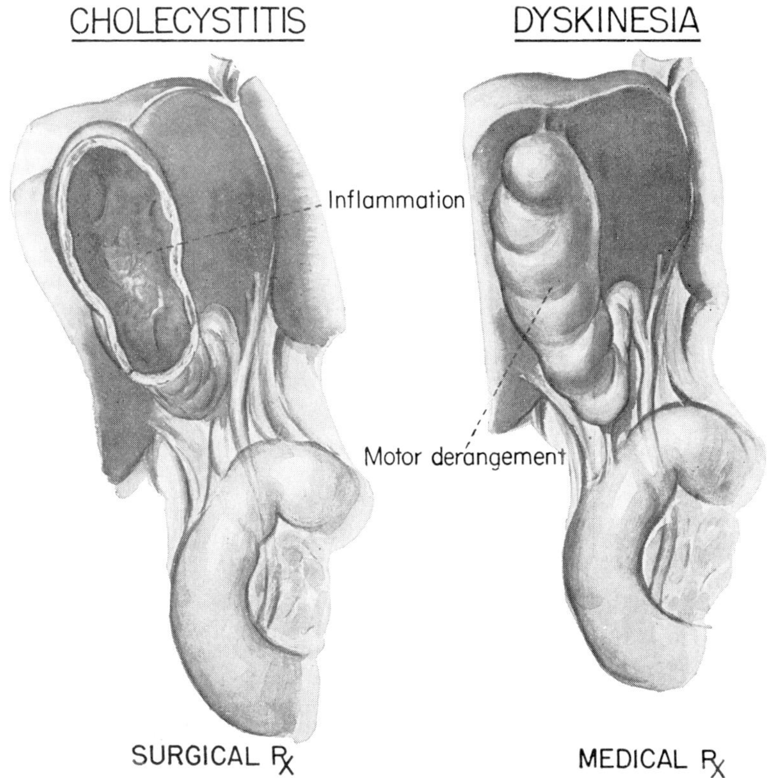

Fig. 225. Cholecystitis or biliary dyskinesia? Cholecystitis is the diseased gallbladder which results from inflammation and infection of the organ. It is associated with systemic signs and symptoms. It should be treated surgically. The biliary dyskinesia is the functionally deranged gallbladder which is unassociated with fever, elevated white blood count and other signs and symptoms of inflammation. It responds well to medical treatment and therefore should *not* be removed.

cucumbers and cabbage. When these foods are eaten, the patient complains of the 2 "B's"—bloating and belching. She further states that she feels more comfortable if she abstains from eating. This is in contrast with the peptic ulcer patient, who takes food to obtain comfort. *Jaundice,* when present, usually is associated with hepatitis or a stone in the common or the hepatic duct (p. 212).

Diagnosis. *Physical examination* may reveal tenderness in the right upper quadrant; however, this is lacking unless an acute exacerbation is present. When the acute phase subsides, the patient may be symptom-free.

The roentgenographic study reveals a poorly functioning or nonfunctioning gallbladder.

Differential Diagnosis. Numerous conditions may present the complaint of "dyspepsia"; however, 3 outstanding diseases must be differentiated. They are peptic ulcer (p. 127), coronary disease (p. 81) and esophageal hiatus hernia (p. 85).

Biliary Dyskinesia (Dyssynergia)

These terms refer to a motor dysfunction of the gallbladder. The etiology is unknown. and there is no discernible lesion. It is believed to be due to a neuromuscular derangement.

The symptoms suggest organic gallbladder disease (cholecystitis). Pain in the right upper quadrant of the abdomen, which radiates to the tip of the right scapula, is present, and selective dyspepsia is complained of. However, the roentgenographic report reveals a well-concentrating and functioning gallbladder. At times delayed filling and emptying of the viscus may be reported.

These patients respond exceedingly well to

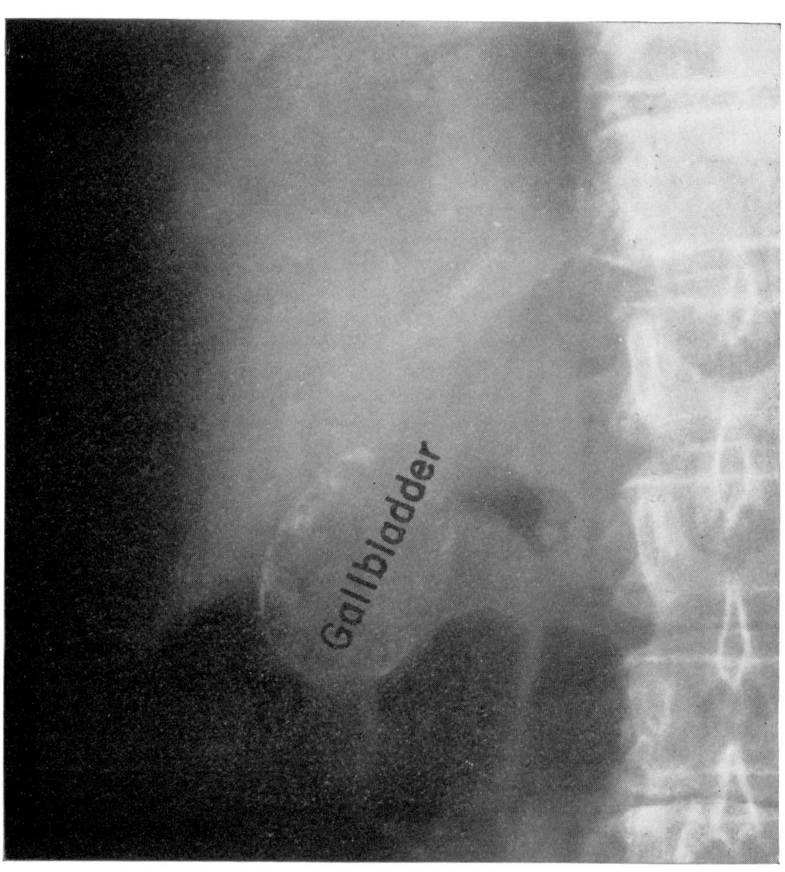

Fig. 226. Roentgenogram of a calcified gallbladder. No contrast medium has been given.

diets that are high in fats. Likewise, they are relieved by nitrites, other antispasmodics and mild sedative therapy.

The patient with cholecystitis should submit to surgical therapy, but the patient with dyskinesia should avoid surgery at all costs, since she can be relieved by a proper medical and dietary regimen (Fig. 225).

Calcification of the Gallbladder

This organ, when inflamed, is a common site for the deposition of calcium (Fig. 226). The calcium may be precipitated onto the surface of gallstones or might lie free in the lumen of the viscus as a paste. Roentgenograms may be interpreted erroneously as concentrated dye within the organ. Unless the condition is kept in mind, the stony hardness can give rise to an erroneous diagnosis of carcinoma.

Tumors of the Gallbladder

Carcinoma of the gallbladder is not uncommon, since it represents about 5 per cent of all carcinomas. It is 4 times more common in women. Calculi are present in almost every case of primary carcinoma of this organ. The signs and symptoms are those of chronic or acute cholecystitis and the presence of a typical mass. This mass is located in the right upper quadrant, it is hard, moves with respiration and is *irregular* (p. 218). Jaundice may or may not be present, depending on the location of metastases or extension by contiguity. Definite diagnosis is made during surgery.

The gallbladder may be involved by direct extension or metastases from primary carcinomas elsewhere.

Primary sarcoma of the gallbladder is a rare disease; when present, it usually is associated with long-standing cholecystitis and cholelithiasis.

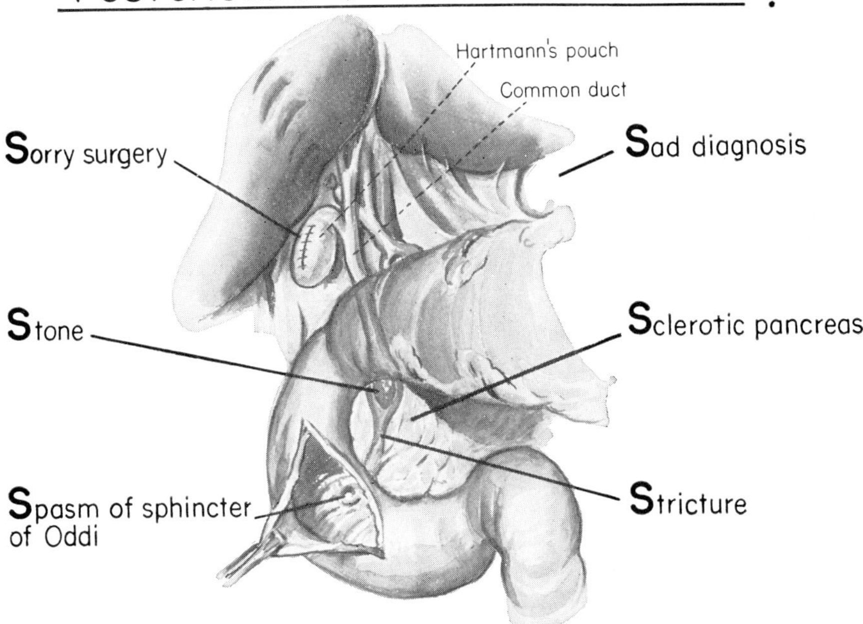

Fig. 227. The term "postcholecystectomy syndrome" is a misleading one and should not be used. The causes of symptoms following cholecystectomy have been enumerated with the "S" mnemonic. "Sorry surgery" refers to an operation that is incomplete or unnecessary. "Sad diagnosis" implies a diagnostic error. Particularly in this latter instance must be mentioned an overlooked hiatus hernia.

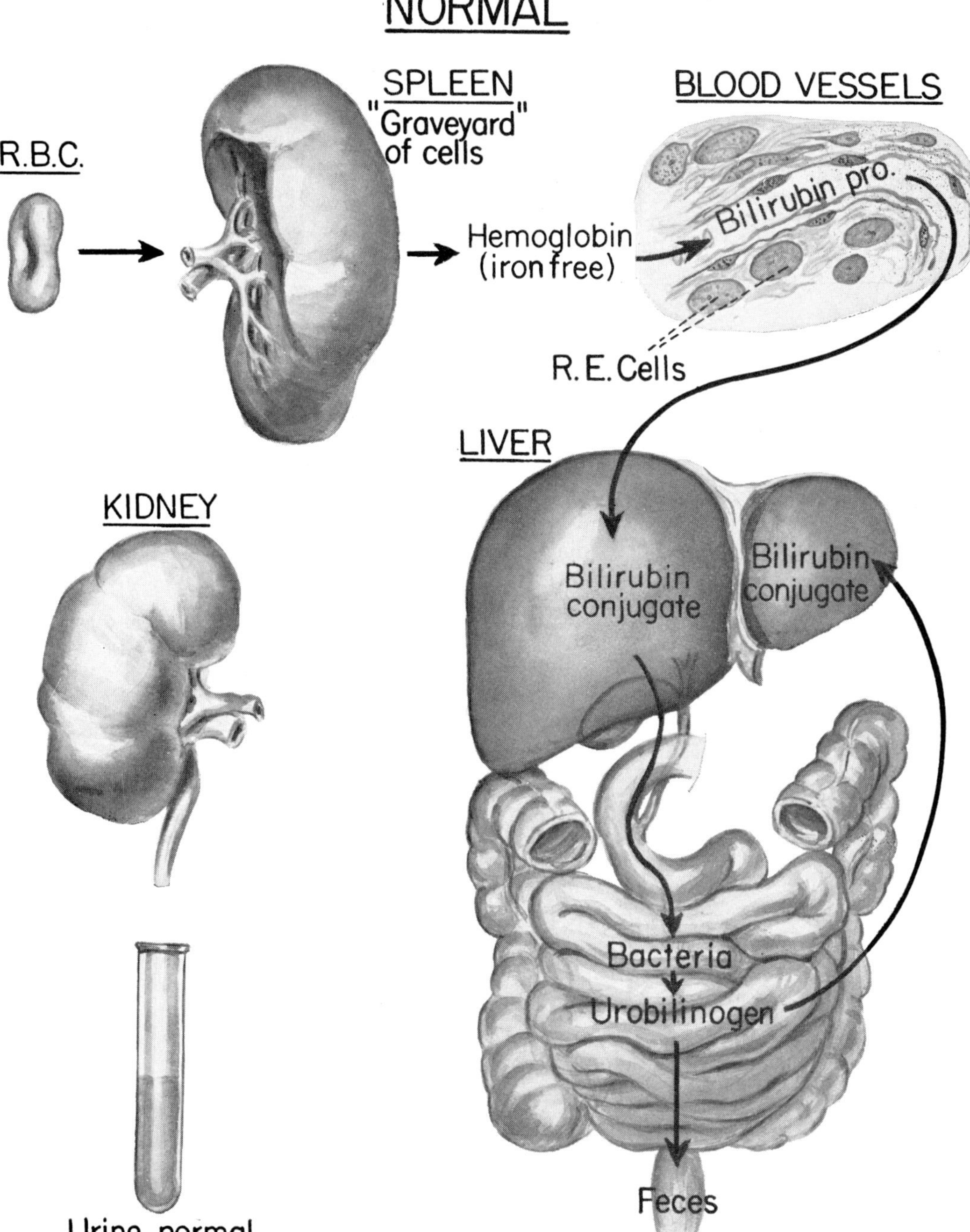

Fig. 228. The normal metabolism of bilirubin and urobilinogen. If there is no excess of these metabolites, they do not overflow into the blood stream and the urine and therefore do not appear in abnormal amounts.

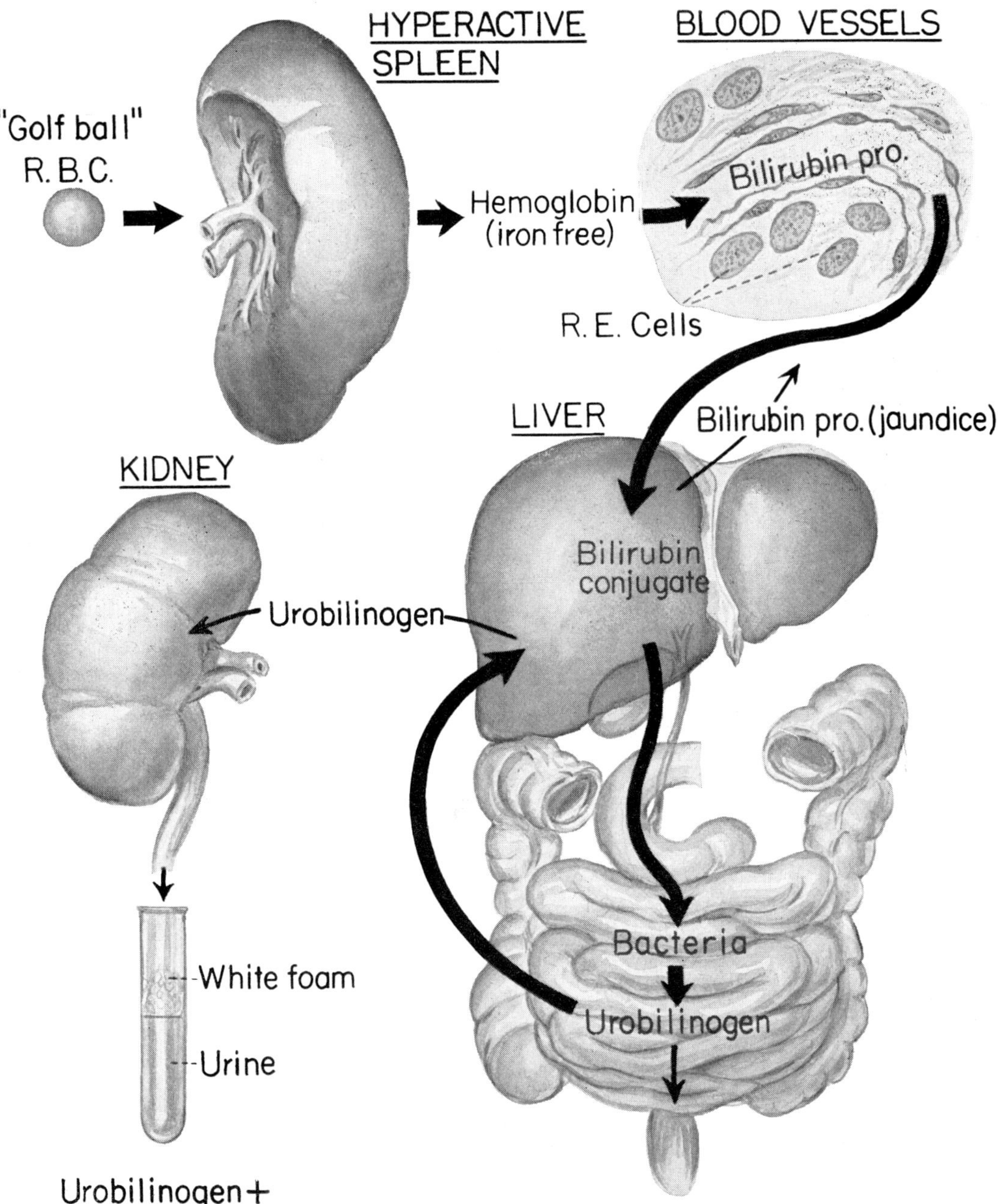

FIG. 229. Prehepatic jaundice. The heavy arrows denote excessive production of the bile pigments. The light arrows denote overflow of these substances.

Choledochitis

Inflammation of the common bile duct has not received the attention that it deserves. It may be associated with infection of the intrahepatic biliary radicals or may occur in conjunction with acute cholecystitis. It is usually a complication of a stone impacted in the common duct. Cases are reported in which marked inflammation of this duct is present without choledocholithiasis. It is impossible to diagnose this condition preoperatively. It is characterized by edema, hyperemia and at times suppurative inflammatory changes in the duct which may extend upward into the liver. Removal of the obstruction, if present, and adequate drainage of the duct are mandatory if the patient's life is to be saved.

Congenital Biliary Obstruction

When jaundice is due to a malformation of the biliary tract, it appears shortly after birth, progresses relentlessly and intensifies with each passing day. When other causes of jaundice have been excluded (p. 212), exploration should be carried out, preferably before the 4th week of life.

Carcinoma of the Extrahepatic Bile Ducts

This has been discussed elsewhere (p. 218).

Postcholecystectomy Syndrome

This term is misleading, since one does not know to what it refers. The letter "S" used in Figure 227 enumerates some of the conditions that cause symptoms following the removal of the gallbladder.

JAUNDICE

To understand the subject of jaundice one must comprehend the physiopathology of the bile pigments (Fig. 228).

Physiology

A review of the life cycle of a normal red blood corpuscle is a logical beginning. According to current concepts, following the destruction of red cells by the spleen, iron-free hemoglobin is liberated. Hemoglobin is converted to bilirubin by the reticuloendothelial system of the liver, the spleen and the bone marrow. The bilirubin is loosely attached to plasma proteins as it is transported to the liver. In the hepatic polygonal cell the bilirubin "proteinate" is conjugated with glucuronic acid by the enzyme, bilirubin transferase, to form bilirubin diglucuronide. The conjugated bilirubin is excreted by liver cells via the intrahepatic and the extrahepatic bile ducts into the duodenum, where it is converted by bacterial action into a metabolite, urobilinogen. Some urobilinogen passes out and colors the feces, and the remainder is absorbed from the intestinal tract and returned to the liver via the portal system. The liver converts urobilinogen back to bilirubin. Based upon this, a most useful way of classifying the symptom of jaundice is:

1. Prehepatic jaundice
2. Intrahepatic jaundice
3. Posthepatic jaundice

With this classification the clinician automatically asks himself: "Is the lesion *before* the liver, *in* the liver or *after* the liver?

Prehepatic Jaundice (Fig. 229)

Conditions producing this type of icterus are associated with an increased destruction of red blood cells (icterus neonatorum), increased fragility of these cells (hemolytic anemia), or those conditions in which the spleen is overactive and destroys the cells (hypersplenism). The physiopathology in all of these conditions is essentially the same, namely, excessive destruction of erythrocytes; this results in an overproduction of hemoglobin, the mother substance of bile. It follows, therefore, that an excessive amount of bilirubin "proteinate" will be produced and delivered to the liver. The liver, although normal, cannot excrete this excess, and it overflows into the blood stream. The jaundice which results is caused by bilirubin "proteinate," a substance that is too heavy to filter over the renal threshold; hence, there is no bile pigment in the urine. This produces an *acholuric jaundice*; in other words, this jaundiced patient has no bilirubin in his urine. This is diagnosed readily if one examines the

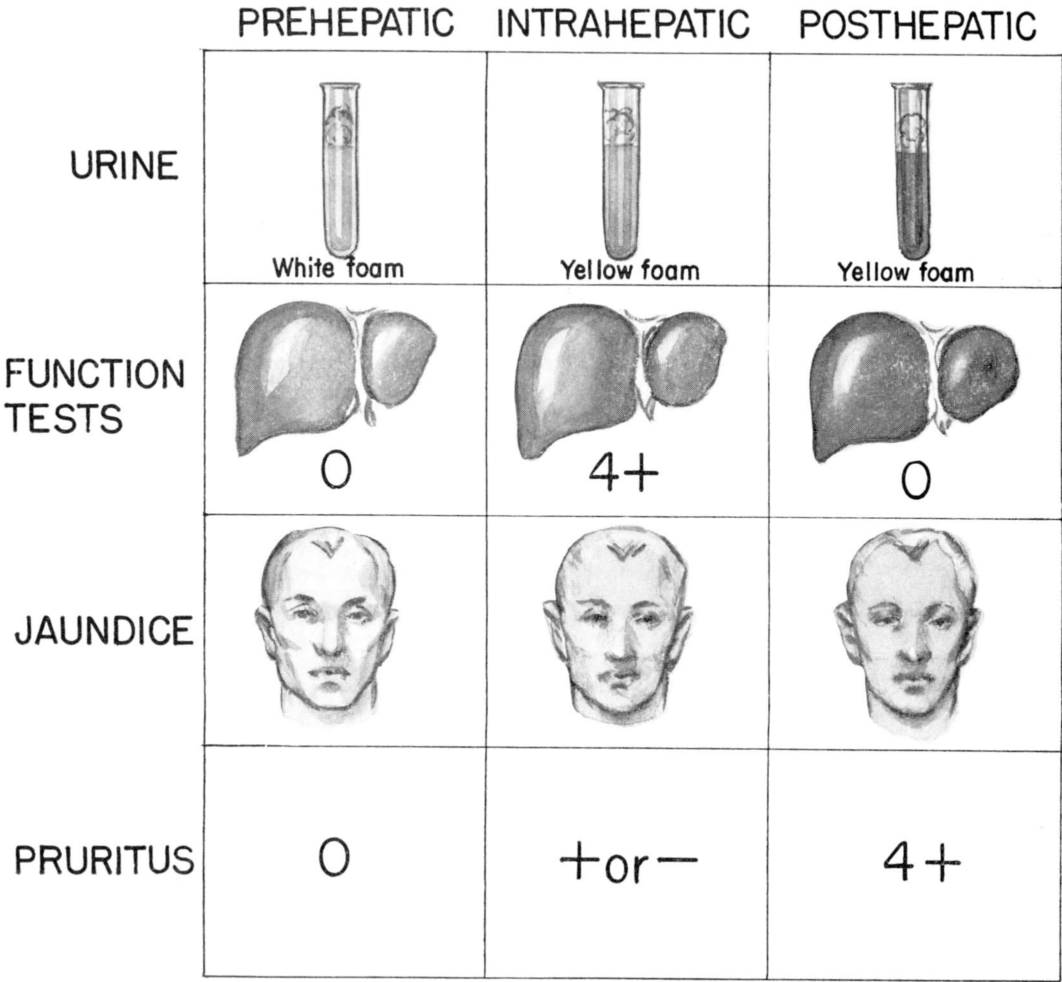

FIG. 230. Diagrammatic presentation of the differential diagnosis of the 3 types of jaundice. As a rule, the degree of jaundice is mild in the prehepatic type, moderate in the intrahepatic type, and marked in the posthepatic type. The latter 2 types may overlap.

urine in a test tube; it is light, and the urinary foam is white. The liver function tests (p. 192) are negative, since there is no damage to the liver. This is a light type of jaundice and may be overlooked. In summary, then, it may be stated that a patient with a prehepatic jaundice presents a light type of icterus, a light urine with a white foam, and negative liver function tests (Fig. 230).

INTRAHEPATIC JAUNDICE (FIG. 231)

In this type of jaundice, the lesion is *in* the liver; this also has been referred to as parenchymatous jaundice. It must be assumed that the entire liver has not collapsed if the patient is still alive; the amount of damage in given cases varies. Many toxins and/or organisms can injure this organ and interfere with one or more of its many functions; hence the liver function tests should indicate such damage (p. 192).

Liver function tests are legion. Various authors have their favorite battery of tests. The clinician should take a *few* of these in which he has most faith and let this constitute the "liver profile." The following table has been helpful in the differentiation of intrahepatic and posthepatic jaundice.

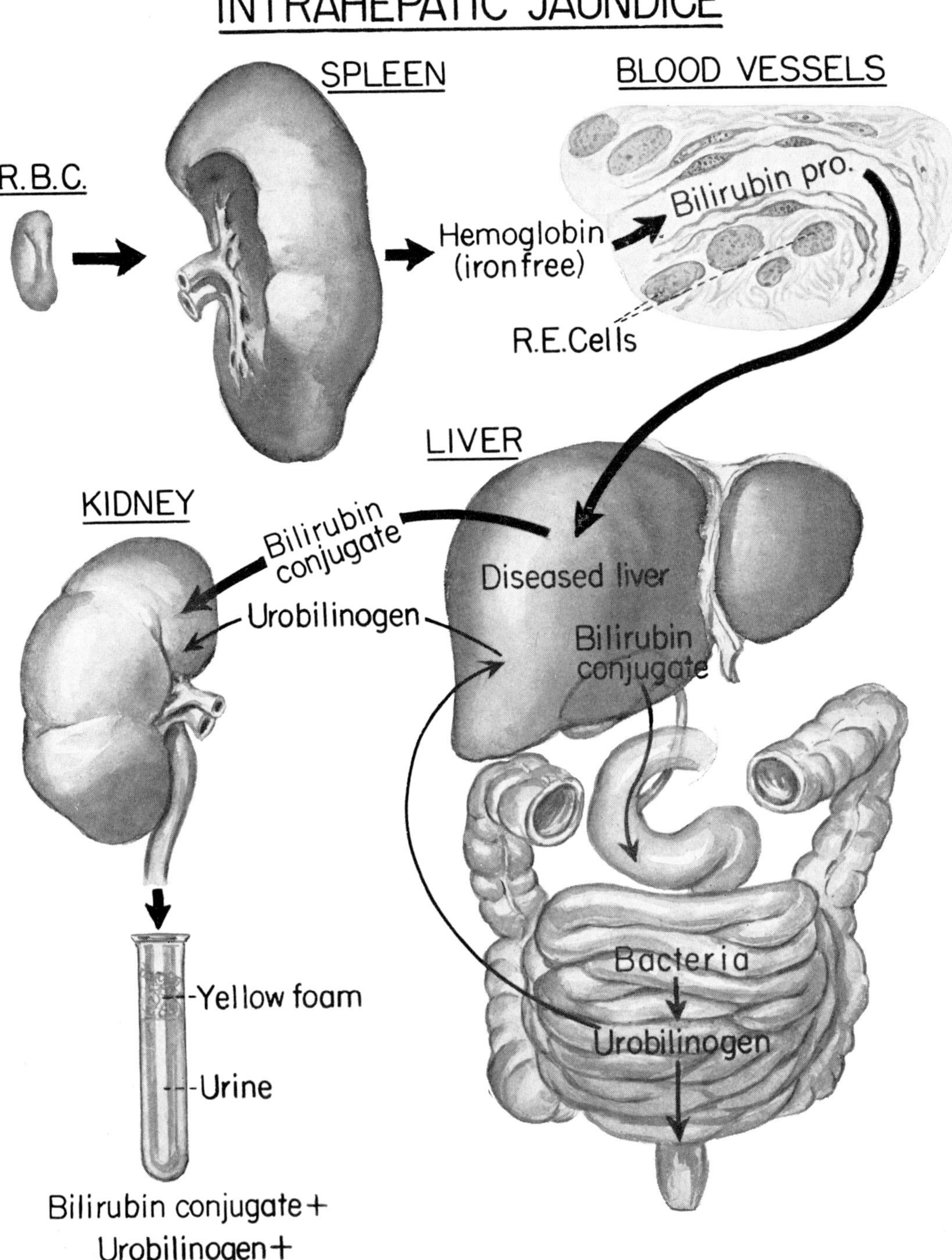

FIG. 231. Intrahepatic jaundice. In this instance the lesion is in the liver. The heavy arrows indicate excess and the light arrows indicate overflow of the pigments. Note that the urine contains both bilirubin and urobilinogen.

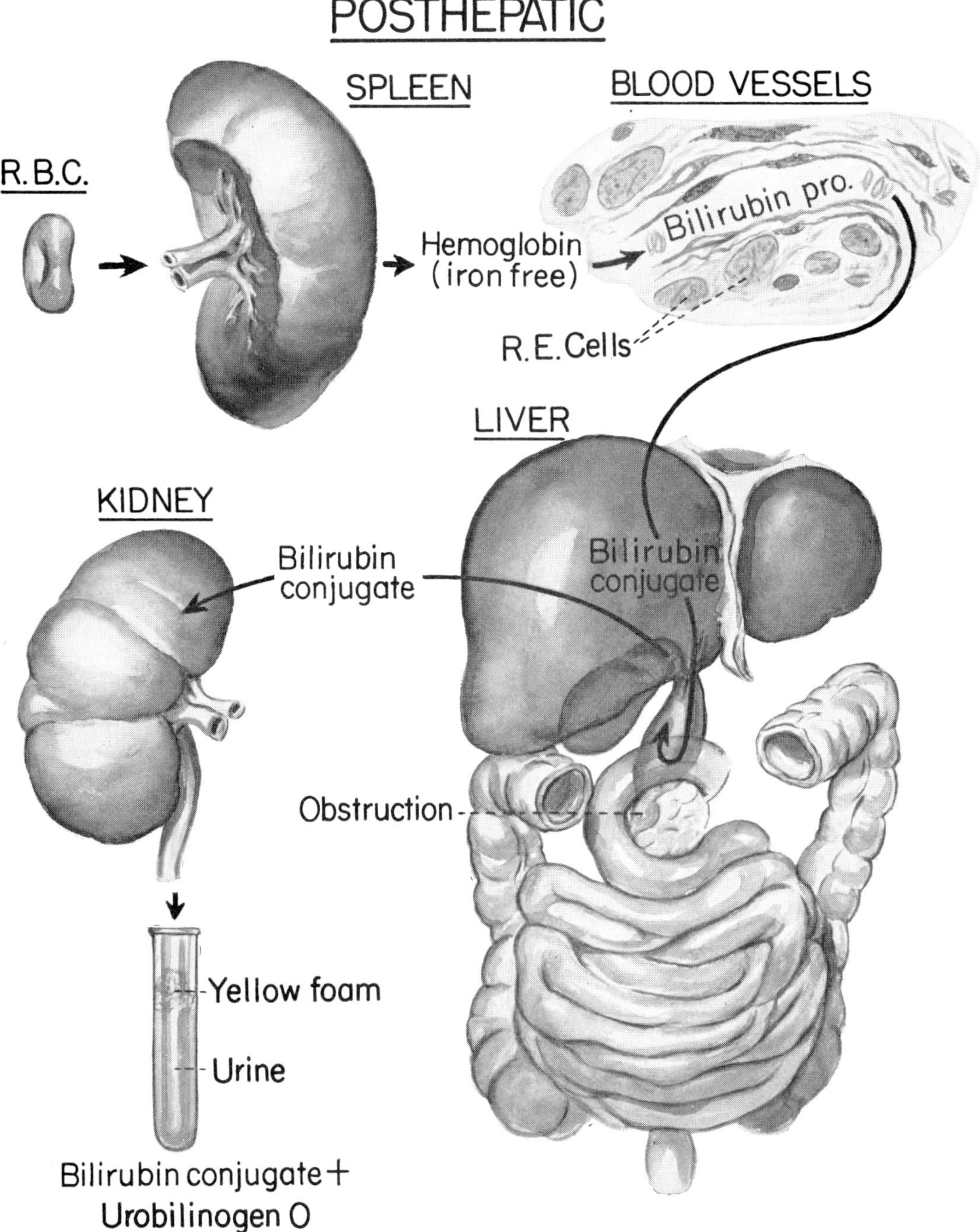

FIG. 232. Posthepatic jaundice. The lesion is usually in the common duct, the ampulla of Vater or the head of the pancreas. The urine contains bilirubin but no urobilinogen.

TABLE 6. DIFFERENTIATION OF INTRAHEPATIC AND POSTHEPATIC JAUNDICE

TESTS	INTRA-HEPATIC JAUNDICE (Liver Cell Damage)	POST-HEPATIC JAUNDICE
Transaminase (SGOT)	High	Normal
Thymol turbidity	High	Normal
Cephalin flocculation	High	Normal
Alkaline phosphatase	Normal	Very high
Cholesterol	Low	High
Serum albumin	Low	Normal
Urinary urobilinogen	High	Low

If the results of the liver tests are equivocal, utilization of the following procedure has been suggested: administration of 40 to 60 mg. of prednisone daily for 4 to 6 days. If the serum bilirubin decreases 50 per cent or more during this time, then intrahepatic jaundice (liver cell damage) is most likely. No tests are infallible, and none is pathognomonic; tests merely suggest the location of the lesion.

In summary, then, one can state that in intrahepatic jaundice, the skin discoloration is deeper, the urine is dark, and its foam is yellow (bilirubin); the liver function tests are positive (Fig. 230).

POSTHEPATIC JAUNDICE (FIG. 232)

In this type, the lesion is distal to the liver (as bile flows). This has also been referred to as obstructive jaundice. Examples should include: stones in the common and the hepatic bile ducts, tumors of the common and the hepatic ducts, tumors of the head of the pancreas, and metastases to the porta hepatis.

In such cases the icterus is much deeper, varying from brown to bronze or even black-yellow. The obstruction to the flow of bile can be either partial or complete. Stones may have a ball-valve action, and tumors may ulcerate; hence, the degree of jaundice may vary from time to time. If the obstruction *is complete*, no bilirubin will enter the duodenum, and no urobilinogen will be formed; the aldehyde test will be negative. If the obstruction is *incomplete*, that bilirubin which enters the duodenum is converted to urobilinogen, which is returned to the liver and converted back to bilirubin as long as the

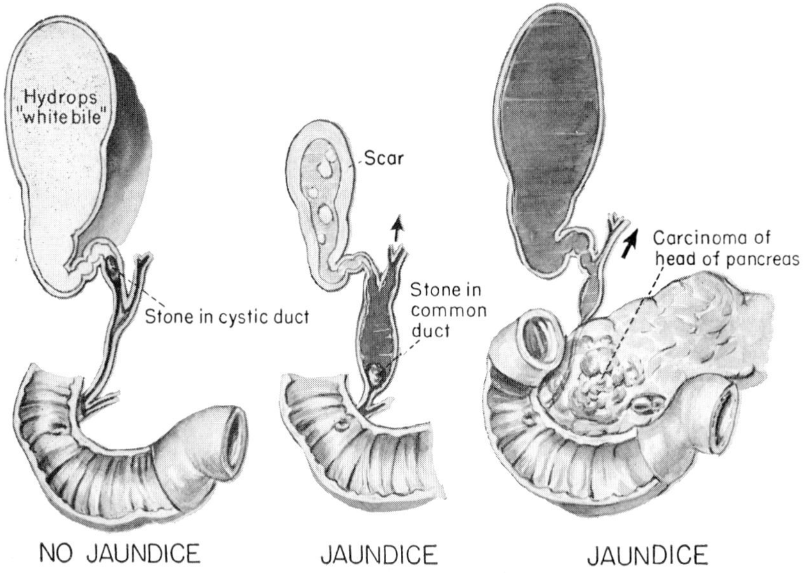

FIG. 233. Courvoisier's law. When a stone is in the cystic duct, the gallbladder is distended and large, but no jaundice is present; when a stone is in the common duct, the scarred gallbladder is shrunken and small, and jaundice is present; with a carcinoma of the head of the pancreas, the gallbladder is distended, and jaundice is present.

FIG. 234. Carcinoma of the common hepatic duct. This is suspected when jaundice is present, plus a small empty noncicatrized gallbladder.

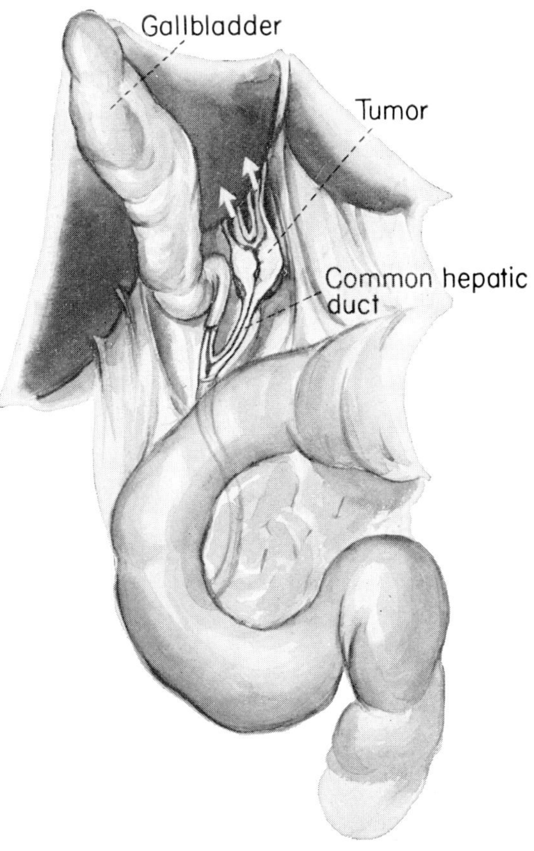

liver is normal. Those patients who have been jaundiced by an obstructing lesion for 4 to 6 weeks develop a biliary cirrhosis. These patients originally have a posthepatic jaundice but later develop the intrahepatic type, and the liver function tests become positive. This should not cause confusion if a careful history is elicited.

In summary, one can state that in posthepatic jaundice the jaundice is deep in color, the urine is very dark (Coca-Cola), the urinary foam is yellow (bilirubin), and the liver function tests are negative (Fig. 230).

DIAGNOSIS

Courvoisier's law (Fig. 233) states that in the presence of a large gallbladder unassociated with jaundice, a cystic duct obstruction must be suspected (mucocele or hydrops of the gallbladder); a small gallbladder in the presence of jaundice usually indicates a stone in the common bile duct; and a large gallbladder in the presence of jaundice indicates

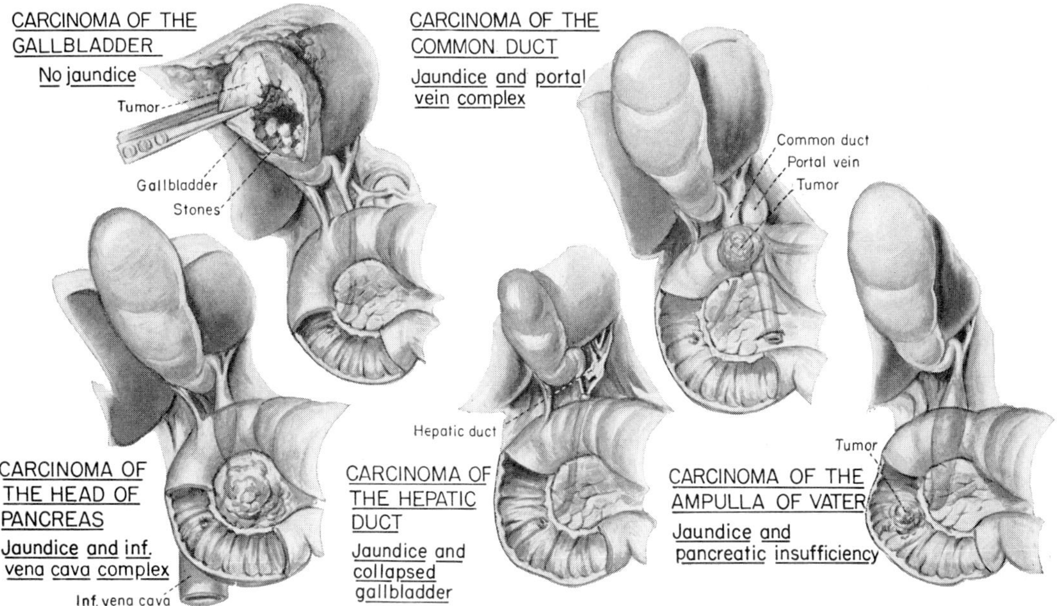

FIG. 235. The differential diagnosis of carcinomas involving the biliary tract. The 5 outstanding conditions are included in this illustration.

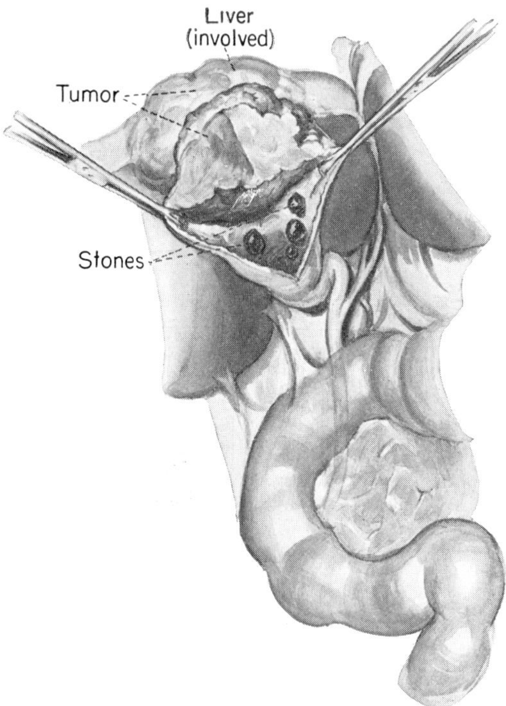

FIG. 236. Carcinoma of the gallbladder usually involves the fundus and is almost always associated with gallstones. Jaundice is absent unless metastases cause obstruction to the outflow of bile.

a malignancy (head of the pancreas or common duct). To this must be added the possibility of a carcinoma of the common hepatic duct with complete obstruction (Fig. 234). In the latter instance jaundice is present, but since no bile reaches the gallbladder, this organ is small, shrunken and practically empty except for some mucoid material.

When the cystic duct is obstructed, bile cannot enter the gallbladder, nor can the mucoid material which originates in the gallbladder escape. For this reason "white bile" is present. The word "bile" is in quotes, because the contained material is truly not bile; the bile pigment which was entrapped in the gallbladder is gradually absorbed. Stones in the common bile duct produce repeated bouts of cholecystitis which result in scar tissue formation; as a result of this the gallbladder is shrunken, thick and small. The gallbladder is large in the presence of a carcinoma of the head of the pancreas or the common duct, because the organ is not inflamed and retains its elasticity; the bile that cannot enter the duodenum is forced up into this noncicatrized organ.

The differential diagnosis of carcinomas involving the biliary tract should include (Fig. 235):

1. Carcinoma of the gallbladder
2. Carcinoma of the common bile duct
3. Carcinoma of the head of the pancreas
4. Carcinoma of the ampulla of Vater
5. Carcinoma of the common hepatic duct

In *carcinoma of the gallbladder* jaundice is not present at the onset, because the mass usually is located in the region of the fundus and does not interrupt the flow of bile (Fig. 236). It is rare to find a carcinoma of the gallbladder that does not contain gallstones. The malignant mass is characteristic in that it is located in the right upper quadrant, is hard, moves with respirations and is *nodular*. The nodularity differentiates it from a hydrops of the gallbladder. Metastases to the porta hepatis may produce jaundice, but this appears late.

Carcinoma of the common duct should be suspected when jaundice is associated with a portal vein complex (Fig. 237). By portal vein complex is meant the clinical picture of portal hypertension; this results from extension of the malignant growth to the portal vein. One recalls the close anatomic relations of the portal vein and the common bile duct. Portal hypertension produces ascites, splenomegaly and dilated veins (esophageal varices, hemorrhoids). An accurate history will reveal that the jaundice preceded the portal hypertension picture, whereas in cirrhosis of the liver the jaundice appears late and is mild.

Carcinoma of the head of the pancreas has been discussed with Courvoisier's law (Fig. 233). To this can be added the fact that since the pancreas is retroperitoneal, a sizable mass involving it not only obstructs the common bile duct but also can attack the inferior vena cava (Fig. 235). An inferior vena cava complex is characterized by dependent pitting edema of the inferior extremities which is associated with dilated superficial veins. Since this is unassociated with dyspnea or orthopnea, a cardiac dependent edema should not cause confusion.

Carcinoma of the ampulla of Vater is suspected when jaundice is associated with pancreatic insufficiency (Fig. 238). The latter results from an absence of pancreatic enzymes in the intestinal tract. This can be detected if the patient is fed meat, and the stool is examined 24 hours later; it will be noticed that striated undigested meat fibers are present.

Carcinoma of the common hepatic duct, as stated, must be considered when a jaundice is present, and the gallbladder is small and empty.

The differentiation between a stone in the common duct and a carcinoma of the biliary tract usually can be made preoperatively. It is true that in most instances painful jaundice is associated with a stone, whereas the less painful progressive jaundice suggests a tumor. However, approximately 20 per cent of patients with stones in the common bile duct are not jaundiced. This is due to a ball-valve action of the stones. A tumor usually produces complete biliary obstruction, but such tumors may ulcerate and permit some bile to slip through. This would produce a fluctuating type of jaundice and suggest a stone. The author has found it helpful to check the serum bilirubin or icterus index for 5 consecutive days (Fig. 239). If the readings continually rise or do not fluctuate, this suggests a neoplasm; whereas if there is fluctuation, a stone is more probable. Exploratory surgery may be necessary to arrive at a final diagnosis.

Pruritus is a most helpful symptom in the

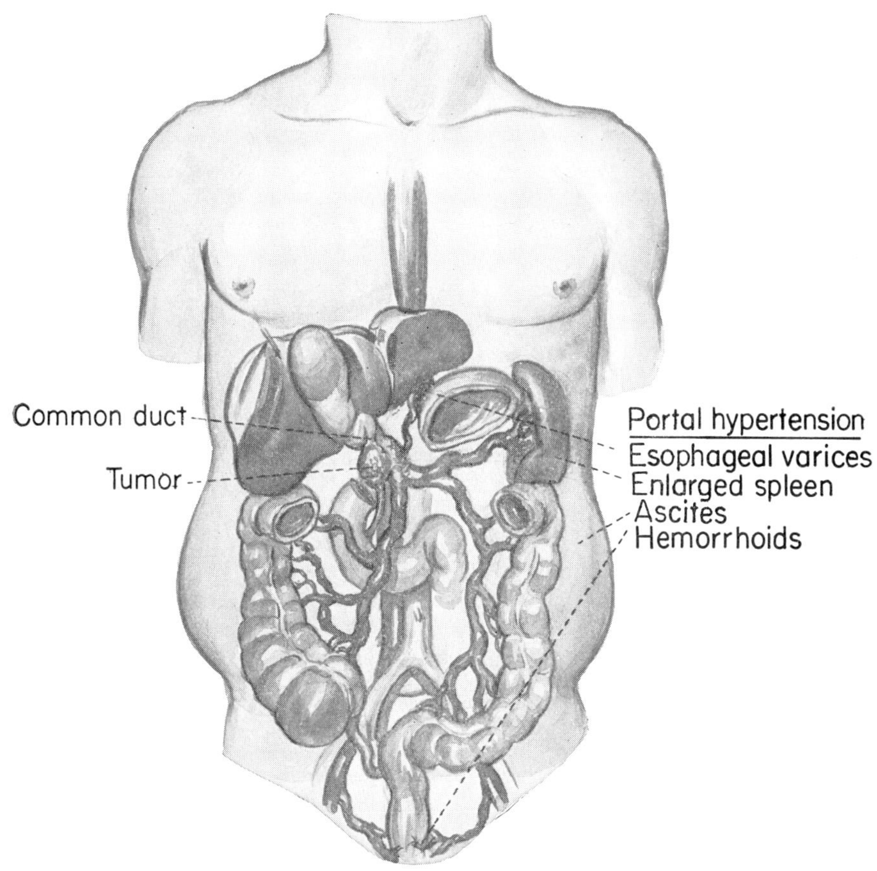

FIG. 237. Carcinoma of the common bile duct is characterized by a jaundice and portal vein complex. The latter produces the signs and symptoms of portal hypertension.

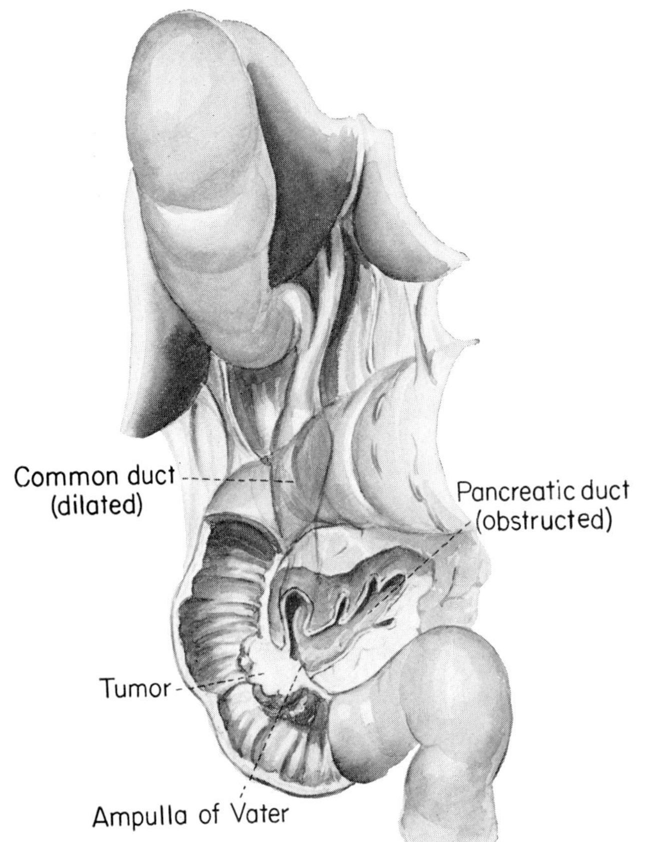

Fig. 238. Carcinoma of the ampulla of Vater produces jaundice and a pancreatic insufficiency.

Fig. 239. A stone in the common duct or carcinoma? If jaundice is due to a stone in the common duct, the gallbladder is small and thick, and the serum bilirubin (icterus index) can fluctuate from day to day. If the jaundice is due to a carcinoma involving the common duct, the pancreas, or the ampulla of Vater, the gallbladder is large, and the serum bilirubin remains high or increases.

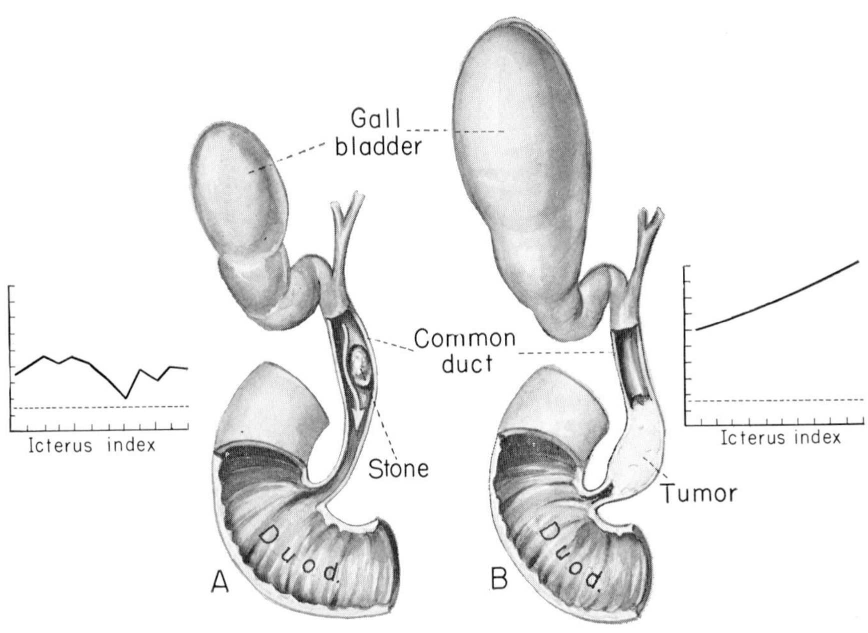

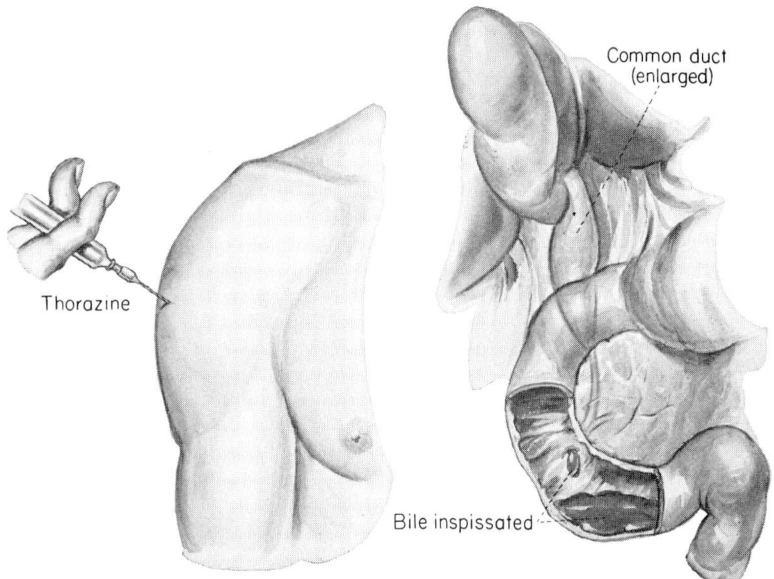

FIG. 240. Jaundice due to Thorazine (chlorpromazine). This is a nonsurgical type of jaundice, and the icterus disappears when the therapy is discontinued.

differential diagnosis. Pruritus is not a symptom of jaundice but is a symptom of posthepatic (obstructive) jaundice, particularly if it is the patient's *primary* complaint. The author never has heard of a case of prehepatic jaundice in which pruritus was present; occasionally, parenchymatous (intrahepatic) jaundice may be associated with mild pruritus, but when the outstanding complaint is pruritus, this is pathognomonic of a posthepatic or obstructive jaundice.

The *pulse* is usually slow in cases of icterus. Bradycardia is a welcome finding, since a tachycardia in the presence of jaundice forebodes liver collapse.

Recently, cases of jaundice have been reported following the use of Thorazine (chlorpromazine) (Fig. 240). The exact mechanism is unknown; hence, it is difficult to classify at this time. It seems it is associated with some dilatation of the common duct and inspissated bile. These are nonsurgical cases, and apparently these patients recover when the medicament is discontinued. Drug-induced jaundice does not always mean chlorpromazine jaundice. Some authorities prefer to classify these drug jaundices as those which mimic viral hepatitis, those which resemble obstructive jaundice and those which produce a mixed type. The agents which produce a jaundice that mimics viral hepatitis belong to the iproniazid group. This is a serious type of jaundice having a mortality rate as high as 15 to 20 per cent. The antiepileptic drugs can produce a similar type of liver damage. An example of a drug producing a "mixed" jaundice is PAS.

8

Pancreas

GENERAL CONSIDERATIONS AND PHYSIOLOGY

The pancreas is one of the smallest and most deeply placed organs in the abdominal cavity. It lies transversely in the epigastrium, crossing the bodies of the 12th thoracic and 1st lumbar vertebrae. It extends from the curve of the 1st part of the duodenum, to which it is firmly attached, to the hilum of the spleen.

Physiologically, the pancreas plays a double role: endocrine (carbohydrate metabolism) and secretory (digestive) (Fig. 241).

The endocrine function is concerned with the production of insulin, which is formed in the islets of Langerhans. Deficiency or absence of this internal secretion produces diabetes mellitus. The islets are diagnostically and surgically important because of the occurrence of adenomas which produce hypoglycemic syndromes (p. 234).

The external secretion is produced by the alveolar tissue. This reaches the duodenum via the ductal system of the pancreas. From 1,500 to 2,000 ml. is secreted in 24 hours. The main enzymes are trypsin, amylase and lipase. Deficiency of the external pancreatic secretion produces a typical *pancreatic triad.* This consists of:

1. Steatorrhea (bulky, gray, frothy stools due to excess fat)
2. Creatorrhea (excess of protein and undigested meat fibers in the stool)
3. Diarrhea (due to imperfect digestion and excessive fermentation)

Pancreatic pain is aggravated when the patient is on his back but is relieved when he is in a sitting position. This applies to both acute and chronic pancreatic conditions (Fig. 242). The importance of pain relief by assuming attitudes of body flexion will be discussed more thoroughly under pancreatic carcinoma (p. 236).

Tenderness may be situated anywhere along the involved viscus. For this reason one cannot exactly pinpoint pancreatic tenderness, but when present it is located supra-umbilically (Fig. 243).

CONGENITAL ABNORMALITIES

Pancreatic Heterotopia

Aberrant pancreatic tissue which has no connection with the main mass of pancreatic gland may occur at any site along the gastrointestinal tract. The most common location, however, is around the pyloric end of the stomach and the duodenum. The presence of such tissue has been recorded also in the jejunum and in Meckel's diverticulum. Usually, ectopic pancreatic tissue causes no symptoms, but those that occur in the region of the stomach or the duodenum may produce pain, hemorrhage, or obstruction and inflammatory changes. When it occurs in the small intestines, particularly in a Meckel's diverticulum, it may act as a spearhead for an intussusception. These are usually confused with tumors, polyps and ulceration. If found during abdominal explorations, they should be excised.

Annular Pancreas

This rare anomaly results from faulty embryologic development. An annular pancreas completely encircles the 2nd part of the duodenum at the level of the major duodenal papilla (Fig. 244). The symptomatology depends on the presence and the degree of duodenal obstruction. This is characterized by colicky abdominal pain, nausea and vomiting as seen with upper gastrointestinal obstruction. If the degree of obstruction is minimal, the symptoms may be delayed until adult life. Peptic ulceration of the first part of the duodenum may be a concomitant finding. Roentgenograms reveal a smooth narrowing of the 2nd portion of the duodenum. Duodenojejunostomy or gastrojejunostomy are curative.

ACUTE PANCREATITIS

Types

This condition has been divided into acute edematous and acute hemorrhagic pancreatitis. Recently, however, it has been divided into gallstone and alcoholic pancreatitis. Either of these may appear as acute edematous or hemorrhagic forms.

Gallstone pancreatitis is characterized by its benign long-term behavior associated with acute relapses which continue until the biliary disease is eradicated. It rarely leads to a replacement of the pancreas by fibrous tissue. Definitive gallbladder and/or common duct surgery cures this type.

Alcoholic pancreatitis leads to pancreatic cirrhosis and gradual destruction of the

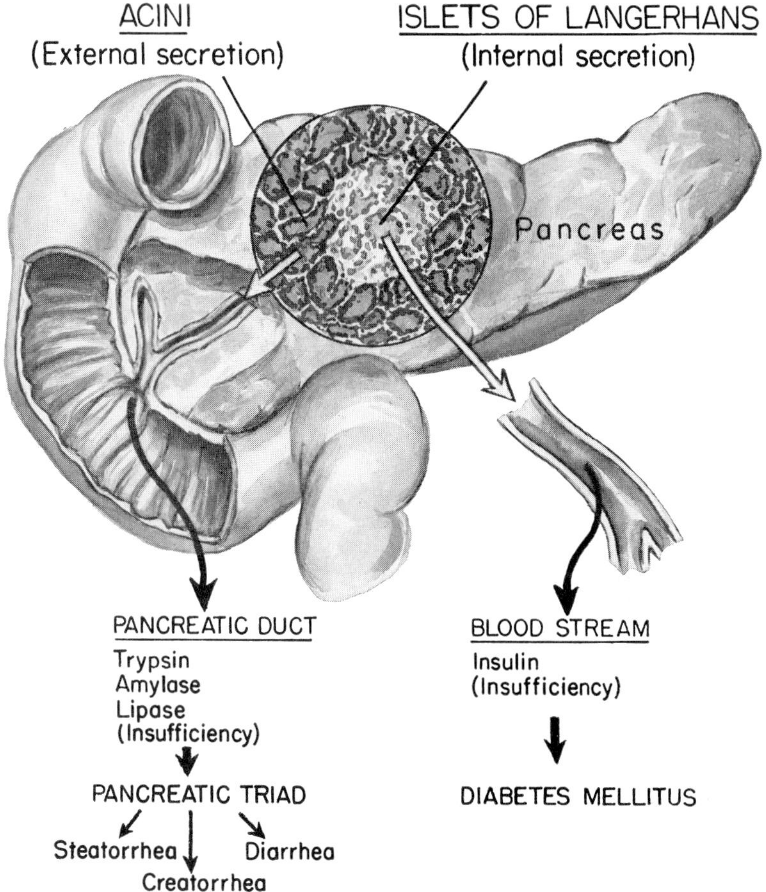

Fig. 241. Physiology of the pancreas. Its internal secretion produces insulin; its external secretion produces digestive enzymes (trypsin, amylase and lipase). Whereas it was formerly believed that the islet cells had only one function, namely, the elaboration of insulin, now it is believed that they also elaborate a gastriclike substance which stimulates gastric secretion and glucagon.

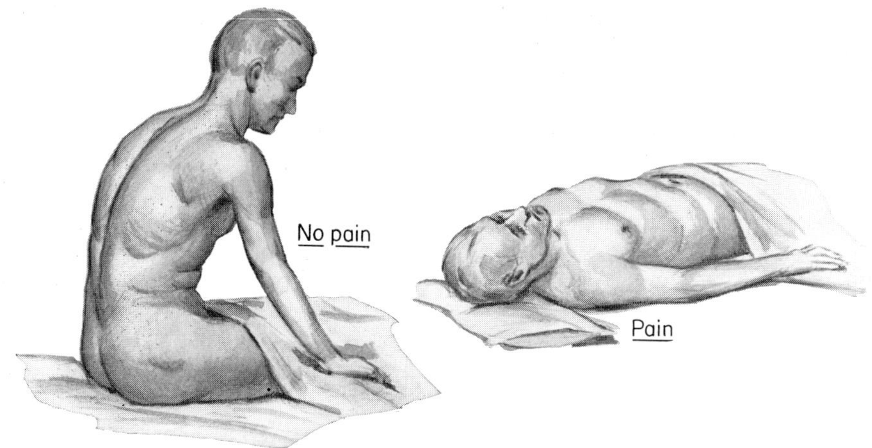

FIG. 242. Pain of pancreatic origin is aggravated by the supine position but is relieved by sitting or the prone position.

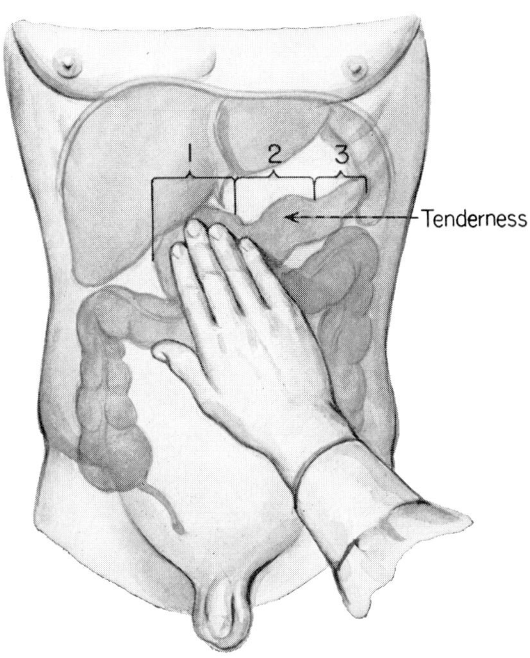

FIG. 243. Pancreatic tenderness is located supra-umbilically.

organ. Exocrine insufficiency (steatorrhea), endocrine insufficiency (diabetes), pancreatic calcification and pseudocysts are the usual sequelae. Alcoholic pancreatitis becomes a serious crippling and disabling condition in contradistinction to the benign course of gallstone pancreatitis. Pancreatic calcification is supposedly diagnostic of alcoholism. It is important to diagnose acute pancreatitis per se whenever possible, since the modern trend toward conservative management lowers both the morbidity and the mortality.

Some patients develop acute pancreatitis following surgery; this has been referred to as *postoperative pancreatitis.* It occurs mainly in upper abdominal surgery, especially gastric and biliary procedures. Diagnosis in the immediate postoperative period is difficult but should be suspected when there is severe abdominal pain and findings of high concentrations of serum pancreatic enzymes.

ETIOLOGY

The etiology may be related to biliary tract disease and the possible presence of a com-

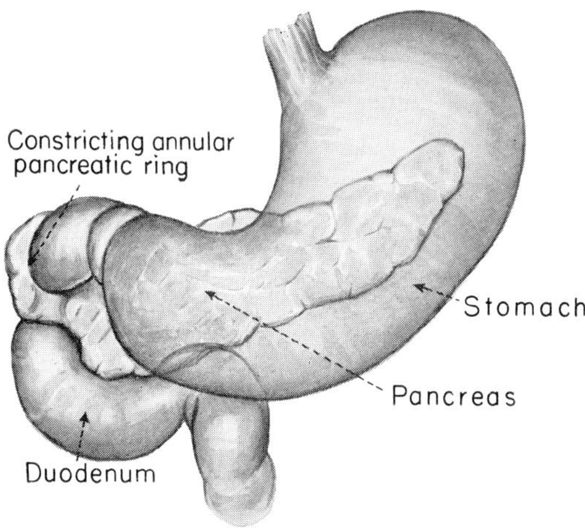

FIG. 244. Annular pancreas.

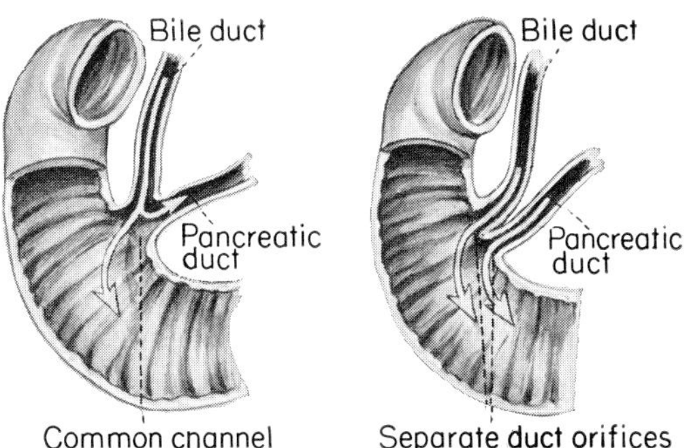

FIG. 245. Some individuals have a common channel for both the common bile and the pancreatic ducts. Such people supposedly are predisposed to pancreatitis, because bile may regurgitate up into the pancreas.

mon channel which exists between the terminal bile and the pancreatic ducts (Fig. 245). Fitz, in 1889, gave an accurate description of the condition; Opie, in 1901, described a case of pancreatitis produced by a stone lodged in the ampulla of Vater; he proposed the "common channel" theory whereby bile regurgitates into the pancreas via the pancreatic duct. It is presupposed that bile salts activate pancreatic ferments, which in turn digest the surrounding tissues. This results in edema, necrosis and hemorrhage.

Other factors have been associated with the etiology, namely, trauma producing interstitial hemorrhage, bacteria, and ingestion of food and alcohol. The author has devised a mnemonic aid showing that the causes of pancreatitis may be associated with the letter "B": *B*acteria, *Bl*ood, *B*ile, *B*ody Juices and *B*ooze (Fig. 246).

SYMPTOMS

Pancreatitis may affect patients of any age, but, it affects predominately those in the middle-age group. Symptoms vary, depend-

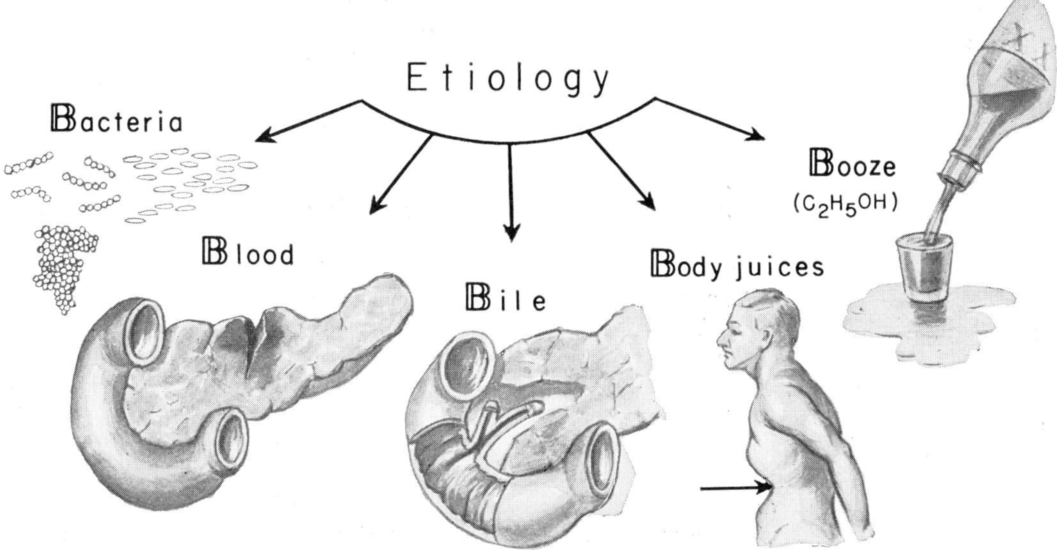

FIG. 246. The etiology of acute pancreatitis.

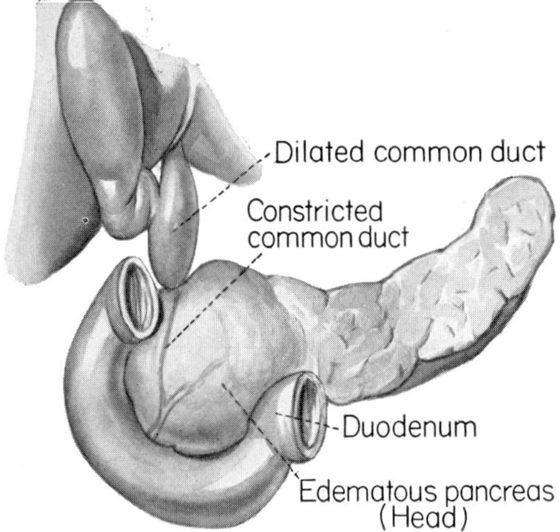

FIG. 247. An edematous head of the pancreas in severe pancreatitis may constrict the pancreatic portion of the common duct and produce jaundice.

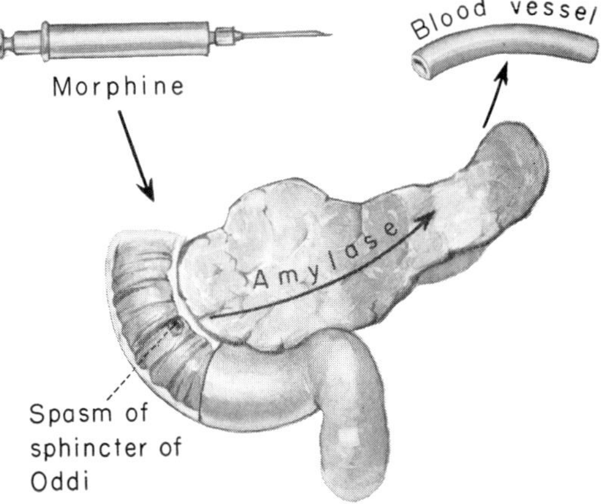

FIG. 248. The serum amylase test may be elevated by injections of morphine. This is supposed to be caused by the smooth muscle contracting effect of morphine on the sphincter of Oddi with resulting regurgitation of amylase into the blood stream.

ing on the extent of the disease; with pancreatic edema the symptoms are mild and vague, whereas in pancreatic necrosis they are violent. The *onset* is sudden and frequently follows the ingestion of a heavy meal and/or alcoholic beverages.

Pain originates in the epigastrium and is constant. It increases to an agonizing severity and is rarely relieved by a single injection of morphine. It tends to radiate through to the back at a level which corresponds to the anterior location of the organ; at times it radiates to the left loin. These patients are relieved in a sitting position and are more distressed when lying on their backs (Fig. 262).

Nausea and vomiting appear shortly after the onset of pain. Rarely does vomiting produce relief.

Physical examination reveals an appearance which leaves no doubt as to the severity of the illness. Whereas *shock* is absent in interstitial (edematous) pancreatitis, it occurs in almost every case of the necrotizing type. There is a striking contrast between the severity of the illness and the paucity of physical findings. The *pulse* is weak and at times increased. The *temperature* is normal in early cases. *Tenderness* is almost always present and is located supra-umbilically. As the disease progresses, *abdominal distention* appears, and the *peristaltic sounds become diminished.* Muscle spasm and rigidity are infrequent. *Jaundice* is present in about 25 per cent of the cases and is due to obstruction of the common duct by edema of the head of the pancreas (Fig. 247); gallstones at the ampulla, or associated hepatitis also may produce jaundice. Cullen's sign (discoloration of the peri-umbilical area) and Grey-Turner's sign (discoloration in the flanks) are supposedly due to extravasation of blood into the retroperitoneal space. These are extremely rare, although it is recorded that they are present in 10 per cent of the cases.

LABORATORY DATA

Leukocytosis usually is present to a moderate degree; however, this is nonspecific. Hemoconcentration as characterized by a high hematocrit and hemoglobin values occur early in the course of the disease.

The *serum amylase* content is almost always elevated early in the course of the disease. A simple laboratory test devised by Somogyi is based on the amylolytic action of blood serum on starch: 180 Somogyi units are considered to be an upper limit of normal, and any figure over 200 is considered to be abnormal. If the disease subsides, or if the necrosis is so severe that no more ferments are produced, the serum amylase drops abruptly. For these reasons the determination must be made, preferably within the first 48 to 72 hours. Morphine also will give an elevated serum amylase test. (Fig. 248). It must be remembered, too, that other conditions, such as peritonitis, pneumonia and perforated ulcers, also may cause an elevated serum amylase test. Therefore, this test is suggestive of pancreatitis but is not pathognomonic.

The *serum lipase test* also has been utilized. This remains elevated longer than the amylase value; however, the test requires additional time and equipment. Values over 2 units per ml. are considered to be abnormal.

Serum calcium determinations also are helpful, because regional fat necrosis becomes the seat of calcification. A diversion of calcium to the pancreas is reflected in a lowering of serum calcium. The normal figures for serum calcium are 8.5 to 10.5 mg. per 100 ml. In this respect one should mention the possible association of hyperparathyroidism and pancreatitis. Cases have been reported in which pancreatitis is obscured by a paradoxically high concentration of serum calcium or low serum phosphate. There are some who support the hypothesis that the simultaneous occurrence of hyperparathyroidism and pancreatitis is due to a common etiologic factor and is not a coincidence.

Hyperglycemia and glycosuria also may be present.

The *roentgenographic findings* are not specific. A segmental ileus has been described; it appears as "a sentinel loop" of jejunum.

Differential Diagnosis

Numerous conditions producing acute abdominal pain could be included herein; however, only the more common ones will be mentioned:

1. Acute cholecystitis (p. 204)
2. Perforated peptic ulcer (p. 132)
3. Small bowel obstruction (p. 180)
4. Acute appendicitis (p. 143)
5. Mesenteric thrombosis (p. 186)
6. Gallstone ileus (p. 186)
7. Coronary occlusion (p. 80)

Complications

Acute pancreatitis should be treated conservatively; however, its complications usually require surgical therapy. The complications are cysts, abscess, pancreatic lithiasis and chronic relapsing pancreatitis (Fig. 249).

Prognosis

Patients with pancreatic edema usually recover, but the mortality of acute hemorrhagic pancreatitis still remains high. Delayed surgery or adequate conservative treatment

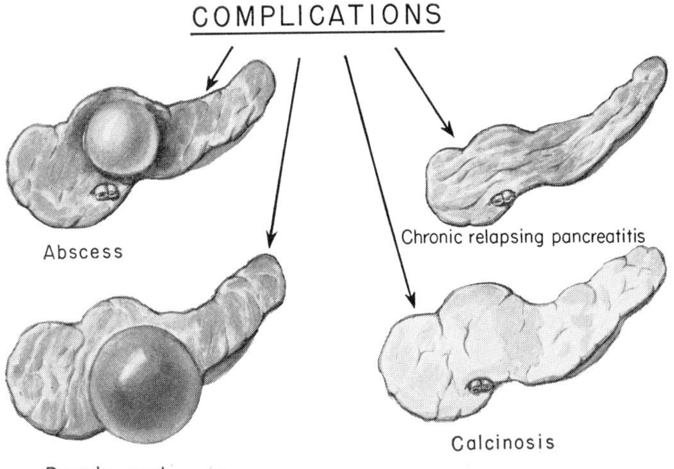

Fig. 249. The complications of acute pancreatitis.

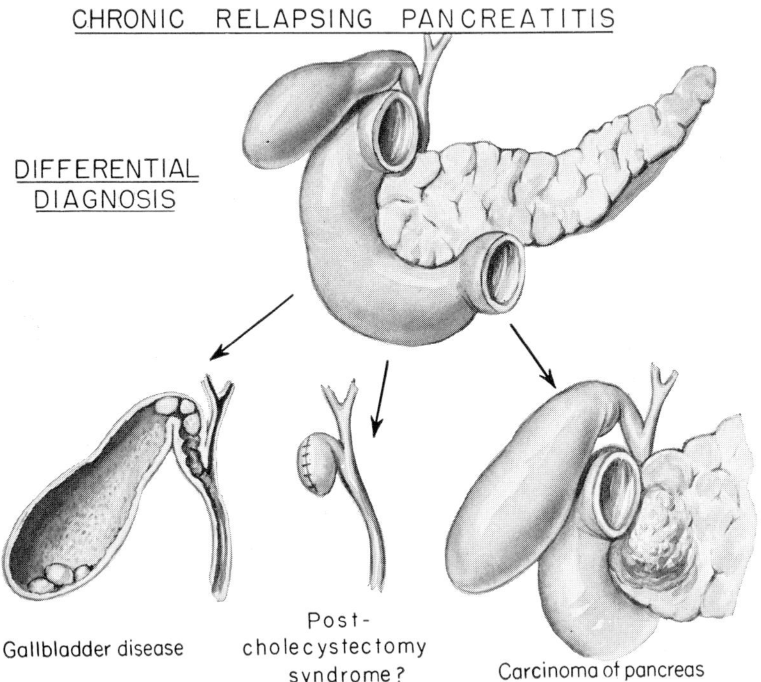

FIG. 250. The differential diagnosis of chronic relapsing pancreatitis.

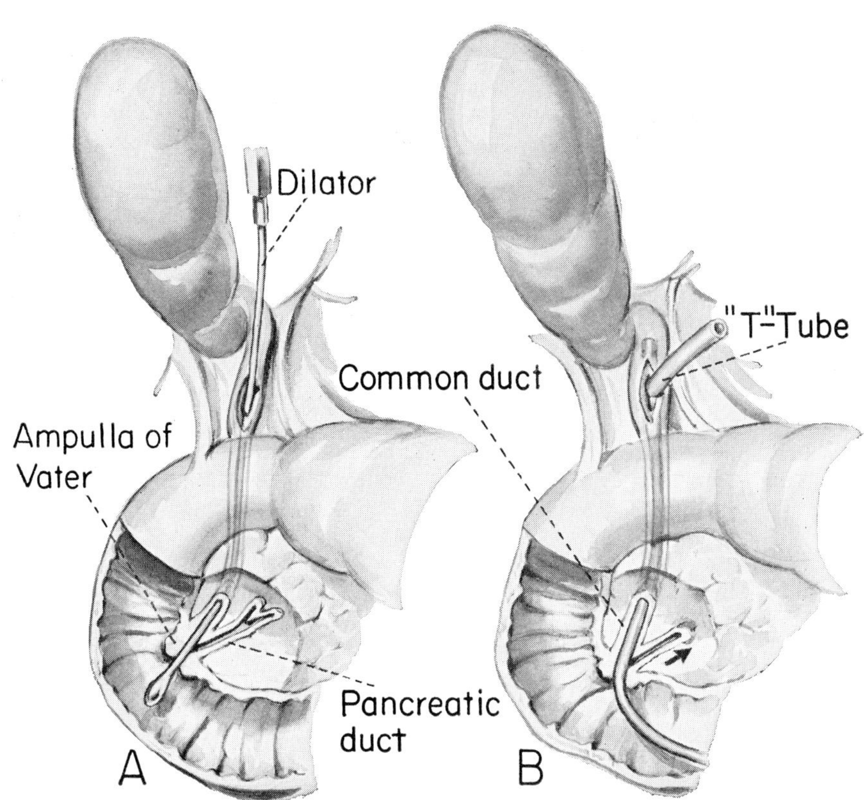

FIG. 251. Dilators may tear the tissue around the ampulla of Vater and produce edema, stasis and inflammation (pancreatitis). Constant pressure by long T-tubes can produce obstruction of the pancreatic duct with resultant inflammation of the pancreas.

has lowered the mortality in this condition from 50 to 15 per cent.

CHRONIC RELAPSING PANCREATITIS

This condition appears to represent recurrent nonlethal or noncatastrophic inflammation of the pancreas. It has assumed considerable significance as it is frequently confused with and at times impossible to differentiate from carcinoma of the pancreas, cholecystitis or so-called postcholecystectomy syndrome (Fig. 250).

Etiology

The etiology is undetermined but appears to be associated with acute pancreatitis. Alcoholism, biliary tract disease, obstruction of the pancreatic duct, all have been suspected of being contributory factors. Obstruction may be due to fibrotic scarring around the outlet of the main pancreatic duct (Wirsung) or calculus obstruction secondary to hyperparathyroidism. The lethal form of pancreatitis usually occurs with the first attack.

The use of large sounds and dilators in the common duct produces trauma to and edema

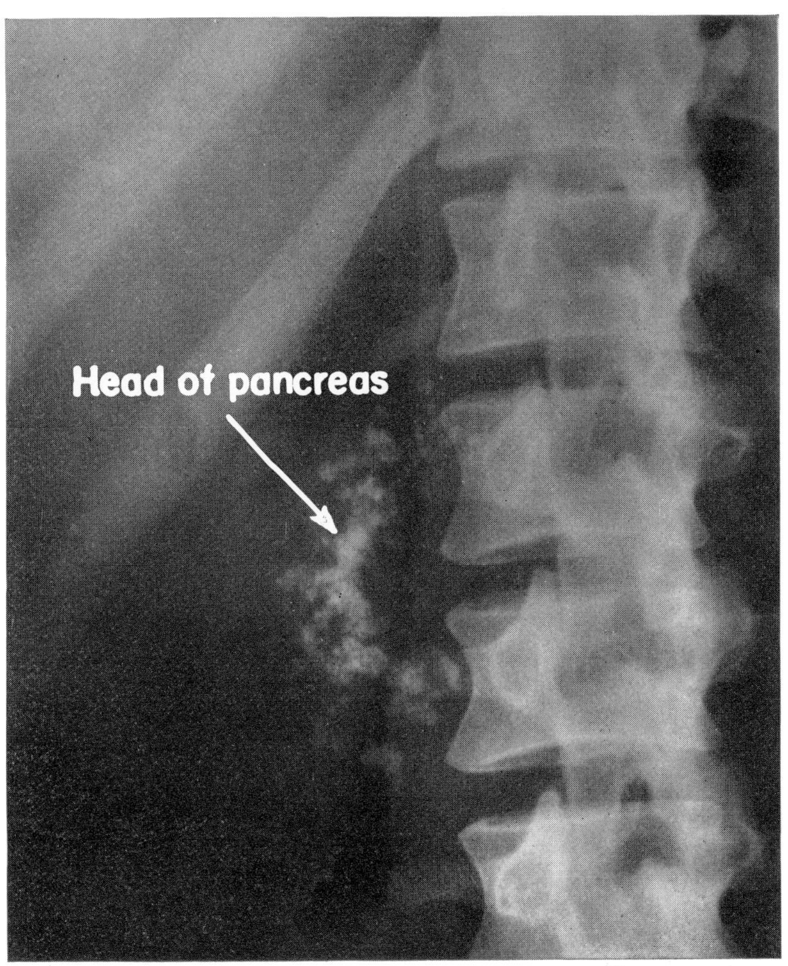

Fig. 252. Roentgenogram revealing calcium deposition in the pancreas.

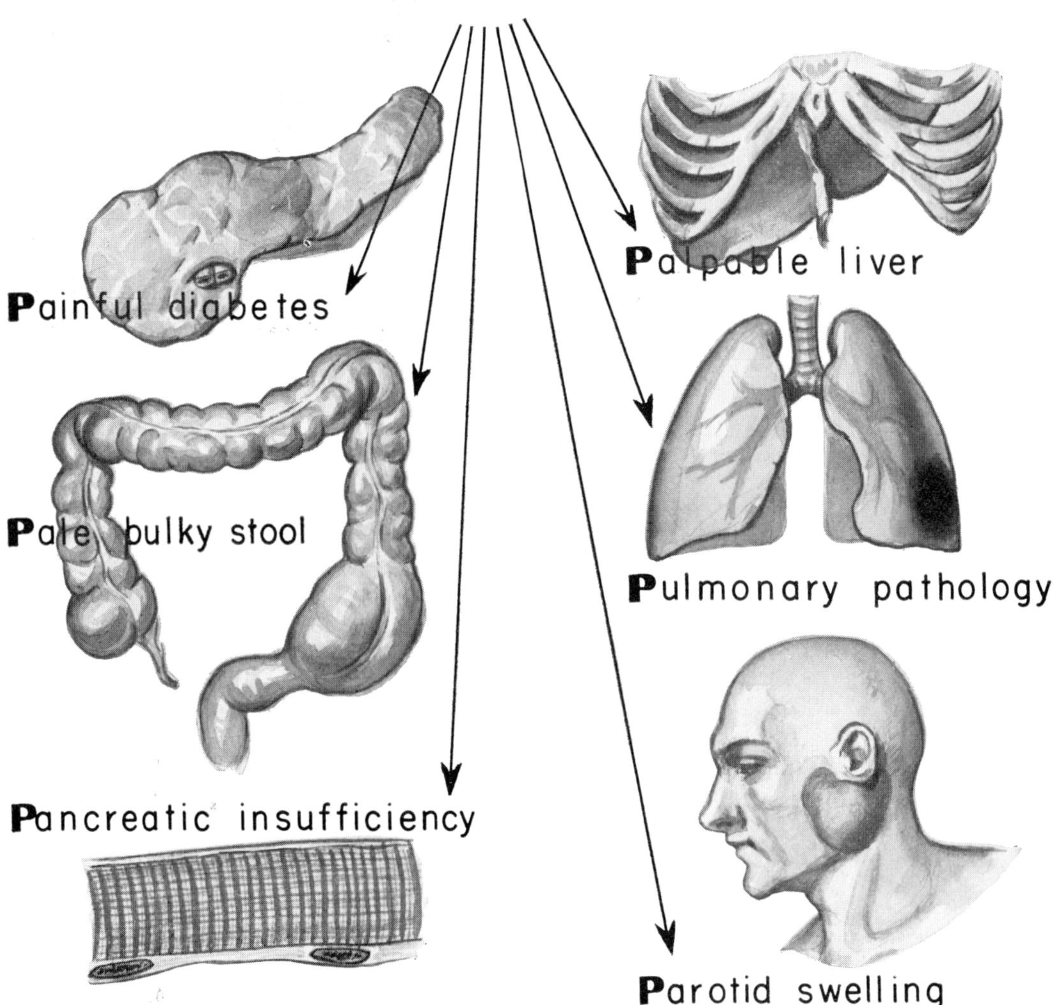

FIG. 253. Some of the signs and symptoms which should suggest chronic relapsing pancreatitis. The letter "P" has been used as a mnemonic.

at the ampulla of Vater, which in turn results in stasis. If a common pancreatobiliary channel is present, this trauma can produce stasis and inflammation in the pancreas (Fig. 251 A). The author is of the opinion that long T-tubes which pass through the common duct and into the duodenum also may produce stasis by constant pressure on or obstruction of the pancreatic duct, which, in turn, results in pancreatitis (Fig. 251 B).

SYMPTOMS

Abdominal *pain*, precipitated by the ingestion of food, is the usual symptom. Frequently it is referred to the back and is aggravated by assuming the supine position. Diarrhea is present in about half of the cases. The pain may be severe enough to require sedation. *Jaundice* may be associated with an acute attack or appear as a painless progressive icterus suggesting a malignant neoplasm. The jaundice is a result of edema of the head of the pancreas which compresses the pancreatic portion of the common duct (Fig. 247). In about one third of the cases the symptoms of diabetes are noted first. The physical examination is essentially noncontributory. At times some tenderness is noted supra-umbilically.

Laboratory Data

Early in the course of the acute phase the serum amylase may be elevated. Following the administration of secretin, a diminished pancreatic excretion can be demonstrated by analysis of the duodenal contents. Glucose tolerance alterations are demonstrable in about one third of the cases; the presence of excess fat and undigested meat fibers in the stool are also suggestive.

The flat roentgenogram may reveal calcium deposits within the parenchyma of the gland which result either from calcium depositions or pancreatic calculi (Fig. 252). No correlation exists between the roentgenographic demonstration of such calcific deposits and the severity of the clinical picture.

The letter "P" has been used as a mnemonic to recall the symptoms and the findings which should suggest this elusive condition (Fig. 253).

Chronic relapsing pancreatitis is one of the conditions which must be kept in mind constantly and included particularly in the differential diagnosis of peptic ulcer, gallbladder disease, hiatus hernia and coronary occlusion.

PANCREATIC CYSTS

Types

Cysts of the pancreas can be divided conveniently into 5 types: (1) congenital, (2) retention, (3) neoplastic, (4) infections and (5) pseudocysts.

They have been divided surgically into true cysts and pseudocysts in that the pseudocysts are not lined with epithelium, whereas the true cystic cavities are (Fig. 254).

The most important type of pancreatic cyst clinically is the *pseudocyst*. These are in reality encapsulated accumulations of fluid in and about the pancreas which occur as a result of trauma or inflammation. Frequently a forceful blow or a severe crushing injury which involves the upper abdomen is revealed in the history. The pseudocyst results from the inflammatory destruction of a part of the pancreatic parenchyma into which there is an escape of pancreatic enzymes (Fig. 255). The cystic fluid is clear or serosanguineous and contains bits of necrotic tissue.

Symptoms

Pain usually is associated with cysts that have attained considerable size. The pain is in the upper abdomen and radiates to the region of the costal arch or the back. Systemic symptoms include weight loss, fatigue, nausea, vomiting and anorexia. The cyst may be palpated more often toward the left subcostal area as a firm tense tumor in the epigastrium. Tenderness is more common in the pseudocyst than in retention or neoplastic cysts. Extrinsic pressure is exerted upon contiguous structures (Fig. 256). Many of these cysts arise in the retroperitoneal

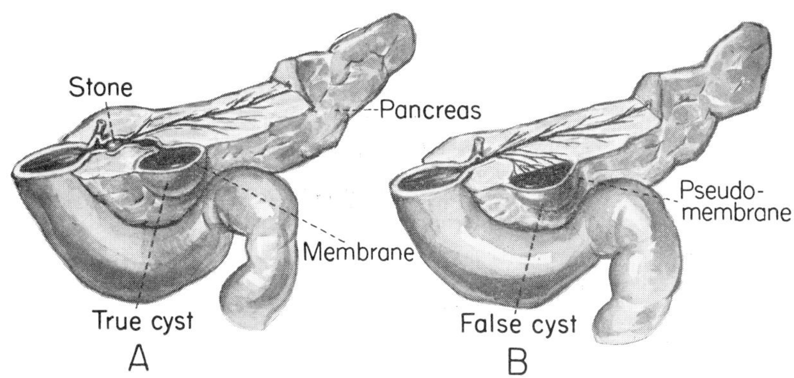

Fig. 254. Pancreatic cysts. The true cyst is rare, is associated with obstruction (retention) and has a well-defined capsule (epithelium). The pseudocyst is common, is associated with trauma or inflammation and has a false capsule (fibrous).

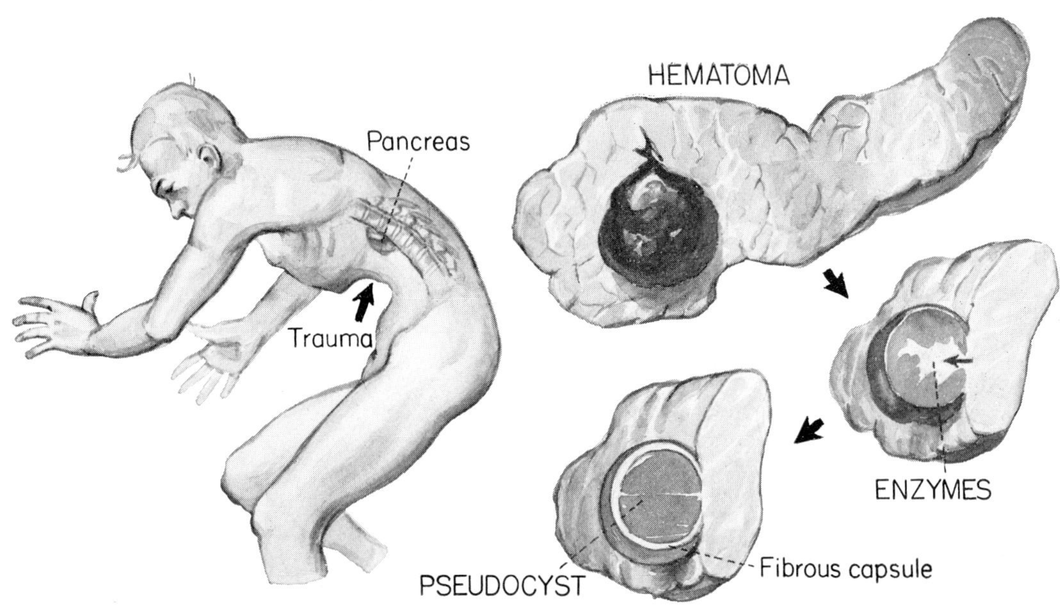

FIG. 255. The physiopathology of a pseudocyst of the pancreas.

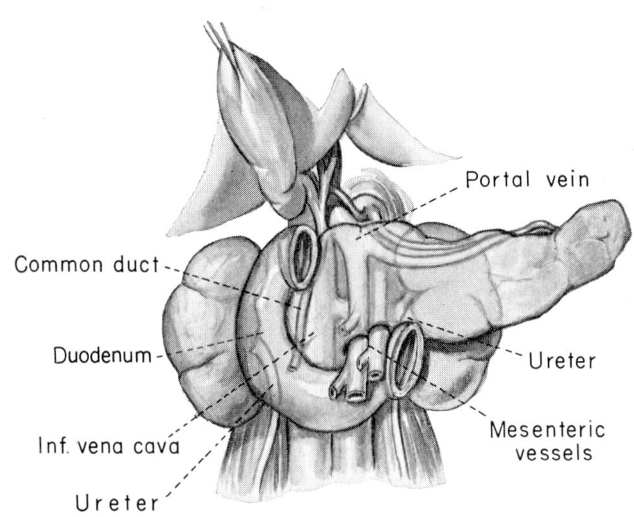

FIG. 256. Some of the structures upon which pancreatic cysts may exert pressure.

space and project forward into the lesser peritoneal cavity; others are intraperitoneal, resulting from a rupture of the pancreatic capsule. They may point through the gastrohepatic or the gastrocolic omenta or may be insinuated between the layers of the transverse mesocolon.

LABORATORY DATA

Specific laboratory tests are available. Elevated serum and urinary amylase, and fasting blood sugars occur more frequently in cysts of inflammatory or neoplastic origin. The *flat roentgenogram* of the abdomen usually reveals a spherical mass in the upper abdomen. Extrinsic pressure on the stomach, the duodenum, the small bowel and the colon may be demonstrable with routine roentgenologic study. Similar displacements may be noted by barium enema or intravenous pyelograms.

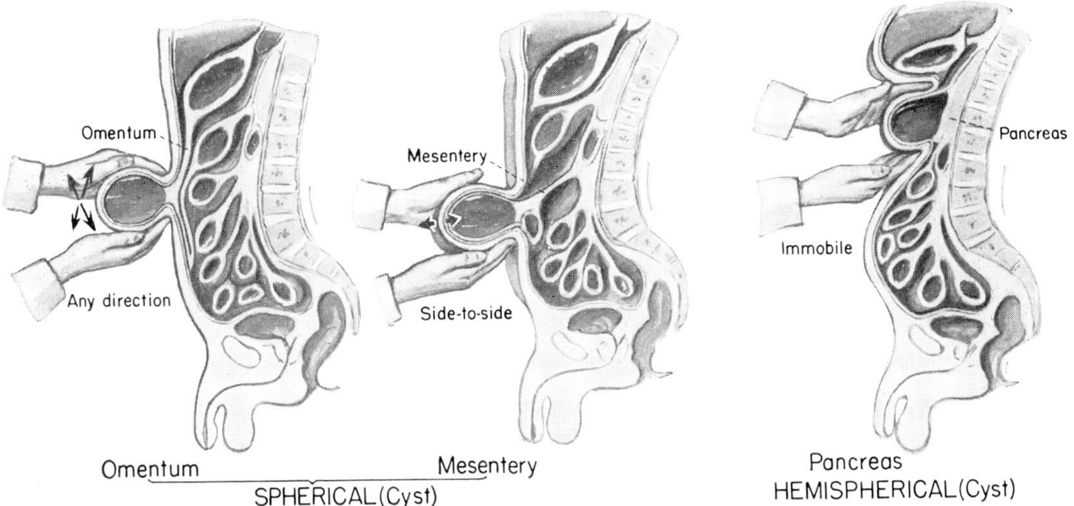

FIG. 257. An omental cyst can be moved in any direction; a mesenteric cyst can be moved from side to side; and a pancreatic cyst is immobile. The former 2 are spherical; the latter is hemispherical.

DIFFERENTIAL DIAGNOSIS

Pancreatic cysts must be differentiated from retroperitoneal tumors, mesenteric cysts, omental cysts, hepatic cysts and renal or perirenal masses. *Splenic cysts* are difficult to distinguish from those involving the tail of the pancreas. *Cysts of the omentum and the mesentery* are suspected by their extreme mobility. Those originating in the greater omentum may be moved in all directions. Cysts or tumors of the mesentery are more mobile in a transverse plane. Omental and

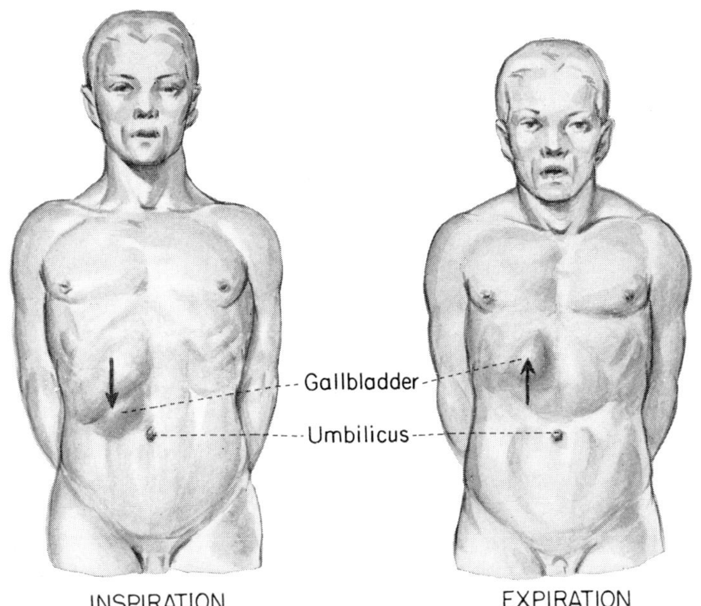

FIG. 258. Differential diagnosis of enlarged gallbladder or pancreas. The gallbladder possesses a greater range of movement with respiration.

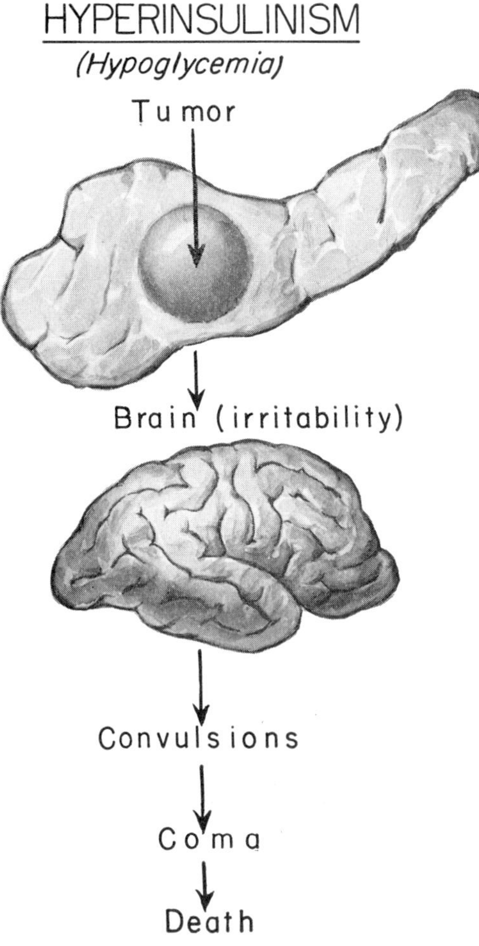

FIG. 259. Islet cell tumors cause hyperinsulinism. If untreated, the condition may become fatal rapidly.

mesenterial cysts tend to be spherical, but the palpable portion of a pancreatic cyst (the exception being the tail of the organ) is hemispherical (Fig. 257). The mobility of pancreatic cysts depends on other locations and the degree of surrounding inflammatory reaction. Cysts located in the pancreatic head or body are essentially immobile, although they may descend slightly on inspiration; those cysts that involve the tail are less fixed; this latter range of mobility might be confusing.

A distended gallbladder may be mistaken for a cyst of the pancreas; however, the gallbladder moves with respirations (Fig. 258).

Congenital cysts are characterized by atresia of the pancreatic ducts, with the formation of numerous minute cysts. A rare condition known as Lindau's disease is the association of renal, hepatic and pancreatic cysts with angiomas of the brain (retina); subnormal mentality completes the picture. A large solitary so-called "congenital" cyst occasionally occurs without evidence of other developmental defects. Such a cyst suggests the existence of retention from a stone or inflammatory process. The rare echinococcic cysts in the pancreas are caused by the tapeworm of dogs (*Echinococcus granulosus*).

ISLET CELL TUMORS

The islet cells secrete insulin, a gastrin-like substance which stimulates gastric secretion and glucagon; the latter promotes glycogenolysis. Therefore, different kinds of tumors can originate in the islet cells.

Insulin-secreting Tumors

These tumors are composed of beta cells and have been referred to as adenomas of the islands of Langerhans or hyperinsulomas. They may be benign or malignant and may occur at any age but are observed most frequently in the 4th and the 5th decades (Fig. 259).

The symptoms are related to the ability of these tumors to produce insulin. The attacks may be intermittent and vary in severity. Usually, they are precipitated by abstinence from food, marked physical exertion or psychic stimuli. The symptoms associated with hyperinsulinism are essentially those of dysfunction of the nervous system. They have been classified as:

1. Involvement of the sympathetic nervous system—dizziness, pallor, perspiration, anorexia, nausea and vomiting
2. Involvement of the central nervous system—tonic and clonic contractions of the extremities, and convulsions
3. Psychic manifestations—mental confusion, maniacal seizures, amnesia and coma

It is unfortunate when such patients are stigmatized by being admitted to psychiatric institutions. Frequent or routine use of blood sugar determinations leads to a correct diagnosis. The disease must be suspected when a history is obtained of intermittent attacks associated with a desire for "sweets," or after an abstinence from food.

Whipple's triad is helpful in making the diagnosis. It consists of:

1. An attack (coma) precipitated by periods of fasting or extreme exertion
2. Fasting blood sugar (12 hours) or during an attack below 50 mg. per 100 ml.
3. Prompt relief of symptoms by the oral or the intravenous administration of sugar (Fig. 260)

The differentiation between benign and malignant islet cell tumors is difficult. Seasoned pathologists have difficulty in differentiating these tumors microscopically. Of clinical significance, however, is the relatively short duration of life when the tumor is malignant. This is in contrast with the long duration of symptoms associated with the benign islet cell neoplasms.

Since the differential diagnosis of spontaneous hypoglycemia embraces a wide variety of conditions, it is helpful to utilize certain tests for insulinomas. Some of the tests being used currently are the glucose tolerance test, the L-leucine test (Flanagan-Schwartz and Ryan), the insulin sensitivity test (Monaco) and the glucagon infusion test (Marks). Although these may prove to be helpful, none is pathognomonic or conclusive.

Differential Diagnosis

Other conditions which produce symptoms referable to hypoglycemia must be considered. Disturbances of the pituitary or the adrenal glands associated with hypoglycemia may be substantiated by thorough studies which include roentgenograms of the skull and specific studies of adrenal function (water test of Kepler, etc.). The eosinophilic response to the injection of epinephrine is helpful. Epinephrine stimulates the pituitary to secrete ACTH, which depresses the eosinophil count. The normal fall should be 50 per cent of the circulating eosinophils. If such a normal depression is present, serious disease of the pituitary or the adrenal cortex may be eliminated.

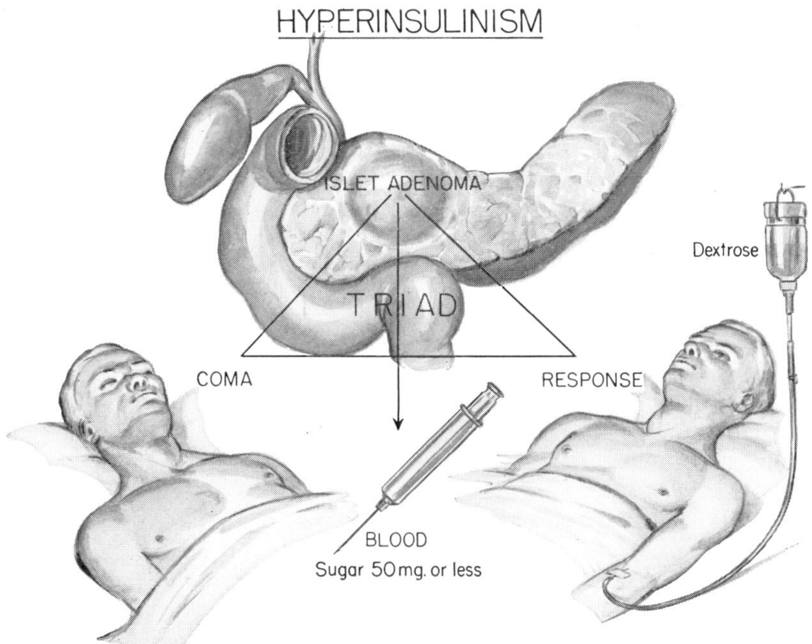

Fig. 260. Whipple's triad is characteristic of hyperinsulinism (islet cell tumor). The triad consists of coma, blood sugar level below 50 mg. and immediate response to dextrose.

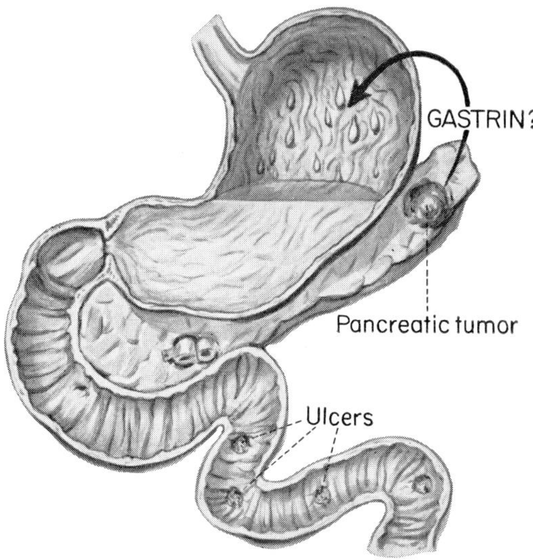

FIG. 261. Ulcerogenic tumors have been found in the pancreas (islet cells) which produce a gastrinlike hormone that produces hypersecretion and peptic ulcer formation.

ULCEROGENIC TUMORS

This condition has been referred to as the Zollinger-Ellison syndrome. It is a fascinating and exasperating type of islet cell tumor. Mann and Williamson produced chronic peptic ulceration experimentally by diverting alkaline pancreatic juices away from the duodenum (1923). In 1955 Zollinger and Ellison recognized and described a syndrome consisting of an ulcer diathesis with marked gastric hypersecretion. It is associated with a nonbeta, noninsulin-producing islet cell tumor of the pancreas. Gregory and others have successfully extracted a histamine-free gastrinlike hormone from the pancreatic islet tumors and their metastases (Fig. 261). Attention has been refocused on the syndrome of multiple endocrine adenomatosis. The endocrine glands most frequently involved include the pancreatic islets, the pituitary, the parathyroids and the adrenals (p. 141). The involved endocrines frequently reveal diffuse hyperplasia.

The **diagnosis** of such tumors will become more frequent as the syndrome becomes better understood. Thus far, most cases have been diagnosed only after a number of serious episodes of perforation, hemorrhage and/or surgical interventions. Control of both the cephalic and the antral phases of gastric secretion by vagectomy and antrectomy or distal gastrectomy is often futile in these cases. A high index of suspicion will help to make the diagnosis, particularly when ulcers are located atypically (jejunum, 2nd, 3rd and 4th parts of the duodenum). Spruelike diarrhea, severe gastric hypersecretion and hypopotassemia suggest such a diagnosis. In these cases the diarrhea may subside when gastric suction is instituted. The tremendous outpouring of gastric acid overwhelms the alkaline secretions of the pancreas, the liver and the upper part of the gastrointestinal tract, inhibiting enzymatic activity of the digestive juices. Because of the severe diarrhea with potassium depletion, regional enteritis has been diagnosed erroneously.

A history of familial endocrine tumors should alert the physician whenever he is confronted with a severe ulcer diathesis. Another suspicious finding is the occurrence of a marginal ulcer a few weeks after competent gastric surgery. Giant rugae have been observed by the roentgenologist and have been referred to incorrectly as Menetrier's disease or gastric polyposis (p. 121).

Approximately 40 per cent of the reported cases have been malignant; metastases occur in regional lymph nodes, liver and lungs. The tumors grow slowly, and the patient is more likely to die of persistent acid peptic disease than of the malignancy.

CARCINOMA OF THE PANCREAS

INCIDENCE

Carcinoma constitutes the most common tumor of the pancreas. It occurs most frequently in the 5th and the 6th decades and is twice as common in diabetics. This follows the general observation that malignant disease is more common in the diabetic.

HEAD AS SITE

The head of the pancreas is the most common site, and tumors that involve this portion may invade the pancreatic portion of the common duct and/or the portal vein. The tumors that involve the body and the tail of the organ usually attain large sizes before clinical signs and symptoms develop.

The signs and symptoms associated with

carcinoma of the head of the pancreas are frequently indistinguishable from neoplasms of the periampullary area (Vater) and from carcinoma of the common bile duct (p. 218). *Pain* is more common than has been thought previously. Contrary to the popular concept that painless jaundice is the outstanding characteristic of this disease, one must re-emphasize the importance of pancreatic pain as an early, if not the earliest complaint. The pain usually is dull, epigastric, radiates to the mid-back region, is aggravated by recumbency and eating, and progresses in severity.

Certain positions afford relief of pain in patients with pancreatic carcinoma (Fig. 262). This was stressed by DaCosta in 1858, who stated that the pain is increased by the erect position, but that patients will seek relief by stooping and curving their bodies forward in order to relax the abdominal parietes. Hence, any body flexion position which relieves the pain should be a diagnostic clue to pancreatic carcinoma, be it in the head, the body or the tail of the organ. The sign is not pathognomonic for pancreas but may be present also in benign and malignant masses that involve the retroperitoneal space.

Jaundice is usually present but is continuous and rapidly progressive. The "P-A-D" triad of biliary obstruction is present, namely, *P*ruritus, *A*cholic stools and *D*ark-colored urine. Weight loss is the most consistent symptom; it is usually rapid and severe. Fatigue is an early and insidious complaint. Anorexia, nausea, vomiting and at times diarrhea are present.

An enlarged liver is present in about 75 per cent of the cases. Despite this enlargement the organ is *not tender*, and its edge remains *relatively sharp* for many weeks. *Nodularity* does not necessarily signify liver metastases or inoperability but may be due to cystic dilatations of the intrahepatic ducts.

An *enlarged gallbladder* is usually present. Courvoisier's law is most helpful in the differential diagnosis (p. 217). The tumor itself is *rarely palpable*.

Laboratory Data. The chief laboratory aids are tests for hyperbilirubinemia, the presence of excess fat and undigested meat fibers in the stool, hyperglycemia, increased alkaline phosphatase, and occult blood in the stool. *Roentgenologic examination* may be helpful if the following can be demonstrated: enlargement and/or displacement of the duodenum and the stomach, an increased duo-

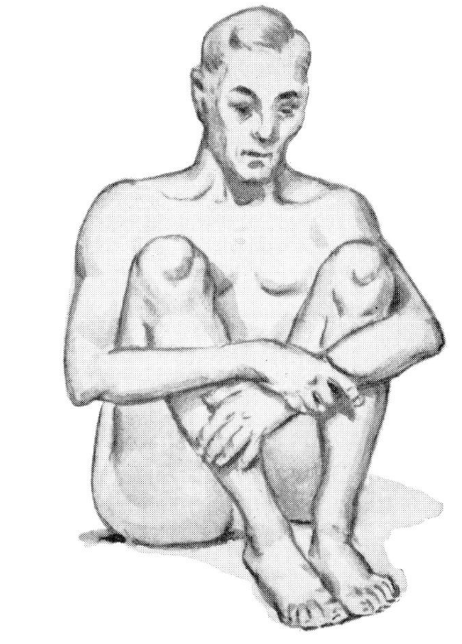

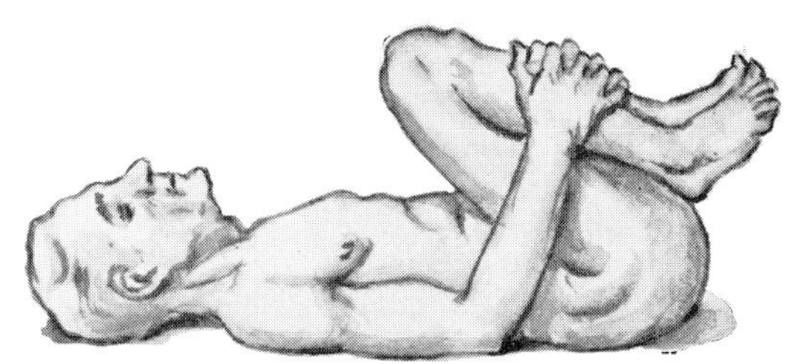

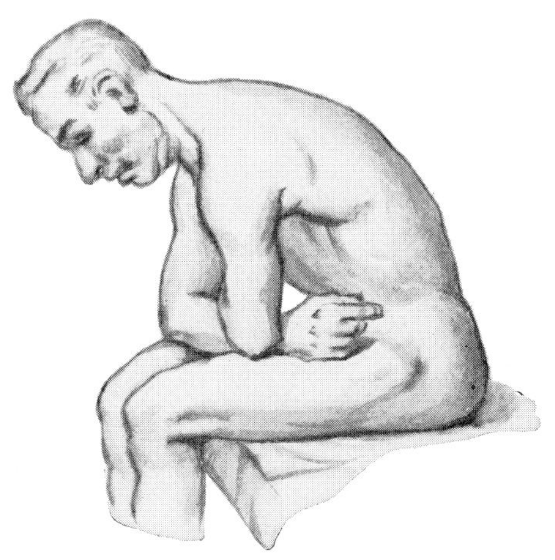

FIG. 262. The positions of body flexion which relieve pain of pancreatic (retroperitoneal) origin.

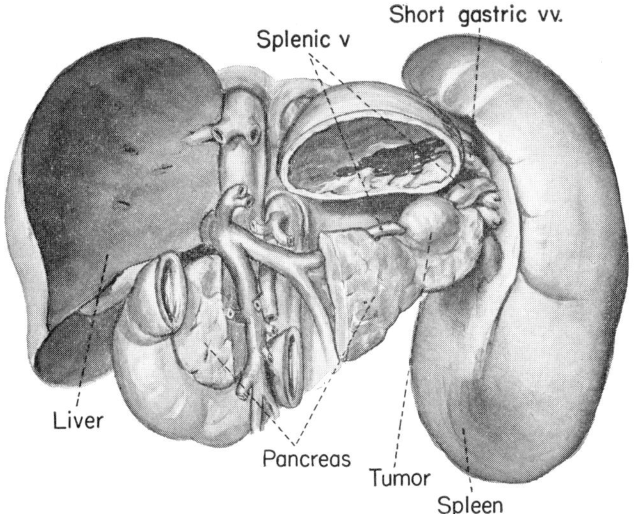

FIG. 263. Benign tumors of the pancreas may cause gastrointestinal hemorrhage because of pressure on the splenic vein and rupture of the short gastric veins.

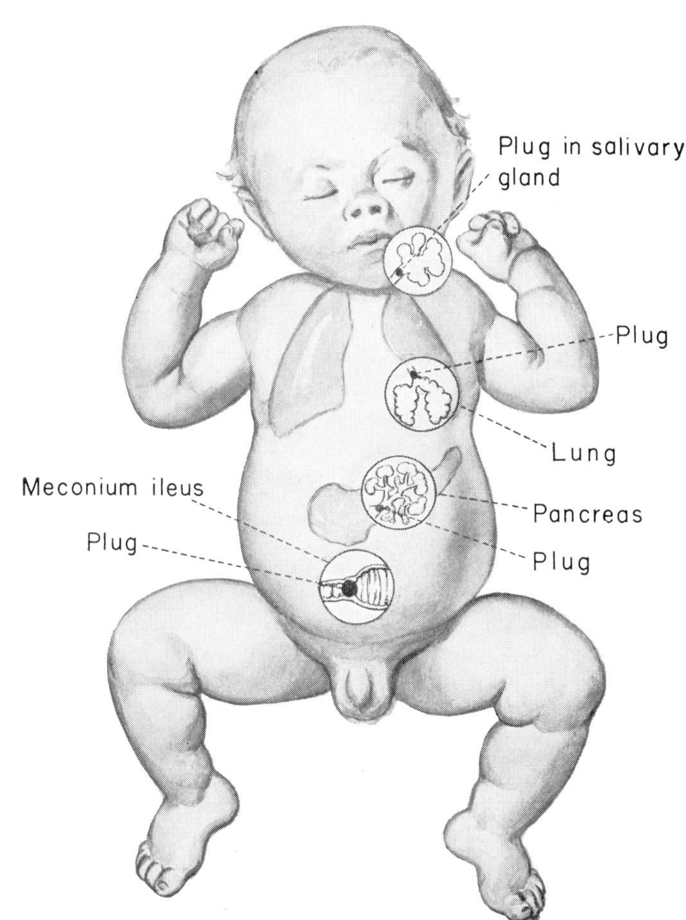

FIG. 264. Fibrocystic disease of the pancreas. The signs and symptoms are caused by plugs of inspissated mucus in various parts of the body.

denal sweep, indentation of the medial aspect of the duodenum, the so-called inverted-"3" sign which is formed by the presence of the 2 adjacent indentures due to a large invasive growth, and actual duodenal obstruction with mucosal irregularity produced by tumor invasion or ischemic ulceration.

Body and Tail as Sites

Carcinoma of the body and the tail of the pancreas usually presents a different clinical picture. The pain, which is in the upper abdominal region, is usually constant. It assumes a girdle pattern around the upper abdomen and the lower thorax. Jaundice is absent or late. Migratory thrombophlebitis and/or multiple venous thromboses may be associated with carcinoma of the body and the tail of the pancreas. This is especially true in elderly patients and is distinguished by its persistence and the great number of veins involved. These tumors can be demonstrated by the roentgenogram only when they have assumed sufficient size to produce extrinsic pressure upon the surrounding structures. The mass may be palpable when the tumor involves the body or the tail.

Sarcoma

Sarcoma of the pancreas is a rare condition; however, this organ may be involved secondarily from retroperitoneal sarcoma.

Benign Tumors or Cysts of the Pancreas

These lesions may encroach upon the splenic vein and produce dilatation and rupture of the short gastric veins (Fig. 263). This must not be overlooked in the diagnosis of so-called "idiopathic" gastrointestinal hemorrhage.

CYSTIC FIBROSIS
(Mucoviscidosis)

This disease is a great masquerader; pulmonary and gastrointestinal symptoms are common (Fig. 264). Two misconceptions concerning the disease are that it is rare, and that it is invariably fatal. It is one of the more chronic diseases of childhood and adolescence and represents the most serious problem in American children. For practical purposes it is the only disease which accounts for pancreatic enzyme deficiency and/or chronic pulmonary (nontuberculous) disease in the pediatric group. Many children with portal hypertension and cirrhosis of the liver are cases of cystic fibrosis. Recent studies suggest that variants are responsible for chronic pulmonary as well as gastrointestinal disorders in adults. The basic physiopathology concerns mucus-producing glands of the body which manufacture an abnormal type of inspissated, viscid mucus.

The disease was recognized about 25 years ago as a condition associated with pancreatic deficiency—hence the name "cystic fibrosis of the pancreas." It is estimated that about 4,000 cases occur each year in the United States. This figure is continually rising with improvements in diagnostic methods. Two to 5 per cent of the general population may be carriers of the cystic fibrosis gene, since it is an inborn error of metabolism. The sweat glands and the parotids also may be involved.

Pancreatic Involvement. Abnormal thick mucus-secretions obstruct the flow of pancreatic digestive enzymes (trypsin, lipase and amylase) and produce enzyme deficiencies. As a consequence, foodstuffs, particularly fats, are poorly digested, and their poor absorption results in characteristic frequent, foul, bulky, fatty stools. Although the child has a good appetite, he fails to gain weight or to grow normally. Signs of malnutrition become manifest, and a protuberant abdomen soon develops. Between 5 and 10 per cent of patients have a meconium ileus. Frequently a flat abdominal roentgenogram reveals the proximal colon and the distal small bowel to be closely packed with bubbly appearing material (Neuhauser's sign). Although a bowel obstruction is present, fluid levels rarely are visible on the roentgenogram. Often rectal prolapse occurs. Frequently, the mother comments that the baby's sweat tastes salty. There is danger of excessive loss of sodium chloride because of the high concentration of salt in the sweat. Pulmonary involvement frequently is associated with a nonproductive cough that is chronic;

asthmatic wheezes, signs of emphysema, bronchiectasis and repeated episodes of respiratory infection are characteristic.

Laboratory tests aid in the diagnosis of cystic fibrosis. The most reliable is the quantitative analysis of sweat for sodium and chloride. There are a number of methods for the stimulation of sweat. One is the pilocarpine iontophoresis test. A sweat chloride concentration above 60 mEq. per liter or sodium above 70 mEq. per liter is consistent with a positive diagnosis. Pancreatic function tests reveal marked or complete pancreatic insufficiency.

9

Spleen

Increased interest in the spleen in recent years is due to a change in concepts concerning the physiopathology and the treatment of splenic diseases. Steroid therapy has modified the role of splenectomy in acquired hemolytic anemia and idiopathic thrombocytopenic purpura. Red cell survival studies have given us a clearer picture of the basic mechanisms, especially in leukemia and myelofibrosis. Better understanding of the physiopathology of congestive splenomegaly may produce a revision of the indications for splenectomy. Splenoportography has become a valuable diagnostic aid in these conditions.

PHYSIOLOGY

This bean-shaped organ contains the largest collection of lymphoid tissue and reticuloendothelial elements in the body. Although many functions have been ascribed to the spleen, none seems to be essential to life. Apparently, the reticuloendothelial system compensates and assumes splenic functions after removal of the organ. In *fetal life* the spleen takes part in the formation of all types of blood cells. In the *adult*, however, the spleen produces only lymphocytes and monocytes. At any period in life it can revert to its fetal function and produce all types of blood cells.

The functions of the spleen (Fig. 265) are believed to be related to:

1. Blood formation
2. Blood destruction
3. Blood storage
4. Iron metabolism
5. Immunity
6. Internal secretion

Blood destruction is brought about by the spleen's ability to select "aged" erythrocytes and reutilize their basic substances (hemoglobin and iron). It has been estimated that this organ can destroy 10,000,000 cells per second (Fig. 266)—a fabulous function, to say the least. A recent concept suggests that

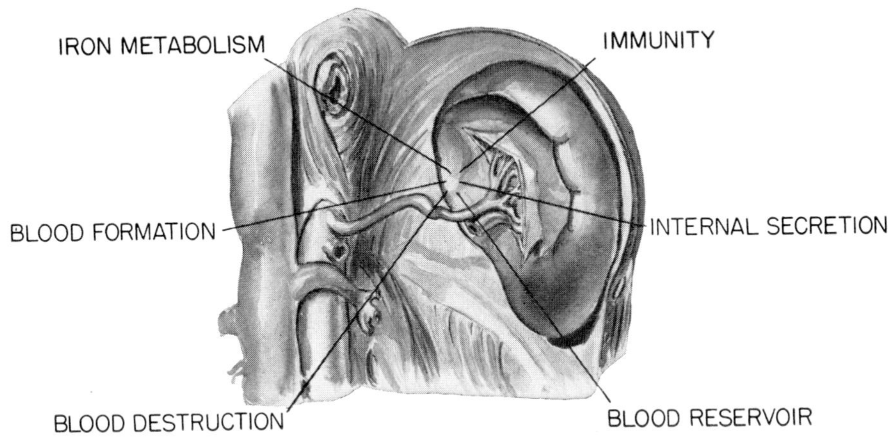

FIG. 265. The supposed functions of the spleen.

the spleen is not the only site of destruction of red cells, since they may undergo intravascular disintegration.

Blood Regulation. The spleen acts as the regulator between the bone marrow (the blood-making factory) and the peripheral blood stream (the blood cell recipient) (Fig. 267). In this way the spleen will maintain the peripheral count of red cells between 4,000,000 and 5,000,000; the white cells between 5,000 and 10,000; and platelets between one quarter and one half million. Should this function become abnormal, hypersplenism and hyposplenism may result.

The storage or reservoir function of this organ can supply blood to the circulation. Splenic contractions are increased by exercise and stress (increased production of adrenalin). Following any hemorrhage, the spleen contracts and attempts to autotransfuse the patient. A spleen which might have been enlarged and palpable prior to the hem-

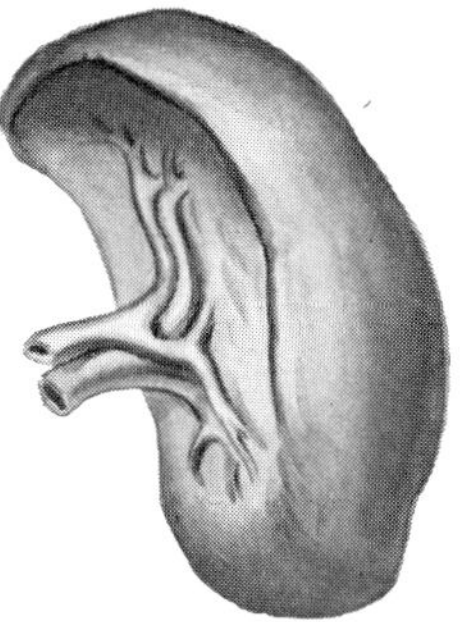

FIG. 266. Blood cell production, destruction and storage are apparently important splenic functions. It should be noted that the spleen may revert to its fetal function of making all types of blood cells.

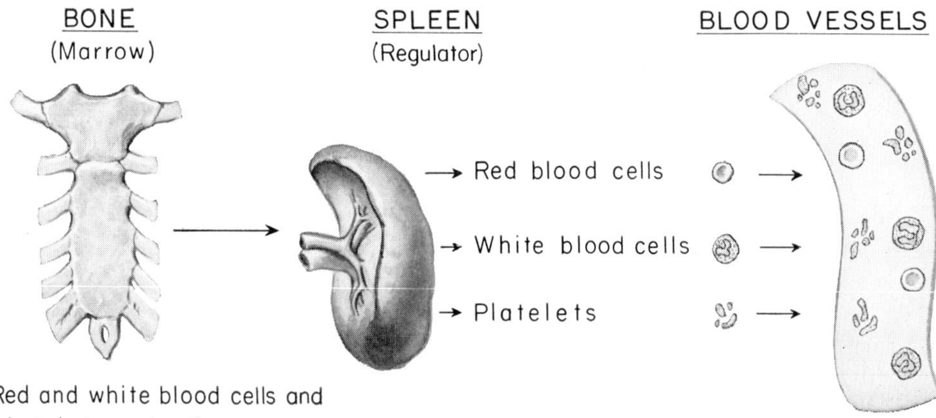

FIG. 267. The spleen acts as a regulating mechanism which is placed between the bone marrow and the peripheral blood stream.

orrhage becomes difficult or impossible to feel after a severe hemorrhage (Fig. 268).

The iron metabolism function is believed to be carried on by the reticuloendothelium of the spleen; this converts hemoglobin into bilirubin.

Immunity is a probable function through the formation of antibodies. However, removal of this organ does not appear to interfere with the well-being of an individual.

Internal secretion is another questionable function. Its relationship to the endocrine system is under critical study.

The removal of an organ with so many functions should be avoided whenever possible.

ANOMALIES

Splenic anomalies include lobulation, congenital absence, accessory spleens and ectopic positions. The 2 last conditions are of particular importance.

Accessory spleens are numerous in the embryo but involute after birth. In congenital hemolytic icterus and thrombocytopenic purpura the number of such spleens is supposedly increased. They are easily confused with hemolymph nodes. They are found most frequently in the splenic hilum, the gastrosplenic ligament and in the region of the upper border and the tail of the pancreas. They are clinically important, because they can perpetuate symptoms of hypersplenism following splenectomy. Their removal is as necessary as is the removal of the spleen proper in cases of hypersplenism, if recurrence of symptoms is to be avoided.

Ectopic spleen (wandering, floating, or movable spleen) is due in part to elongation of the splenic ligament. Symptoms vary with the position of the organ; ptotic spleens are particularly prone to torsion. If splenic torsion is complete, the symptoms are acute, severe and dramatic; if incomplete, a subacute or chronic history may be elicited (Fig. 269). A correct preoperative diagnosis of torsion is a rarity; it is confused clinically with torsion of the ovary or intestinal obstruction.

Of particular interest is the ectopic position of a spleen or accessory spleens to the gonad. It is to be recalled that the splenic bud develops close to the embryonic gonad (Fig. 270). As the ovary or the testis descends, a few splenic cells may become attached to the sex gland and descend with it. Whenever recurrent symptoms of hyper-

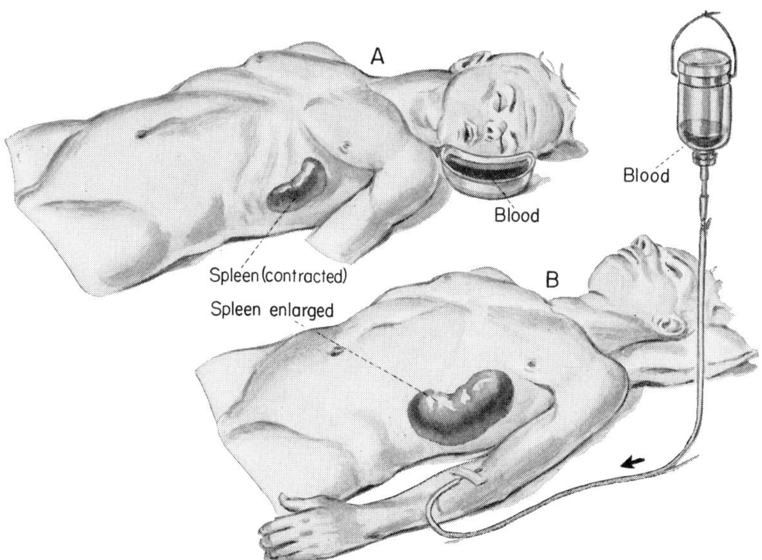

FIG. 268. The spleen contracts and diminishes in size following any severe hemorrhage because it attempts to return blood to the body and autotransfuse the patient.

splenism appear after splenectomy, such accessory spleens must be considered.

HYPERSPLENISM

This term refers to splenic hyperactivity which results in a decrease in one or more of the blood-forming elements. Hematologists differ as to the mechanism. Hypersplenism is classified as primary or secondary, the latter being a complication of some other disease.

Four conditions are directly related to hypersplenism (Fig. 271):

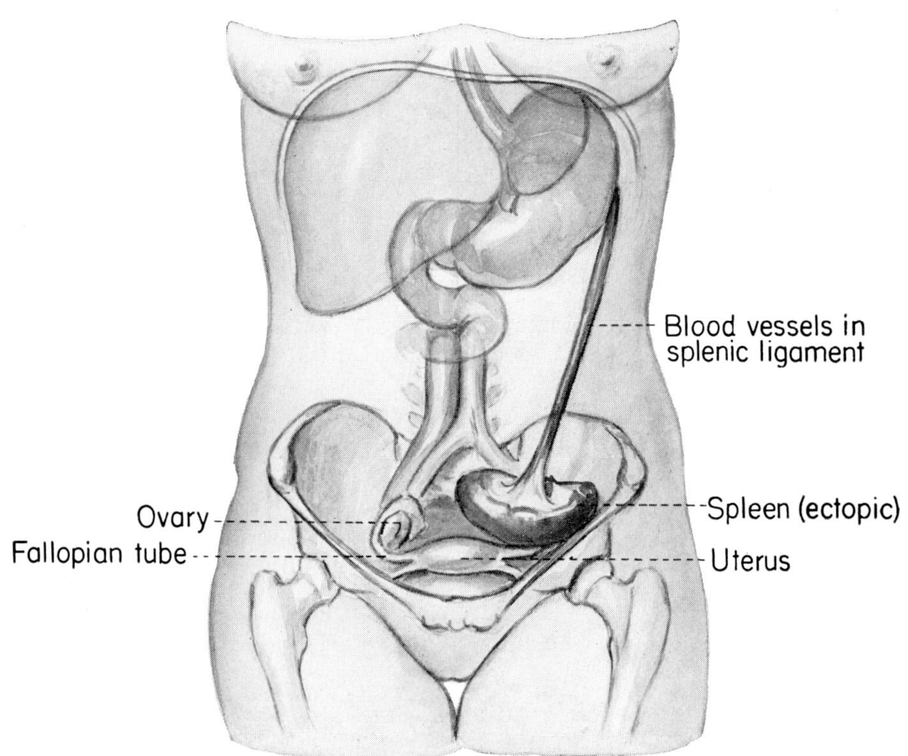

FIG. 269. So-called wandering spleen in relation to the left ovary (author's case).

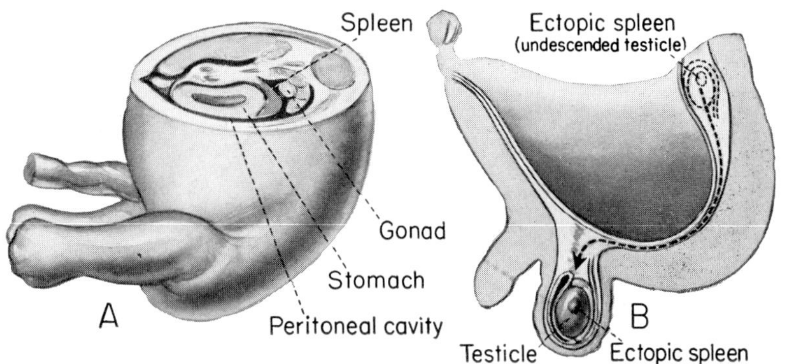

FIG. 270. Ectopic spleens may be situated on the left testicle or the left ovary, because these structures are closely related to each other in the early developmental period.

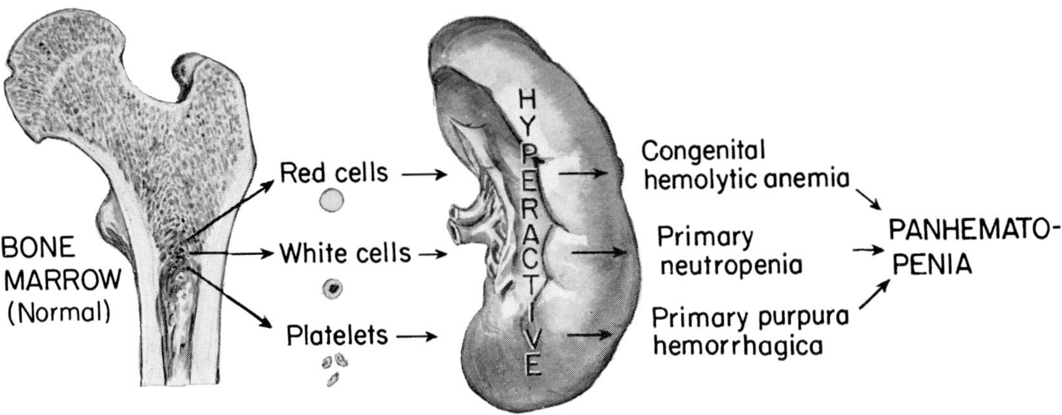

FIG. 271. Hypersplenism refers to an overactive spleen. Four conditions are directly related to it. The type of blood cell destroyed determines the name of the condition.

1. Congenital hemolytic anemia—excessive destruction of red blood cells
2. Essential thrombocytopenic purpura—excessive destruction of blood platelets
3. Primary splenic neutropenia—excessive destruction of neutrophils
4. Panhematopenia—excessive destruction of all blood elements

Congenital hemolytic anemia (congenital hemolytic icterus, spherocytic icterus, acholuric jaundice, Chauford-Minkowski anemia). This is a familial disease that commonly occurs in several members of a given family. Since the symptoms are mild, unless hemolytic crises are present, the case may be undiagnosed. There is a tendency toward exacerbations and remissions. Some authorities are of the opinion that this condition is not a result of hypersplenism per se but rather a defective production of sphero-

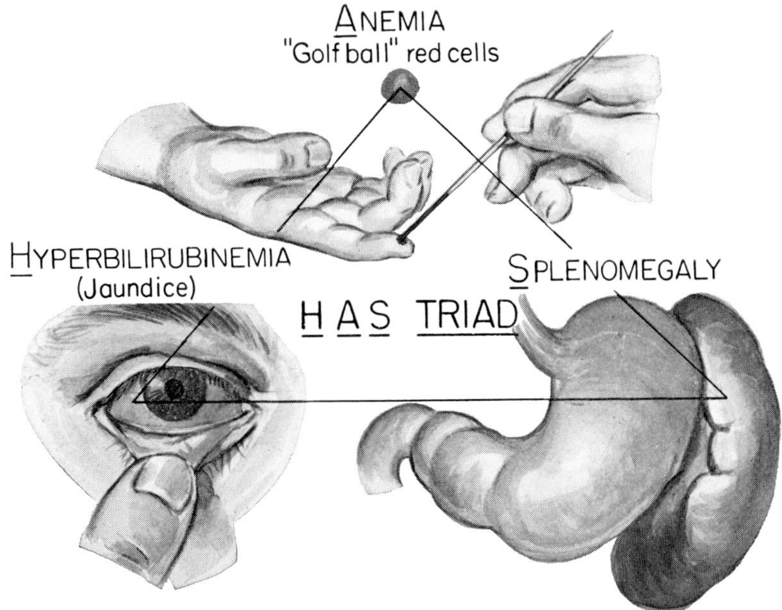

FIG. 272. The H-A-S triad (hyperbilirubinemia, anemia and splenomegaly) associated with congenital hemolytic anemia.

cytic erythrocytes with the spleen acting only to destroy these defective cells.

DIAGNOSIS. The diagnosis should be made when the triad of hyperbilirubinemia, anemia and splenomegaly is present—the H-A-S triad (Fig. 272). *Jaundice* (hyperbilirubinemia) is the cost common symptom but may be overlooked, since it is usually mild or may be subclinical. The *anemia* is moderate, of microcytic type which is characterized by the so-called "golf-ball" red blood cells (microcytic spherocytosis). *Splenomegaly* is common, the enlarged spleen producing pressure and symptoms on surrounding structures. Other findings that should suggest this condition are multiple small bilirubin gallstones, particularly in the young, individuals with an *elongated tower head*, and *ulcers* on the inferior extremities (Fig. 273). The last have been diagnosed erroneously as varicose ulcers; one should not diagnose a varicose ulcer unless varicose veins are present.

HEMOLYTIC CRISIS. This is a critical episode in which the icterus and the anemia increase, and the patient becomes severely ill. During such crises there is a rapid depression of red blood cells and a marked increase in hemolysis. The red blood cell count may drop below 1 million.

LABORATORY DATA. This information can be particularly helpful. *Bone marrow* studies reveal an erythroid hyperplasia. The *red blood cells* represent the characteristic spherocytes with an increased fragility, the hemolysis beginning in 0.7 to 0.5 per cent saline solution (normal, 0.45% saline). An increase in the number of reticulocytes is noted in the peripheral blood. The *blood van den Bergh test* is elevated and indirect. *Urobilinogen* is increased in the urine and the stool. No bile (bilirubin) is present in the urine (acholuric jaundice).

It is imperative to diagnose congenital hemolytic anemia, since the administration of blood transfusions may produce or aggravate a hemolytic crisis. Blood cannot be administered to these patients until the spleen is removed or until the splenic artery has been ligated. Since this condition has been referred to also as a *primary* hemolytic anemia, splenectomy is indicated and gives excellent results.

SECONDARY HEMOLYTIC ANEMIA

This is thought to be a form of hypersplenism in which the hemolytic anemia develops during the course of another disease process. The symptoms may resemble those of congenital hemolytic anemia but are usually overshadowed by the chronic disease. Frequently, the spleen is enlarged. Patients with leukemia, lymphoma and other debilitating diseases often have secondary hemolytic anemia. At times the removal of the spleen may produce dramatic hematologic re-

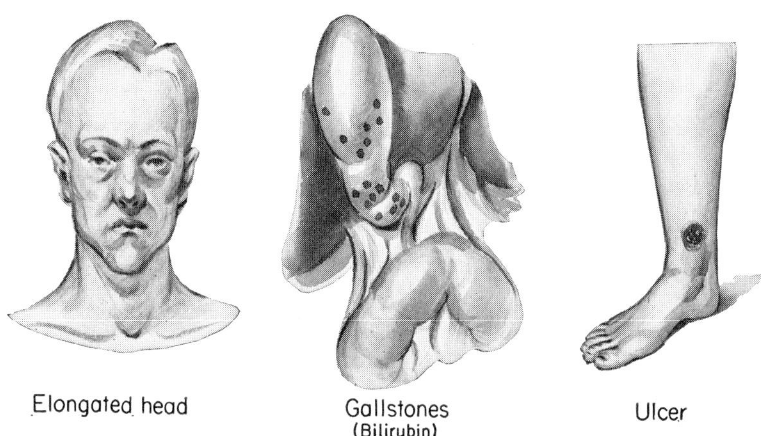

FIG. 273. Individuals with elongated heads, bilirubin gallstones and nonvaricose ulcers might be congenital hemolytic anemia patients.

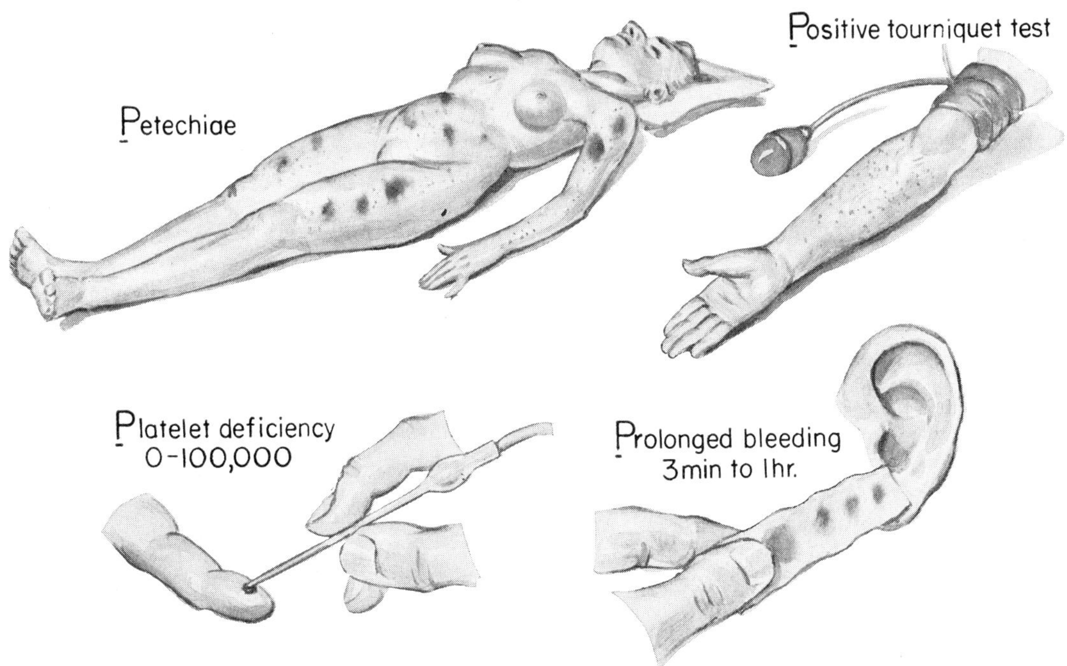

FIG. 274. The cardinal findings in essential thrombocytopenic purpura. The letter "P" has been used as a mnemonic.

sults, thereby affording opportunity for the treatment of the specific primary disease.

ACQUIRED HEMOLYTIC ANEMIA

This type of hemolytic anemia differs from both the primary (congenital) and the secondary types. There is no familial history. Researchers have found that red cells transfused from patients with hereditary anemia into normal recipients survive 20 to 50 days. However, erythrocytes from patients with acquired anemia transfused into normal recipients survive the normal length of time (100 to 120 days). When no other cause for increased hemolysis can be found, hemolytic anemia is referred to as idiopathic acquired hemolytic anemia. In other cases autoantibodies, autohemolysins, auto-agglutinins and isohemolysins may be discovered by special immunologic studies.

The symptoms resemble those of primary congenital hemolytic anemia, occur later in life and frequently are more severe. Spontaneous recovery occurs occasionally; this has not been encountered in primary hemolytic anemia. The spleen may be palpable but is not particularly enlarged. The *Coombs' test*, which is positive for auto-agglutinins in acquired hemolytic anemia, is the best confirmatory test. About half of these patients have a good hematologic response following splenectomy.

Essential Thrombocytopenic Purpura. Known also as idiopathic thrombocytopenic purpura, purpura hemorrhagica, and Werlhof's disease, this is a hemorrhagic disorder that occurs more frequently in children and young adults. In children the sex incidence is approximately equal, but in adults it is predominantly a disease of females. The cardinal findings are (Fig. 274):

1. *P*etechiae
2. *P*ositive tourniquet test
3. *P*latelet deficiency
4. *P*rolonged bleeding time

Petechial hemorrhages usually appear first; they occur most commonly on the extremities and the abdomen. Bleeding from mucous membranes is common (nose, gums, bowels, kidneys and vagina). The most serious complication is *intracranial hemorrhage*; it constitutes the most frequent cause of death in these patients.

The *tourniquet test* is positive during the active phase of the disease. It demonstrates the tendency for blood capillaries to rupture and produce petechial hemorrhages. It is performed by occluding the *veins* of the superior extremity, not the arteries, for 5 minutes. It has also been referred to as the Rumpel-Lead phenomenon.

The *blood platelets* are usually reduced below 100,000 per cu. mm. (normal platelet count is between one quarter and one half million). During the quiescent stage, the platelets may number 60,000 to 100,000; however, during an exacerbation the platelet count may drop to zero. There is no disturbance in the leukocyte or the erythrocyte count unless leukocytosis and/or anemia result from an associated hemorrhage or intercurrent infection. *It is mandatory to do a platelet count on every case of bleeding regardless of the age of the patient or the source of the hemorrhage.*

Prolonged bleeding time is present (normal, 1 to 3 minutes). In these cases the bleeding time is over 3 minutes and may be increased to 1 hour. This time is the period that elapses between capillary puncture and cessation of bleeding. The clotting time remains normal. The clot retraction is totally absent or markedly delayed (normal, usually from 30 to 60 minutes). Splenomegaly is *uncommon*; if present, it suggests some other disease.

Purpura hemorrhagica may be acute or chronic. The chronic form runs a cyclic course, being associated with remissions and exacerbations.

DIFFERENTIAL DIAGNOSIS. This condition must be differentiated from secondary thrombocytopenic purpura and hemophilia. Of particular value is a study of the bone marrow. If the condition is one of essential thrombocytopenic purpura a megakaryocytic hyperplasia will be found. There may be a striking resemblance between idiopathic thrombocytopenic purpura and acquired hemolytic anemia in onset, course, prognosis and response to splenectomy and steroid therapy. Evans has suggested a common etiology for both conditions. He has emphasized the facts that some patients with acquired hemolytic anemia have thrombocytopenia without purpura, and some patients with idiopathic thrombocytopenic purpura, while not having hemolytic anemia, nevertheless do have a positive Coombs' test. Like acquired hemolytic anemia, idiopathic thrombocytopenic purpura can be the first manifestation of lupus erythematosus.

PROGNOSIS. The results following splenectomy are favorable in over 70 per cent of the patients. Relapses occur more commonly in females. Infants, children, and individuals over 40 years may have remissions induced by blood transfusions and conservative treatment. The need for immediate splenectomy has diminished since the advent of steroid therapy and the transfusion of fresh blood that is collected in plastic bags which preserve the blood platelets. A platelet count over 50,000 per cubic mm. almost always relieves the danger of bleeding. Most authorities are of the opinion that patients with essential thrombocytopenic purpura should be treated by corticoid therapy and, if necessary, platelet transfusion. The controversy existing today is how long one should wait between corticoid therapy and eventual definitive splenectomy.

Primary Splenic Neutropenia. This condition, first described by Wiseman and Doan, also belongs to the primary hypersplenic diseases.

It is associated with frequent infections, particularly those involving the oropharynx. The diagnosis is confirmed hematologically by a severe specific neutropenia and a myeloid hyperplasia of the bone marrow. A diagnostic triad may be utilized which consists of:

1. Splenomegaly
2. Peripheral neutropenia
3. Bone marrow hyperplasia

The differential diagnosis includes Banti's syndrome, Felty's syndrome and particularly the toxic neutropenias in which there is *an absence* of bone marrow hyperplasia.

Primary Splenic Panhematopenia. In this condition there is an indiscriminate elimination of all the circulating cellular elements. Although leukopenia is the most persistent feature, thrombocytopenia and erythropenia are also demonstrable. The signs and symptoms usually include weakness, icterus, repeated bouts of infection (oropharyngeal) and bleeding tendencies. The diagnostic triad of this condition includes: splenomegaly, panhematopenia (reduction of all 3 elements of the blood), and hyperplasia of the bone marrow.

SECONDARY HYPERSPLENISM

In this condition the overactivity of the spleen is associated with some other disease. The following 4 criteria are diagnostic:

1. Splenomegaly
2. Evidence in the peripheral blood of a reduction of one or more of the cellular elements
3. Bone marrow hyperplasia
4. The presence of some other disease

Such conditions as portal hypertension (Banti's syndrome), acquired hemolytic anemia, Boeck's sarcoidosis, chronic leukemia, Hodgkin's disease and tuberculosis are a few of the diseases that are related to the syndrome of secondary hypersplenism.

Recent reports suggest beneficial effects of splenectomy for conditions associated with secondary hypersplenism. The indication may be to relieve the patient of discomfort because of the size and the weight of the organ and/or to improve the hematologic status.

HYPOSPLENISM

It is the opinion of some authorities that hypofunction of the spleen is as distinct an entity as is overactivity (hypersplenism). Whether or not such conditions as *polycythemia vera* should be considered under this heading is still debatable. A condition called *agnogenic myeloid metaplasia* has been suspected of being the end-result of polycythemia vera. In this myeloid metaplasia state the spleen and other organs attempt to take over the functions of a sclerosing and inadequate bone marrow. The spleen becomes enlarged, supposedly the result of a compensatory mechanism. The removal of such enlarged spleens, theoretically at least, is contraindicated.

Gaucher's disease is a rare familial disease characterized by splenomegaly, enlarged lymph glands, and peculiar pigmentations which develop on the face, in the conjunctivae and on the lower legs. Hemorrhagic diathesis and positive roentgenographic findings are helpful in confirming the diagnosis. The roentgenograms may reveal areas of bone destruction due to so-called "Gaucher's cells." The diagnosis can be confirmed if these cells are demonstrated in the bone marrow smear. The condition may be associated with secondary hypersplenism.

MYELOFIBROSIS

This has been referred to as myelosclerosis and agnogenic myeloid metaplasia. Fortunately, it is uncommon, affects both sexes equally and occurs usually in the 6th and the 7th decades. It is associated with diffuse fibrosis of the bone marrow, splenomegaly and leukoerythroblastic anemia. The spleen may become tremendously enlarged, often extending below the umbilicus. At times it is accompanied by hepatomegaly, which, when present, frequently follows leukemia (treated with irradiation) or polycythemia vera. Since marrow smears are difficult to obtain by puncture, a marrow biopsy becomes necessary. The prognosis varies from a few months to a few years. Although the spleen is a source of extramedullary hematopoiesis, in some instances it may become hypersplenic with a production of hemolytic anemia and/or thrombocytopenic purpura. It then becomes a major decision whether or not to remove a compensatory source of hematopoiesis.

CONGESTIVE SPLENOMEGALY

Banti was the first to describe a disease which we now refer to as congestive splenomegaly. In Banti's disease or Banti's syndrome splenomegaly, anemia, gastrointestinal hemorrhage, cirrhosis of the liver, jaundice and ascites are present. It took approximately a half century to appreciate the fact that splenomegaly and hypersplenism were due to *portal* hypertension. Splenectomy has been performed alone or in combination with portacaval and splenorenal shunts for this condition.

INFECTIONS

The incidence of splenitis and splenic abscesses has diminished since the advent of the antibiotics. Abscesses are most commonly located in an area of devitalized splenic pulp that is infected. The diagnosis is suspected when there is pain in the splenic region which is referred to the left shoulder or the left chest, a tender enlarged spleen and a septic syndrome (fever, chills, sweats and leukocytosis). It has been suggested that a susceptibility to infection, especially in infants and children, is present after splenectomy. The most common severe infections reported have been meningitis due to the pneumococcus and the meningococcus. It has been advised to postpone splenectomy for congenital hemolytic anemia, if possible, until after the 1st year of life.

Chronic splenitis is suspected if symptoms of infection persist, and a large spleen is demonstrable. Occasionally, this is associated with secondary hypersplenism, tuberculosis, Boeck's sarcoid, syphilis, malaria and leishmaniasis.

Felty's syndrome is characterized by splenomegaly, neutropenia and polyarthritis. Splenectomy has been beneficial, even afflicting the arthritic manifestations in some instances.

TUMORS

Neoplasms of the spleen are benign, malignant or metastatic. Exclusive of the lymphomas, splenic neoplasms are infrequent. The spleen is rarely the site of metastatic tumors. It has been suggested that this organ possesses some protective element

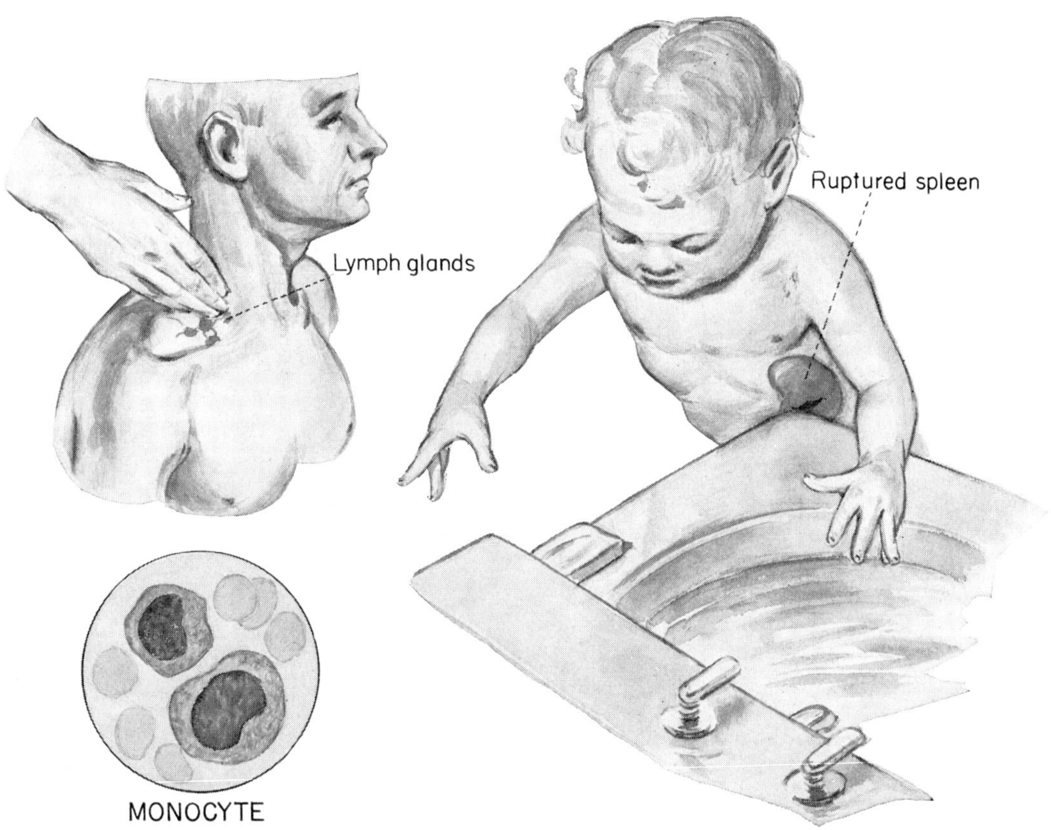

FIG. 275. Infectious mononucleosis is seen most frequently in younger individuals. It should be suspected in cases which are associated with unexplained fever; enlarged cervical lymph glands and splenomegaly are characteristic. These enlarged spleens are susceptible to trauma and rupture. The blood examination reveals an increase in monocytes.

against malignant diseases. The diagnosis is rarely made preoperatively, since the symptoms are vague. Splenomegaly, if detected, is the one finding that attracts attention. The 2 most frequent tumors encountered are those associated with lymphosarcoma and Hodgkin's disease.

CYSTS

Exclusive of hydatid cysts, the most commonly encountered cystic involvement of the spleen is the retention type. If it attains a large size, symptoms result from pressure on surrounding organs. The splenic enlargement is suspected when the roentgenogram reveals the stomach displaced to the right, the splenic flexure antero-inferiorly and the kidney inferiorly. If the cysts have been present for months or years, evidences of calcium deposits are noted. The specific skin test and the complement fixation test are of value in determining whether or not the mass is of echinococcic origin. Less common are the dermoid and the epidermoid varieties of cysts.

Splenic puncture, although advocated by some, has too great a calculated risk to be utilized with any degree of frequency. The author personally fears the procedure. When indicated, and this probably would be most infrequent, one versed in this technic should be permitted to conduct the procedure. However, the attending physician must assume the risk of a probable death.

RUPTURED SPLEEN

This condition should be considered in all patients who have sustained traumatic injuries, particularly those involving the left side of the abdomen or the chest. The spleen is particularly vulnerable because of its fixation by ligaments, its close proximity to the ribs and its consistency. Malaria, syphilis, tumors and other conditions that result in splenomegaly increase its susceptibility to injury. Particularly in the latter instance must be mentioned infectious mononucleosis (Fig. 275). Early and accurate diagnosis of splenic rupture is imperative, because these patients succumb if proper treatment is not instituted rapidly.

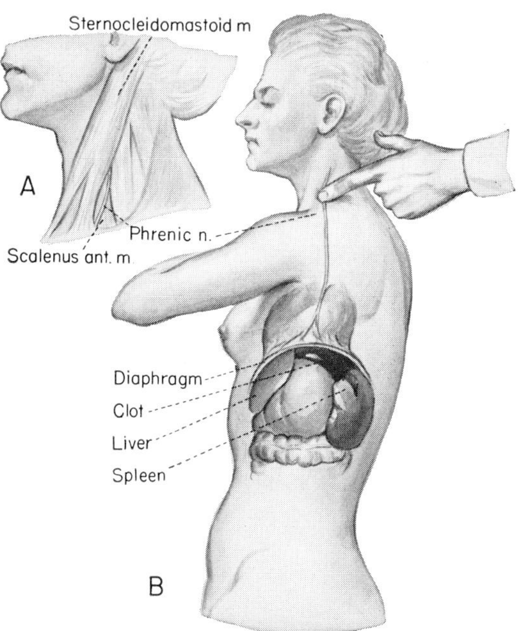

FIG. 276. When a ruptured spleen results in a subdiaphragmatic hematoma, pain can be elicited by pressing the left phrenic nerve. Pressure on the nerve should be made supraclavicularly in an angle formed by the sternocleidomastoid and the scalenus anticus muscles.

Because of the close anatomic relationship between the spleen, the lower left ribs and the kidney (Fig. 317), any injury to the latter 2 structures should suggest the possibility of splenic involvement. Any patient with a history of trauma and a *hematuria* should have a careful evaluation of the spleen. Two types of splenic injury occur: one associated with an intact capsule and the other in which the capsule is torn. It is best to consider these separately, since their clinical pictures differ.

When the *capsule is intact,* the bleeding is not intra-abdominal. The peritoneal reaction is minimal; however, tenderness may be elicited in the left upper abdominal quadrant. As the hemorrhage progresses, it is accompanied by a gradual enlarging of the organ, which eventually becomes palpable. Subcapsular bleeding has been known to distend the splenic capsule to such a degree that it contains 1 liter or more of blood. Serial blood counts are particularly helpful in confirming the diagnosis of subcapsular hematoma in that they reveal a progressive secondary anemia and neutrophilic leukocytosis. Straining at stool, coughing, overeating or vomiting frequently results in a capsular tear. When the tear occurs, signs of intraperitoneal hemorrhage and shock develop.

When the capsule is torn, the diagnosis should be made early, because a definite clinical picture is present. The trauma that precipitates the injury is followed by a "latent period" (symptomatic silence) which usually lasts from 6 to 10 hours. Later the patient develops a sudden collapse from hemorrhage. The signs and symptoms depend on the degree of hemorrhage. Peritoneal irritation produces pain in the left upper abdominal quadrant. If the bleeding continues, tenderness and rigidity appear and may involve the entire abdomen. Because of the ability of the vascular system to accommodate itself to alterations in blood volume, the changes in blood pressure and pulse rate may not be present; this gives the clinician a sense of false security. Shock (p. 281) becomes apparent as the hemorrhage progresses. Pain referred to the left shoulder or the left supraclavicular area is quite common. If there is a splenic hematoma, digital pressure made between the *left* sternocleidomastoid and the scalenus anticus will produce severe pain. This phenomenon is explained by the fact that sensory branches from the splenic capsule travel to the left phrenic nerve (Fig. 276). This sign has been found to be positive in some cases of subcapsular hematoma with an intact capsule. Saegesser is of the opinion that whenever the sign is present, it justifies surgical exploration for an injured spleen. Another diagnostic aid that can be used with caution is the roentgenogram taken in the Trendelenburg position after the patient has had a small swallow of barium. If free fluid (blood) is present in the lesser peritoneal sac or in the upper left abdominal quadrant, there will be an area of separation between the barium in the cardiac end of the stomach and the diaphragm. The flat roentgenogram may reveal medial displacement of the splenic flexure and the proximal descending colon, a distorted air bubble (*magenblase*) in the stomach and possibly an enlarged "splenic" shadow (Fig. 277). The psoas muscle shadow is helpful in differentiating such displacement from a retroperitoneal mass. If the suspected lesion is retroperitoneal, the psoas shadow usually is obliterated. Further roentgenographic evidence reveals an elevation of the left hemidiaphragm and serration of the greater curvature of the stomach.

Percussion elicits an increased area of splenic dullness and obliteration of gastric tympany (Traube's space).

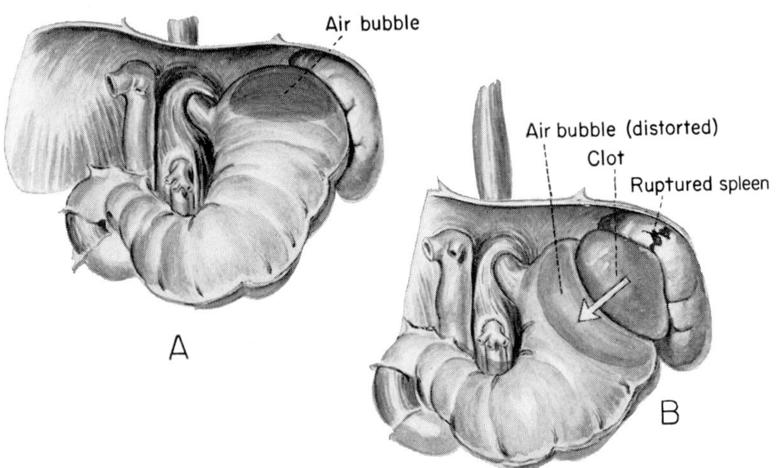

FIG. 277. Medial displacement of a gastric air bubble (*magenblase*) by a splenic hematoma. If present, this is readily demonstrated by the flat roentgenogram.

Abdominal ascultation reveals a diminution in intestinal sounds as the hemorrhage progresses. When the peritonitis becomes diffuse, these sounds are absent.

Laboratory data may be helpful; however, the red blood cell count and hemoglobin do not decrease until later despite the severity of the hemorrhage. The white blood cell count becomes elevated early, often reaching 18,000 to 20,000; therefore, it is of greater diagnostic significance. *"Abdominal tap"* as a diagnostic aid is mentioned to be condemned. A negative tap does not rule out the diagnosis of a ruptured spleen. Some authorities advocate such taps in each of the 4 abdominal quadrants. Apparently, those who advocate such peritoneal harpooning do not realize the safety with which an exploratory operation can be conducted.

Peritoneal autotransplantation of splenic tissue after an extensive injury to the spleen is referred to as *splenosis*. Splenic autotransplantation has been known to follow traumatic rupture of the spleen during the course of a splenectomy. The term implies multiple small splenic transplants in the peritoneal cavity. The condition represents a definite clinical and pathologic entity.

THROMBOSIS OF THE SPLENIC VEIN

This may be a primary condition due to a congenital anomaly; however, it can be associated with various types of infection. Bleeding esophageal varices are associated with this condition and must be differentiated from portal hypertension. If the hypertension is intrahepatic, the liver function tests will be positive. The diagnosis is important, because splenectomy is curative in splenic vein thrombosis.

10

Hernia

The varieties of hernia can be differentiated as to time, location, causation, contents and reducibility. Unfortunately, there is no simpler way to discuss the subject.

A *hernia* (rupture) is an abnormal protrusion of a viscus and its sac through the walls of the cavity that it normally occupies. *Prolapse* also refers to the escape of a viscus through an anatomic opening; however, the protruding part is not covered by a sac.

CLASSIFICATIONS

1. **As to Time**

A. *Congenital*, a hernia that exists at birth

B. *Acquired*, one that develops after birth

2. **As to Location**

A. *External* hernias protrude through the parietes, the underlying sac and its contents being situated under the skin.

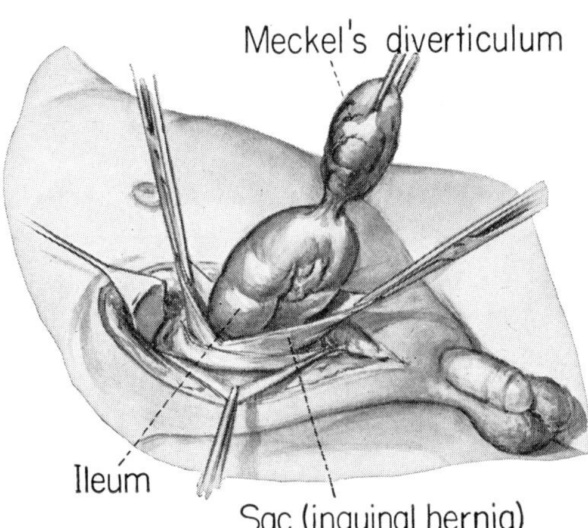

FIG. 278. Littre's hernia. This inguinal hernia contains a Meckel's diverticulum.

B. *Internal* hernias lie within the abdomen (intersigmoid fossa, pericecal fossae, foramen of Winslow, etc.).

C. *Inguinal* hernias involve the inguinal region.

D. *Femoral* hernias traverse the femoral canal.

E. Miscellaneous locations, such as ventral, obturator, lumbar, perineal, sciatic, vaginal, pudendal and diaphragmatic

F. *Interstitial* hernias are located between the layers of the abdominal wall.

3. **As to Contents**

A. *Epiplocele* contains omentum.

B. *Enterocele* contains small intestine.

C. *Cystocele* contains urinary bladder.

D. *Cecocele* contains the cecum.

E. *Richter's* hernia contains only a part of the circumference of the bowel.

F. *Littre's* hernia as described by Alexis Littre: the hernial sac contains a Meckel's diverticulum (Fig. 278).

4. **As to Causation**

A. Traumatic

B. Postoperative (incisional)

5. **As to Reducibility**

A. Reducible when the contents are returned to the abdominal cavity, either spontaneously or by manipulation (taxis)

B. Irreducible when the contents cannot be returned to the abdomen

ETIOLOGY

Hernias occur commonly during infancy and between the ages of 15 and 50. Umbilical hernias of childhood are seen equally in the sexes but after middle life are more frequent in females. Heredity plays a part in that there is a history of similar herniations in about 25 per cent of the cases.

Those specific hernias which are considered to be most important and most common will be discussed:

- Inguinal
- Sliding
- Femoral
- Ventral
  - Median
  - Lateral
  - Incisional
- Internal

INGUINAL HERNIA

These hernias constitute about 85 per cent of all hernias. They *are more common in men* than women, because the descent of the testicle makes the inguinal canal larger and more vulnerable. *Hernias occur more frequently on the right side*, probably because of the later descent of the right testicle. Inguinal hernias may be of 2 types: indirect or direct. They should be considered as 2 entirely different conditions and will be discussed as such.

Indirect Inguinal Hernia

This has been referred to as an oblique or lateral inguinal hernia.

Indirect inguinal hernia is an *embryologic* hernia, since it is related to the descent of the gonad (Fig. 279). Therefore, this type of hernia follows the course of the spermatic cord as far as the scrotum, or the round ligament into the labium majus. As the hernia leaves the internal abdominal inguinal ring, it traverses the inguinal canal and emerges at the external (subcutaneous) inguinal ring.

As the testicle descends, it pushes together the 2 leaves of peritoneum which extend downward toward the scrotum. If descent of the testicle fails, the peritoneal prolongation remains open (Fig. 279 B). Therefore, in *every* case of undescended testicle there must be an associated indirect inguinal hernia. The 2 peritoneal layers which form the vaginal process may not fuse firmly despite the normal descent of the testicle; a potential embryologic weakness then exists, and a hernia may develop (Fig. 279 C). If such a hernia is present at birth, it is referred to as *congenital*. If it develops after birth, it cannot be called congenital; however, it is nevertheless embryologic.

Age plays an important role in the diagnosis, because an indirect inguinal hernia appears in younger individuals. These hernias are seen more frequently before middle life (40 to 50).

This hernia (slow to appear) does not im-

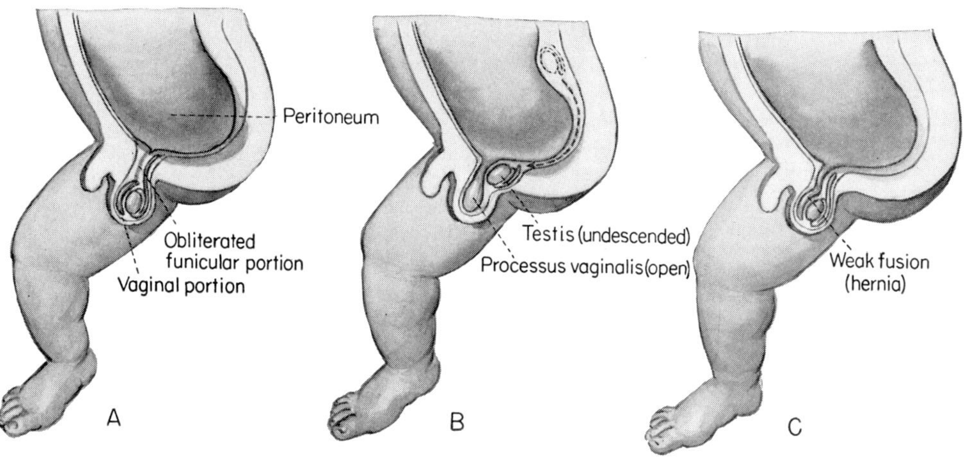

Fig. 279. Indirect inguinal hernia. (A) Normal descent of the testicle and obliteration of the processus vaginalis. (B) In every case of undescended testicle there is an associated indirect inguinal hernia. (C) When the fusion of the layers of the processus vaginalis is weak, an indirect inguinal hernia can develop.

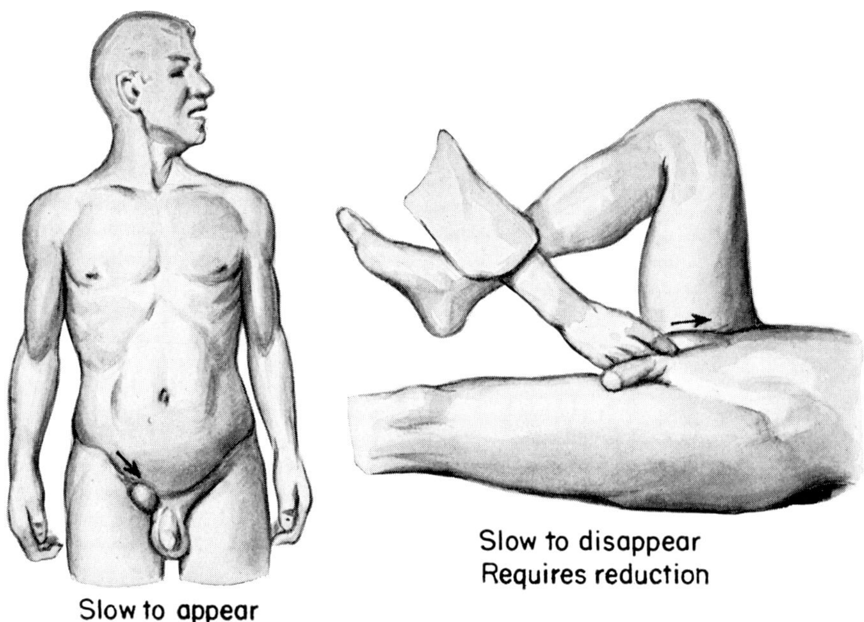

FIG. 280. An indirect inguinal hernia is slow to appear and slow to disappear. Frequently, it requires reduction. This is explained by the small caliber of the internal inguinal ring.

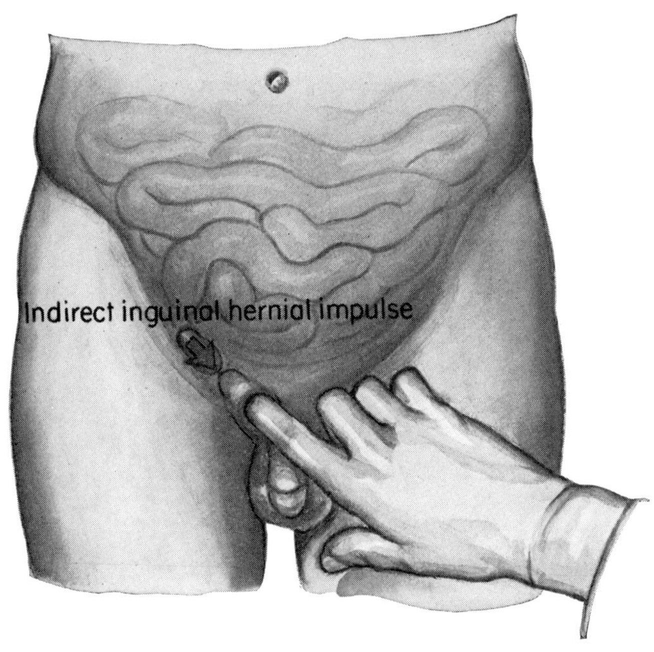

FIG. 281. The impulse transmitted from an indirect inguinal hernia touches the *tip* of the examining finger.

mediately "pop out" when the patient stands (Fig. 280). The patient states that it usually reduces itself *slowly* or disappears while he is asleep. This is explained by the fact that this type of hernia has to find its way gradually through the *small* internal inguinal ring. The smallness of this ring also explains the need for reduction (taxis).

Scrotal hernias are a type of indirect inguinal hernias. They must be differentiated from scrotal masses (testicular tumors, hydroceles, etc.). (See p. 267.)

Strangulated inguinal hernias are practically always *indirect*. This also is explained by the fact that the internal inguinal ring is narrow and predisposes to constriction around the hernial contents. The term "strangulated" should not be confused with "incarcerated," since the latter refers to irreducibility. When a hernia becomes strangulated, it is irreducible to be sure, but its blood supply is also interfered with.

A specific impulse is transmitted to an examining finger placed in the external inguinal ring if an inguinal hernia is present. In the indirect inguinal variety the hernia descends along the inguinal canal traveling from lateral to medial. Therefore, this type of hernia would touch the *tip* of the examining finger (Fig. 281). This can be demonstrated readily if the patient is asked to cough or strain.

Direct Inguinal Hernia

Direct inguinal hernia is an *acquired* type of hernia. It is not related to the embryologic descent of the testicle but is dependent on the weakening of the transversalis fascia in Hesselbach's triangle. Such tissue weakness usually occurs later in life (40 to 60 years).

These hernias *appear rapidly*; as the patient assumes an erect posture, the hernia "pops out." The bulge appears at the middle of Poupart's ligament. Direct hernias *disappear* rapidly and spontaneously (Fig. 282). The explanation for such rapid appearance and spontaneous disappearance is the fact that there is no narrow ring to form a constricting neck. Hesselbach's triangle, through which this hernia protrudes, is a wide, fossa-like space.

Direct hernias do not become scrotal, because they do not follow the path of the descending testicle. They merely bulge toward the inguinal canal, approaching it from the medial side.

These hernias *do not strangulate*, because they are associated with a wide-mouthed fossa (Hesselbach's triangle) and not with a constricting ring.

An *impulse* is transmitted when patients with direct inguinal hernias cough or strain (Fig. 283). However, this impulse contacts

DIRECT HERNIA

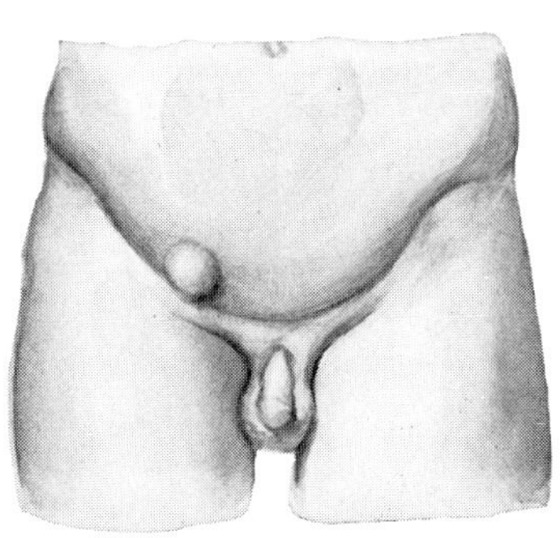

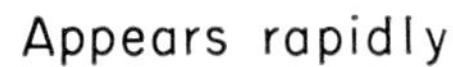

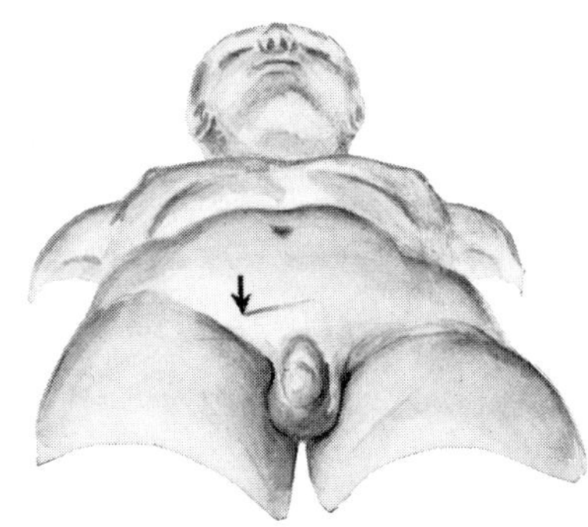

FIG. 282. Direct inguinal hernias appear rapidly (pop out) and disappear without requiring reduction when the patient is supine.

the *pulp* of the examining finger, lifting the distal end of the digit upward.

Differentiation of these 2 types of hernias is important, because the recurrence rate in direct hernia is greater, surgery is imperative in the indirect variety, and the treatment of each is entirely different. They cannot be differentiated clinically by feeling the pulsations of the deep epigastric artery, because this vessel is not palpable under normal circumstances. The differential diagnostic points are tabulated in the next column.

The author has found it helpful to liken inguinal hernias to a pair of pants (Fig. 284). The indirect inguinal variety is like the new (young) pair of pants in which the seam (vaginal process) is the predominant weak point. Should such a torn seam be taken to a tailor, the defect is corrected readily by merely suturing it. The same applies to the surgical correction of an indirect inguinal hernia by high ligation of the sac (seam). A direct inguinal hernia would be represented by an older pair of pants in which the seam (vaginal process) has held for many years, but the cloth (transversalis fascia) is getting threadbare and tearing. If such a pair

Differential Diagnosis

Indirect Inguinal Hernia	Direct Inguinal Hernia
Embryologic	Acquired
Young man's hernia (under 50)	Older man's hernia (over 50)
Appears slowly	Appears rapidly
Disappears slowly (requires reduction)	Disappears rapidly (spontaneous reduction)
May become scrotal	Not scrotal
May strangulate	Strangulation very rare
Impulse touches *tip* of examining finger	Impulse touches *pulp* of examining finger

of pants were taken to a tailor, he would attempt to find a cloth similar to the torn one and patch it. This is what should be done in correcting direct hernias, in which cases a patch (rectus sheath) is placed over the weakened part of transversalis fascia.

SLIDING HERNIA

This is a variety of indirect inguinal hernia in which a viscus (sigmoid, cecum, or blad-

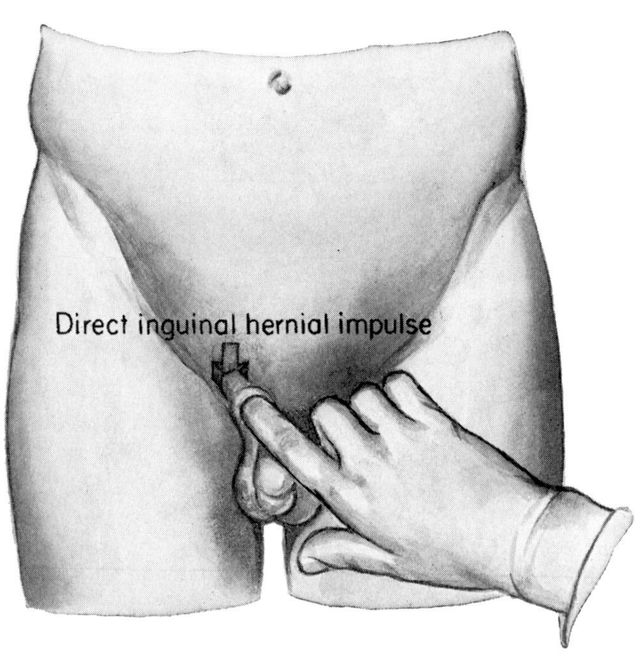

Fig. 283. The impulse transmitted from a direct inguinal hernia touches the *pulp* of the examining finger.

der) "slides" into the sac and forms part of it (Fig. 285).

Sliding hernias have the following characteristic triad (Fig. 286):

1. They are scrotal.
2. They are irreducible.
3. They rarely strangulate.

Since the inguinal canal and the internal inguinal ring are widely dilated in this type of hernia, strangulation is rarely to be feared. It is impossible to ligate the sac high, because a viscus constitutes part of the sac. These hernias must be included in the differential diagnosis of scrotal masses (see p. 267).

FEMORAL HERNIA

This hernia is *below* the inguinal ligament in contradistinction to inguinal hernia, which is above the ligament. It occurs more commonly in women because of the wider pelvis, the broader femoral canal and the poorly developed iliopsoas muscle. However, it is less frequent in women than inguinal hernia.

It must be emphasized that a femoral hernia may travel downward through the femoral canal, come out the femoral ring beneath Poupart's ligament and then change its course, turning upward over Poupart's

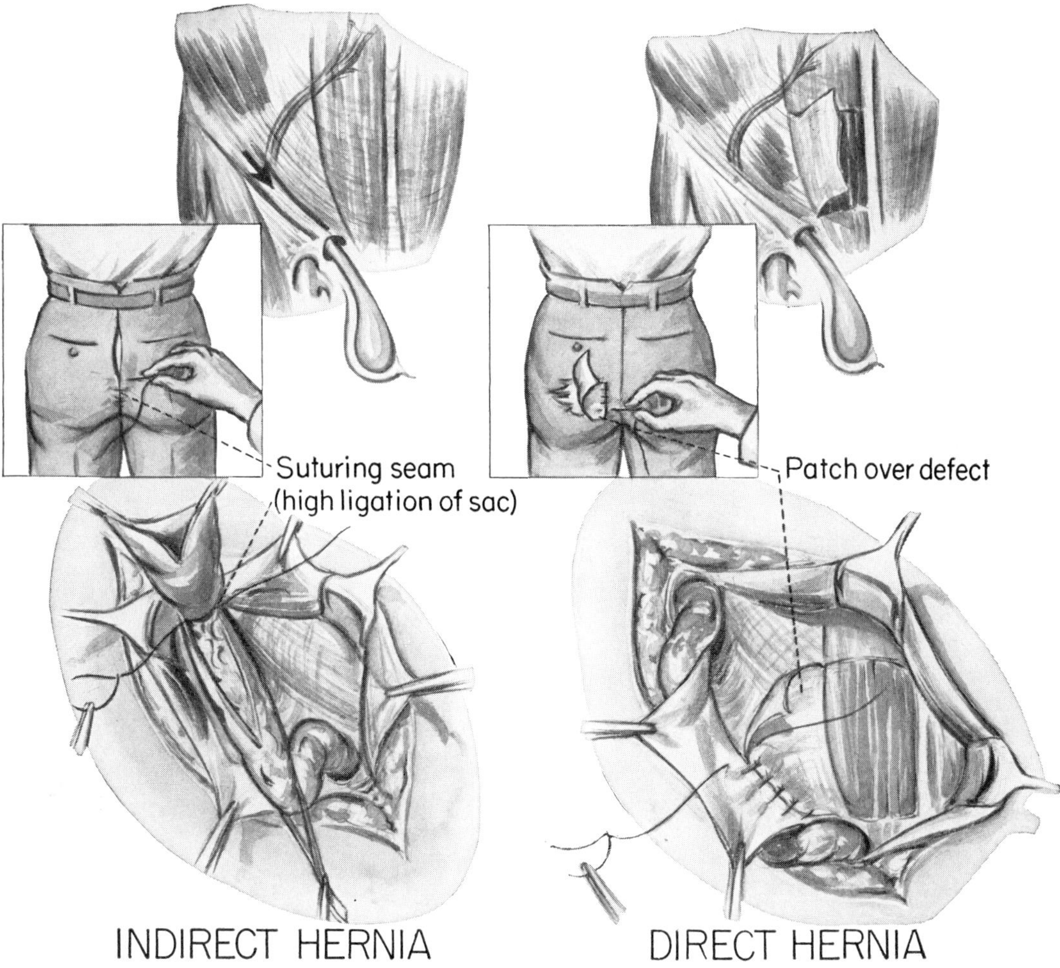

FIG. 284. Comparison of inguinal hernias to a pair of pants. The indirect variety is a defective seam (vaginal process) which must be resutured (high ligation of the sac). The direct variety is a worn out piece of cloth (transversalis fascia) which must be patched.

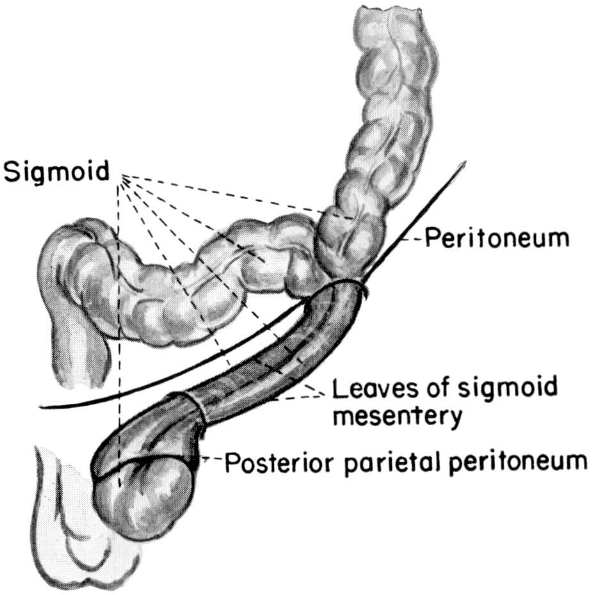

Sigmoid
Peritoneum
Leaves of sigmoid mesentery
Posterior parietal peritoneum

FIG. 285. A sliding hernia in which the sigmoid makes up part of the sac.

No strangulation
TRIAD
Bowel
Scrotal
Irreducible

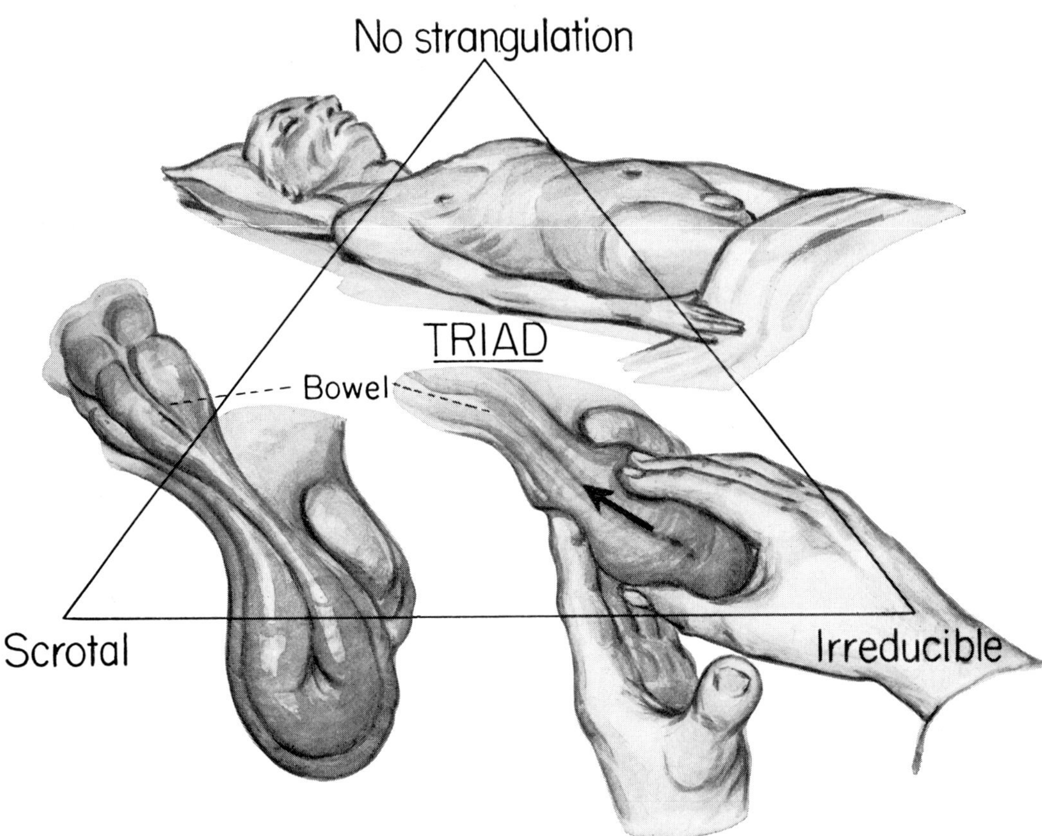

FIG. 286. The diagnostic triad of sliding hernia; they are scrotal, irreducible and rarely strangulate.

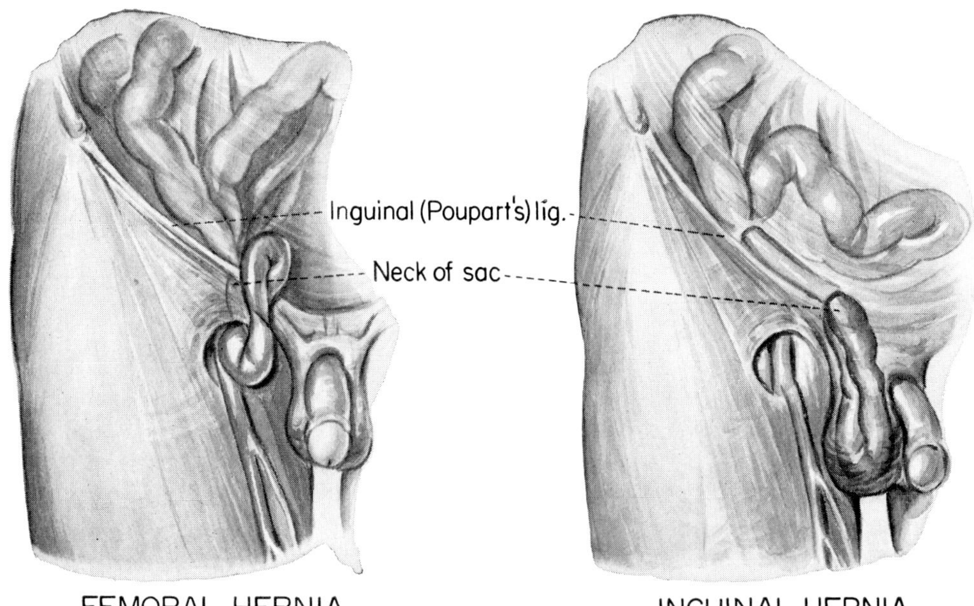

FIG. 287. The *neck* of the sac of a femoral hernia is *below* the inguinal (Poupart's) ligament; the neck of the sac of an inguinal hernia is *above* the inguinal ligament.

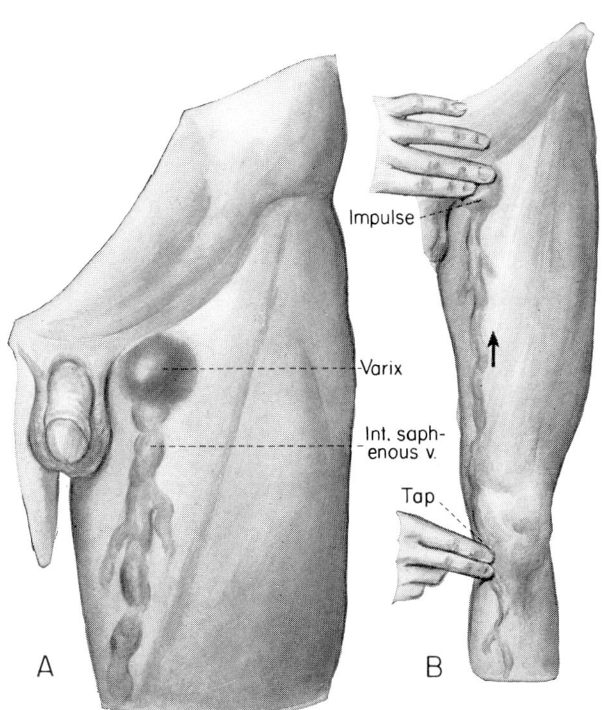

FIG. 288. A saphenous varix at the fossa ovalis can be differentiated from a femoral hernia by the presence of varicose veins leading to the varix and the demonstration of an impulse when tapping a lower vein.

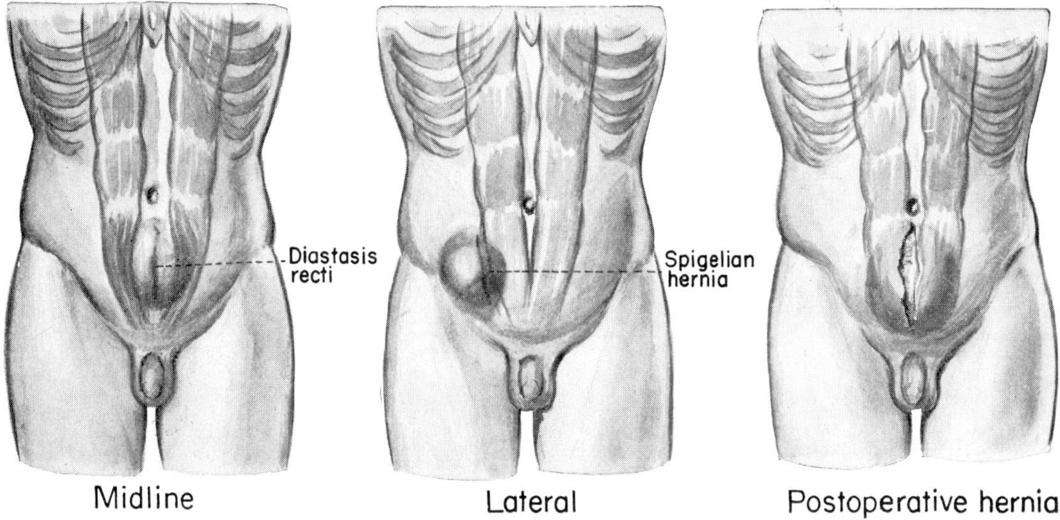

FIG. 289. Ventral hernias may be divided into midline, lateral and postoperative.

ligament. This explains why a femoral hernia is readily confused with an inguinal hernia. It is the relation of the *neck* of the sac to Poupart's ligament rather than the fundus of the sac which avoids confusion with inguinal hernia. In the case of a femoral hernia the neck of the sac is below Poupart's ligament; in inguinal hernia the neck of the sac is above Poupart's ligament (Fig. 287).

To differentiate an inguinal hernia from a femoral hernia one should place the examining finger in the external inguinal ring of the suspected side; if the bulge is a femoral hernia, the inguinal ring and canal will be empty. Since the femoral ring is a narrow one, and since the lacunar (Gimbernat's) ligament is an unresisting band, strangulation is frequent. The femoral canal is not

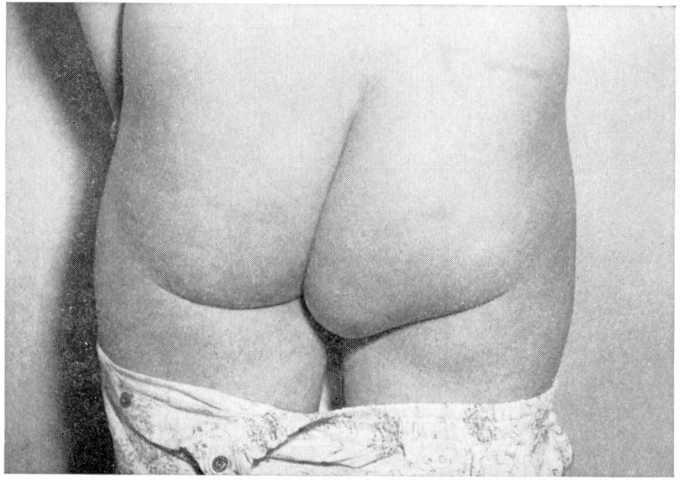

FIG. 290. This asymmetry of the buttocks is produced by a gluteal hernia. If the gluteal mass is a hernia, it transmits an impulse on coughing or straining, and frequently it can be reduced.

open at birth; hence this type of hernia is rarely seen before the 2nd decade.

The *differential diagnosis* must include subperitoneal lipoma, aneurysm of the femoral artery, saphenous varix and enlarged lymph nodes.

A saphenous varix at the fossa ovalis closely resembles a femoral hernia, because it forms a soft swelling, it is reducible on pressure or recumbency, and transmits an impulse on coughing. Two things, however, should call attention to the varix: the presence of other varicosities on the thigh or the leg and a percussion impulse transmitted to the varix (Fig. 288).

Enlarged lymph nodes in the region of the fossa ovalis may press on the genitofemoral nerve and produce reflex vomiting which suggests a strangulated hernia. The so-called suppurating gland of Cloquet, when reddened and inflamed, may closely resemble a strangulated femoral hernia. It is important to examine the entire extremity, particularly the foot and the area between the toes, for the primary source of infection.

VENTRAL HERNIA

In a broad sense any hernia which involves the abdominal wall can be considered to be a ventral hernia. Inguinal, femoral and umbilical hernias are treated as specific varieties. The ventral hernias per se are divided into 3 types (Fig. 289): (1) midline, (2) lateral and (3) postoperative.

Midline Ventral Hernias

Midline ventral hernias have been referred to as divarications of the recti, linea alba (epigastric) hernia, and diastasis of the recti muscles. *Divarication* of the recti is a separation of these muscles which occurs usually between the navel and the xiphoid and is present frequently in children. As the child strains, a supra-umbilical protrusion in the midline is noted. This is usually transient and disappears as soon as the muscles develop. Rarely is any surgical therapy indicated; however, the parents require reassurance.

Linea alba (*epigastric hernia*) also occurs between the navel and the xiphoid; it is found more commonly in adults, particularly males in the 3rd decade who are engaged in strenuous labor. This hernia is composed of extraperitoneal fat which protrudes through a meshwork of interlacing fibers in the midline. This mass is small, globular and usually irreducible; it becomes extremely painful if it strangulates. This must be differentiated from lipomas and other tumors and cysts in

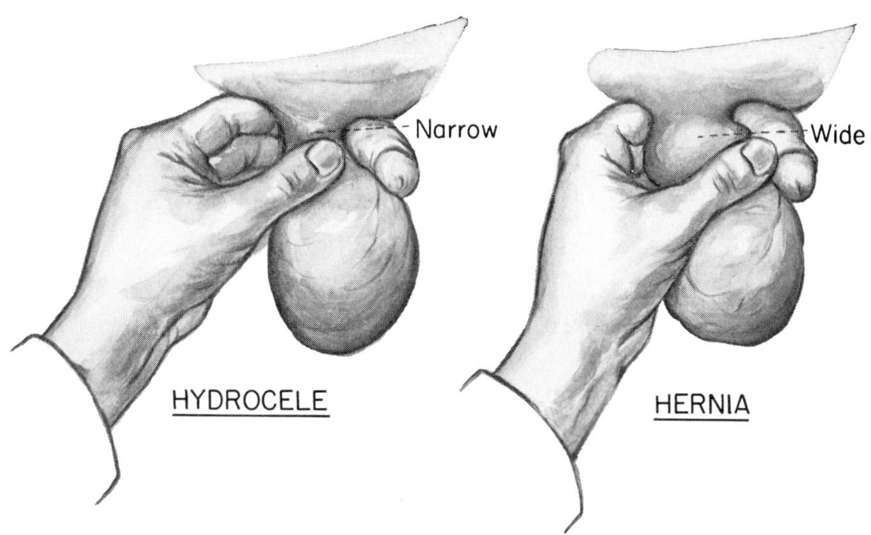

Fig. 291. A scrotal mass per se does not affect the width of the spermatic cord in the region of the external inguinal ring. A scrotal hernia, however, is associated with a marked increase in the width of the spermatic cord.

the midline. *Diastasis of the recti muscles* can occur anywhere along the linea alba but is found most frequently infra-umbilically. Multiparous women who present a marked relaxation of the anterior abdominal wall are particularly predisposed. One can test for a diastasis by having the patient, who is supine, raise the body upward from the hips and watch for a bulging between the recti.

Lateral Ventral Hernias

Lateral ventral hernias (spigelian hernia) are not frequent. They occur at the linea semilunaris, which marks the lateral border of the rectus abdominis muscle. The weakest point is usually at the site where the inferior epigastric artery enters the rectus muscle. These hernias should not be confused with tumors or cysts, since the hernia is usually reducible and transmits an impulse on coughing or straining.

Postoperative Hernias

Postoperative hernias may follow any operative procedure; it is particularly common in males who have had upper abdominal surgery or females who have had pelvic surgery. Predisposing factors to the development of such hernias are wasting of the muscles, nerve paralysis, faulty abdominal wall closures, infection, drains and malnutrition. The hernial sac is usually adherent to the abdominal wall; it may be lobulated and therefore confused with lipomas. They may strangulate and produce intestinal obstruction (p. 176).

Such hernias as obturator, sciatic, retroperitoneal and internal are rare. *Gluteal hernias* are rare; however, they must be suspected whenever an asymmetry is discovered in the buttocks (Fig. 290). Such masses must be differentiated from tumors and cysts; however, the hernia can frequently be reduced, and it transmits an impulse on coughing or straining. Roentgenograms may be helpful.

SCROTAL SWELLINGS

The differential diagnosis between an indirect inguinal scrotal hernia and a hydrocele may cause confusion. A hydrocele transilluminates light; however, if an appreciable amount of blood is present in the tunica vaginalis, transillumination will not be demonstrable. If a scrotal hernia contains large bowel (cecum or sigmoid), these gas-containing viscera may transilluminate light. Although helpful in most instances, translucency is not pathognomonic. A more certain method of differentiating these 2 con-

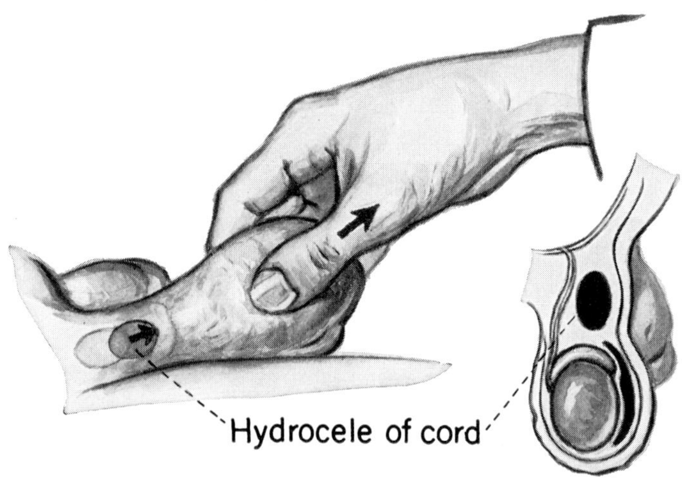

Fig. 292. To differentiate a hydrocele of the cord from an indirect inguinal hernia gentle traction should be made on the testis caudally. If the mass is a cord hydrocele, it will move with the cord.

ditions is the relationship of the size of the spermatic cord to the scrotal mass (Fig. 291). If the scrotal mass is a hydrocele, the examiner's fingers can be placed around a normal spermatic cord at the external inguinal ring. However, if the scrotal mass is due to a hernia, it is difficult to get above the swelling, since the fingers must incorporate the spermatic cord, the hernia and its contents, which are very wide. Another helpful method, although not as accurate, is "weighing" the scrotal mass. Hydroceles are heavier than hernias.

Nontranslucent chronic swellings of the scrotum should call to mind malignant disease of the testes, tuberculosis of the epididymis and gumma of the testicle. Acute testicular swellings usually are caused by epididymitis or torsion of the testicle (Fig. 297).

An encysted hydrocele of the cord may be confused with an indirect inguinal hernia. The former does not transmit an impulse on coughing, and it is not reducible unless a communication with the abdominal cavity exists. A simple method of differentiating the 2 is to place gentle traction caudally on the testis; it will be noted that if the mass is a hydrocele of the cord, it will move with the testis with traction (Fig. 292).

11

Genitourinary Conditions

Under this heading will be included only those conditions which more commonly fall into the realm of general surgery. Therefore, this section is divided into:

1. Urologic conditions causing abdominal pain
2. Hematuria
3. Scrotal enlargements

Trauma involving the genitourinary tract is discussed in Chapter 13.

UROLOGIC CONDITIONS CAUSING PAIN

Renal and ureteral pain is due to an increase in pressure within the kidney capsule, the renal pelvis or the ureter. Such obstructions produce referred abdominal pain which follows the course of the kidney, the ureter and the bladder. Some authorities believe that involvement of various segments of the ureter result in different locations of referred pain. Hence, they state that upper ureteral lesions produce pain radiating over the crest of the ilium, whereas involvement of the lower segments of the ureter is associated with pain which passes into the groin, the genitalia, and the medial aspect of the thigh (Fig. 293). The pain may radiate to the right upper abdominal quadrant and cause diagnostic confusion. Such exceptions are difficult to explain.

If a ureteral obstruction is complete, the pain is more severe and colicky, and the referred pain pattern is more typical. However, if the obstruction is partial, renal tenderness is frequently absent, and the pain may not appear in the costovertebral angle. In the latter instance the pain approximates the segmental distribution.

When the right kidney or ureter is involved, the pain and the tenderness can simulate acute appendicitis. The history and the physical findings usually will differentiate the 2. The term "Murphy punch" suggests a pugilistic approach to surgical diagnosis. Rough or punching maneuvers have no place in diagnostic armamentarium. Specific tenderness and spasm of the erector spinae muscle group can be demonstrated by gentle palpation which will give adequate information. A patient suffering with colicky pain moves about, but one affected with peritonitis lies perfectly quiet (Fig. 294). Examination of the urine may reveal pus, blood or clumping. However, if the obstruction is complete, the urine on the involved side will be blocked, and the urinalysis will be normal.

The importance of emergency intravenous urograms, *without* cleansing enemas (if such enemas are contraindicated) cannot be overemphasized. Such urograms frequently reveal the site of the lesion.

The flat roentgenogram is also helpful, since it reveals a calculus in about 85 per cent of the cases.

Bradycardia is particularly suggestive of a renal or a ureteral block.

HEMATURIA

All the causes of hematuria are too numerous to present. Some of the more common ones, however, are depicted in Figure 295. One must never forget the possibility of a blood dyscrasia. An acutely inflamed appendix which is in direct contact with the ureter also may cause hematuria.

If blood appears at the beginning of micturition and then disappears, a urethral lesion must be suspected; if blood is present throughout the entire act of micturition, a lesion of the kidney is probably present; if the urine is clear at the beginning of micturition and becomes bloody at the end, a lesion involving the bladder must be sought (Fig. 296).

The differential diagnosis must include *retroperitoneal tumors*. These may be divided, in a broad sense, into 3 categories:

1. Tumors arising in organs which are located in the retroperitoneal space
2. Primary or metastatic tumors which involve the retroperitoneal lymph nodes
3. Unattached tumors (lipomas, cysts, fibromas, dermoids, malignant tumors, etc.)

Some of the more specialized methods used in the differential diagnosis of these lesions are pyelography, pneumography (gas introduced into the retroperitoneal space either by the lumbar or the presacral route), and arteriography. Some of these methods are not without danger.

SCROTAL ENLARGEMENTS

Although the scrotum contains few structures, enlargements in this region may present diagnostic difficulties. Four outstanding points must be established in the history:

1. Onset—acute or chronic
2. Presence or absence of pain
3. History of trauma
4. The duration of the enlargement

It has been found helpful to divide such swellings into painful and painless lesions (Fig. 297). The *painful* enlargements include epididymitis, acute orchitis, and torsion of the testicle. The *painless* enlargements include hydrocele, hematocele, tumors of the testicle, spermatocele, varicocele and *nonstrangulated* indirect inguinal hernias. The differential diagnosis of these conditions has been discussed under their respective headings.

Varicocele is a common congenital swelling of the spermatic cord that usually occurs on the left side (Fig. 297). It results from varicosities of the pampiniform plexus and presents a characteristic "bag of worms" sensation to the examining fingers. A varicocele on the right side suggests a malignant

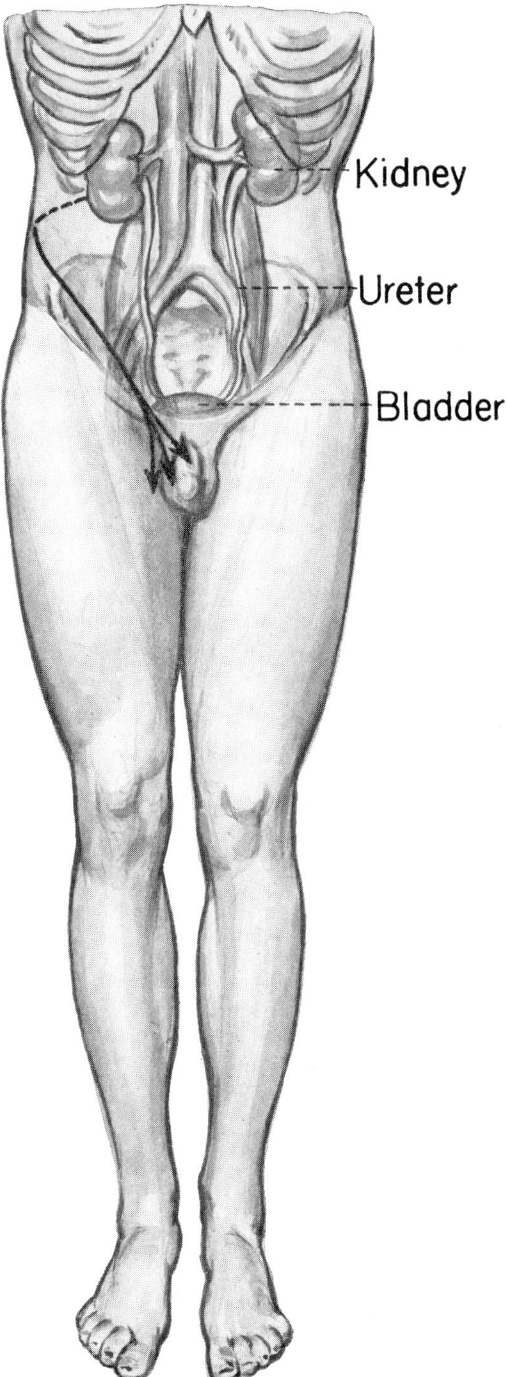

FIG. 293. Renal (ureteral) pain is referred downward along the course of the kidney, the ureter and the bladder.

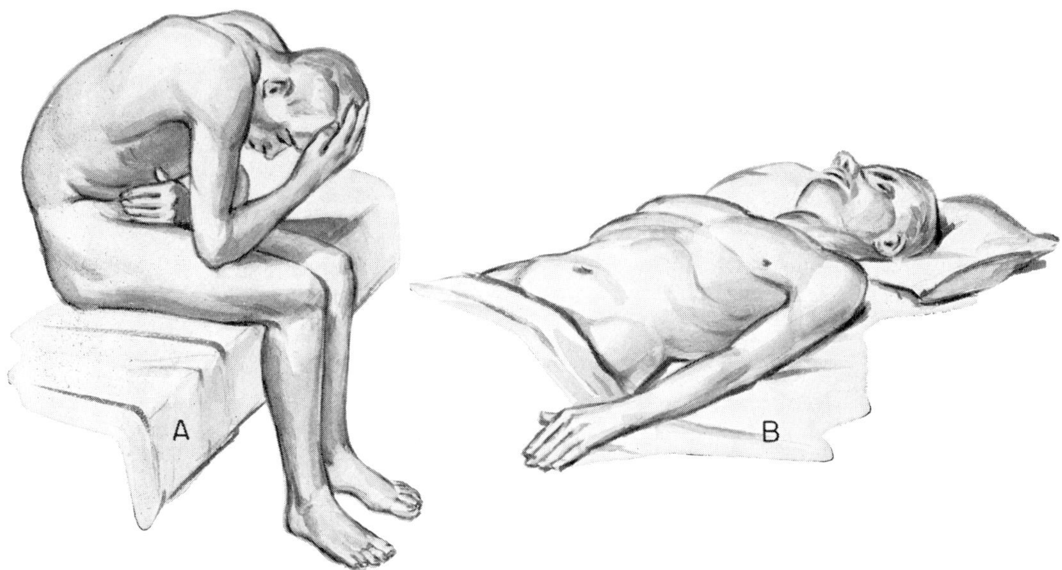

FIG. 294. Colic or peritonitis? (1) The patient with colic moves about or sits. (2) The patient with peritonitis lies perfectly quiet.

process obstructing the right spermatic veins. Another suggestion of malignancy is sudden venous engorgement within the spermatic cord after maturity. Metastases from testicular or renal carcinoma are the usual causes.

Acute funiculitis is a diffuse swelling with marked tenderness of the spermatic cord. It is generally a complication of acute prostatitis, cystitis and/or urethritis.

Torsion of the spermatic cord usually occurs before puberty but may commence at any age. Trauma or exertion is the general precipitating factor. The first symptom is severe and acute testicular pain, nausea and, at times, mild shock. A reddish-blue cystic swelling on one side of the scrotal contents is suggestive. If the patient is seen soon after the onset, the cord or the testicle may be detorted by gently elevating and rotating the testicle; this gives immediate relief. Since the testicle may twist in either direction, detorsion should be attempted accordingly. Should the torsion be complete, strangulation and gangrene of the testicle results in a few hours, necessitating orchiectomy. It is frequently difficult to differentiate torsion from acute epididymitis or orchitis. J. C. Angell of London suggests that 2 anomalies predispose to testicular torsion: (1) the 2 layers of tunica vaginalis which normally invest the testis alone extend higher to cover the epididymis and the cord and (2) frequently the testis is separated from the epididymis by a lengthened mesorchium. This occurs bilaterally (Fig. 298). The patient should be examined while standing. The affected testicle is drawn up by the torsion, but the *"normal"* testicle lies in a vertical position. If differentiation is impossible, surgical exploration is indicated. Torsion also must be differentiated from a strangulated inguinal hernia.

Tumors are more common in the spermatic cord than in the epididymis or the testicular tunics. They are usually benign, and the most common variety is a lipoma. Sarcoma is the most common malignant tumor of the spermatic cord.

Hydrocele is the most frequent intrascrotal swelling (p. 267). It is a collection of serous fluid within the tunica vaginalis which may be congenital, traumatic, inflammatory or secondary to a testicular tumor. Congenital hydroceles may disappear shortly after birth. A persistent communication between the peritoneal cavity and the tunica vaginalis results in a hydrocele which changes its size (reducing hydrocele). Often it disappears

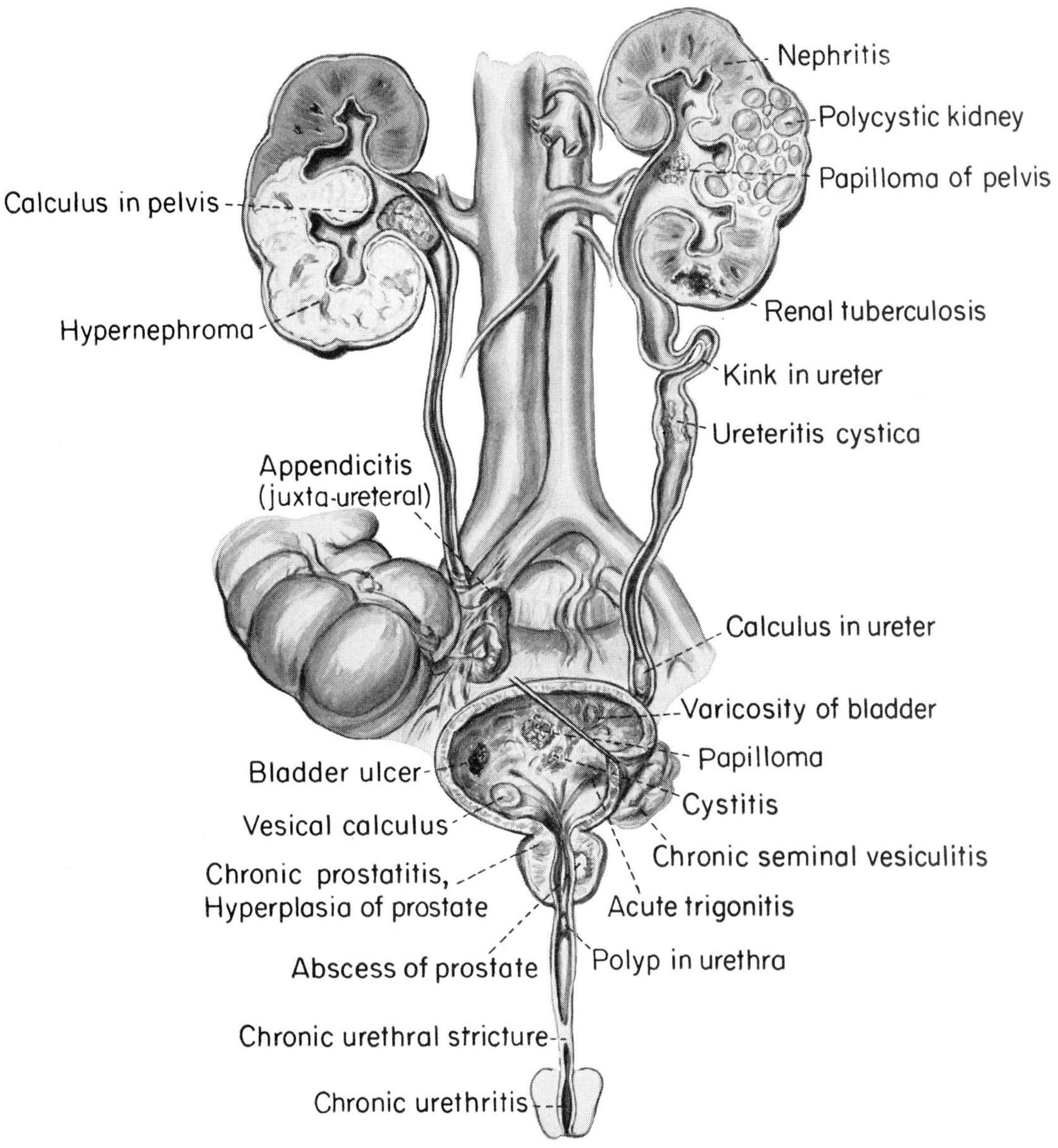

FIG. 295. Some of the more common causes of hematuria.

when the patient is recumbent, and frequently it accompanies a hernia. Hydroceles must be differentiated from scrotal hernias, spermatoceles and tumors. A spermatocele may become large enough to resemble a hydrocele, but the former is posterior to the testicle. Small spermatoceles are isolated cystic swellings associated with the epididymis. Their contents are milky and include spermatozoa, whereas hydrocele fluid is serous.

Acute epididymitis is the most common inflammatory lesion involving the scrotal contents. It may be due to any pathogen which infects the urinary tract, but usually it is a complication of urethritis, cystitis and/or prostatitis. Trauma is a questionable etiologic factor. It is characterized by pain, tenderness, scrotal redness, swelling of the epididymis and toxic symptoms. Tuberculous epididymitis lacks the tenderness and the other evidences of acute inflammation.

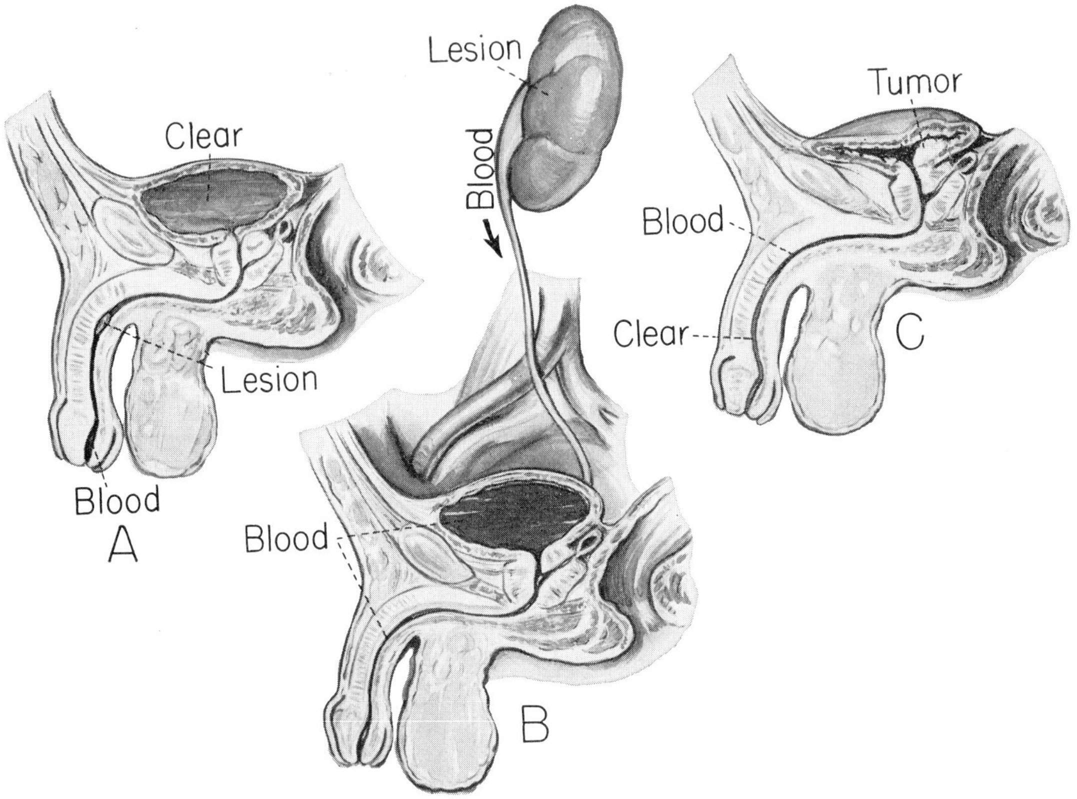

FIG. 296. If blood appears at the beginning of micturition and then disappears, a urethral lesion is suspected; if blood is present throughout the entire act of micturition, a kidney lesion is probably present; if the urine is clear at the beginning of micturition and then becomes bloody, a bladder lesion is the probable cause.

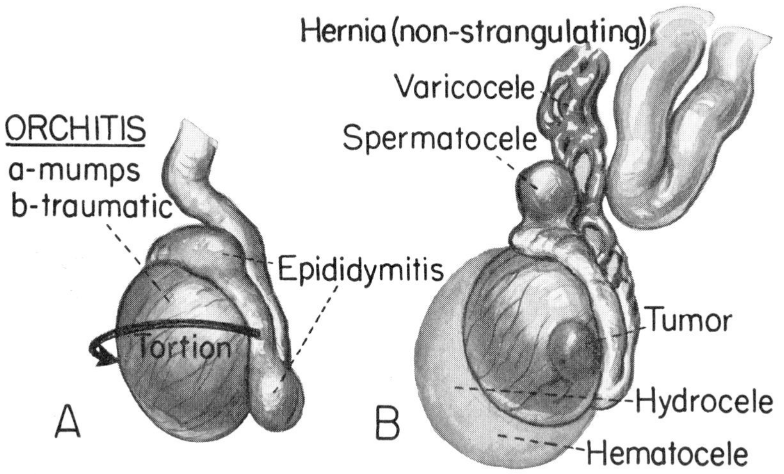

FIG. 297. Differential diagnosis of scrotal swellings.

Acute epididymo-orchitis is due to gonococcal infection, mumps, or nonspecific pyogenic infections. It may be associated with instrumentation.

Tumors of the testis must be considered to be malignant until they are proved to be otherwise. The exceptions to this are the rare fibroma of the tunica albuginea and the so-called adenomatoid tumor that is found in the epididymis. Although testicular neoplasms may be found at any age, they occur predominantly between the ages of 20 and 35 (the age of greatest sexual activity). To attempt to classify these tumors to everyone's satisfaction is an almost impossible task. A simple classification has been suggested.

1. Seminoma
2. Teratoma
3. Interstitial cell tumors

Seminoma is the most common testicular malignancy and the least malignant. *Teratoma* (mixed tumor) may reproduce any type of tissue. They are highly malignant, metastasize hematogenously and lymphogenously, and can contain both differentiated and undifferentiated tissues (bone, cartilage, nervous tissue, teeth and hair). The *interstitial cell tumors* arise from the Leydig cells. They cause virilization and enlargement of breasts before puberty. They are usually benign. It is unfortunate that testicular tumors produce symptoms so late; too often the first symptoms are due to the metastatic lesions. The metastases of these tumors tend to skip past the regional lymph glands and to cross to the opposite side. They often spread to mediastinal glands and the supraclavicular nodes; blood-borne metastases to the lungs and the liver are common.

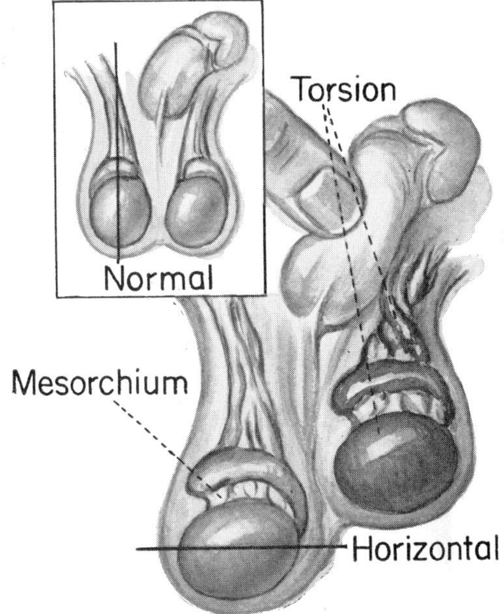

FIG. 298. The normal testicle assumes a vertical position. Testes which lie in a horizontal position are predisposed to torsion.

IDIOPATHIC RETROPERITONEAL FIBROSIS

This condition is being recognized more frequently and brought to the attention of the clinician. It has become an intriguing and fascinating diagnostic challenge. Other names assigned to it are periureteral fascitis, perirenal (Gerota's) fascitis, nonspecific retroperitoneal inflammation, periureteral fibrosis and periureteritis plastica. It is probably more prevalent than the literature suggests. Undiagnosed annoying "backache," gynecologic disturbances, unexplained gastrointestinal symptoms and unilateral extremity edema are examples of overlooked idiopathic retroperitoneal fibrosis.

J. K. Ormand published the first accurate description and recognized this entity in 1948. His patient was a 45-year-old man who died of bilateral ureteral obstruction due to an "inflammatory retroperitoneal process" of unknown origin. Although the etiology is not known, it is interesting that cases were not reported in the preantibiotic era; whether or not this fact is coincidental has not been determined. Practically everything ranging from allergy, malignancy and viruses has been suspected. The basic histopathologic processes are those of fibrosis with variable degrees of inflammatory reaction. Biopsies of these lesions work a great hardship on the diagnostic ability of qualified pathologists.

Symptomatology. Any patient with an un-

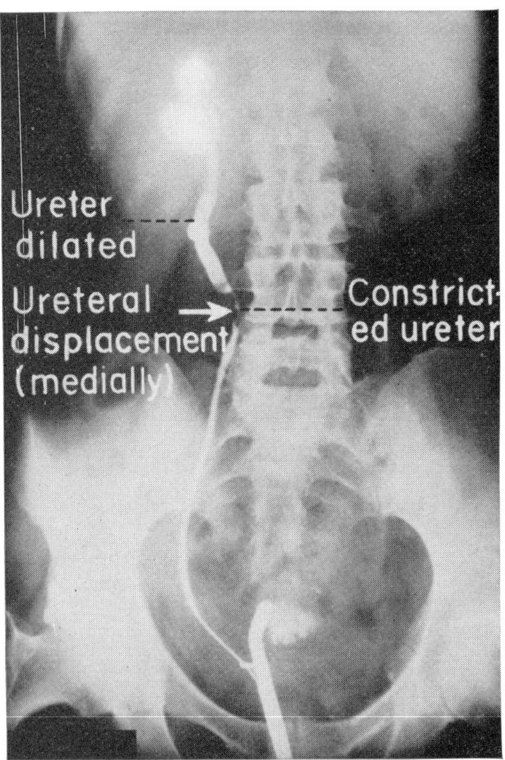

FIG. 299. Idiopathic retroperitoneal fibrosis. Retrograde pyelogram revealed the typical constricted and medially deviated segment of ureter on the patient's right side. Slight dilatation is noted above this point of constriction. Medial deviation of the ureter is almost pathognomonic of this condition.

explained *backache* or vague *epigastric distress* and/or *gastrointestinal complaints* should be suspected of having idiopathic retroperitoneal fibrosis. The urinary symptoms are conspicuous by their absence. Obstruction of the internal spermatic vessels may produce testicular pain; obstruction of the abdominal aorta, the vena cava and/or the iliac vessels may give rise to vascular symptoms and possible occlusion. The fibrotic plaques often form over the presacral plexus and produce unexplained impotency and loss of libido. Obstruction of the common bile duct with jaundice has been reported. The process can extend upward to the region of the diaphragm and is not solely localized to the true pelvis. In the preanuric phase the symptoms may be so vague that it is impossible to recognize the condition as urologic. Most of these patients are referred to the orthopedic, neurologic, medical, surgical and/or psychiatric services before they reach the urologist. The condition has been known to cause intestinal obstructions, especially when the large bowel is involved. It is extremely difficult to differentiate this from carcinomatous infiltration. Physical examination is only slightly contributory. The commonest finding is tenderness over one or both kidneys, and occasionally there is mild abdominal tenderness unassociated with rectus defense or rigidity. The roentgenographic findings usually give the first clue (Fig. 299). An involved segment of ureter is noted medial to its normal position. Since the ureter below the pelvic rim rarely is involved, it usually remains normally placed. Above the constricted area the ureter is somewhat dilated, but the dilatation in most instances is surprisingly slight. In early cases, when one or both kidneys are still functioning, the diagnosis may be made by an intravenous pyelogram; however, it is the retrograde pyelogram that is diagnostic. If the condition is permitted to progress, hydroureter, hydronephrosis and final renal damage result.

12

Gynecologic Conditions

A few gynecologic conditions warrant discussion in a text dealing with surgical diagnosis because of the differential diagnostic problems which arise. These conditions include:

1. Gonorrhea and its complications
2. Ectopic pregnancy (ruptured and unruptured)
3. Twisted pedicles (ovarian cysts and fibroids)
4. Endometriosis

GONORRHEA AND ITS COMPLICATIONS

This condition accounts for a high percentage of infections in the fallopian tubes. The gonococcus is a fragile organism; nevertheless, it spreads rapidly through the endometrium and into the tubes. Suppuration occurs, and frank pus exudes from the fimbriated ends of the tubes, resulting in a pelvic peritonitis. Because of the deep position of the pelvic peritoneum and the low virulence of the organism, the infection remains somewhat localized; however, the tubes, the ovaries, the omentum and the bowel are involved frequently. This tendency to involve more than 1 structure permits one to consider this subject under the heading of "pelvic inflammatory disease."

Pelvic inflammatory disease usually is associated with other stigmata of gonorrhea; hence, such sites of infection should

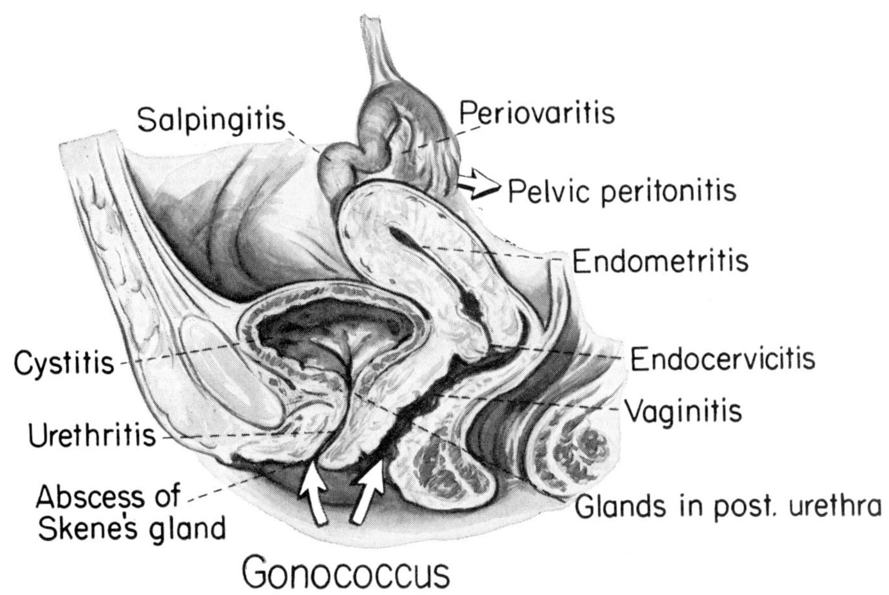

FIG. 300. Sites of gonorrhea in the female.

be sought for. They are represented by infections of the Bartholin glands, abscess of Skene's gland, vaginitis, endocervicitis, endometritis, salpingitis, tubo-ovarian abscess and pelvic peritonitis (Fig. 300). The lesions just enumerated are found in adult women; the exception is vaginitis, which appears only in childhood (juvenile vaginitis). The *onset* of an attack of pelvic inflammatory disease is related to the menstrual period, appearing immediately before, during or after menstruation. The *pain* is quite constant and characteristically starts in the lower abdomen, this being an important differential diagnostic point, since most cases of appendicitis start in the epigastrium. *Backache* is a common complaint. Disturbances in appetite (anorexia, nausea and vomiting) are not as frequent as in appendicitis. Although a pelvic peritonitis may be present, the patient does not appear to be seriously ill. In acute salpingitis the fever may reach 101° to 103°, and the pain may be bothersome, but the patient's general appearance is good. In contrast to this, by the time a patient with acute appendicitis has severe pain and fever she usually appears to be seriously ill. If pelvic inflammatory disease localizes to the right lower quadrant, and tenderness is present in the region of McBurney's point, the differential diagnosis between it and acute appendicitis is most taxing. Localization in the right lower quadrant in cases of salpingitis is explained by the "watershed" action of a redundant sigmoid which directs the pus and the exudate to the right (Fig. 301).

The *vaginal and rectal examinations* are particularly helpful in the differential diagnosis. If a vaginal discharge is present, it may contain gonococci; however, this organism disappears rapidly and may be difficult to demonstrate. Positive smears may be found in Bartholin or Skene's glands. Bimanual vaginal examinations are conducted if the hymen is not intact; rectal examinations are conducted; but of more value than either of these is the so-called bidigital examination (Fig. 172). This is accomplished by placing the index finger in the vaginal orifice and the middle finger in the anal orifice. One can immediately differentiate a fecal mass from the cervix and the adnexae. The examiner should attempt carefully to elicit pain on moving the cervix. This is one of the most characteristic and constant findings of pelvic inflammation. Induration, bulging, or distinct masses may be identified in the lateral fornices. The posterior cul-de-sac, if involved, also may present a distinct

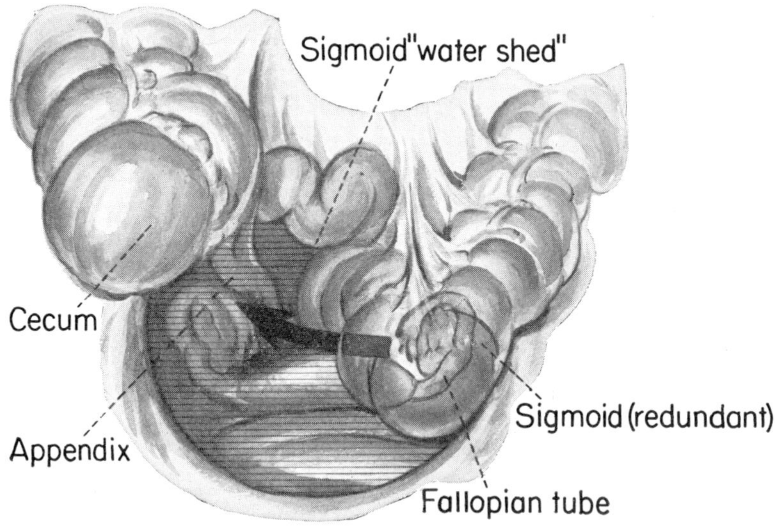

Fig. 301. Pus from an infected left fallopian tube is directed to the region of the appendix by the "watershed" action of a redundant sigmoid.

bulging. Although tenderness is present over the abdomen, muscle spasm is not marked. Unlike neoplasms, inflammatory masses do not present a sharply defined margin but rather a bulge or resistance.

Signs of small-bowel, nonstrangulated, complete or incomplete intestinal obstruction appear when loops of ileum become attached to the inflamed area (p. 176).

If a *pelvic abscess* develops, the examining finger can detect immediately whether this mass is bulging or pointing. Bulging is, as the name signifies, a forward resistance; however, if this mass is fluctuant, it will point; the latter resembles the soft over-ripened spot on an apple or a pear (Fig. 302). If the latter is present, the mass is ready to be opened.

The direct diagnosis of pelvic inflammatory disease is important, because in most

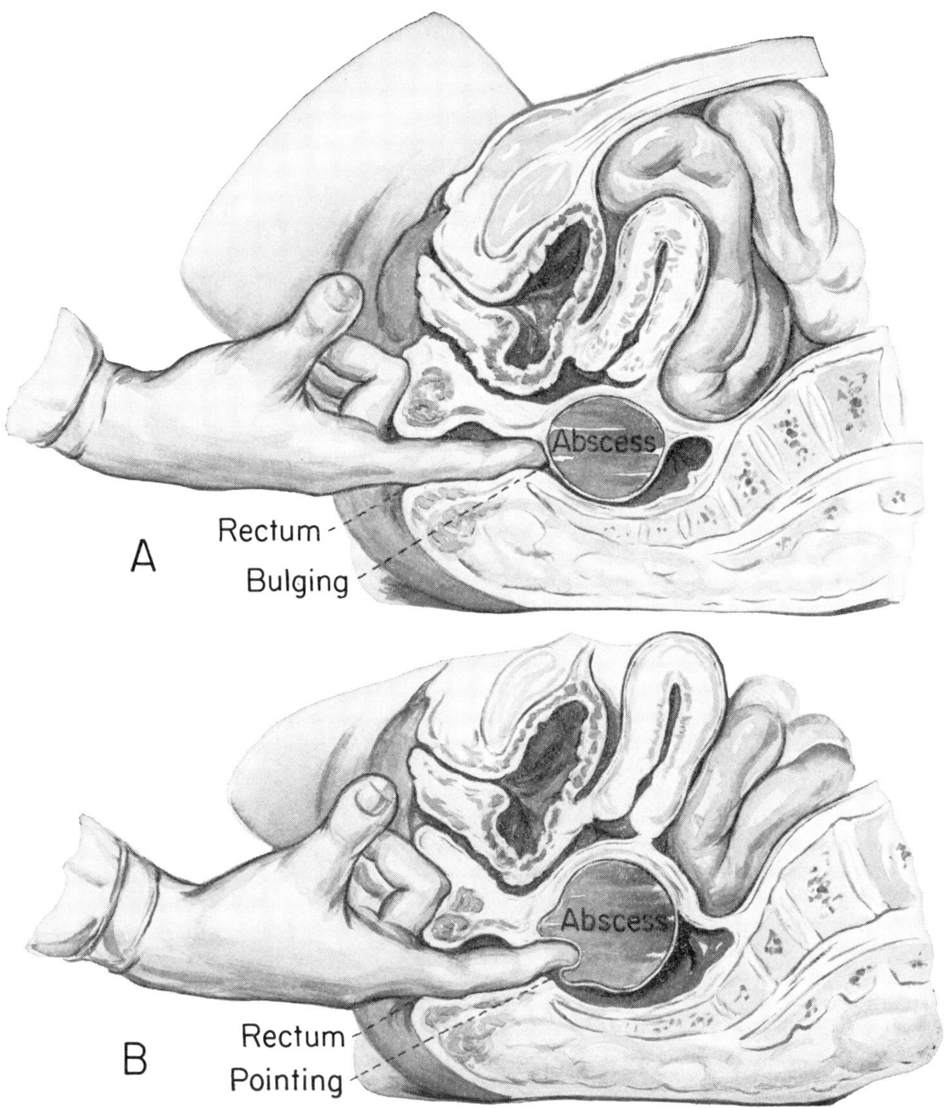

FIG. 302. Bulging or pointing? Bulging masses present a firm rounded resistance. Pointing is produced by a fluctuant mass and presents a "soft spot" in the rounded mass.

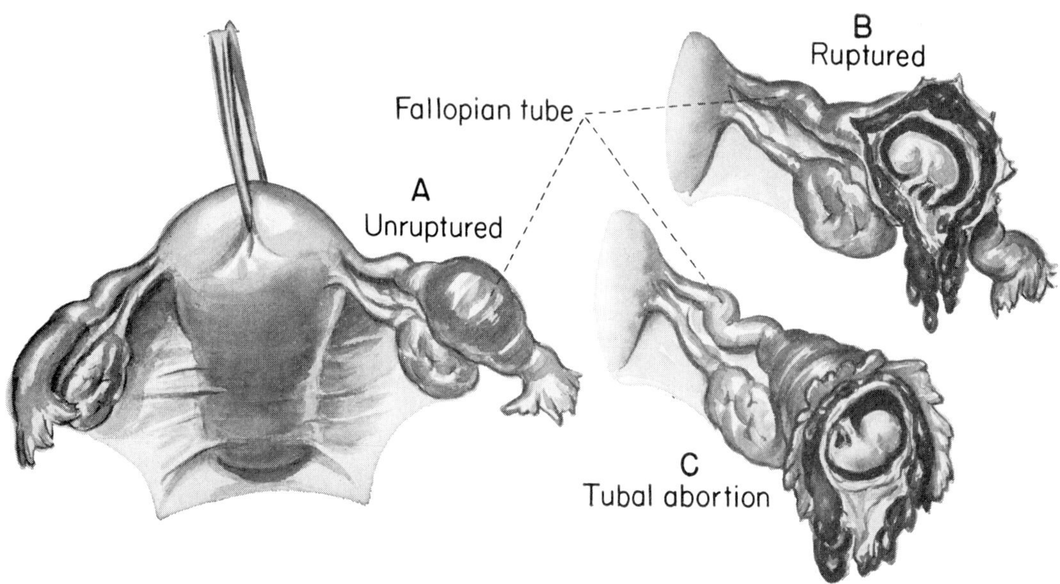

FIG. 303. Ectopic (tubal) pregnancy can be divided into (1) unruptured, (2) ruptured and (3) tubal abortion.

instances this condition may be treated conservatively; elective surgery can be delayed or frequently avoided. Despite all of our differential diagnostic acumen, the seasoned physician knows that in some instances it is impossible to differentiate acute salpingitis from acute appendicitis. If such a dilemma exists, it is better to err on the side of safety and explore.

Ruptured graafian follicle (so-called mittelschmerz) may simulate pelvic inflammatory disease or acute appendicitis. It occurs in the intermenstrual phase at that time when the graafian follicle ruptures. The degree of hemorrhage will determine the extent of peritoneal irritation. If the diagnosis is in doubt, exploration is advised. Unless a well-developed peritonitis is present, these cases lack signs of inflammatory disease and rarely, if ever, present an appreciable elevation in fever or in the white blood count.

ECTOPIC (TUBAL) PREGNANCY

By ectopic pregnancy is meant the development of a fertilized ovum in any place other than the uterine cavity. When such fertilized ova develop in the fallopian tube, we refer to this as a tubal pregnancy. In tubal gestation growth of the ovum produces tubal distention; the eroding action of the villi results in a thinning and tearing of the tubal wall. This condition should be differentiated into:

1. Unruptured tubal pregnancy
2. Ruptured tubal pregnancy
3. Tubal abortion (Fig. 303)

UNRUPTURED TUBAL PREGNANCY

In an unruptured tubal pregnancy there is a gradual oozing of blood in to the peritoneal cavity as the tube slowly distends and tears. This condition is associated with an insidious onset but requires immediate and accurate diagnosis. Constant pain, although not severe, is a result of tubal distention.

TUBAL ABORTION

Peristalsis of the tube during the course of a tubal abortion may give rise to cramping pain (coliclike) and some localized tenderness.

RUPTURED TUBAL PREGNANCY

Ruptured tubal pregnancy is a comparatively common condition with fairly characteristic signs and symptoms.

The diagnosis should not be difficult if

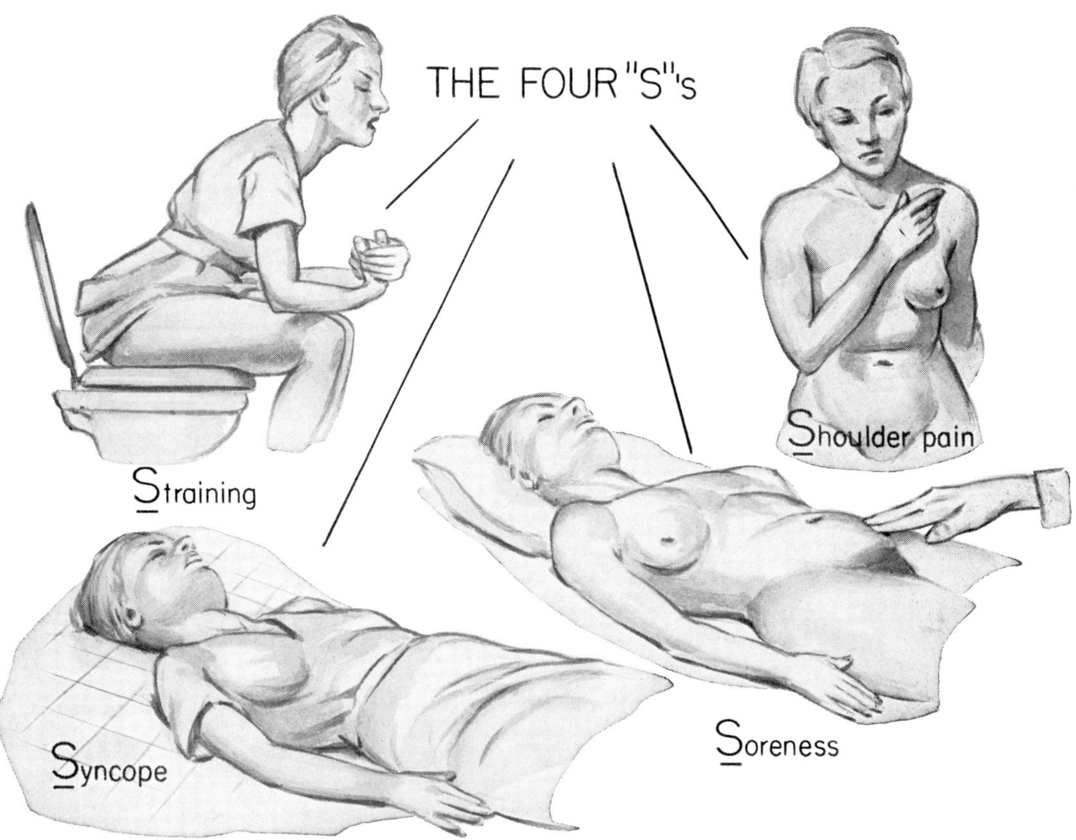

FIG. 304. In the diagnosis of ruptured tubal pregnancy the 4 "S's" constitute a helpful mnemonic.

the case is typical. The severity of the clinical picture depends on the amount of blood loss and the acuteness of the rupture. Sudden lancinating pain is always present. Often it is precipitated by such exertion as is associated with defecating, voiding, lifting or copulating. The patient frequently relates the story that while straining at stool this severe pain struck like "a bolt out of the sky." Following this onset, which frequently is associated with "fainting," a generalized soreness and tenderness develop over the entire abdomen. The pain and tenderness are greater in the lower abdomen and frequently center in the right lower abdominal quadrant regardless of which tube has ruptured. This is explained by the watershed action of a redundant mesosigmoid which guides the escaping blood to the region of the appendix (Fig. 301). Rarely do the symptoms subside enough to permit the patient to continue her usual daily routine. About 20 per cent of these patients complain of pain in the region of the shoulder or the supraclavicular area. This is explained by the fact that blood moves under the diaphragm and irritates the phrenic nerve (Fig. 304).

Shock, or a shocklike picture, probably prostration, is present in about 25 per cent of these patients.

The menstrual history of such patients usually reveals some irregularity. Normal menses may be absent, or abnormal uterine bleeding may occur. Over half of these women give a history of having amenorrhea followed by a spotty type of uterine bleeding; however, there is no characteristic type of menstrual irregularity.

Secondary signs of pregnancy, such as the presence of colostrum and enlargement of the breasts and the uterus, are helpful if present.

Physical examination reveals *abdominal tenderness* in all cases with the exception of those patients who are prostrate. The tenderness is found more frequently on the right, because more ectopic pregnancies involve the right tube, and, as stated, the path along the mesosigmoid directs blood from ruptured tubes to the right side. Rigidity is mild and not too significant. The author has yet to see a positive Cullen's sign (bluish discoloration in the umbilical region) in his 25 years of practice. It must be very rare.

Pelvic examination is most helpful. The cervix feels soft and appears bluish. Any movement or manipulation of it results in excruciating pain. This is noted in over 80 per cent of the cases; it must be elicited gently. In well over half of the cases a definite tender mass or bulging can be felt in the fornices or the posterior cul-de-sac. Some enlargement of the uterus also may be present. The gloved examining fingers should be inspected for the presence of a dirty brownish discharge which is characteristic of tubal pregnancies; this is in contrast with the copious bright-red blood seen in threatened uterine abortions. Gynecologists and obstetricians have stressed the importance of aspiration of the posterior cul-de-sac. They state that the demonstration of a hemoperitoneum is an accurate method of diagnosing ectopic pregnancy (Fig. 305).

Laboratory aids are not completely reliable or specifically diagnostic. The red blood cell count is rarely under 3,000,000 unless the hemorrhage has been massive. The various hormonal tests, sedimentation rate, white blood count, or diagnostic curettage may give contributory evidence but are not thoroughly reliable.

The differential diagnosis is essentially that of the "acute abdomen."

TWISTED PEDICLES

Any intra-abdominal mass that is pedunculated may twist; the most common are ovarian cysts and uterine fibroids (Fig. 306). The nature and the degree of pain varies with the degree of torsion. If the torsion is complete, the pain is so severe that it is difficult to control with opiates. If, however, it is incomplete, or if detorsion takes place, the onset is gradual, and the pain is negligible. Torsion of any viscus is associated with vomiting. This occurs almost as soon as the pain appears, so that there is a short interval or no interval between the initial pain and vomiting. The pain is located in the lower abdomen, and tenderness frequently is uni-

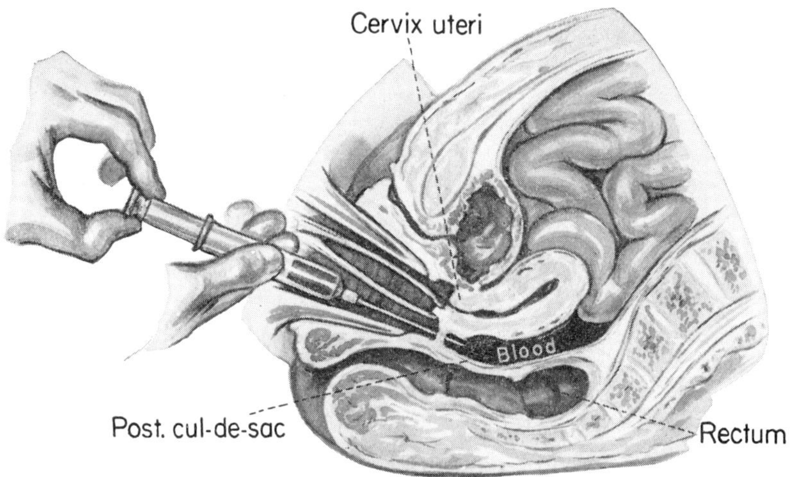

FIG. 305. The demonstration of a hemoperitoneum by aspiration of the posterior cul-de-sac.

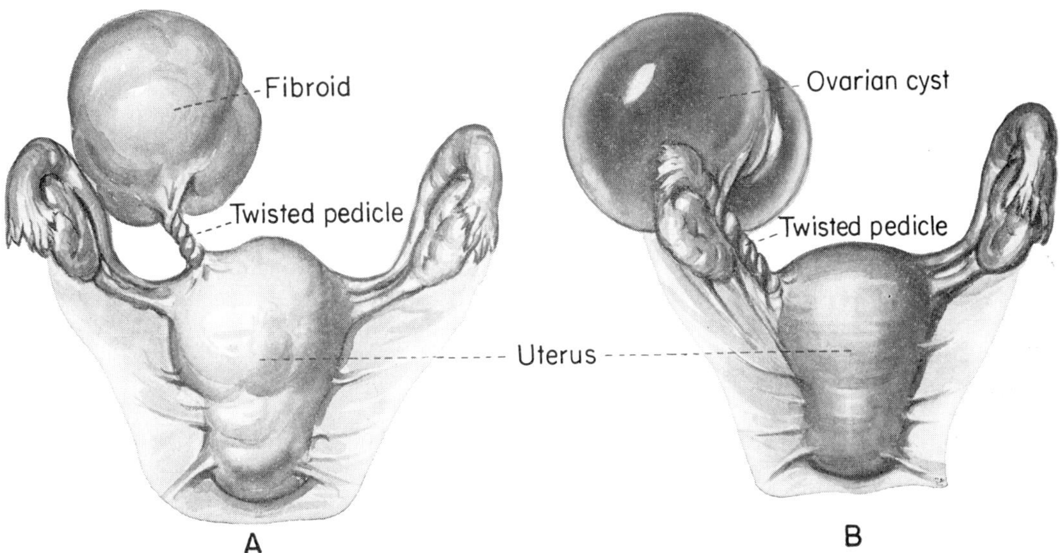

FIG. 306. The most common pelvic masses that may twist are pedunculated uterine fibroids and ovarian cysts.

lateral until a spreading peritonitis sets in. The pain has a tendency to radiate down the thighs. If the torsion is complete, and the blood supply to the viscus is occluded, shock or a shocklike picture becomes evident. Fever and leukocytosis increase as the twisted viscus becomes necrotic. In most instances a mass is palpable, abdominally, vaginally, or by means of a bidigital examination (Fig. 172). When rigidity is marked, it becomes difficult to outline the mass.

ENDOMETRIOSIS

This condition implies invasion by the endometrium of tissues and areas that are foreign to it. The most common sites are the uterus, the ovaries and the pouch of Douglas. Extragenital locations include the bowel, the umbilicus, the bladder, or the ureter (Fig. 307). Although this condition is common, it frequently is undiagnosed or misdiagnosed, because the history is either not properly taken or interpreted.

Acquired dysmenorrhea and/or progressive dysmenorrhea should make one suspicious of endometriosis. When the complaint of painful periods is elicited, it must be determined whether or not such periods have been present since menarche. It will be found that these patients state that their periods were normal and painless until a given time when pain became apparent.

The dysmenorrhea becomes progressively worse with succeeding cycles. When endometriosis affects the ovary, it frequently produces the so-called "chocolate" or "tarry" cyst (retained menstrual blood). If such a cyst ruptures, severe peritoneal irritation results.

Acquired dyspareunia is a frequent complaint. These patients state that sexual intercourse has become painful, whereas prior to a given time it was not. Other causes may be responsible for this symptom; however, it should suggest the possibility of endometriosis.

Other symptoms include pelvic pain, infertility and abnormal (usually excessive) menstruation. Cyclic bleeding from the rectum, periodic attacks of intestinal obstruction at the time of the menstrual period, backache, and pain in the region of the groin and the umbilicus may be present. If backache is due to a retro-displaced uterus, it is readily relieved by a well-fitted pessary. This would not be so in endometriosis.

Physical examination frequently reveals a shotty sensation posterior to the cervix; this can be felt per rectum. Some authorities believe that shotty nodules in the region of the uterosacral ligaments are the earliest and most frequent findings. Such nodules are dependent on the location of the endometrial implants; they may be felt in the region of the ovary or the anterior and the posterior cul-de-sacs. Cystoscopy may reveal involvement of the bladder. The final diagnosis rests with the microscopic demonstration of endometrial tissue.

RUPTURED GRAAFIAN FOLLICLE

This condition must be included in the differential diagnosis of acute abdominal conditions. This diagnosis should be considered in any woman who gives a history of acute abdominal pain that occurs in the intermenstrual period. The severity of the symptoms is dependent on the amount of intraperitoneal hemorrhage. Tenderness and bulging may be present in the posterior cul-de-sac. Adnexal tenderness is most marked on the side on which the rupture occurred. This condition is most frequently confused with acute appendicitis, ruptured ectopic pregnancy, or salpingitis.

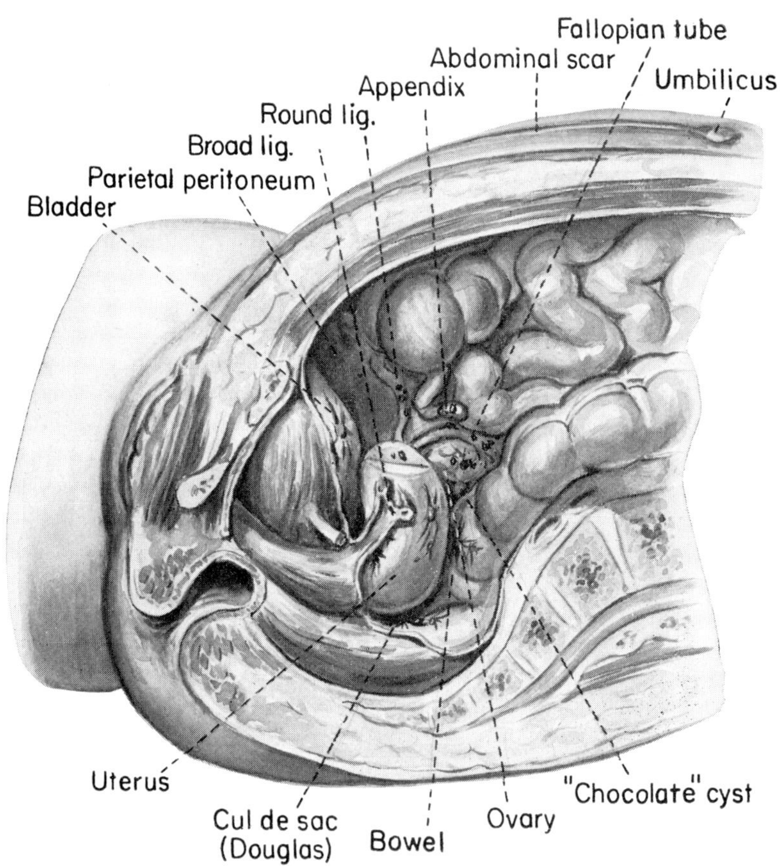

Fig. 307. Some sites of endometrial implants.

13

Abdominal Injuries

The diagnosis of a serious intra-abdominal injury is not always possible immediately after the accident. Frequently, trauma without visceral injury causes enough disturbance to the nervous system to produce an initial period of collapse. An injury to the *deep epigastric vessels* with hemorrhage into the anterior abdominal wall may be equally confusing. To add further to the diagnostician's dilemma is the fact that retroperitoneal hemorrhage and/or a fracture of the spine are frequently followed by ileus. It is a truism that delay encourages deterioration; however, watchful expectancy (3 to 6 hours) is permissible when the diagnosis is doubtful. It is incumbent on the clinician to be on guard for signs and symptoms of *shock, hemorrhage* and *infection.*

Any injury to the abdominal wall, however slight, may be accompanied by serious lesions of the contained viscera. Since the signs and symptoms of intraperitoneal mischief are often equivocal for some hours, it becomes mandatory to examine the abdomen at *half-hour intervals.* These examinations should be done by the *same individual.*

A plan must be followed in evaluating a patient who has sustained trauma to the abdomen. When one possesses such a definite plan, valuable time is saved, no organs are overlooked, and proper therapy is instituted readily. The plan that has been most suc-

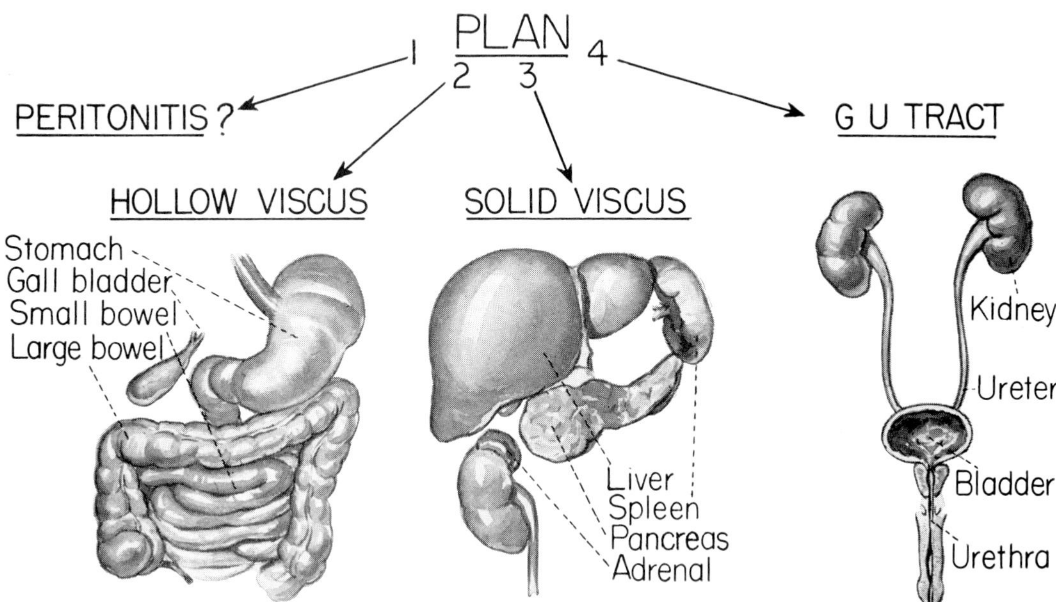

FIG. 308. A workable plan which aids the clinician in evaluating the "traumatic abdomen."

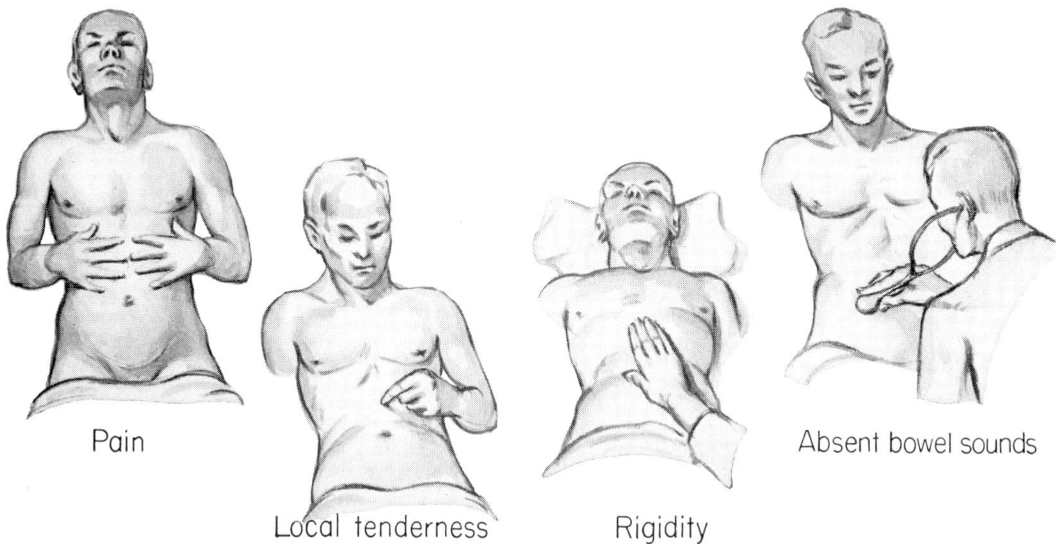

Fig. 309. Early signs and symptoms of peritonitis are depicted. These are dependent on the degree of peritoneal soiling.

cessful in the author's hands is one in which 4 questions are considered (Fig. 308):

1. Are signs of peritonitis present?
2. Is a hollow viscus injured?
3. Is a solid viscus injured?
4. Is the genitourinary tract injured?

It is possible that multiple injuries may be present.

ARE SIGNS OF PERITONITIS PRESENT? (Fig. 309)

The more important and earlier signs of peritonitis are:

Abdominal pain
Localized tenderness
Muscular rigidity
Diminution and/or absence of bowel sounds

Elevation of pulse, distention, pelvic peritoneal tenderness, shifting dullness and vomiting are signs of far-advanced peritonitis (Fig. 310). If the signs subside, surgical intervention rarely is indicated; however, if they remain stationary or increase, surgical exploration is warranted. Exceptions will be discussed subsequently.

IS A HOLLOW VISCUS INJURED?

The hollow viscera that must be considered in abdominal trauma are the stomach, the duodenum, the jejuno-ileum, the colon, the rectum and the biliary tract.

Stomach

Rupture usually occurs when this organ is full, or if some pre-existing lesion produces a point of weakness. Since the stomach usually contains an air bubble (magenblase) a spontaneous pneumoperitoneum is present in most cases. The air bubble escapes into the peritoneal cavity and can be seen under the fluoroscope or on a flat roentgenogram (Fig. 153). The patient should be examined in the sitting position or in a left lateral decubitus. If free air is present, it will be seen between the right hemidiaphragm and the liver. No contrast media should be given; the absence of free air does not rule out a ruptured stomach. The other signs of spreading peritonitis that have been enumerated are present. A rare type of rupture is one in which the tear has taken place on the posterior wall of the stomach, and the contents leak into the lesser peritoneal cavity (Fig. 311). In such cases the early signs of peritonitis are lacking. A flat roentgenogram usually discloses a hydropneumoperitoneum (fluid level) in the lesser omental sac.

Small Bowel and Colon

These can be considered together. The intestinal wall is sensitive only to distention;

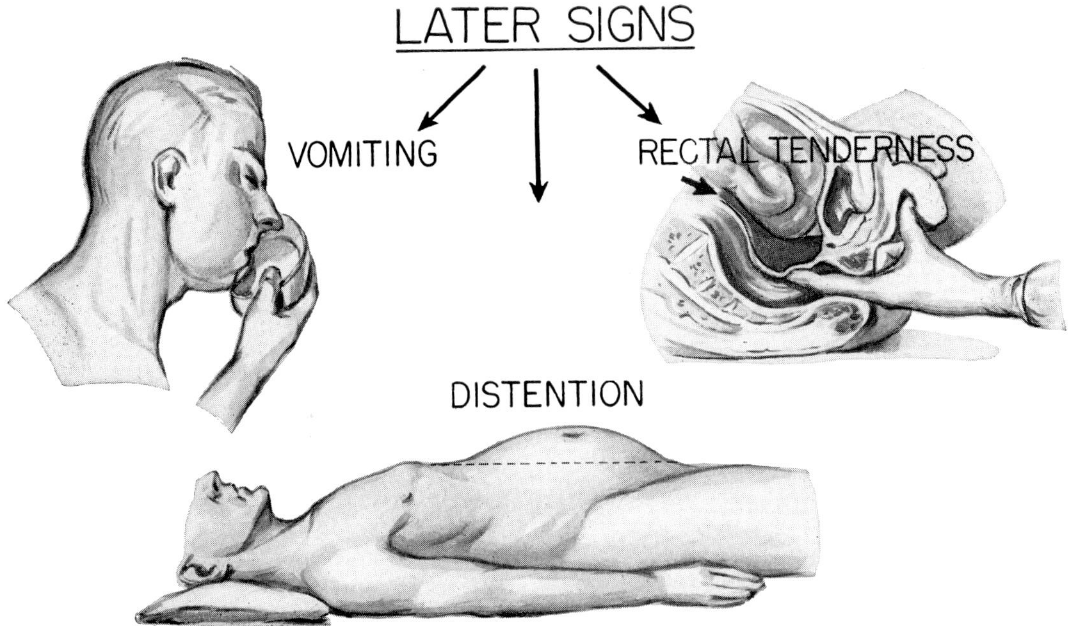

FIG. 310. Signs of later and/or far-advanced peritonitis.

therefore, pain does not occur until peritonitis develops. The clinical picture may be delayed or confused, because it is dependent on the size of the leak, the nature of the leaking contents, and whether or not the leakage takes place into the general peritoneal cavity. The tear may involve only a portion of the circumference of the bowel. If the rent is small, the edges of the mucous membrane pout and plug the gap, resulting in a negligible leak (Fig. 312). A lull in the symptoms produces a sense of false security. If food is permitted, peristaltic activity is increased, and the rent in the bowel is reopened. Spreading peritonitis then becomes apparent. If the bowel is divided completely, peritoneal soiling is marked, and the signs and symptoms are present early (Fig. 313). Perforation may occur at any point where the blow impinges the bowel against the vertebral

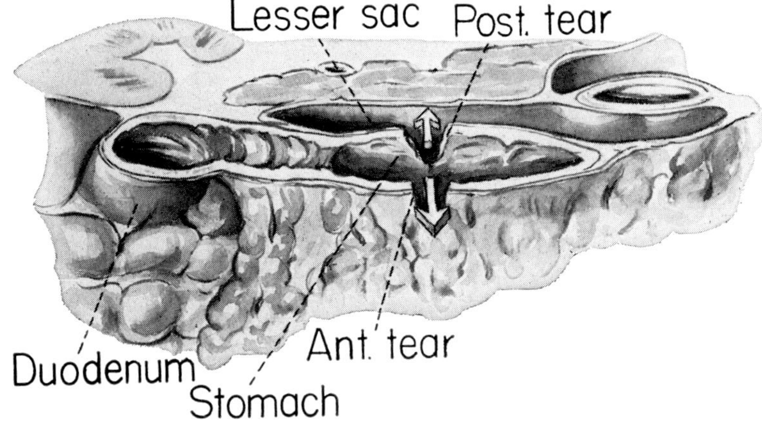

FIG. 311. Traumatic rupture of the stomach may take place anteriorly or posteriorly, as the arrows indicate. Posterior ruptures leak into the lesser peritoneal cavity.

column, and where it is more or less fixed. Such fixed points of the small bowel most commonly occur at the duodenojejunal junction and in the region of the terminal ileum (Fig. 314). Most perforations are found 6 or 8 inches distal to the ligament of Treitz. Spontaneous pneumoperitoneum is rarely demonstrated with the roentgenogram in small bowel perforations, whereas, in cases of ruptured colon, a spontaneous pneumoperitoneum can be demonstrated frequently. The reason for this is that gas is normally present in the large bowel. The exact site of the lesion can be determined only by celiotomy. If the colon is perforated, clinical evidence of peritonitis occurs with rapidity, owing to the extremely irritating quality of colonic contents.

Retroperitoneal rupture of the duodenum requires special mention (Fig. 315). The mortality is unusually high because of the difficulty in locating and repairing the rent. In over half of the cases the tear is retroperitoneal; as a result of this, signs of peritonitis are wanting, and treatment is delayed. These patients frequently have pain which is referred to the right loin; although they appear ill, they are usually ambulatory, and the seriousness of their injury is overlooked. Bowel sounds are usually normal or slightly diminished, and tenderness can be elicited only on deepest pressure. The flat roentgenogram may reveal scattered air in the retroperitoneal tissue or around the right kidney. Such findings are quite pathognomonic. Although the early symptoms are deceptively mild, the later ones are tragically grave.

Biliary Tract (Fig. 316)

These injuries are rare; they usually result from a vehicle passing directly over the abdomen. It is unlikely that a correct preoperative diagnosis will be made, since the signs and symptoms are identical with those of rupture of the small intestines. If the leak is great, chemical irritation from bile will result in rather rapid spreading and severe peritonitis. The presence of bile in the peritoneal cavity is not pathognomonic, since intraperitoneal rupture of the duodenum also may be associated with biliary peritonitis. Jaundice appears after a few days. Peritoneal aspiration in search for bile is not advocated. Such peritoneal "taps" are not without danger.

IS A SOLID VISCUS INJURED?

The abdominal cavity contains 5 solid viscera; they are the liver, the spleen, the kidney, the pancreas and the adrenals. Four of these will be considered here; the kidney is discussed under the heading of genitourinary tract.

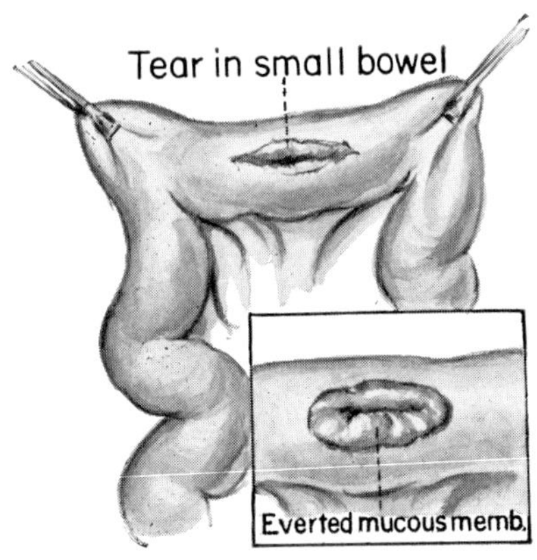

Fig. 312. A small tear in the bowel. The insert shows the everted pouting mucous membrane plugging the rent and preventing leakage.

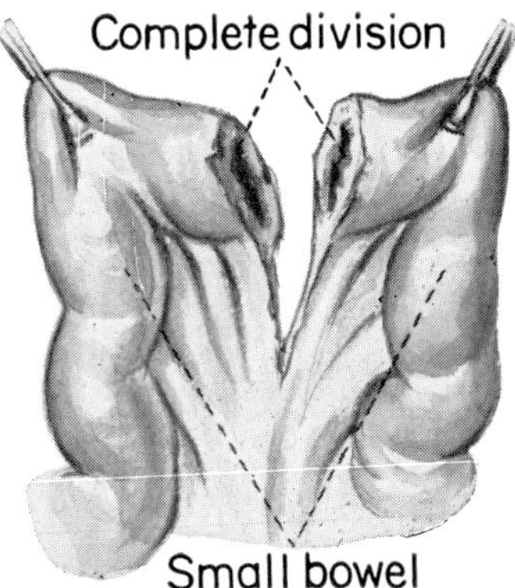

Fig. 313. The small bowel may be completely divided. It is difficult for the mucous membrane to plug such orifices.

Spleen

Trauma to this organ must be diagnosed early if these patients are to be saved. The classic picture presents no diagnostic difficulties; however, atypical splenic ruptures may lead to serious errors. Three types of rupture must be kept in mind, namely, rupture with hemorrhage into the peritoneal cavity; rupture of the splenic parenchyma with subcapsular or retroperitoneal hematoma; and delayed rupture of the spleen.

Injury to this viscus must be suspected when there is tenderness in the left upper quadrant, evidences of shock and internal hemorrhage, and injuries to the lower left ribs, particularly the 10th. The spleen may

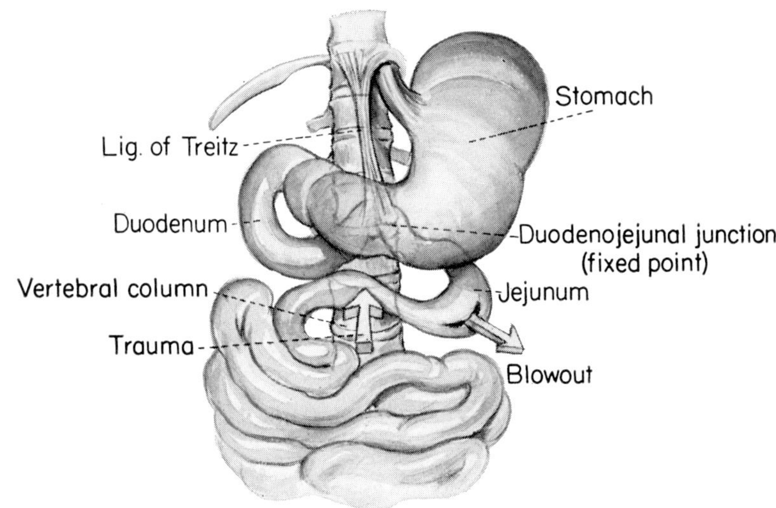

Fig. 314. The mechanism of a ruptured jejunum following trauma.

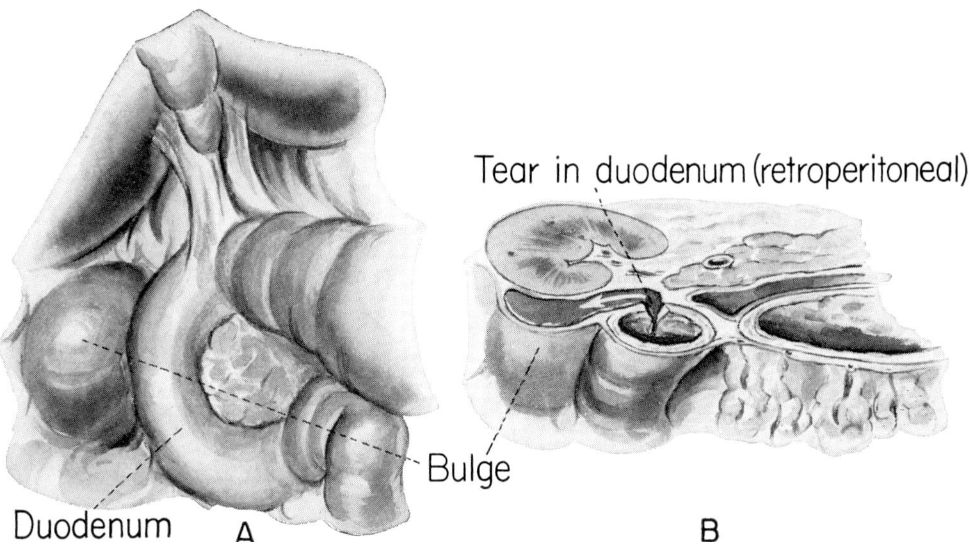

Fig. 315. Retroperitoneal rupture of the duodenum may be overlooked because of the late appearance of signs and symptoms of peritonitis.

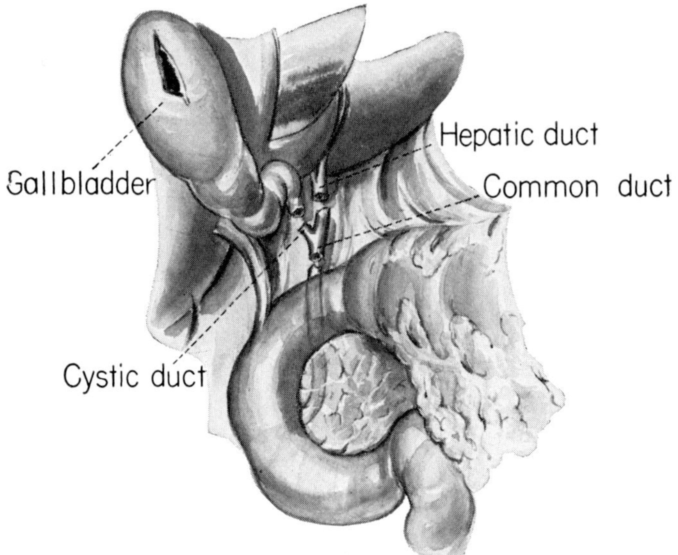

FIG. 316. Possible structures involved in an injury to the biliary tract.

be injured at the same time that the left kidney has sustained trauma; hence, whenever a hematuria is present, a splenic rupture should be considered also (Fig. 317). Auscultation of the abdomen usually reveals diminished amount or absence of bowel sounds. When the classic type with diffuse hemorrhage is present, a massive perisplenic hematoma results. The author has found it particularly difficult to palpate a normal or even somewhat enlarged spleen; however, it is easy to percuss the spleen, be it normal or enlarged. The normal spleen is approximately the size of the palm of the hand. If one percusses downward along the midaxillary line, splenic dullness is located in the

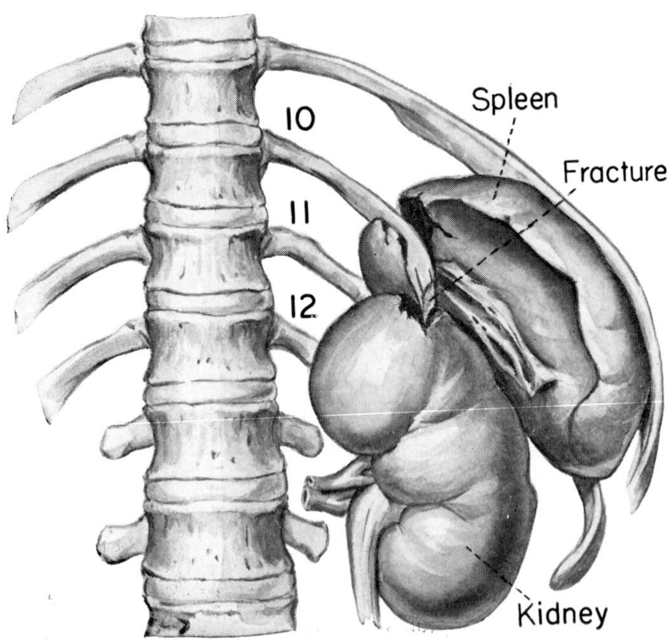

FIG. 317. Because of the close anatomic relationships of the spleen, the kidney and the 10th rib, a combination of injuries must be suspected when one of these structures is injured.

region of the 8th or the 9th rib; this dullness continues to the 10th rib or slightly below. In the event of splenic rupture with massive bleeding this area of normal splenic dullness is increased because of the surrounding clot. Organs in the immediate vicinity may be displaced. This displacement can be identified by means of a flat roentgenogram (Fig. 318). The splenic hematoma displaces the gastric air bubble to the right, and the splenic flexure downward and medially. If there is insufficient air in the stomach, this may be introduced through a Levin tube; this procedure is safer than producing dilatation by means of a carbonated drink, since there may be associated gastrointestinal damage. Obliteration of Traube's space is present. Traube's space is bounded above by the lower border of the lung, on the right by the liver, below by the costal margin, and on the left by the spleen. Normally, when percussed, this space produces a tympanitic note. If the patient's condition warrants, fluoroscopic examination might reveal limitation of motion, or elevation of the left hemidiaphragm. Complaint of left shoulder pain is suggestive of a splenic injury; this results from an irritation of the left phrenic nerve, which is transmitted up-

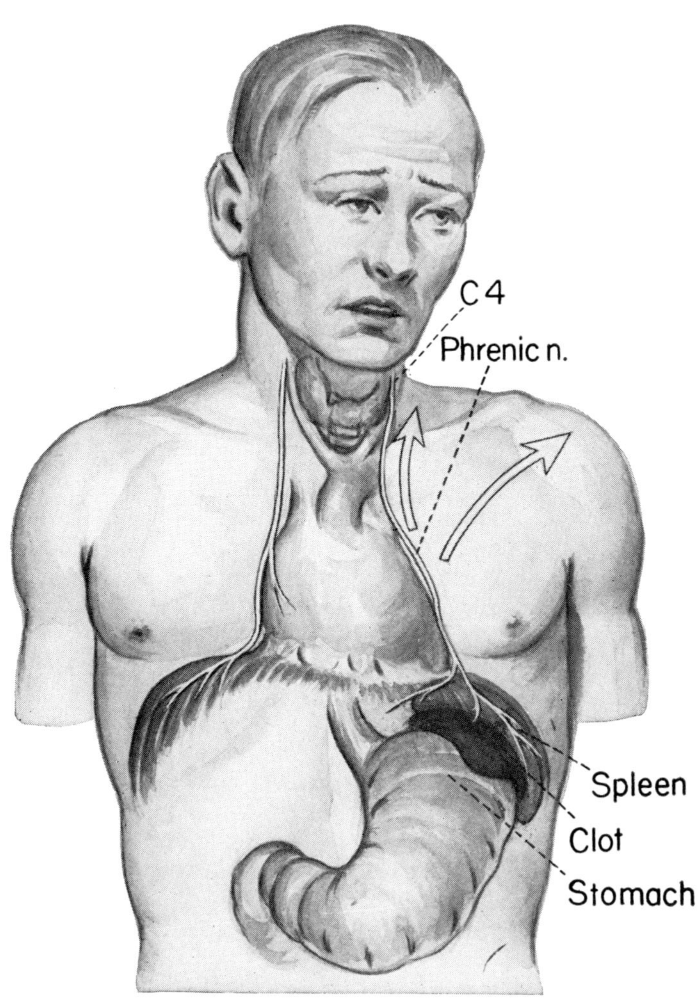

FIG. 318. A splenic hematoma produces pain in the left shoulder because of pressure on the left phrenic nerve. The displacement of the stomach should be noted.

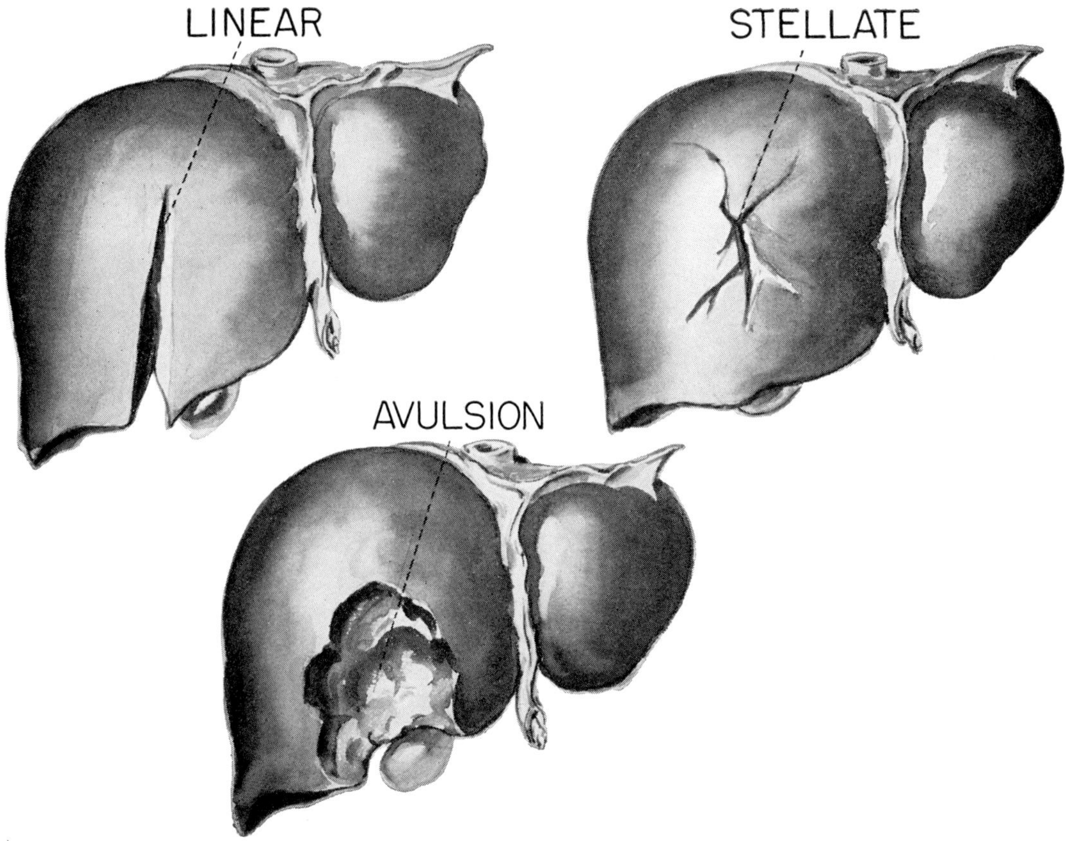

FIG. 319. Types of injury that may affect the liver following trauma.

ward to its origin at C4 (Fig. 318). Of particular diagnostic value is the production of splenic pain when pressure is maintained behind the sternocleidomastoid on the scalenus anticus muscle immediately above the left clavicle (Fig. 318). The chemical and irritating action of blood in the peritoneal cavity causes an ileus and absence of bowel sounds. Blood loss is revealed by pallor, a falling hematocrit and increased pulse; the heart sounds are heard clearly over the midabdomen since fluid acts as a conductor.

With subcapsular hemorrhage no blood escapes into the peritoneal cavity, and pain and tenderness, if present, are minimal and in the left upper abdominal quadrant. A persistent unexplained anemia might be the most prominent sign; however, enlargement of the spleen is also significant.

Delayed rupture of the spleen results from hemostasis or trifling leakage into the peritoneal cavity. The quiescent period may vary from days to weeks, at the end of which time the capsule tears, and a sudden dramatic hemorrhage occurs. The clinical picture becomes the classic one of ruptured spleen. Failure to elicit the history results in delayed diagnosis.

LIVER

This organ usually fractures in a stellate fashion; however, the injury may be a simple linear one or a severe avulsion (Fig. 319). The right lobe is involved 6 times as often as the left. Since the force necessary to rupture the liver is more severe than that for the spleen, associated injuries are common and add to the diagnostic difficulties. Sixty per cent of patients with ruptured livers have other injuries; 20 per cent involve the right kidney or lung; and 35 per cent have fractures of the lower right ribs. Diagnosis of a ruptured liver is difficult, because the clinical manifestations depend almost entirely on internal hemorrhage. If the capsule is torn, bleeding is profuse and produces a marked peritoneal reaction. This is accompanied by right upper abdominal pain, tenderness and rigidity of the abdominal muscles. If the bleeding continues, the symptoms of progressive hemorrhage and spreading peritonitis become apparent. In bleeding from the dome of the liver, blood accumulates in one of the subphrenic spaces and may give rise to right shoulder pain. If the diaphragm is torn, blood accumulates in the right pleural cavity. Jaundice usually appears in several days. It is expedient to do repeated icterus indices or serum bilirubin determinations to discover a subclinical jaundice. The author has been particularly fearful of needle aspiration of the abdomen in search of blood or bile. Roentgenograms with the patient erect are especially helpful to determine the position of the diaphragm, the evidence of injury to overlying ribs, and the possibility of fluid in the right pleural cavity.

Pancreas

The position of the pancreas within the upper abdomen usually affords it excellent protection from injury. However, its fixed position in front of the spine makes it vulnerable to those injuries associated with great force applied to the anterior abdominal wall. As in all other injuries, one must be aware of the variations of intensity of signs and symptoms which are dependent on the degree of injury. Trauma to surrounding organs further adds to the diagnostic difficulties. The pain is usually located supra-umbilically, depending on whether the head, the neck, the body or the tail of the organ is involved; it also may involve the lumbar region. A characteristic complaint is that the pain is exaggerated when the patient is on his back but is relieved when he is in a sitting or a prone position (Fig. 242). Traumatic pancreatitis may result; autodigestion gives rise to the familiar picture of acute hemorrhagic pancreatitis with its associated sanguineous peritonitis and fat necrosis (p. 223). The hemorrhage and the peritonitis that result may involve the lesser and/or the greater peritoneal cavities. The main complication to be considered is pseudocysts (p. 231). These are differentiated from the true cysts in that the pseudocyst has no true capsule.

Adrenal Gland

Traumatic involvement of this organ is rare. There are no diangostic signs; usually it is associated with injury to surrounding organs. The trauma is discovered coincidentally upon exploration.

IS THE GENITOURINARY TRACT INJURED?

Since the kidney is a solid viscus, and the ureters, the bladder and the urethra are hollow viscera, it is best that the genitourinary tract be considered as a unit. It is with a degree of anatomic license that the urethra is included with the abdominal organs. In any injury to the genitourinary tract hematuria is the outstanding finding. This necessitates an evaluation of each one of the organs in this tract. Meteorism, which frequently accompanies retroperitoneal injuries, requires careful evaluation.

Kidney

Hematuria, pain and/or tenderness in the renal area, and a mass in the flank suggest an injury to the kidney. To demonstrate such a mass is difficult; however, if one looks for a flattening of the normal contour of the loin, renal involvement on that side must be considered (Fig. 320). This is accomplished readily if one merely lowers the bed covers and compares both loin outlines. It is helpful to divide kidney injuries into 3 major groups. Group 1 consists of a simple contusion with or without minor parenchymal damage. Group 2 reveals major parenchymal damage often associated with rupture of the true kidney capsule and extravasation of blood and urine into the perirenal tissues. Group 3 includes the shattered kidney with gross disruption of the normal architecture and loss of a recognizable pelvis. The clinical picture of Group 3 is similar to that of Group 2 except that the signs and symptoms or blood loss and shock are more marked. In Group 1 the clinical symptoms are minimal. Of immense diagnostic aid are the excretory urogram and the retrograde pyelo-

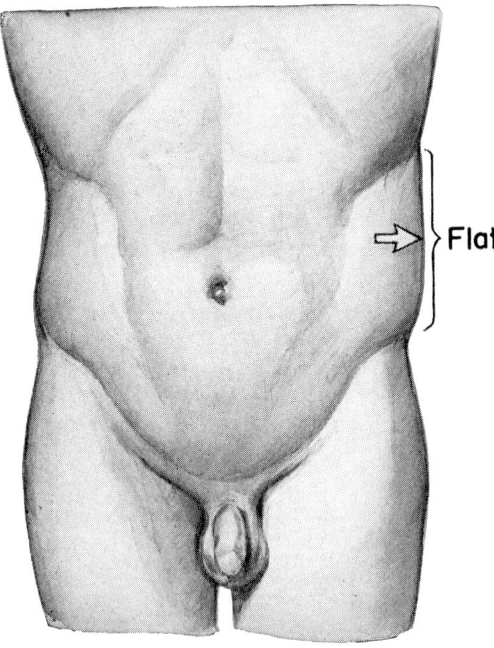

FIG. 320. Flattening of the normal contour of the loin suggests an injury (hematoma) or mass involving the kidney.

gram. If injury to the kidney is suspected, a flat roentgenogram should be obtained. This may be helpful in that it may reveal distortion and an obliteration of the psoas shadow on the involved side. However, this is not sufficient and should be combined with pyelography as soon as possible. Opinions differ concerning the value of intravenous pyelography; however, the consensus suggests that this should be the first step in the urologic examination. Although it may be inadequate and disappointing in some cases, it frequently furnishes the necessary information; this is particularly true of the Group 1 lesions. The procedure is easily executed and often replaces cystoscopy. It can be repeated at periodic intervals and carried out at the bedside. If the results of intravenous pyelography are inconclusive, or if doubt exists, then retrograde studies must be made. In the Group 2 lesions, urography study reveals evidence of parenchymal fracture and perirenal hematoma. In the Group 3 lesions, in which the kidney is shattered, the roentgen studies reveal the gross disruption and loss of a recognizable kidney pelvis.

URETER

Fortunately, the ureters are well protected, are mobile and have elastic walls that resist ordinary trauma; hence, injury from external trauma is rare. Intravenous pyelography or retrograde pyelo-ureterography usually clinches the diagnosis. If the injury is mild, few or no symptoms are present. If the ureter is severely traumatized, denuded or torn, extravasation of urine results. This is detected readily by means of dye studies.

BLADDER AND URETHRA

Although the urethra is not an abdominal organ, it cannot be separated in a discussion of injury to the genitourinary tract. It is permissible to include it as an appendage of the bladder.

In both ruptured bladder and ruptured urethra, a hematuria is usually present. There is frequently a desire to urinate but an inability to do so. If the patient is able to void, the urine should be collected in 2 portions. An equally bloody urine in both specimens is indicative of trauma to the bladder or the upper urinary tract. Blood in the first specimen and not in the second is indicative of injury to the genital tract.

Bladder injuries have been classified as simple contusion, intraperitoneal rupture and extraperitoneal rupture. The intraperitoneal type is seen commonly in patients who have had blows to the lower abdomen; it occurs most commonly when the bladder is full. The extraperitoneal rupture is associated more commonly with fractures of the bony pelvis. In these cases recovery is directly dependent on prompt recognition and treatment. Because of this, many authorities have abandoned the early routine usage of catheterization, irrigation tests and cystoscopies. The most reliable diagnostic procedure is *cystography*.

A satisfactory program is the following: A scout roentgenogram of the abdomen and the bony pelvis is taken. This is followed by an intravenous urogram; this supplies information regarding the presence of 2 kidneys and some evaluation as to their function. After the 30-minute film, even though the bladder shadow suggests no evidence of extravasation, the patient is catheterized, and a retrograde cystogram is done.

If the sterile catheter cannot be passed into the bladder, and there is bleeding from the external urethral meatus, then one must rule out a rupture of the membranous or prostatic urethra. To demonstrate such a lesion a urethrogram is done. This will reveal the location and the extent of the rupture.

14

Superior Extremity: The Hand

Only *the hand* will be considered in this chapter. Numerous specialized texts dealing with the superior extremity, particularly orthopedic conditions, are available.

Because of its prehensile function the hand and the fingers are exposed to injury. Although such injuries may be slight, they permit the introduction of microorganisms. If such infections are not diagnosed and treated early, loss of limb or life may result.

PERIPHERAL NERVE INJURY

This lesion must be detected immediately. It would be a rare clinician who remembers the minute details of the nerve supplies to the extremities, to say nothing of the numerous anomalies. When one examines a hand, one must have at his disposal simple tests that detect injuries to the 3 main nerves, namely, the median, the ulnar and the radial. The

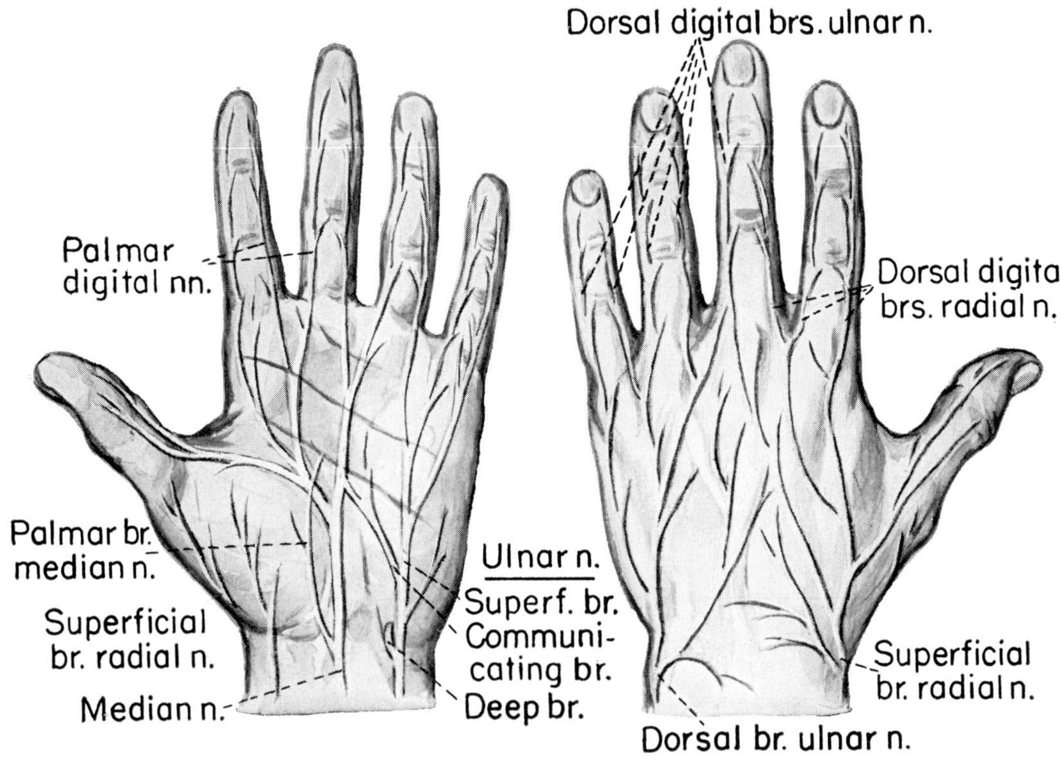

FIG. 321. The sensory nerve supply of the hand.

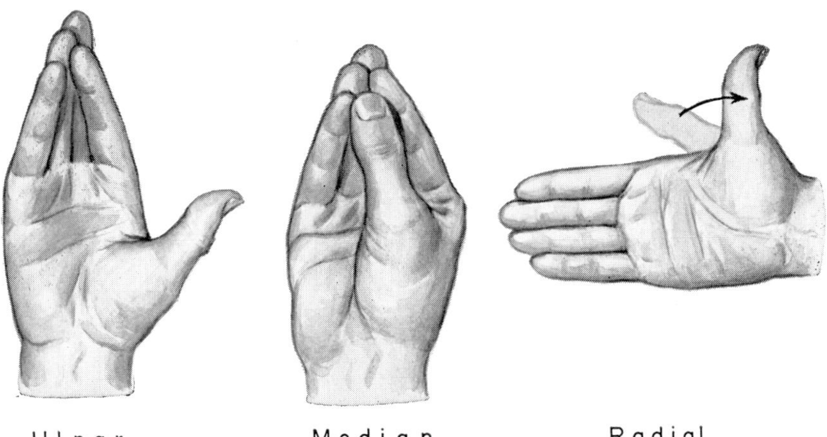

FIG. 322. Rapid testing of the hand for nerve injury. If the patient can make a "4-fingered cone," the ulnar nerve is intact. The ability to approximate the thumb and to make a "5-fingered cone" implies a normal median nerve. The radial nerve is the "extensor" nerve. The "trigger" test of the thumb is pathognomonic of its normalcy.

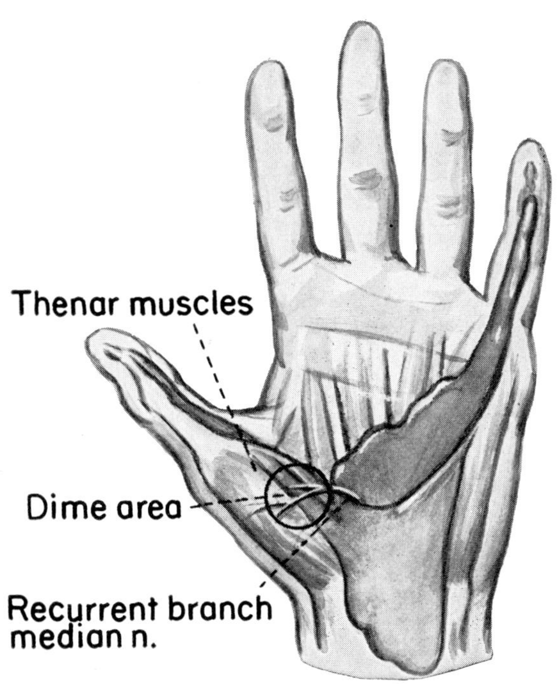

FIG. 323. The "dime area." If a dime is placed over the summit of the thenar eminence, the area is readily outlined. The recurrent branch of the median nerve lies very superficially in this area.

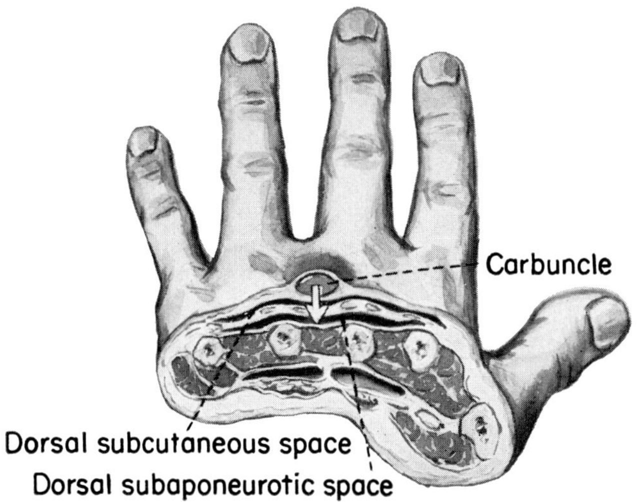

FIG. 324. Carbuncle of the dorsum of the hand. These infections may burrow deeper to the dorsal subcutaneous and/or the dorsal subaponeurotic spaces.

sensory nerve distribution to the hand is depicted in Figure 321. In the vast majority of cases an injured nerve may be diagnosed by testing one function. When a single test is used for a major nerve, the most distal functions should be tested. If these suggest nerve injury, then all functions of the involved nerve should be analyzed and the extent of the injury determined.

Tests for the ulnar nerve are accomplished readily in the following way:

1. Sensory: pinprick sensation over the palmar surface of the distal phalanx of the 5th finger
2. Motor: the ability to make a "4-fingered cone" (Fig. 322)

Tests for median nerve injury:

1. Sensory: pinprick sensation over the palmar surface of the distal phalanx of the index finger
2. Motor: the ability to make a "5-fingered cone" (Fig. 322)

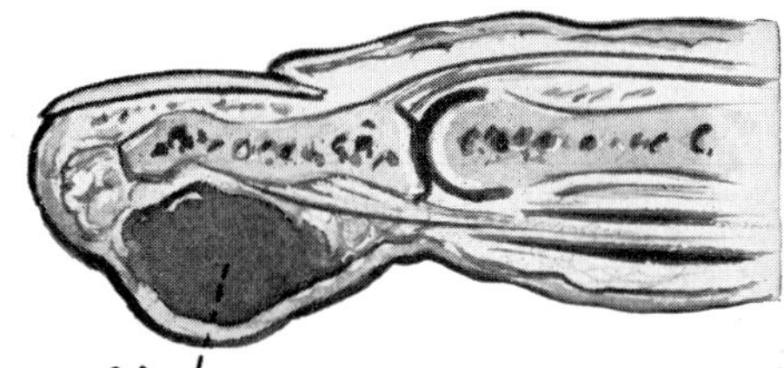

FIG. 325. A felon is an infection of the anterior closed space of the finger.

Radial nerve tests:

1. Sensory: pinprick sensation over the dorsum on the radial side of the hand
2. Motor: extend the thumb in "trigger" fashion (Fig. 322).

The *dime area* must be kept in mind whenever there is an injury involving the thenar eminence (Fig. 323). If a dime is placed over the summit of the thenar eminence, the area is outlined. Within it the recurrent branch of the median nerve enters and supplies the 3 important thenar muscles (flexor pollicis brevis, abductor pollicis brevis and opponens pollicis). If this nerve is injured (it lies very superficially), the thumb becomes paralyzed, and the hand loses the greater part of its usefulness.

INFECTIONS

Serious hand infections may result from trivial skin injuries. The most common hand infections encountered are carbuncles, felon, paronychia, tenosynovitis, space infections and infections of the bursae.

CARBUNCLES

Carbuncles of the hand are found most frequently on the dorsum because of the presence of hair follicles and sweat glands. The diagnosis is simple. It should be treated adequately and early, because, if neglected, it burrows deep and involves the 2 dorsal spaces of the hand, namely, the subcutaneous space (between the skin and the extensor

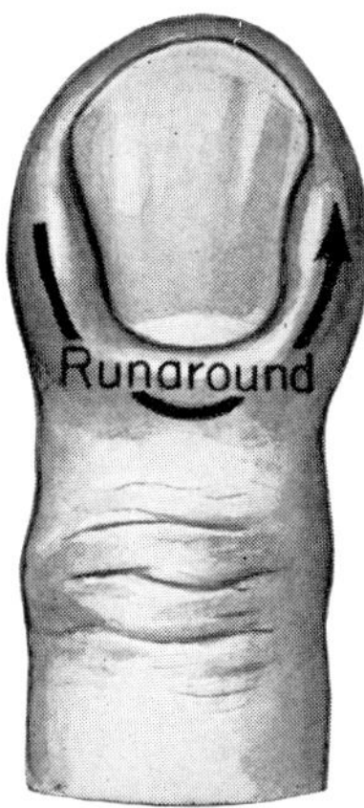

FIG. 326. Paronychia (runaround) may progress to a stage of abscess formation under the nail root. These infections become chronic if not treated adequately.

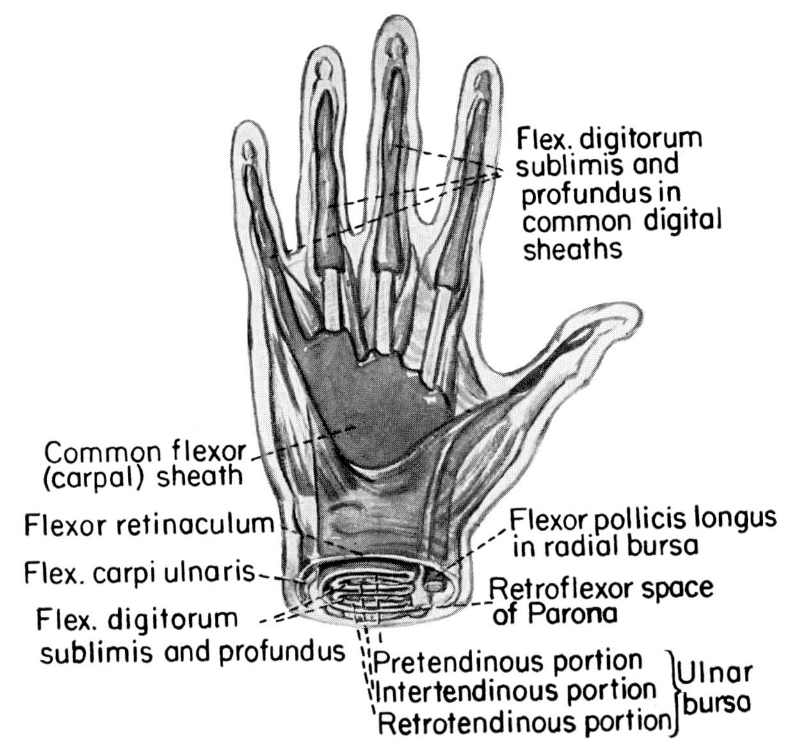

FIG. 327. The most common arrangement of the flexor tendon sheaths of the fingers.

tendons) and the dorsal subaponeurotic (between the extensor tendon and the metacarpal bones) (Fig. 324).

FELON

A felon is an infection that involves the closed space of the terminal phalanx. If this is not diagnosed and treated early, osteomyelitis occurs (Fig. 325). Extension of such closed space infections shuts off the blood supply to the diaphysis of the terminal phalanx. This causes aseptic bone necrosis, which may become infected secondarily. There are some who challenge this concept of occlusion of the digital vessel and believe that bone involvement is due to direct extension of the infection. Both mechanisms no doubt play a role. No clinician should treat a felon without having a roentgenogram of the distal phalanx first, to rule out osteomyelitis. Of diagnostic importance is the fact that the pain is so severe that the patient "walks the floor" and is unable to obtain relief unless a large dose of a narcotic is given. One must *not* wait for suppuration or fluctuation before instituting surgical therapy. The involved distal phalanx is tight, tense and reddish. The patient can demonstrate the point of exquisite tenderness.

PARONYCHIA

A paronychia has been called a "runaround." If left untreated, it may travel completely around and under the nail and form a horseshoe-shaped abscess (Fig. 326). These infections usually appear spontaneously; however, there is frequently a history of injury or "hangnail" or some trauma produced in the course of a manicure. In contradistinction to a felon, although the paronychia appears to be more inflamed, the pain is much less. It rarely, if ever, requires sedation. Therefore, its location and different type of pain immediately differentiate it from a felon. Adequate therapy results in rapid cure; however, *chronic paronychia* should make one suspect fungous infections,

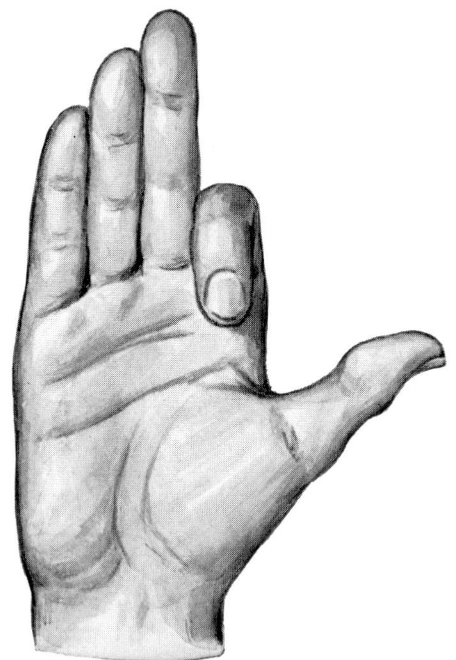

FIG. 328. Flexion of the involved finger (tenosynovitis) produces the "crochet-hook" sign.

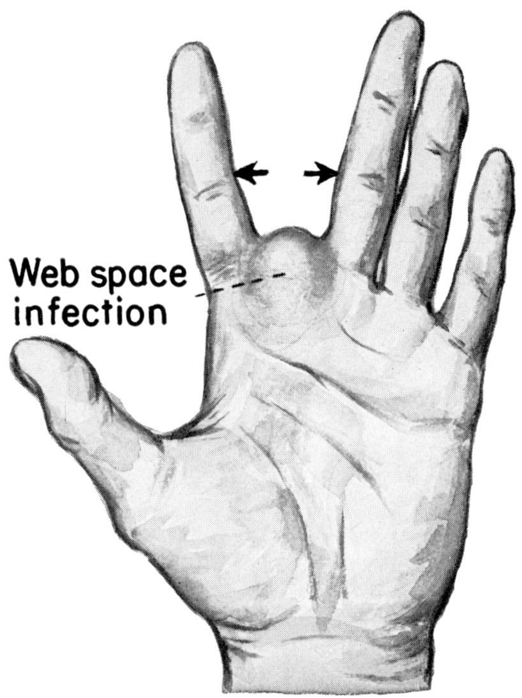

FIG. 329. When the interdigital (web) space is infected and swollen, the fingers to either side of the space are pushed apart.

which are commonly found in people whose hands are frequently immersed in water.

TENDON SHEATH INFECTIONS (TENOSYNOVITIS)

Infections of the flexor tendon sheaths usually follow trauma, especially injuries which occur to the transverse skin creases. It is not necessary that the injury penetrate the tendon sheath. This is a dangerous infection, since it leads to early necrosis of the tendon and permanent disability. The infection may extend directly along the sheath into the hand and the forearm. Particularly is this so in the case of the little finger and the thumb. Figure 327 demonstrates the usual pattern of tendon sheaths; however, varieties do exist.

The essential signs of an infected tendon sheath are:

1. Flexion of the involved finger (crochet-hook sign) (Fig. 328)
2. Swelling and loss of function
3. Tenderness over the infected sheath

The slightest attempt at extension produces exquisite pain; however, it is rarely necessary to submit the patient to such torture. If the little finger is infected (tenosynovitis), the ulnar bursa may be involved; similarly, if the thumb is infected, the radial bursa must be examined carefully. Infected tendon sheaths may rupture into the interdigital web spaces. If a web space is involved, the fingers to either side of this space are pushed apart (Fig. 329). Web-space infections may also be present in the absence of a tenosynovitis.

Tenosynovitis must not be mistaken for lymphangitis and lymphadenitis; the latter presents the usual red streaks and glands (Fig. 330). Lymphangitis requires nonoperative treatment, whereas acute tenosynovitis frequently requires surgical intervention.

SPACE INFECTIONS

The fascial spaces of the hand are 2 in number, namely, the middle palmar and the thenar.

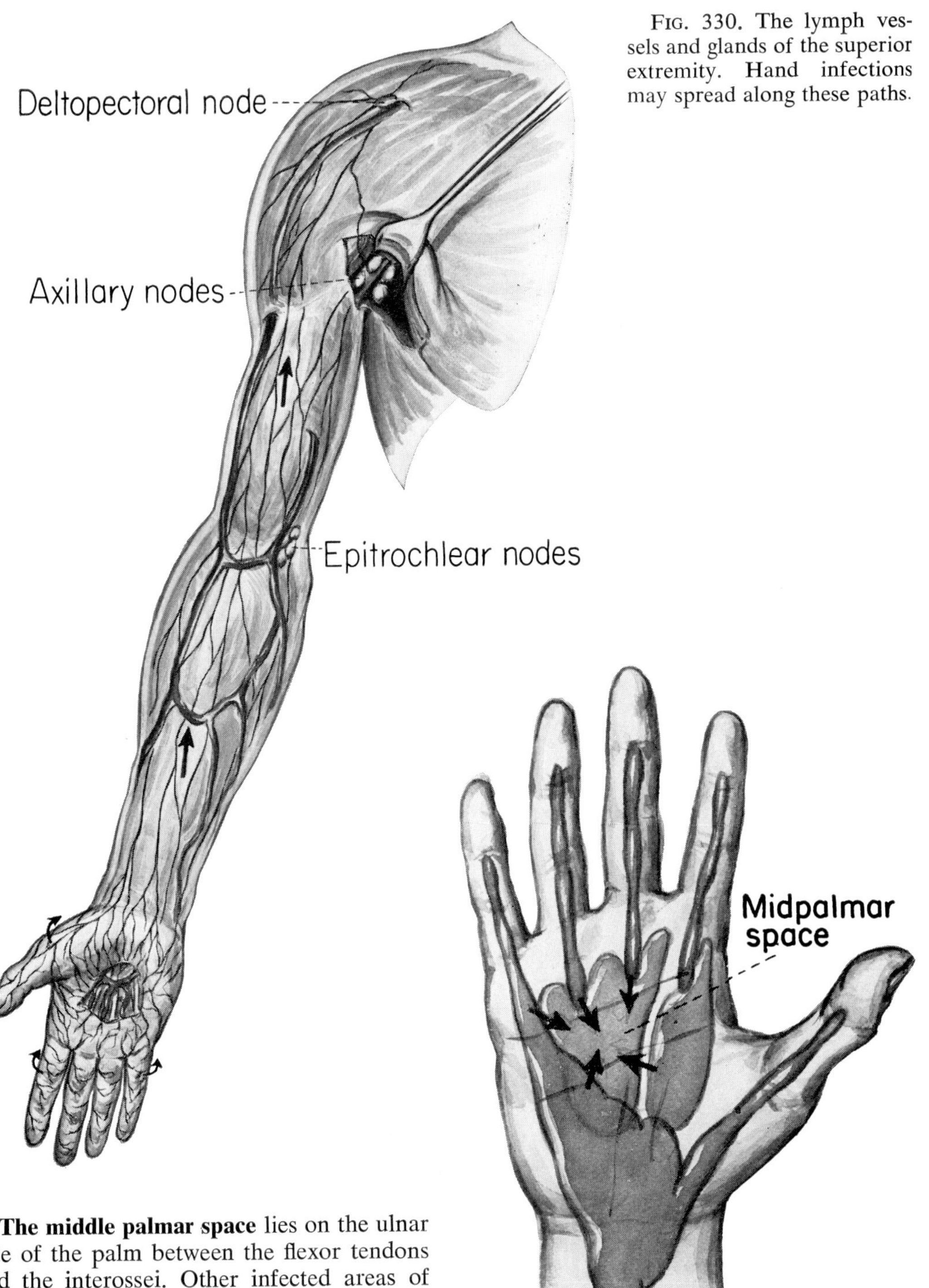

FIG. 330. The lymph vessels and glands of the superior extremity. Hand infections may spread along these paths.

FIG. 331. The midpalmar space may become infected from other foci of infection in the hand. These have been indicated by arrows.

The middle palmar space lies on the ulnar side of the palm between the flexor tendons and the interossei. Other infected areas of the hand may drain into it. These have been indicated in Figure 331. Diagnostic signs that suggest infection of this space include the usual signs of inflammation plus obliteration of the normal concavity of the palm

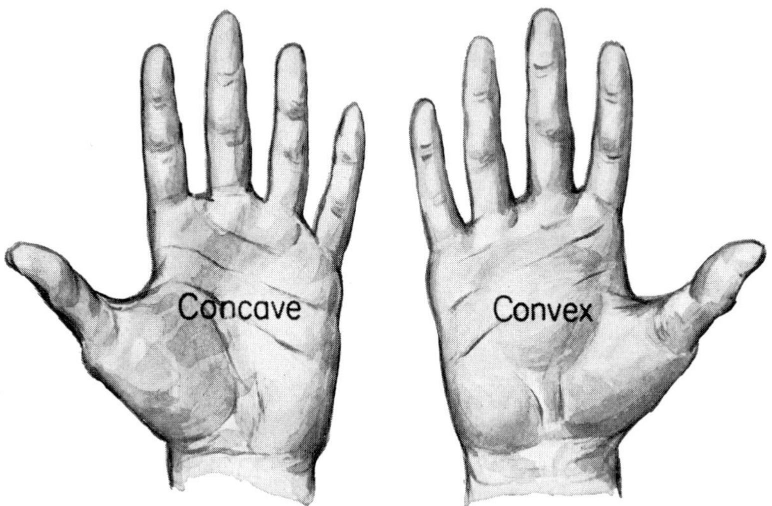

FIG. 332. In midpalmar space infection the normal concavity of the palm of the hand is replaced by a slight bulging.

(Fig. 332). There is tenderness in the central part of the palm, and the 3rd, the 4th and the 5th fingers may be held in partial flexion. Massive dorsal edema (which is frequently confusing) is also present.

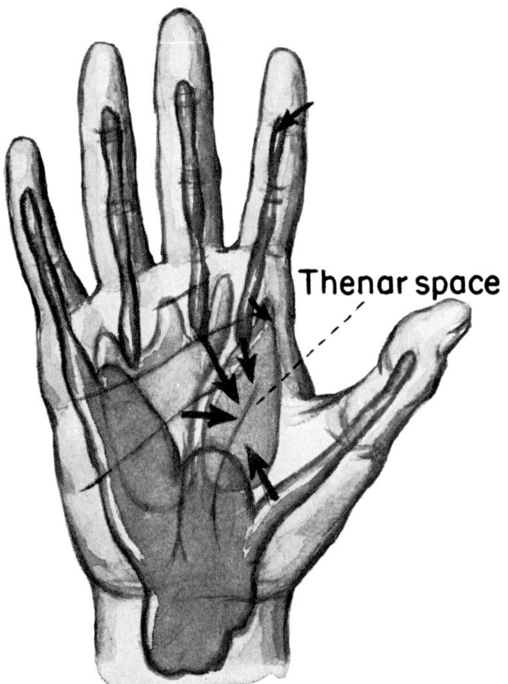

FIG. 333. The possible paths of extension of infection to the thenar space are indicated by arrows.

The thenar space is on the radial side of the palm and partly covered by the thenar muscles. The possible paths of extension into this space are demonstrated in Figure 333. Involvement of this space can be diagnosed by the typical ballooning of the space between the thumb and the index finger (Fig. 334). It is helpful to have the patient hold up both hands and then compare both thumb-index finger spaces to compare the normal concavity with the obliteration on the opposite side. The usual signs of inflammation are present.

Infections of the radial and the ulnar bursae are secondary to the involvement of the tendon sheath of the thumb and the little finger, respectively. The palmar spaces, when involved, may also involve these bursae. Infections of the bursae tend to spread rapidly into the forearm and produce a necrosis of the flexor tendons.

INFECTIONS OF THE BURSAE

Involvement of the ulnar bursa is suspected when the following signs can be elicited:

1. Fullness in the palm of the hand; however, the concavity remains
2. Fullness above the anterior annular ligament
3. Tenderness along the course of the tendon sheath of the little finger and the ulnar bursa

4. Marked edema of the dorsum of the hand

Involvement of the Radial Bursa. When this bursa is involved, the following signs should be sought:

1. Flexion of the distal phalanx of the thumb
2. Swelling above the anterior annular ligament
3. Tenderness over the flexor pollicis longus tendon sheath

It cannot be overemphasized that in most hand infections the dorsum of the hand swells early and massively. This is explained by the fact that the areolar tissue here is loose. Such swelling may attract the attention of the clinician, and a misplaced incision results.

Carpal Tunnel Syndrome

The term *carpal tunnel syndrome* is associated with motor, sensory and/or autonomic disturbances of the median nerve as it passes through the carpal tunnel. The transverse carpal ligament is a heavy fibrous band which stretches from the pisiform and the hamate bones medially to the scaphoid and the trapezium laterally; with the posterior concave carpal bones a canal is formed (Fig. 335). The median nerve and the flexor tendons pass through this canal on their way to the hand; the nerve lies in front of the tendons and immediately behind the transverse carpal ligament. Involvement of the median nerve may be due to trauma (occupational), tenosynovitis or anything that increases the volume of the structures in this tunnel. It has been referred to also as a "median neuritis."

This syndrome is found most commonly in women, usually those who are middle-aged or in the 5th or the 6th decade. The onset is insidious, and it persists for months or years before the patient seeks medical aid.

The most prominent symptoms are sensory, such as paresthesias, numbness, and pain which follows the course of distribution of the median nerve. A feeling of "needles and pins" or fullness is frequent. The pain is cutting, burning, sharp or dull and is most severe at night or upon rising. Paroxysmal attacks occur which last 15 to 30 minutes, even awaking the patient from a sound sleep. Relief may be obtained by a change of posture. Motor involvement is characterized particularly by weakness and clumsiness of thumb movements (picking up small objects or writing). Discoloration of the skin and cold hands suggest vasomotor disturbances. Muscle involvement becomes obvious with the development of thenar atrophy and decreased power in opposition and abduction of the thumb. Tapping over the nerve at the wrist may produce sensory phenomena (Teinel's sign). The maintenance of forced hyperflexion for a minute or so may precipi-

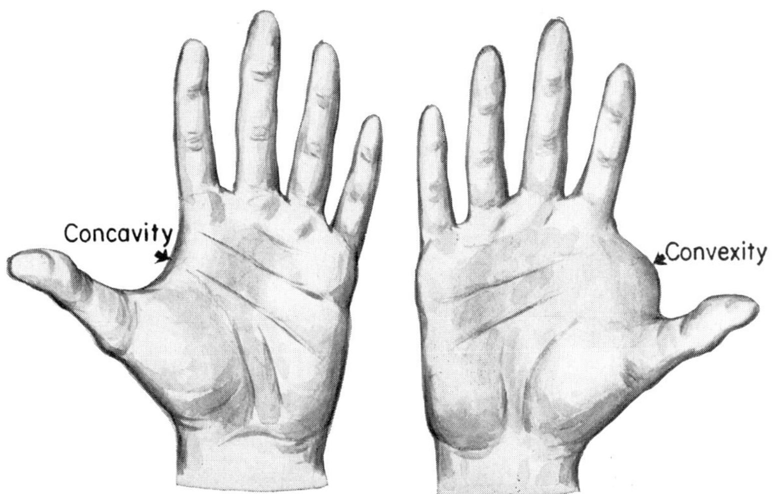

Fig. 334. In thenar space infection the normal concave curve (web) between the thumb and the index finger is replaced by a convex bulging.

tate pain and paresthesias (Phalen's sign). Roentgenograms of the wrist, sweat tests, nerve conduction studies and electromyography have been used as diagnostic aids.

The injection of hydrocortisone at times gives dramatic relief, particularly during acute episodes. Definitive treatment requires division of the transverse carpal ligament.

Human Bites of the Hand

These lesions deserve special mention because of some unusual features. Wounds contaminated with human mouth organisms produce the most destructive infections seen in the hand. The particular organisms responsible for this condition are spirochetes and fusiform bacilli, which grow in symbiosis under anaerobic conditions. A darkfield examination will reveal their presence. Because of the bacterial flora of the human mouth, which also includes the streptococcus, the staphylococcus and *E. coli*, these bites are more serious than tooth wounds inflicted by other animals. Most of these wounds appear over the knuckles, resulting from fist fights.

Penetrating wounds (caused by teeth), involving subcutaneous and subaponeurotic tissues, are ideal for anaerobic infections. The onset and the progress of bite infections is dramatically rapid, the wound becoming red and swollen within 24 hours. A watery, foul discharge appears first. Pain is present and aggravated severely by the slightest degree of motion. The temperature usually is elevated. Untreated cases reveal early gangrene of the superficial tissues and thick, putrid pus exuding from the wound. Any or all of the spaces of the hand may be involved. One attempts to prevent serious local complications, such as suppurative arthritis (metacarpophalangeal joints), osteomyelitis and ankylosis. Septicemia and death may occur.

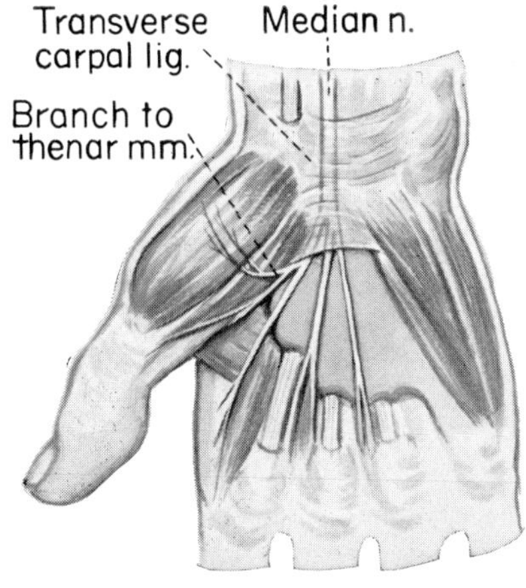

Fig. 335. The median nerve passes beneath the transverse carpal ligament in front of the flexor tendon and sends motor branches to the thenar muscles.

RAYNAUD'S DISEASE

The cause of this disease is unknown. Arguments still exist as to whether it is due to hyperactivity of the sympathetic nervous system or to local arteriolar defects. The "typical" cases of Raynaud's disease usually appear in emotionally unstable young women. The attack is brought on by emotion or cold. First, severe blanching appears and then cyanosis (in the fingertips and occasionally the toes). If the attack is prolonged, true ischemic pain and anoxia result. Ischemic ulcers and soft tissue atrophy may ensue. A sclerodermalike condition develops in which the skin becomes involved by fibrous tissue growth. Excessive sweating is a common but not a constant complement.

So-called *Raynaud's phenomena* are chronic arteriospastic states which may be associated with many other causes. Usually, the phenomena are less severe than those of the typical Raynaud's disease and are not confined to young women; the feet may be affected as frequently as the hands. These phenomena are not progressive and do not cause ulceration.

In the later cases of Raynaud's disease the pathologic changes are obliterating endarteritis, tortuous dilated capillary loops, subcutaneous fibrosis and ulceration.

TUMORS OF THE HAND

Fortunately, malignant tumors of the hand are rare. If a malignant neoplasm occurs here, it is usually of the melanotic group. Many of these, fortunately, are preceded by benign lesions which, if diagnosed promptly, can be removed and cured. Among the more common of such precursors may be:

1. Pigmented moles and/or nevi
2. Irradiation burns
3. Keloids
4. Senile keratoses
5. Chemical burns
6. Foreign body granulomas
7. Pyogenic granulomas

When diagnosed, these should be removed by wide excision.

The malignant lesions, as stated, travel rapidly along the lymphatics (Fig. 330). It should be noted that the lymphatic drainage from the thumb, the index finger and half of the 3rd finger usually drains directly into the axillary nodes. The lymphatic drainage from half of the third, the ring and the little fingers drains by way of the superficial cubital nodes. This does not imply that every enlarged node is a metastatic one; these may be inflammatory; however, it is safer to consider them as malignant until proved to be otherwise.

A ganglion may be considered as a mucoid tumor that occurs in the tendons (sheaths) of the hand. It is found most frequently over the dorsal or the volar aspect of the wrist, where it attaches to the tendons and frequently to the synovia of the joints. It is characterized by its mobility with a given tendon, its smoothness and its cystic consistency. It is benign.

DUPUYTREN'S CONTRACTURE

The diagnosis of this condition is usually easy. The condition is not too uncommon; heredity plays a part. It is not a contracture of the tendons but of the palmar fascia, usually on the ulnar side and most frequently involving the 4th and the 5th fingers. The disability is due to the inability to extend these fingers; there is no pain or tenderness. The condition is benign, and recurrences following therapy are quite common.

15

Inferior Extremity

VARICOSE VEINS

This condition is the penalty that man pays for having assumed the upright posture. Other etiologic factors are weakness of the venous wall and/or valves, thrombosis of the deeper veins, childbirth, prolonged rest, and trauma. Associated with uncontrolled venous stasis are edema, induration, cellulitis and fibrosis. Phlebitis and recurrent attacks of cellulitis are late symptoms and may lead to ulceration.

The term *primary* varicosed veins implies that the deep system of veins is normal. The term *postphlebitic syndrome* by contrast suggests interference with the normal function of the deep veins. This condition is discussed on page 305.

The inferior extremity has 3 systems of veins, namely, superficial, communicating and deep (Fig. 336). All of these have valves which prevent venous reflux. The patency of the veins and the competence of the valves assure successful return of blood in the proper direction. When the valves become incompetent, and the veins dilate, the blood flow reverses its course; this retrograde flow produces the pathologic changes associated with increased pressure, stasis and hypoxia.

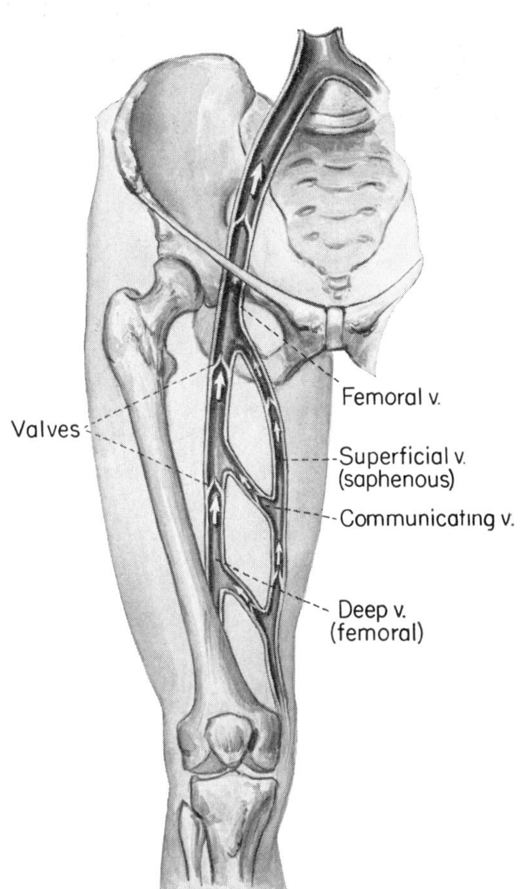

FIG. 336. The normal venous circulation of the inferior extremity. The arrows indicate the normal blood flow toward the heart and from superficial to deep veins.

The *superficial venous system* is made up of the greater saphenous system (anteromedially) and the lesser saphenous system (posteromedially). The greater saphenous empties into the deep venous system at the common femoral vein, and the lesser saphenous into the popliteal veins.

The *deep system of veins* is made up of the anterior and the posterior tibial veins, which become the popliteal vein; this in turn becomes the common femoral vein.

The *communicating set of veins,* as the name implies, communicates with the superficial and the deep systems and by means of its valves conveys blood from the superficial to the deep set.

Primary varicosed veins are dilated, elongated and tortuous veins which occur in the absence of any acquired mechanical obstruction. The common type involves the superficial veins (saphenous system) of the lower extremity. They are referred to as congenital or idiopathic varices; frequently, a familial history can be elicited. They may occur at an early age, even before the 2nd decade. The veins are clearly visible and filled with blood which flows in a retrograde direction. Most frequently involved is the long (internal) saphenous vein; next in frequency is the short (external) saphenous. Although the valves in the involved segments are not diseased, they become incompetent because of venous dilatation. The deep system of veins usually is normal, the symptoms are mild, and for many years a benign course is followed. The most common complaint is a cosmetic one. The veins gradually enlarge, and a "tired feeling" develops. Mild to moderate edema gradually ensues, which in turn is followed by dermatitis and ulceration. Another annoying and at times disabling complication is hemorrhage. Thrombosis is characterized by sudden pain, redness and local swelling over a vein which previously was collapsible and painless. Hemorrhage usually occurs when a small varix is exposed to trauma. Although the injured varix is small, the hemorrhage may be profuse and threatening. Such dramatic hemorrhage is con-

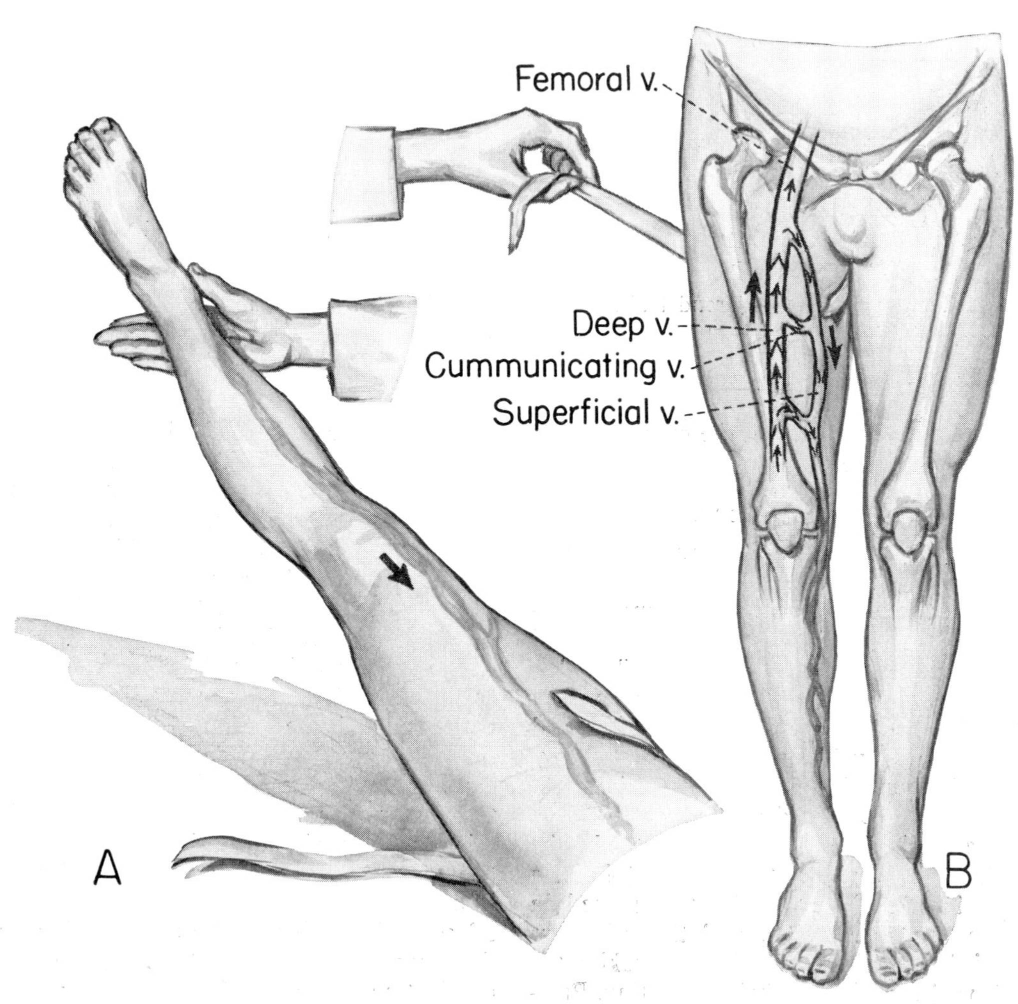

FIG. 337. The single Trendelenburg test for testing the superficial set of veins (see text).

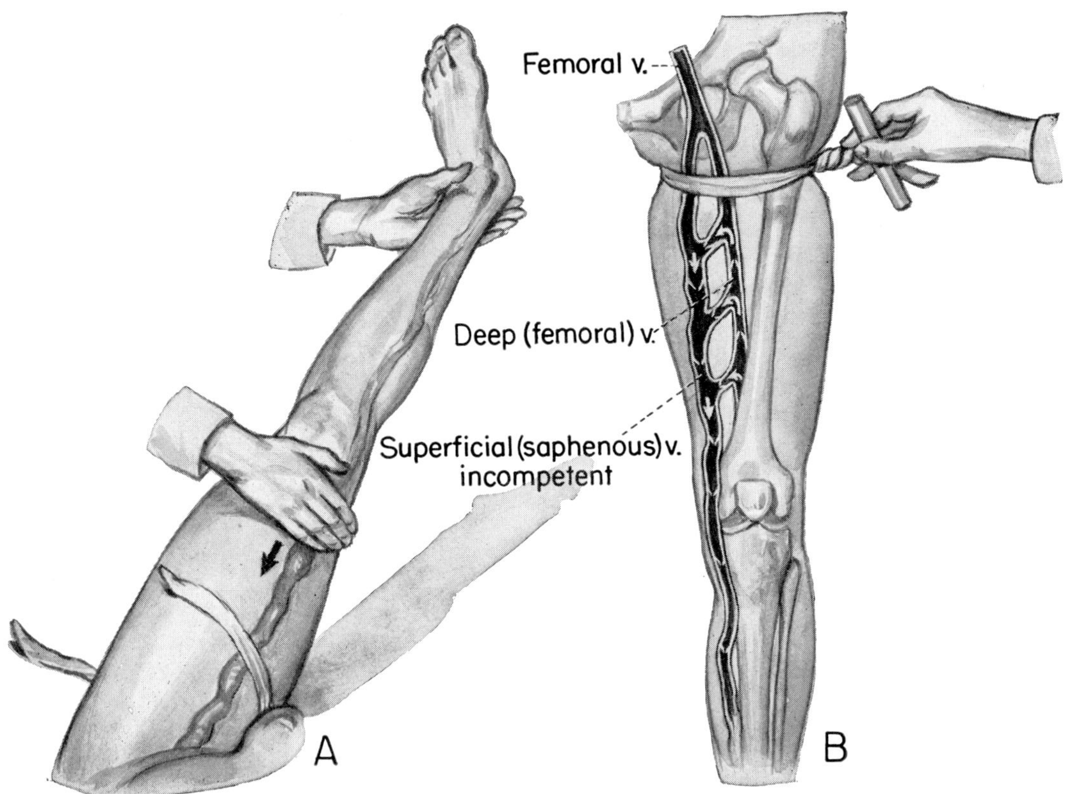

FIG. 338. The double Trendelenburg test for testing the communicating set of veins (see text).

trolled easily by elevating the extremity and applying pressure.

TESTS OF VEINS

In deciding the proper therapy for these varicosities it becomes essential to know which of the veins, superficial, communicating or deep, are incompetent. The superficial set of veins is tested by the single Trendelenburg test; the communicating veins are tested by the double Trendelenburg test; and the deep set of veins is tested by the Perthes' test. Many modifications and variants of these tests have been described.

The **superficial set of veins** is tested by the single Trendelenburg test in the following way (Fig. 337). The patient is placed in the recumbent position, and the veins are emptied by raising the limb and stroking the varicosed veins in a cephalad direction. Pressure is applied over the termination of the long saphenous vein, and with this pressure maintained, the patient is asked to stand. The pressure then is released, and if rapid filling of the saphenous from above appears, this indicates a positive test, which signifies incompetency of the valves.

The **communicating set of veins** is tested by the double Trendelenburg test (Fig. 338). This is conducted essentially the same way as the single Trendelenburg test in that the patient again is placed in the recumbent position, the superficial veins are stroked and emptied, digital pressure is applied over the termination of the long saphenous, and with this pressure maintained, the patient is asked to stand. However, the pressure in this test is maintained and not released for at least 30 seconds. Filling of the veins during this time suggests an incompetency of the communicating veins which connect the deep and the superficial sets. Should this occur,

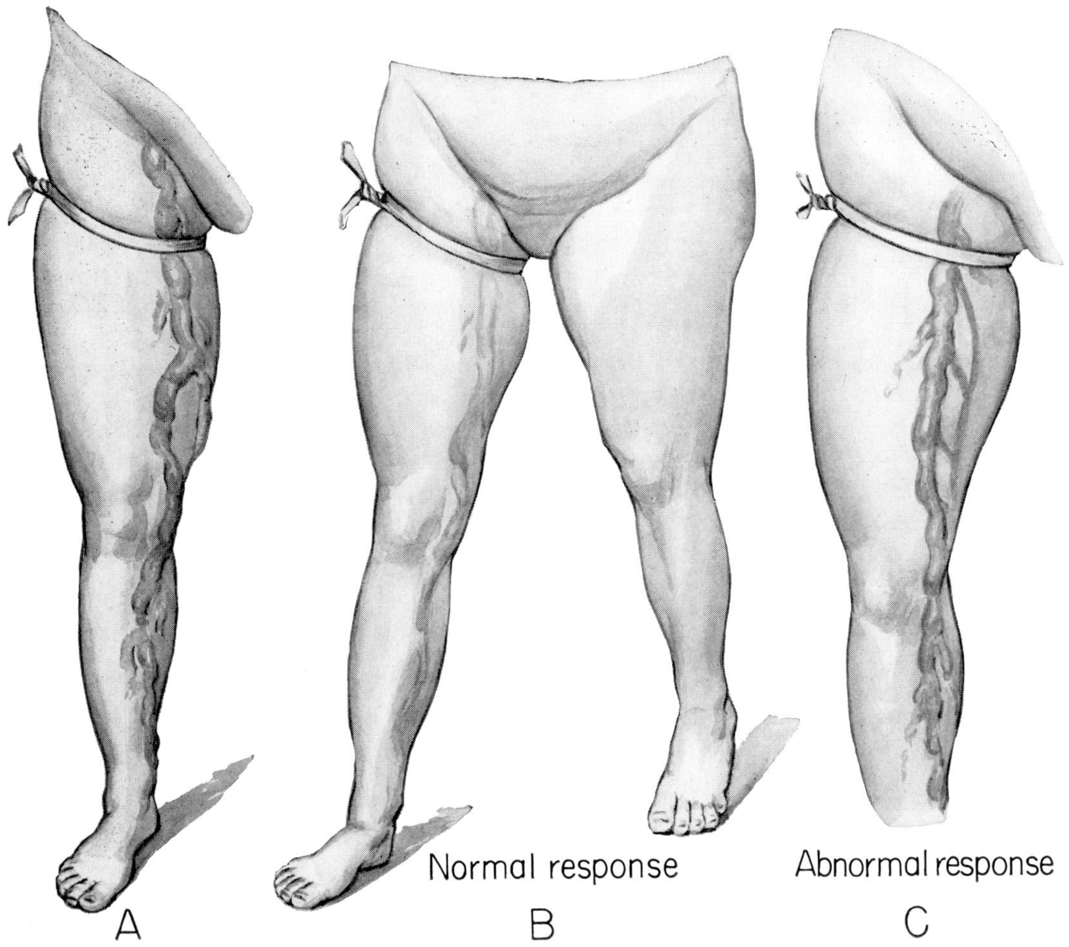

FIG. 339. Perthes' test is used to test the deep set of veins (see text).

the test is considered as positive and indicates the necessity for multiple ligations or stripping procedures.

The **deep set of veins** is tested by Perthes' test (Fig. 339). This is conducted in the following way. With the patient standing and the superficial veins dilated, a tourniquet is applied to the middle of the thigh. As the patient walks, these dilated superficial veins should empty if the deep set is patent (Fig. 339 B). However, if the superficial veins become more prominent and produce pain while walking, this is a positive Perthes' test and indicates obstruction to the deeper set (Fig. 339 C). If the superficial veins are compensatory for a nonfunctioning deep set, great caution must be observed if any surgery is attempted on such veins.

Other tests, such as the Ochsner-Mahorner and double tourniquet test, are helpful but rarely necessary. A battery of elaborate tests involving venograms, manometric determinations and radioactive solutions has been suggested. These are not only expensive but may result in annoying complications. They are rarely necessary. It is well to remember that any patient who can wear an elastic stocking which collapses his superficial veins and thereby receives relief can be considered as having a competent set of deep veins.

POSTPHLEBITIC SYNDROME

This term implies an interference with the deep veins of the extremity which results from thrombophlebitis. It usually is a severely disabling condition. Recanalization of the thrombosed segments may occur, but the injured valves result in functionless and at times occluded veins. Chronic venous stasis (venous hypertension) follows a rather stereotyped course in that edema appears first and then dilatation of the superficial veins; dermatitis usually makes its appearance later, and ulceration may occur rapidly thereafter.

VENOUS THROMBOSIS

The occurrence of spontaneous blood clotting in the veins of the inferior extremity is quite common. It may occur in either the deep or the superficial set of veins; however, it is more common in the former. Venous thrombosis may result from stasis of blood flow, change in the intimal lining, or an alteration in the clotting mechanism of blood. This is particularly true of deep venous thrombosis. The condition frequently is associated with trauma, postpartum or postoperative periods, blood dyscrasias, carcinomas and cardiac disease.

Phlebothrombosis (bland thrombus) refers to a clot which is loosely adherent to the vein wall and prone to break loose, thereby causing pulmonary embolus and infarction. The first indication that this type of deep venous thrombosis exists may be sudden death from a massive pulmonary embolus. There are milder forms in which the patient complains of coughing, chest pain and hemoptysis. A flat roentgenogram of the chest some hours later reveals findings consistent with the diagnosis of pulmonary infarction. Phlebothrombosis may be totally unaccompanied by signs or symptoms in the involved extremity, or the patient may complain of mild tenderness in the calf muscles, particularly on moving or walking. Occasionally, slight swelling of the foot and the ankle with minimal dilatation of the superficial veins may be noted. Although the local phlebothrombosis has been referred to as "bland," the lethal potential is tremendous.

Thrombophlebitis, on the other hand, when involving the deep venous system, refers to a clot that is firmly adherent to the venous wall. It irritates the wall and produces a massive deep sterile venous inflammation, which in older terminology has been referred to as phlegmasia alba dolens (milk leg of pregnancy). In this condition the onset is relatively acute, and the involved extremity becomes swollen, painful, cold and blanched; it may extend from toe to groin (iliofemoral venous thrombosis). Early in the disease the inflammatory irritation results in reflex vasospasm which involves the arterial tree. It is not unusual to find an absence of the popliteal or the dorsalis pedis pulsations. As the disease progresses, the extremity becomes warm and red. The patient frequently runs a febrile course. Whether phlebothrombosis and thrombophlebitis are manifestations of the same disease or are different entities still is moot.

ARTERIAL OCCLUSIONS

Acute Arterial Occlusions

These are usually produced by emboli or thrombi. In many cases it is difficult to distinguish between the 2, but if the onset is associated with extreme suddenness, embolic occlusion usually is present. It has been stated on page 307 that arterial spasm may be associated with venous thrombosis.

Arterial emboli are frequently associated with rehumatic heart disease. Other cardiac conditions can produce intracardiac thrombus formation, which in turn results in peripheral emboli. Such diseases include hypertensive or atherosclerotic heart disease, auricular fibrillation and so-called thyrocardiac disease (hyperthyroidism).

When an arterial embolus occludes a major vessel in an extremity, the onset is dramatic and sudden. The involved part becomes cold and numb, and the patient complains of a loss of function. The part distal to the embolus is whitish, yet cyanotic, and there is anesthesia. Pain as a rule is transitory and not the chief complaint. The most common sites where emboli lodge are the bifurcation of the common iliacs, the femoral and the popliteal vessels. Pallor, paralysis, pain and coldness are not present proximal to the level of occlusion. Oscillometric readings are particularly helpful in determining the level of obstruction. Associated reflex arterial spasms occur regionally and result in further thrombosis, both above and below the obstruction. Such spasms reduce the effectiveness of the collateral circulation. Diagnosis is vitally important, since the earlier the condition is recognized, the better the 2 main complications, arterial spasm and intra-atrial thrombosis, can be combated. It is the belief of many that as soon as the diagnosis is made, heparin and papaverine should be administered, and embolectomy should be considered.

Arterial Thrombosis. This condition can

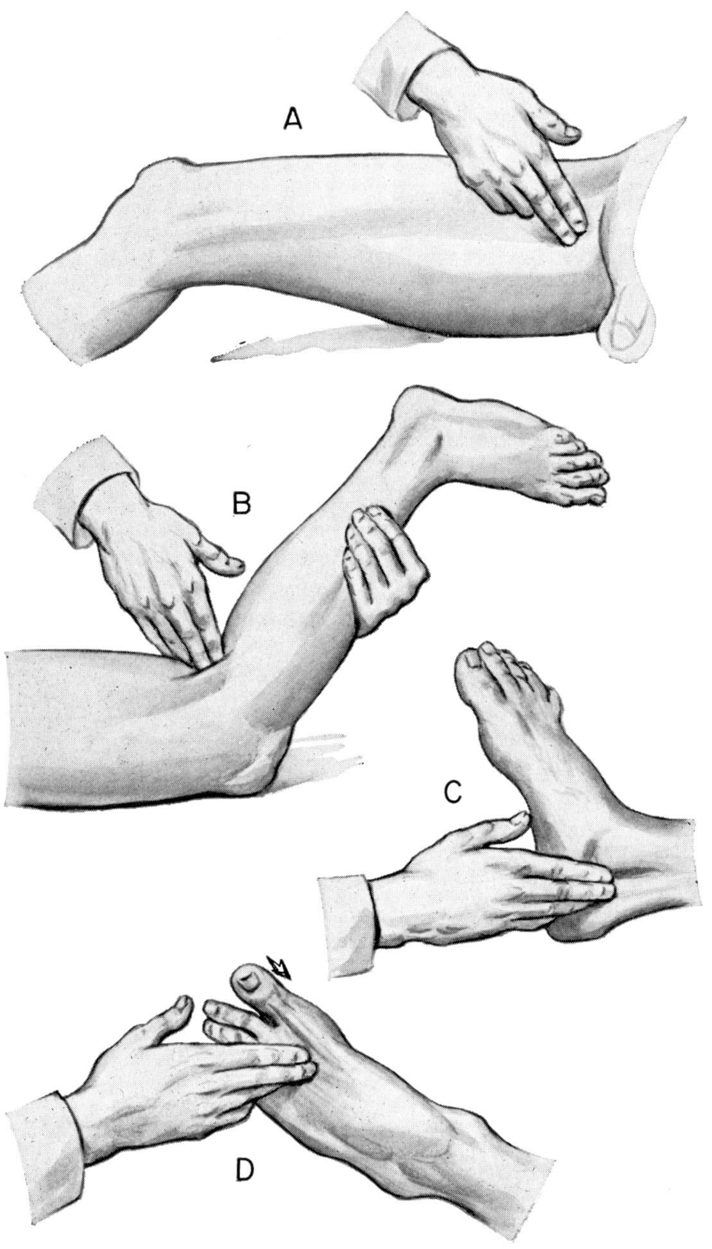

FIG. 340. Palpation of arteries of the inferior extremity: (A) femoral artery, (B) popliteal artery, (C) posterior tibial artery and (C) the dorsalis pedis.

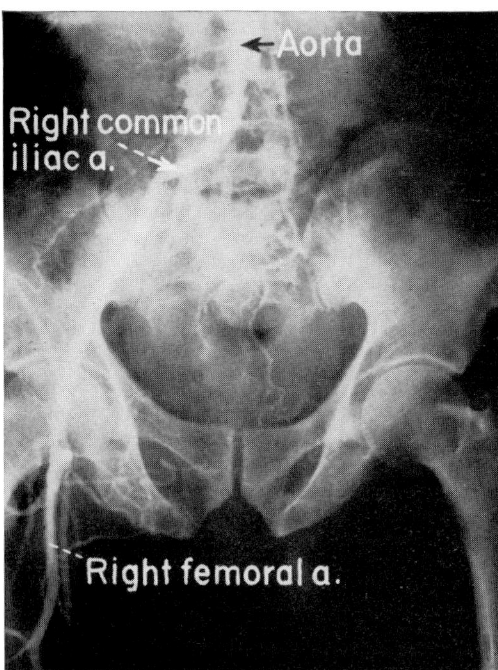

FIG. 341. Aortograph, showing obstruction of the left common iliac artery due to atherosclerosis.

be differentiated from arterial embolus. In thrombosis the onset may be more gradual, and there is an antecedent history of intermittent claudication in the lower extremity. Thrombosis frequently is associated with atherosclerotic vascular disease, in which there are intimal thickening and gradual reduction in the size of the vessel lumen. Collateral circulation is somewhat enhanced by this gradual occlusion, so that complete obstruction does not cause the severe ischemic symptoms seen in embolus. The changes associated with atherosclerotic disease are discussed subsequently.

CHRONIC ARTERIAL INSUFFICIENCY

The 2 main conditions associated with structural changes in the inferior extremity are atherosclerosis and Buerger's disease (thromboangiitis obliterans).

ATHEROSCLEROSIS

The etiology is still moot. Some etiologic factors heatedly discussed are heredity, metabolic defects (hypercholesterolemia and diabetes), hypertension, high fat diets and trauma.

Intermittent claudication is one of the more important symptoms; it signifies that the working muscles of the extremity need oxygen. The patient relates a typical history of being able to walk only a short distance before developing cramps in the calf, the thigh or the buttock; this condition is relieved when he ceases walking. Examination of the limb at this "early" stage will reveal an extremity which appears to be essentially normal except for an absence of pulsations in the femoral and/or the popliteal vessels; oscillometric readings are either diminished or absent. During the early stage *capillary circulation*, as measured by the lack of excessive redness of the foot on dependency, usually is absent.

As the disease progresses, and arterial impairment becomes more severe, one notes evidence of an inability to heal minor lacerations, blister formations and a susceptibility to infection. *Rest pain* becomes prominent as the disease progresses. This is a burning type of pain, characteristically worse at night; frequently it is relieved by hanging the foot over the side of the bed or by movement. There is a distinct abnormal redness on dependency. Often the patient states that he sleeps with the feet in a dependent position.

The final stage is gangrene. Examinations for pulsations of the femoral, the popliteal, the posterior tibial and the dorsalis pedis arteries should be conducted in a systematic way (Fig. 340). The *femoral artery* is palpated midway between the anterior superior iliac spine and the pubic spine just below the midpoint of the inguinal ligament. The *popliteal artery* is felt best between the hamstring tendons slightly lateral to the midplane of the popliteal space; the patient is positioned face down, and the knee is flexed to a position a little less than 90°. The examiner supports the patient's leg with one hand while he palpates the popliteal space with the other. The *posterior tibial artery* is felt between the tendon of Achilles and the internal malleolus.

TABLE 7. DIFFERENTIAL DIAGNOSIS OF ATHEROSCLEROSIS FROM BUERGER'S DISEASE

ATHEROSCLEROSIS	BUERGER'S DISEASE (Thromboangiitis Obliterans)
1. Older people (5th-7th decade)	1. Younger people (3rd-4th decade)
2. Migratory phlebitis rare	2. Migratory phlebitis frequent (50%)
3. Upper extremity involvement rare	3. Upper extremity involvement frequent
4. Femoral and popliteal artery pulsations absent or diminished	4. Femoral and popliteal artery pulsations present
5. Larger vessels involved at onset of symptoms	5. Usually involves medium-sized vessels below the knee
6. Diabetes more common	6. Diabetes rare
7. Coronary heart disease fairly common	7. Coronary heart disease not common
8. Relationship to smoking questionable	8. Relationship to smoking definitely established
9. Prognosis poor	9. Prognosis somewhat better

The *dorsalis pedis artery* is felt midway between the ankle and first toe web. Often it is located lateral to the tendon of the extensor hallucis longus, which stands out when the patient dorsiflexes his great toe.

BUERGER'S DISEASE

Buerger described this condition in 1908 as a peculiarly painful insufficiency of the peripheral arteries noted particularly in males who were given to heavy smoking. It was found that veins were involved as well as arteries (50% of reported cases), with the phlebitis migrans which appeared as inflammatory streaks following the linear course of veins usually located below the knee. So-called "Buerger's of the veins" has been discussed. There are some who believe that these painful inflammatory venous nodules indicate that the condition eventually will involve the arteries. Even in far-advanced Buerger's disease in which gangrene is present, popliteal artery pulsations may remain palpable. Table 7 presents 9 diagnostic points in differentiating atherosclerosis from Buerger's disease.

Aids in diagnosing vascular occlusions are currently available to the clinician. Aortography (Fig. 341) and arteriography can aid the diagnostician in determining the level as well as the degree of obliteration present in any given vessel or vessels.

Index